Bellet's

ESSENTIALS OF CARDIAC ARRHYTHMIAS

Second Edition

RICHARD H. HELFANT, M.D., F.A.C.P., F.A.C.C.

Director, MidAtlantic Heart and Vascular Institute, and
Chief, Division of Cardiology,
Presbyterian–University of Pennsylvania Medical Center;
Professor of Clinical Medicine,
University of Pennsylvania School of Medicine,
Philadelphia, Pennsylvania

1980

W.B. SAUNDERS COMPANY   Philadelphia   London   Toronto

W. B. Saunders Company: West Washington Square
Philadelphia, PA   19105

1 St. Anne's Road
Eastbourne, East Sussex BN21 3UN, England

1 Goldthorne Avenue
Toronto, Ontario M8Z 5T9, Canada

Library of Congress Cataloging in Publication Data

Bellet, Samuel, 1899–

Bellet's Essentials of cardiac arrhythmias.

Includes bibliographies.

1. Arrhythmia.   I. Helfant, Richard H.   II. Title.
III. Title: Essentials of cardiac arrhythmias. [DNLM:
1. Arrhythmia – Diagnosis.   2. Arrhythmia – Therapy.
WG330 B442]

RC685.A65B43 1980   616.1'28   79–3919

ISBN 0–7216–4626–3

Bellet's Essentials of Cardiac Arrhythmias   ISBN   0-7216-4626-3

Last digit is the print number: 9   8   7   6   5   4   3   2   1

Contributors

VIDYA S. BANKA, M.D., F.A.C.P., F.A.C.C.

Director of Cardiac Catheterization Laboratories, Presbyterian—University of Pennsylvania Medical Center; Associate Professor of Medicine, University of Pennsylvania School of Medicine, Philadelphia, Pennsylvania.

Arrhythmias Related to the Sinus Node (with Richard H. Helfant). *Ventricular Arrhythmias* (with Richard H. Helfant). *Digitalis* (with Richard H. Helfant). *Defibrillation and Electric Countershock.*

MONTY M. BODENHEIMER, M.D., F.A.C.P., F.A.C.C.

Director of Nuclear Cardiology, Director of Cardiology Research, Presbyterian—University of Pennsylvania Medical Center; Associate Professor of Medicine, University of Pennsylvania School of Medicine, Philadelphia, Pennsylvania.

General Discussion of Arrhythmias (with Richard H. Helfant). *Coronary Heart Disease and Sudden Death* (with Richard H. Helfant). *Valvular, Myocardial, and Pericardial Disease* (with Richard H. Helfant). *Arrhythmias in Infants, Children, and the Fetus* (with Richard H. Helfant). *Brain and Heart Relationships. Infectious Diseases and other Disease States* (with Richard H. Helfant). *Cardiac Arrest.*

MICHAEL S. FELDMAN, M.D., F.A.C.P., F.A.C.C.

Director, Graphics Laboratory, Presbyterian—University of Pennsylvania Medical Center; Assistant Professor of Clinical Medicine, University of Pennsylvania School of Medicine, Philadelphia, Pennsylvania.

An Approach to Arrhythmia Analysis (with Richard H. Helfant). *Disturbances of Electrolyte Balance* (with Richard H. Helfant). *Anesthesia and Surgery* (with Richard H. Helfant). *Antiarrhythmic Agents* (with Richard H. Helfant). *Cardiac Pacing* (with Richard H. Helfant).

RICHARD H. HELFANT, M.D., F.A.C.P., F.A.C.C.

Director, MidAtlantic Heart and Vascular Institute and Chief, Division of Cardiology, Presbyterian—University of Pennsylvania Medical Center; Professor of Clinical Medicine, University of Pennsylvania School of Medicine, Philadelphia, Pennsylvania.

General Discussion of Arrhythmias (with Monty M. Bodenheimer). *An Approach to Arrhythmia Analysis* (with Michael S. Feldman). *Arrhythmias Related to the Sinus Node* (with Vidya S. Banka). *Paroxysmal Supraventricular Tachycardia* (with Robert I. Katz). *Atrial Flutter* (with Robert I. Katz). *Atrial Fibrillation* (with Robert I. Katz). *Junctional Rhythms* (with Robert I. Katz). *A-V Dissociation* (with Robert I. Katz). *Ventricular Arrhythmias* (with Vidya S. Banka). *A-V Heart Block* (with Benjamin J. Scherlag). *Stress Testing, Ambulatory Monitoring, and Physiological Testing: Clinical Uses and Limitations. Coronary Heart Disease and Sudden Death* (with Monty M. Bodenheimer). *Valvular, Myocardial, and Pericardial Disease* (with Monty M. Bodenheimer). *Arrhythmias in Infants, Children, and the Fetus* (with Monty M. Bodenheimer). *Digitalis* (with Vidya S. Banka). *Disturbances of Electrolyte Balance* (with Michael S. Feldman). *Anesthesia and Surgery* (with Michael S. Feldman). *Infectious Diseases and other Disease States* (with Monty M. Bodenheimer). *Antiarrhythmic Agents* (with Michael S. Feldman). *Cardiac Pacing* (with Michael S. Feldman).

ROBERT I. KATZ, M.D., F.A.C.P., F.A.C.C.

Director, Vectorcardiography, Presbyterian—University of Pennsylvania Medical Center; Assistant Professor of Clinical Medicine, University of Pennsylvania School of Medicine, Philadelphia, Pennsylvania.

Paroxysmal Supraventricular Tachycardia (with Richard H. Helfant). *Atrial Flutter* (with Richard H. Helfant). *Atrial Fibrillation* (with Richard H. Helfant). *Junctional Rhythms* (with Richard H. Helfant). *A-V Dissociation* (with Richard H. Helfant).

RALPH LAZZARRA, M.D., F.A.C.C.

Professor of Medicine, Chief of Cardiology, University of Oklahoma Health Sciences Center, Oklahoma City, Oklahoma.

Anatomy. Basic Electrophysiology. Anomalous Atrioventricular Conduction and the Pre-Excitation Syndromes.

BENJAMIN J. SCHERLAG, Ph.D., F.A.C.C.

Professor of Medicine, University of Oklahoma Health Sciences Center; Cardiovascular Physiologist, Veterans Administration Medical Center, Oklahoma City, Oklahoma.

A-V Heart Block (with Richard H. Helfant).

Preface

The Second Edition of Bellet's *Essentials of Cardiac Arrhythmias* recognizes the considerable advances made during the past decade that contribute to our understanding of the prevalence and etiology of cardiac arrhythmias and to our ability to diagnose and treat them. Our understanding of the mechanisms of supraventricular and ventricular arrhythmias as well as the pre-excitation syndromes has been drastically altered. Our recognition of the prevalence of sinus node disturbances has become such that they are now among the most common indications for permanent cardiac pacemaker implantation! The increasing use of long term electrocardiographic monitoring to detect arrhythmias has virtually revolutionized our appreciation of their prevalence and severity. Considerable new information also has become available concerning abnormalities of the trifascicular conduction system as precursors of heart block. And the uses and limitations of His-bundle electrocardiography and newer programmed stimulation techniques has been further refined.

Important progress has also been made in the therapy of cardiac arrhythmias. Our understanding of clinical pharmacology now allows for more rational use of digitalis and of old and new antiarrhythmic drugs. We have seen major changes in the design and flexibility of programming of cardiac pacemakers, and the longevity of newer power sources has dramatically increased.

These advances are presented in a context that was developed by Dr. Bellet to emphasize the *essential* information and make it readily accessible to internists, house staff, and medical students as well as clinical cardiologists. Thus, this book is a concise yet inclusive reference for what the clinician needs to know about the diagnosis, clinical significance, and therapeutic implications of cardiac arrhythmias.

It has been a privilege and a pleasure to have the opportunity to edit this edition of Bellet's *Essentials of Cardiac Arrhythmias.* Dr. Bellet was a source of professional inspiration to me. I admired him professionally and I deeply appreciated the personal kindness, thoughtfulness, and sage advice offered by this legendary figure upon my arrival at the University of Pennsylvania ten years ago.

RICHARD H. HELFANT

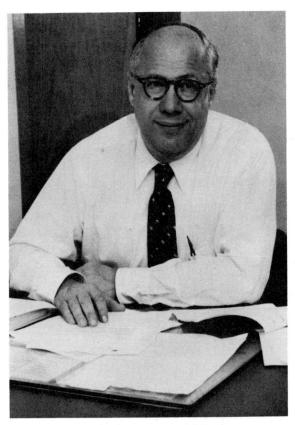

SAMUEL BELLET, M.D.

Contents

ANATOMY

RALPH LAZZARRA, M.D.

Traditionally, anatomy has guided electrophysiology by providing provocative leads and clues to specific sites of impulse generation and routes of impulse transmission. More recently, the exploration of cellular ultrastructure with methods such as electron microscopy and histochemistry has clarified important linkages between anatomy, biochemistry, and physiology, illuminating the relationship between the structure and function of myocardial cells.

When the electrophysiology of the heart is considered, it has become customary to distinguish two categories of cardiac cells. The first is the *ordinary myocardium* of the atria and ventricles, also termed "undifferentiated" or "working" myocardium. This tissue, making up the largest portion by far of the cardiac cells, performs the contractile function of the heart. The second category comprises a diverse group of cells and structures referred to as the *specialized conduction system* of the heart (Todd, 1932; Truex, 1961, 1974; Viragh and Challice, 1973). Distinctive anatomic components of the specialized conduction system include the SA node, the AV node, the His bundle, and the bundle branches, including the arborizations of peripheral Purkinje fibers. The inclusion of specialized atrial fibers in the specialized conduction system, organized in preferential conduction pathways, is in dispute.

The His bundle, bundle branches, and Purkinje networks may be referred to as the *ventricular conduction system* or the *His-Purkinje system* (Fig. 1–1).

ORDINARY MYOCARDIUM

The bulk of the atrial and ventricular walls is made up of ordinary myocardium. Although some investigators have noted differences between atrial and ventricular cells, it is useful to consider a prototype ordinary myocardial cell without regard to its location. Some of the histologic and ultrastructural features of ordinary myocardium are shown in Figure 1–2. These cells are branched cylinders with diameters of 5 to 15μ, which are separated by fibrous tissue septae into bundles with parallel orientation. This orientation has specific regional patterns in the heart that may be important in the temporal sequence of impulse distribution, since conduction is more rapid in a direction parallel to the long axes of the fibers in the bundles.

Ordinary myocardial cells stain relatively deeply and show cross striations because of their myoglobin content. The cell membrane, the *sarcolemma*, encloses the *sarcoplasm* and intracellular substructures (Simpson et al., 1973). It has a thickness of approximately 90 Å and an external glycoprotein coat that may influence the ionic environment

Text continued on page 5

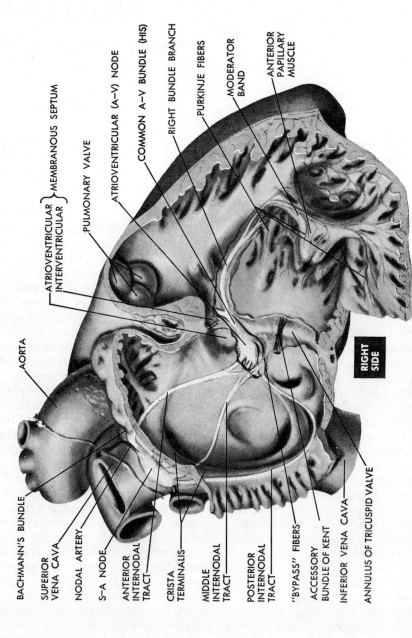

BACHMANN'S BUNDLE

SUPERIOR VENA CAVA

NODAL ARTERY

S-A NODE

ANTERIOR INTERNODAL TRACT

CRISTA TERMINALIS

MIDDLE INTERNODAL TRACT

POSTERIOR INTERNODAL TRACT

"BYPASS" FIBERS

ACCESSORY BUNDLE OF KENT

INFERIOR VENA CAVA

ANNULUS OF TRICUSPID VALVE

AORTA

ATRIOVENTRICULAR INTERVENTRICULAR } MEMBRANOUS SEPTUM

PULMONARY VALVE

ATRIOVENTRICULAR (A-V) NODE

COMMON A-V BUNDLE (HIS)

RIGHT BUNDLE BRANCH

PURKINJE FIBERS

MODERATOR BAND

ANTERIOR PAPILLARY MUSCLE

RIGHT SIDE

Figure 1-1. *See legend on opposite page.*

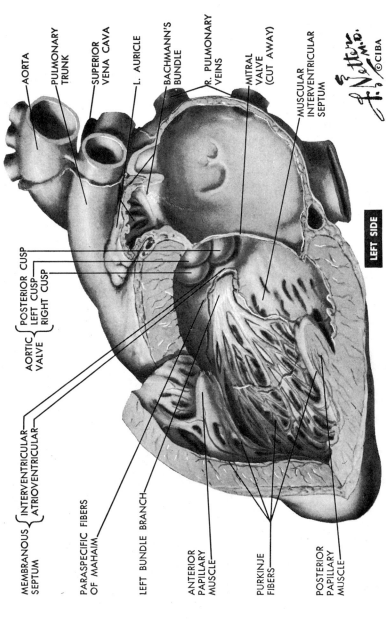

AORTA

PULMONARY TRUNK

SUPERIOR VENA CAVA

L. AURICLE

BACHMANN'S BUNDLE

R. PULMONARY VEINS

MITRAL VALVE (CUT AWAY)

MUSCULAR INTERVENTRICULAR SEPTUM

LEFT SIDE

AORTIC VALVE { POSTERIOR CUSP / LEFT CUSP / RIGHT CUSP

MEMBRANOUS SEPTUM { INTERVENTRICULAR / ATRIOVENTRICULAR

PARASPECIFIC FIBERS OF MAHAIM

LEFT BUNDLE BRANCH

ANTERIOR PAPILLARY MUSCLE

PURKINJE FIBERS

POSTERIOR PAPILLARY MUSCLE

Figure 1-1. Drawings of the heart with chambers open and the specialized conduction system highlighted. (© Copyright 1969 CIBA Pharmaceutical Company, Division of CIBA-Geigy Corporation. Reproduced with permission from The CIBA Collection of Medical Illustrations, by Frank H. Netter, M.D. All rights reserved.)

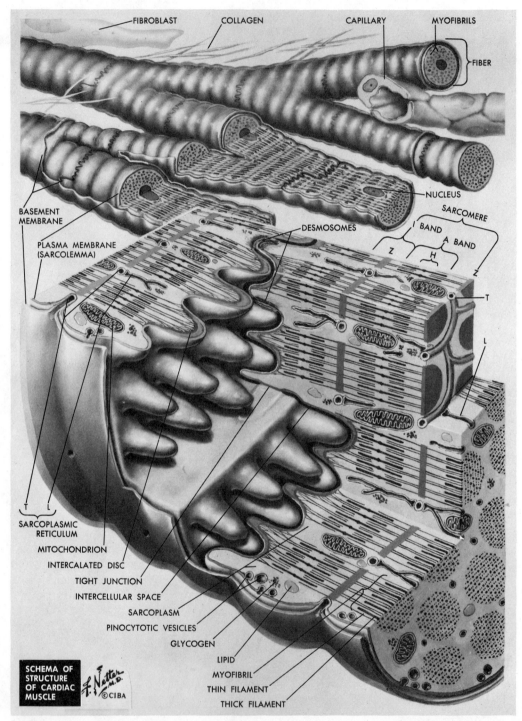

Figure 1–2. Drawing of myocardial fibers illustrating architecture and substructures. (© Copyright 1969 CIBA Pharmaceutical Company, Division of CIBA-Geigy Corporation. Reproduced with permission from The CIBA Collection of Medical Illustrations, by Frank H. Netter, M.D. All rights reserved.)

adjacent to the membrane. The sarcolemmas of adjacent cells abut the long axis of the cylinders perpendicularly at the *intercalated discs,* which are interdigitated appositions of the sarcolemmas at the ends of the cylinders (Fig. 1–2). The sarcolemmas of adjacent cells form distinctive loci of contact at the ends or side which are of several types: 1) the *desmosome* (macula adherens), 2) the fascia adherens, and 3) the nexus (zonula adherens). The nexus, a region where adjacent sarcolemmas appear to fuse in a dense membrane, is thought to have a low resistance to electrical current flow; that is, high conductance to certain mobile ions. The desmosomes and fasciae adherens are thought to provide mechanical adhesion between cells and between the cell membranes and myofibrils.

The sarcolemma also has tubular invaginations perpendicular to the surface, called T tubules (0.2 μ in diameter), which bring the extracellular fluid and the impulse closer to the myofibrils. There is another system of tubules and cisternae that is entirely intracellular called the *sarcoplasmic reticulum.* It sequesters calcium during diastole, thus keeping the sarcoplasmic concentration of calcium low. The sarcoplasm of working myocardial cells is packed with myofibrils, composed of orderly arrays of thin actin and myosin filaments in repeating units called *sarcomeres* (about 2.5μ in length). These structures compose the cross striations seen on light microscopy. The nucleus is central, and mitochondria are numerous (Fig. 1–2). Mitochondria have specialized membranes capable of creating electrochemical gradients.

THE SPECIALIZED CONDUCTING SYSTEM

The SA node

The SA node is located at the junction of the right atrium and superior vena cava in the vicinity of the sulcus terminalis (Fig. 1–1) (Keith and Flack, 1907; Truex, 1976). It is an ovoid structure with a broad body and tapering ends, approximately 15 mm long, 5 mm wide, and 1.5 mm thick. A portion of it is subendocardial. The cells in the sinus node have a loose, irregular arrangement interspersed with fibrous tissue, vessels, and numerous adrenergic and cholinergic nerve endings. The mesh of cells and collagen surrounds the SA nodal artery.

The SA node is composed of several cell types (James, 1961b; Tranum-Jensen, 1976). Pacemaker cells are small (3 to 10μ in diameter) and pale, with a central nucleus and few myofibrils. The sarcoplasmic reticulum is poorly developed, and mitochondria are sparse. There are few or no intercalated discs or T-tubules and few nexuses.

At the margin of the SA node are typical atrial myocardial cells. Transitional cells with intermediate structural characteristics are interposed between the pacemaker cells and the ordinary myocardial cells. They appear to form intercalated discs with ordinary myocardial cells at the margin of the node. Another cell type, which is large (15μ in diameter) and pale because of the poor myofibrillar content, has been likened to Purkinje fibers in the ventricles. The existence of this pale cell is disputed. Histologic sections of the SA node containing these cell types are shown in Figure 1–3.

Atrial Conducting Tracts

Few issues have generated more controversy than that of the specialized conducting tracts in the atria (Janse and Anderson, 1974). The controversy began with the observation in 1909 by Thorel (1910) of large, pale, Purkinje-like cells in the atria, intermingled with ordinary myocardial cells. The existence of cells with a larger diameter and fewer myofibrils than those of ordinary

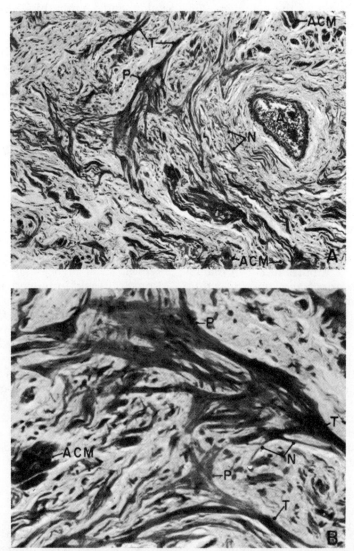

Figure 1–3.   Microscopic appearance of the central region of the sino-atrial node surrounding the nodal artery *(A)*. Typical ordinary atrial myocardial cells (ACM), transitional cells (T), nodal cells (N), and pale cells (P) are labeled. The complex network of cells surrounding the nodal artery is shown at lower magnification at top (× 42). *B,* The microscopic appearance and interconnections of the cells are shown at higher magnification (× 356 cm). (Reproduced by permission from Truex, R.C., *in* Wellens, H.J.J., et al.: The Conduction System of the Heart. Philadelphia, Lea & Febiger, 1976.)

atrial myocardium has not, however, been the focus of the dispute. The primary issue is the formation of continuous tracts of such cells connecting the SA and AV nodes; that is, it is argued that these pale cells do not form continuous tracts but are dispersed rather randomly among ordinary atrial myocardial cells with which they freely interconnect.

Internodal tracts (anterior, middle, and posterior) as well as an anterior interatrial tract (Bachmann's) have been described. There is no evidence of fibrous ensheathment of these atrial tracts, as is the case for the bundle of His and bundle branches. The evidence indicates that the putative tracts connect throughout their course with ordinary atrial muscle. There are apparent ridges, crests, and bands of parallel bundles that could provide preferential pathways of conduction even without special structural and functional properties of the individual fibers. Electrophysiological studies have intensified rather than diminished the controversy. It is agreed that there are automatic cells in the atria outside the SA and AV nodes, that there are preferential pathways of high velocity, and that there are certain differences in the electrophysiological characteristics of atrial cells in different locations. However, the question of *tracts* composed entirely of specialized cells remains unresolved. This hinges somewhat on the definition chosen for the term "tract," since some investigators have made insulation from ordinary myocardium a prerequisite.

The AV Node

The AV node resides in a strategic location in the lower atrial septum anterior to the orifice of the coronary sinus, superior to the tricuspid ring, posterior to the fibrous trigone, and inferior to the tendon of Todaro (Tawara, 1906), a thin posterior extension of the fibrous trigone. These landmarks are shown in Figure 1–4. Full agreement concerning the proximal and distal limits of the node proper in relation to atrial muscle, the bundle of His and transitional regions has not been reached. The node is approximately 5 to 7 mm long and 2 to 5 mm wide. Its central region, referred to as the "compact node" and "mid-node" (Becker and Anderson, 1976; Anderson et al., 1974), is distinctive in its composition of densely packed interwoven and tangled cells. There is some evidence that the compact node bifurcates into limbs with tricuspid and mitral orientations. Mid-nodal cells are often described as small, but their irregular shape makes accurate determination of size difficult. The relative lack of interspersed fibrous tissue contrasts with the SA node. The AV nodal cells, like SA nodal cells, are poor in myofibrils and mitochondria. Nexuses are infrequent. Typical intercalated discs are absent, but myofibrils of different cells join through fasciae adherens in an irregular network. The histologic appearance of the AV node is seen in Figure 1–5.

Transitional cells join atrial myocardium to the AV node in relatively discrete zones called intermediate areas or nodal approaches. Recently, posterior superficial and deep groups of transitional fibers have been described (Fig. 1–6). The posterior group enters from the sinus septum and from a muscular tract extending beneath the coronary sinus into the posterior atrial wall. The superficial cells extend forward from the sinus septum and inferiorly from the anterior limbus. The deep cells connect from the left side of the septum to the deep node and its mitral horn. Distally, the relatively tangled cells of the compact node assume a more parallel arrangement of fibers and blend into the penetrating bundle of His. Cholinergic and adrenergic nerve fibers are copious. Large, pale cells, similar to those found in the SA node, have also been described.

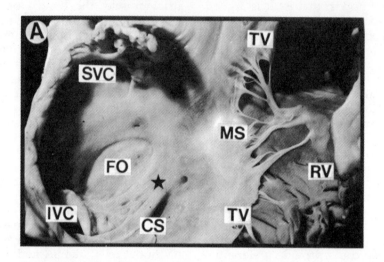

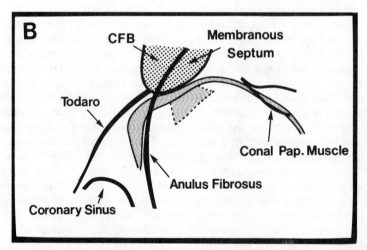

Figure 1–4. Topographical relationships of the atrioventricular junctional area viewed from the right side. At top is a heart specimen in which the right atrium has been opened. The membranous septum (MS) is transilluminated. SVC = Superior vena cava; FO = fossil ovalis; CS = coronary sinus; RV = right ventricle. The eustachian ridge is indicated by an asterisk. For comparison at bottom is a drawing of the main structures involved viewed from a similar angle. The tendon of Todaro, which runs in the eustachian ridge, inserts into the central fibrous body. The area of the compact node is delineated by the tendon of Todaro, the central fibrous body, and the tricuspid valve base. The apex of this triangle is a landmark to the position of the compact node. This is a better landmark for the position of the "node" than the ostium of the coronary sinus. (From Becker, A. E., and Anderson, R. H., *in* Wellens, H.J.J., et al.: The Conduction System of the Heart. Philadelphia, Lea & Febiger, 1976.)

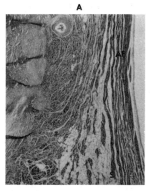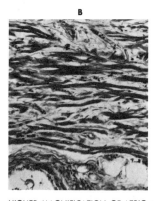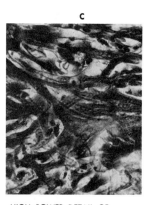

ATRIOVENTRICULAR NODE, SHOWING ARTERY, ANNULUS FIBROSUS (AF), INTERVENTRICULAR SEPTUM (S), AND OVERLYING ATRIUM (GOLDNER TRICHROME STAIN, X 10)

HIGHER MAGNIFICATION OF ATRIO–VENTRICULAR NODE: INTERLACING, LOOSELY PACKED FIBERS, AND SEGMENTS OF SMALL ARTERY AND VEIN (HOLMES SILVER STAIN)

HIGH–POWER DETAIL OF ATRIOVENTRICULAR NODAL FIBERS (MASSON TRICHROME STAIN)

Figure 1–5. Microscopic appearance of the atrioventricular node. In panel *A* at lower magnification, the AV nodal artery, annulus fibrosus (AF), the interventricular septum (S), and overlying atrium are shown. In panel *B,* at higher magnification, interlacing, loosely packed fibers and segments of a small artery and vein are shown. Detail of atrioventricular fibers is shown at higher magnification in panel *C.* (© Copyright 1969 CIBA Pharmaceutical Company, Division of CIBA-Geigy Corporation. Reproduced with permission from The CIBA Collection of Medical Illustrations, by Frank H. Netter, M.D. All rights reserved.)

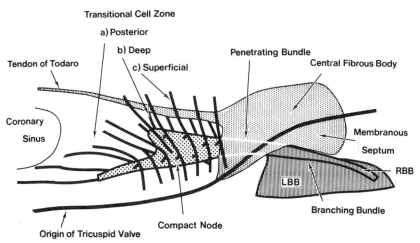

Figure 1–6. Diagrammatic representation of the atrioventricular junctional area. The specialized area is divided into four different zones: the branching bundle, the penetrating bundle, the compact node, and the transitional cell zone. The compact node, which is composed of leftward and rightward going components, continues anteriorly with the penetrating bundle. The compact node is contacted by three groups of transitional cells: superficial, passing superficially to the tendon of Todaro and partly extending over the compact node and into the tricuspid valve base; deep, connecting with the left side of the septum; and posterior. The posterior group connects with the myocardium both above and below the ostium of the coronary sinus. LBB = left bundle branch; RBB = right bundle branch. (From Becker, A.E., and Anderson, R.A. *in* Wellens, H.J.J., et al.: The Conduction System of the Heart. Philadelphia, Lea & Febiger, 1976.)

The His Bundle

The His bundle emerges as a discrete bundle of fibers from the compact node. It leaves the atrial septum and enters the membranous ventricular septum by crossing the inferior and rightward aspect of the fibrous trigone (Lev, 1968). This portion of the bundle, called the *penetrating bundle,* is shown in Figure 1–7. This structure is distinguished by its encirclement by fibrous tissue and the parallel organization of its fiber bundles.

Some of the cells may resemble nodal cells, particularly in the proximal portion of the bundle. However, most take on some of the characteristics of ordinary myocardial cells: larger size, more myofibrils, more glycogen, intercalated discs, and more frequent nexuses. Large, pale Purkinje fibers are not common in the His bundle.

At the lower margin of the membranous septum, the His bundle rides the crest of the muscular ventricular sep-

tum. Here a sheet of fibers making up the origin of the left bundle branch peels off to the left. Distal to the relatively broad origin of the left bundle branch, the bundle turns rightward and downward over the right septal surface to form the origin of the right bundle branch (Fig. 1–7). The portion of the bundle giving off the fibers of the left bundle branch is called the "branching portion," while the asymmetrical bifurcation into right and left bundle branches has been termed a "pseudobifurcation" (Rosenbaum, 1970). The His bundle courses close to the aortic, mitral, and tricuspid valves. It is, therefore, especially susceptible to disease processes extending inferiorly from the aortic valve, which attaches to the membranous septum. The length of the bundle is variable, averaging 1 cm, and the width is 1 to 3 mm. Within the His bundle, fibrous septae separate parallel fascicles of fibers which have infrequent interconnections (James and Sherf, 1971). This has led some ob-

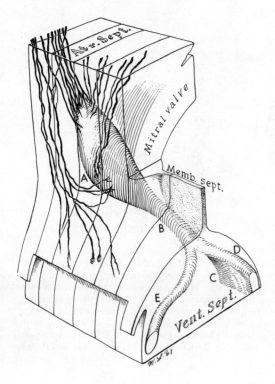

Figure 1–7. Diagrammatic representation of the atrioventricular node and proximal conduction system. The atrial septum (Atr Sept), mitral valve, membranous septum (Memb Sept), and muscular ventricular septum (Musc Sept) are shown in relationship to the A-V node (A), the penetrating His bundle (B), the fibers of the left bundle branch (C and D), and the right bundle branch (E). (From James, T.N.: Amer. Heart J. 62:756, 1961.)

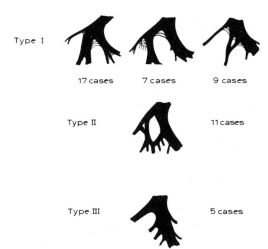

Type I

17 cases   7 cases   9 cases

Type II

11 cases

Type III

5 cases

Figure 1–8. Distribution of left bundle branch fibers in 49 human hearts. Representative examples of each type are shown. (From Kulbertus, H.E., and Demoulin, J.C.L., *in* Wellens, H.J.J., et al.: Conduction System of the Heart. Philadelphia, Lea & Febiger, 1976.)

servers to postulate that these fascicles may function independently, transmitting impulses like nerve fibers in a trunk. However, electrophysiological studies indicate that normally the interconnections prevent such "longitudinal dissociation."

The Bundle Branches

The right and left bundle branches differ strikingly in their function and anatomy. The right bundle branch emerges from the right septal surface, anterior to the insertion of the septal leaflet of the tricuspid valve on the membranous septum. It usually courses as a compact bundle just below the muscle of Lancisi, forming an arc with anterior convexity (Fig. 1–1). At the level of the lower third of the right ventricular septal surface, it arborizes into the subendocardial peripheral Purkinje network that connects with the ordinary myocardial cells of the free wall and lower septum.

Recently, our knowledge of the structure and function of the left bundle branch has undergone considerable change. The bundle has been depicted as bifurcating in the upper portion of the left ventricular septal surface into

anterior (superior) and posterior (inferior) divisions which diverge and proceed to the respective papillary muscles of the left ventricle. At this point, the bundle ramifies into Purkinje networks. According to this view, the two divisions interconnect only at levels of the distal network formed by the arborizations. The arborizations form a lacework of interconnecting subendocardial Purkinje fibers covering the lower septum and free wall. These Purkinje fibers connect with ordinary myocardial cells through transitional fibers. This description contrasts with that of early anatomists, who considered the left bundle branch to be a diverging fan of interconnected fibers on the left septal surface. Both views agree that the left bundle branch fibers in the upper septum are ensheathed by fibrous tissue and do not connect with ventricular myocardium.

Recent painstaking histologic studies (Demoulin and Kulbertus, 1972) of the left bundle branch suggest that the bifascicular representation is an oversimplification in man and that a septal ramification exists between the diverging borders of the bundle. Reconstructions of the left bundle branch from recent studies are shown in Figure 1–8. There seem to be considerable variation and complexity in the architecture of the left bundle branch, but the simple bifascicular representation is uncommon.

The Purkinje fibers tend to be larger in diameter than ordinary myocardial fibers, although their size varies in different species. They are clear because of their sparsity in myofibrillar and mitochondrial content. While lacking T-tubules (Sommer and Johnson, 1968), they do have intercalated discs, well-developed nexuses, and more abundant glycogen than other types of cardiac cells. Their high glycogen content permits them to be visualized grossly with iodine stain. However, in specimens from human autopsies, iodine staining is ineffectual because of postmortem glycogenolysis. This practical problem has prolonged the controversy concerning the architecture of the human left bundle branch. Some investigators believe that Purkinje fibers penetrate into ventricular myocardium in a direction perpendicular to the endocardial surface for one third to one half the thickness of the wall.

The nerve supply to the ventricular conduction system in man is uncertain. In some species, both adrenergic and cholinergic fibers are discernible with histochemical techniques in the vicinity of the fibers of the ventricular conduction system.

Bypass Fibers

Kent Bundles. Fibers crossing the AV ring to connect atrial and ventricular working myocardium have been detected in the human heart at various locations on its right and left sides (Lev and Lerner, 1955). They may be free wall or septal in location. They are found more commonly in hearts of young individuals (Truex et al., 1958).

James Tracts. Fibers connecting to the distal portion of the compact node or the proximal bundle of His have been described (James, 1961C). This connection is said to approach from ordinary atrial myocardium of the posterior portion of the atrial septum, bypassing much of the compact node. Other anatomists have questioned these findings (Becker and Anderson, 1976).

Paraspecific Fibers of Mahaim. Fibers connecting the distal AV node or His bundle with the ordinary working myocardial fibers of the upper ventricular septum have also been described (Mahaim, 1947). Their functional significance is uncertain, since there is a poor correlation between the histologic demonstration of such fibers and appropriate electrocardiographic findings or arrhythmias (see Chapter 13).

THE CORONARY CIRCULATION

In the human heart, the right coronary artery courses in the right atrioventricular sulcus to the crux of the heart, (the point at which the right and left atrioventricular sulci cross the posterior sulci of the interatrial and interventricular septa). In the approximately 90 per cent of hearts having right dominant circulation, the artery turns inferiorly to descend in the posterior intraventricular sulcus as the posterior descending coronary artery (James, 1961a; Helfant and Banka, 1978). The left main coronary artery divides after a short course into the anterior descending coronary artery, which descends in the anterior interventricular sulcus, and the left circumflex artery, which circles in the left AV sulcus to the posterior region of the heart. In approximately 10 per cent of hearts, the circumflex artery proceeds to the crux, where it provides the posterior descending coronary artery (left dominant circulation).

The *artery of the SA node* arises from the proximal right coronary artery in about 60 per cent of cases and from the proximal circumflex artery in about 40 per cent. Collateral circulation is relatively abundant in the region of the SA node. The *AV nodal artery* arises from the superior portion of the posterior descending coronary artery at the crux of the heart and penetrates anteriorly to supply the AV node and, in some hearts, the His bundle and proximal bundle branches (Figure 1–9). The ventricular septum is supplied in its anterior two thirds by perforating branches of the anterior descending coronary artery and in its posterior third by branches of the posterior coronary artery (Fig. 1–9). The His bundle and bundle branches receive their blood supply from both anterior and posterior septal vessels. The proximal portions of the ventricular conduction system are supplied by the *first septal perforator* of the anterior descending coronary artery and branches of the AV nodal artery. However, the ventricular conduction system may receive some blood supply directly from the ventricular chambers, since the fibers are in the subendocardium in direct proximity to the chambers. The extent of collat-

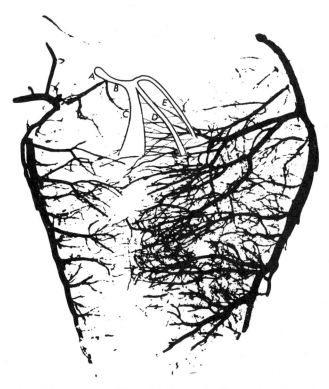

Figure 1–9. Drawing of the proximal atrioventricular conduction system shown in relationship to the coronary arteries in the anterior and posterior interventricular sulci. The anterior descending coronary artery on the right provides penetrating branches which supply the His bundle (B), the right bundle branch (C), and the left bundle branch (D and E). The posterior descending coronary artery on the left supplies the A-V nodal artery to the atrioventricular node (A) and the His bundle. The penetrating branches of the posterior descending coronary artery supply parts of the bundle branches. (From Rotman, M., et al.: Circulation 45:703, 1972.)

eral circulation to the AV node is unclear.

It is known that ordinary myocardium is very susceptible to ischemic damage when the coronary circulation is compromised. The endocardial layers are particularly vulnerable because they are most distant from the epicardial major coronary arteries and because they generate the most tension and therefore have higher oxygen requirements. Atrial and right ventricular myocardial cells are relatively more resistant to ischemia than are left ventricular cells, perhaps because less tension is generated in contraction. With reduction of blood flow to the left ventricular myocardium, however, electrophysiological alterations can be detected quite rapidly, usually within a minute. The specialized conducting cells are more resistant to ischemia than is the ordinary myocardium.

The heart is richly innervated by both adrenergic and cholinergic fibers from various receptors located in the vascular free walls and the myocardium. The extent of parasympathetic influence on ventricular myocardial cells and the ventricular conduction system is in doubt. There is persuasive evidence that parasympathetic influences are much less prominent in the ventricles than in the atria.

REFERENCES

Anderson, R. H., Janse, M. J., van Capelle, F. J. L., Billette, J., Becker A. E., and Durrer, D.: A combined morphological and electrophysiological study of the atrioventricular node of the rabbit heart. Circ. Res. 35:909, 1974.

Becker, A. E., and Anderson, R. H.: Morphology of the human atrioventricular junctional area. In Wellens, H. J. J., Lie, K. I., and Janse, M. J. (eds.): The Conduction System of the Heart. Philadelphia, Lea & Febiger, 1976, p. 263.

Demoulin, J. C., and Kulbertus H. E.: Histopathologic examination of concept of left hemiblock. Brit. Heart J. 34:807, 1972.

Helfant, R. H., and Banka, V. S.: A Clinical and Angiographic Approach to Coronary Heart Disease, Philadelphia, F. A. Davis. Co. 1978.

James, T. N.: The Anatomy of the Coronary Arteries, New York, P. B. Hoeber, Inc. 1961a.

James, T. N.: The anatomy of the human sinus node. Anat. Rec. 141:109, 1961b.

James, T. N.: Morphology of the human heart atrioventricular node, with remarks pertinent to its electrophysiology. Am. Heart J. 62:756, 1961c.

James, T. N., and Sherf, L.: Fine structure of the His bundle. Circulation 44:9, 1971.

Janse, M. H., and Anderson, R. H.: Specialized internodal atrial pathways: Fact or fiction? Europ. J. Cardiol. 2:117, 1974.

Keith, A., and Flack, M. W.: The form and nature of the muscular connections between the primary divisions of the vertebrate heart. J. Anat. Physiol. 41:171, 1907.

Lev, M.: The conduction system. In Gould, S. E., (ed.): Pathology of the Heart and Blood Vessels. Springfield, Il, Charles C Thomas, 1968, p. 185.

Lev, M., and Lerner, R.: The theory of Kent. A histologic study of the normal atrioventricular communications of the human heart. Circulation 2:176, 1955.

Mahaim, I.: Kent's fibers and the AV paraspecific conduction through the upper connection of the bundle of His. Am. Heart J. 33:651, 1947.

Rosenbaum, M. B.: The hemiblocks: Diagnosis and clinical significance. Mod. Conc. Cardiovasc. Dis. 39:141, 1970.

Simpson, R. O., Rayns, D. G., and Ledingham, J. M.: The ultrastructure of ventricular and atrial myocardium. In Dalton, A. F., and Haguenen, F. (eds.): Ultrastructure in Biological Systems, Vol 6, Challice, C. E., and Viragh, S., (eds.): Ultrastructure of the Mammalian Heart. New York, Academic Press, 1973, p. 43.

Sommer, J. R., and Johnson, E. A.: Cardiac muscle. Comparative study of Purkinje fibers and ventricular fibers. J. Cell. Biol. 39:497, 1968.

Tawara S: Das Reitzleitungssystem des Saügetierherzens. Jena, Gustav Fischer, 1906.

Thorel C.: Vorläüfige Mitteilung über eine besondere Muskelverbindung zwischen der Cava superior und den Hisschen Bundeln. Münch. med. Wschr. 57:183, 1910.

Todd, T. W.: The specialized system of the heart. In Cowdry, E. V. (ed.): Special Cytology. New York, P. B. Hoeber, Inc., 1932, p. 1175.

Tranum-Jensen, J.: The fine structure of the atrial and atrioventricular (AV) functional specialized tissues of the rabbit heart. In Wellens, H. J. J., Lie, K. I., and Janse, M. J. (eds.): The Conduction System of the Heart. Philadelphia, Lea & Febiger, 1976, p. 55.

Truex, R. C.: Comparative anatomy and functional considerations of the cardiac conducting system. In DeMello, W. C., (ed.): The Specialized Tissues of the Heart. Amsterdam, Elsevier Publishing Co. 1961, p. 22.

Truex, R. C.: Structural basis of atrial and ventricular conduction. Cardiovasc. Clin. 6:1, 1974.

Truex, R. C.: The sino-atrial node and its connections with the atrial tissues. *In* Wellens, H. J.J., Lie, K. I., and Janse, M. J., (eds.): The Conduction System of the Heart. Philadelphia, Lea & Febiger, 1976, p. 55.

Truex, R. C., Bishof, J. K., and Hoffman, E. L.: Accessory atrioventricular muscle bundles of the developing human heart. Anat. Rec. *131*:45, 1958.

Viragh, S., and Challice, C. E.: The impulse generation and conduction system of the heart. *In* Dalton, A. F., and Haguenan, F., (eds.): Ultrastructure in Biological Systems, Vol 6. Challice, C. E., and Viragh, S., (eds.): Ultrastructure of the Mammalian Heart. New York, Academic Press, 1973, p. 43.

2

BASIC ELECTROPHYSIOLOGY

RALPH LAZZARA, M.D.

In order to understand cardiac rhythms fully, it is useful to have a working appreciation of normal cellular electrophysiology and of the abnormalities thought to be responsible for arrhythmias. Electrophysiology can be conceptualized as the use of electrical energy in cellular functions, since it is based on the creation of electrochemical gradients or potentials across cell membranes. These gradients result from an unequal distribution of ions between the interior and exterior of cells and underlie the fundamental cardiac electrophysiological functions of *automaticity* (cardiac impulse initiation) and *conduction* (cardiac impulse propagation). Electrochemical gradients and ionic movements among intracellular compartments relate primarily to metabolic and contractile functions.

THE NORMAL CARDIAC CELL

Membrane Potential

In common with other cells, cardiac cells contain disparately high concentrations of potassium (K^+) and protein anions compared with the extracellular fluid (Hoffman and Cranefield, 1960). Conversely, they contain much less sodium (Na^+), chloride (Cl^-), and calcium (Ca^{++}) (Fig. 2–1).

This unequal ionic distribution results partly from differences in the facil-

ity of movement of specific ions across the sarcolemma; that is, differences in *permeability* (or conductance) of the membrane to specific ions. The membrane has both resistive and capacitive properties, since it both conducts current and stores charge (Fozzard, 1977). At rest, the sarcolemma is far more permeable to potassium than to sodium or calcium. (It is virtually impermeable to the large anionic protein molecules.)

The cell membrane actively transports certain ions against electrochemi-

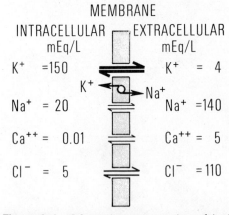

Figure 2–1. Schematic representation of ionic distributions and membrane permeabilities and transport in cardiac cells. The relative sizes of arrows penetrating openings in the membrane represent the relative resting permeabilities. The circle with arrows in the membrane signifies the active transport of sodium and potassium.

16

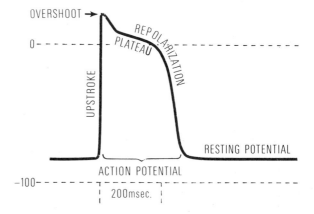

OVERSHOOT →

0

OVERSHOOT

REPOLARIZATION

PLATEAU

UPSTROKE

RESTING POTENTIAL

ACTION POTENTIAL

−100

200msec.

Figure 2–2. Typical resting and action potentials of ventricular myocardial cells. The various components are labelled. A voltage scale in mV is shown to the left and a time scale below.

cal gradients. An energy-dependent ion pump in the sarcolemma identified with the enzyme Na-K, ATPase, transports sodium to the exterior of the cell and potassium to the interior (Thomas, 1972). The *membrane potential* (more precisely called "transmembrane" potential) is determined by the transmembrane concentration gradients of different ions and their relative permeabilities. The electrical potential assumes a magnitude (and a polarity) sufficient to restrain the total number of ions impelled to leave the compartment; that is, a magnitude determined by the concentration gradient.

Since potassium is much more permeable in the resting state than are the intracellular anions or extracellular cations, excess potassium, moving down its concentration gradient from interior to exterior, is not accompanied in the membrane by neutralizing charges. Thus, a negative transmembrane *resting potential* forms in the internal compartment relative to the external compartment. The magnitude of this potential is approximately −90 mV.

Action Potential

Following an appropriate stimulus to the myocardium, *excitation*, the generation of a transmembrane *action potential* occurs. This is initiated by a rapid and marked increase in permeability to sodium (Noble, 1966). A representation of

the action potential for ventricular myocardial cells is shown in Figure 2–2. The upstroke of the action potential represents the switch from the resting state of high permeability to potassium to the active state of high permeability to sodium; that is, a shift from a *potassium equilibrium potential* toward a *sodium equilibrium potential.*

At rest, when the ventricular myocardial cell is in a stage of equilibrium near the potassium equilibrium potential, there is virtually no net flow of current across the membrane. However, if current is driven passively outward across the membrane from a current source elsewhere (e.g., a myocardial cell nearby which has been excited), the membrane will partially depolarize. If the membrane potential is not brought to the *threshold potential* (−60 mV) by this passive current flow, it will return to its resting state when the current stops without generating an action potential. This purely passive response to subthreshold current is called an *electrotonic* response.

The permeability of the membrane to sodium ions depends directly on the transmembrane potential (Weidmann, 1955). When the membrane is fully polarized with a membrane potential of −90 mV, its permeability to sodium is quite low. However, if the membrane is partially depolarized, permeability to sodium increases. At the level of the threshold potential, the permeability to sodium exceeds the permeability to potassium. At this level, the membrane potential will actively shift toward the sodium equilibrium potential and there will be a transient inward flow of current, the source of which is external sodium. The driving force is the potential energy in the electrochemical gradient for sodium, which is attracted to the interior of the cell both by the negative intracellular potential and lower intracellular concentration. The distribution of current flow between excited and resting portions of the membrane in relation to the upstroke along a length of membrane is shown in Figure 2–3.

With excitation, the membrane potential moves to approximately +25 mV, the *overshoot*. Because this change does not depend on current driven from some source elsewhere, it is called a *regenerative* or *active* membrane response. It has been convenient to consider this great increase in sodium permeability as the result of the opening of a *rapid channel* specific for sodium ions. The term "channel" should, however, not be interpreted anatomically.

The increase in permeability to sodium is transient, and within a few seconds it is markedly curtailed. This proc-

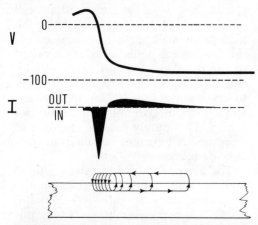

Figure 2–3. Distribution of transmembrane potentials (V) and current (I) along a segment of cardiac fiber. The spatial distribution of potentials (mV) is shown at the top, the transmembrane current in the middle, and a simple representation of a cylinder with local circuits of current below.

ess has been referred to as *inactivation*. Inactivation is maximal at membrane potentials more positive than the threshold potential and is minimal at membrane potentials more negative than −90 mV. Between −90 and −60 mV, there is partial inactivation of the rapid channel. If the membrane potential remains for more than a few milliseconds at levels between −60 and −90 mV, the rapid sodium channel will be partially inactivated; that is, excitation will produce a lesser increase in the sodium permeability than that which occurs in a fully polarized membrane. This affects the upstroke in two ways. First, the upstroke is reduced because the membrane potential falls short of approximating the sodium equilibrium potential. Second, the velocity of the upstroke is reduced because the velocity of the upstroke depends, to a large extent, on the transient inward movement of sodium ions. The way in which inactivation affects the upstroke can be expressed by graphs of the maximal velocity of the upstroke or the overshoot plotted against the membrane potential at excitation. The relationship between the maximal upstroke velocity ($\dot{V}$ max) and membrane potential, called the *membrane responsiveness curve*, has been used most commonly to assess inactivation (Fig. 2–4). It is important to distinguish the process of inactivation from the process of increasing sodium permeability that occurs when a membrane is excited. (That process could be termed *activation*). It was stated previously that activation involves an *increase* in permeability to sodium as the membrane potential is changed from −90 mV to threshold potential (−60 mV). On the other hand, inactivation involves a *decrease* in permeability to sodium as the membrane potential is changed from −90 to −60 mV. These two processes represent opposing responses of the membrane to a change in membrane potential. The two processes differ temporally, since activation occurs within a fraction of a millisecond when the membrane potential is

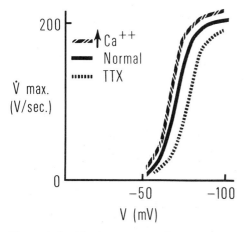

Figure 2–4. Membrane responsiveness curves. The maximal velocity of the upstroke (V max) is plotted against transmembrane potential at excitation (V). Increased extracellular calcium (Ca^{++}) augments upstroke velocity. Tetrodotoxin (TTX), a blocker of the rapid channel, diminishes upstroke velocity at any given membrane potential.

brought to a new level, whereas inactivation requires at least several milliseconds. Inactivation predominates when the membrane potential has remained at a certain level for more than several milliseconds and modulates the intensity of activation.

At the end of the upstroke, the permeability of the membrane to sodium diminishes to a level near that of the resting state; however, the membrane potential does not return to the resting potential. It remains near zero for a period before it repolarizes. This *plateau*, the hallmark of most cardiac cells, is incompletely understood. An important determinant of the plateau is an increase in permeability to calcium which begins during the latter part of the upstroke and persists for much longer than the transient increase in permeability to sodium (Reuter, 1973). Like the increase in permeability to sodium, the increase in calcium permeability generates an inward flow of calcium ions via their electrochemical gradient. Consequently, the membrane potential is prevented from returning to more negative levels. This calcium current is often referred to as the *slow cur-*

rent to distinguish it from the *rapid current* of sodium during the upstroke and is said to flow through the *slow channel*. It is likely that the calcium inflow during the plateau is important in the contractile response.

Electrophysiologically, the plateau is important because it delays *repolarization* and the return to resting potential. Since the cardiac cell cannot be excited again until it has repolarized to a level more negative than the threshold potential, the plateau results in a long *absolute refractory period* — that is, that period of inexcitability which follows an excitation. The duration of the action potential of the ventricular myocardial cell is approximately 250 msec. A decrease in permeability to potassium and a residual small increase in permeability to sodium above the resting level probably also contribute to the plateau (Coraboeuf et al., 1976). Repolarization appears to result from an increase in permeability to potassium and a decrease in permeability to sodium and calcium, restoring the resting state. Certain of the variations in conductance to various ions are shown in Figure 2–5.

There are variations in membrane

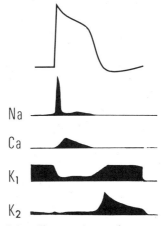

Figure 2–5. Changes in conductance of Purkinje fibers for various ions during the action potential and during slow diastolic depolarization. The potassium conductance has been separated to two components (K_1 and K_2). During diastole, one component (K_1) remains high, while the other (K_2) declines, producing diastolic depolarization.

properties among cell types which lead to differences in their resting and action potentials. Some of these differences are relatively unimportant, but others are crucial for the specific electrophysiological functions of the different cell types.

AUTOMATICITY

Certain myocardial cells do not maintain a stable resting potential, but instead undergo gradual *diastolic depolarization*. When the level of membrane potential depolarizes to threshold, an action potential is generated. The cells that manifest automaticity are located in the sinoatrial node, certain other sites in the atria, such as the crista terminalis, and regions near the ostium of the coronary sinus, the AV node, the His bundle, and the bundle branches, including the peripheral Purkinje network (Hoffman, 1960). Diastolic depolarization may have different mechanisms in different automatic cells. For example, in the SA node, it appears that diastolic depolarization may be strongly dependent on a relatively high resting permeability to calcium, causing drift toward the calcium equilibrium potential (Coraboeuf et al., 1976). On the other hand, the membranes of Purkinje fibers depolarize during diastole primarily because there is decreasing permeability to potassium, causing drift away from the potassium equilibrium potential.

The rate of generation of impulses by automatic foci is determined by 1) the level of membrane potential at the termination of the action potential, called the *maximum diastolic potential*, 2) the rate of diastolic depolarization, and 3) the level of the threshold potential. These relationships are shown in Figure 2–6. Pacemaker dominance of SA nodal cells is a reflection of the more rapid rate of diastolic depolarization and lower levels of maximum diastolic potential of SA nodal cells than of *latent pacemakers* at other sites.

Numerous agents affect automaticity by influencing those factors that determine the rate of pacemaker firing (West, 1972). For example, the sympathetic neurotransmitters increase the rate of diastolic depolarization, whereas acetylcholine slows the rate of diastolic depolarization and produces a more negative maximum diastolic potential. Increased extracellular potassium concentration slows the rate of diastolic depolarization of Purkinje fibers, while increased extracellular calcium concentration makes the threshold potential more positive.

CONDUCTION

Once an action potential is generated at an automatic focus, it is accompanied by a flow of electrical current that depolarizes adjacent membranes to their threshold potentials, in turn producing additional action potentials. Thus, the original action potential propagates to adjoining membranes. Continuation of this process constitutes the process of impulse *conduction*.

Several factors influence the velocity of conduction: 1) the action potential itself, specifically, the upstroke of the action potential, which supplies the generator voltage for the excitatory current that flows down the myocardial

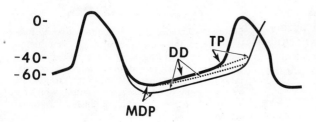

Figure 2–6. Transmembrane potentials of a pacemaker cell. The curves that are thinner or interrupted indicate slowing of the firing rate due to changes in threshold potential (TP), maximum diastolic potential (MDP), or the rate of slow diastolic depolarization (DD).

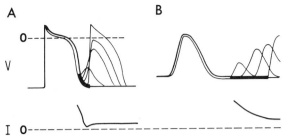

Figure 2-7. The refractory periods of cardiac cells. On the left, are normal myocardial cells activated during repolarization. Double outline of the transmembrane potential curve represents a period of inexcitability, the absolute refractory period. The solid bar on the transmembrane potential curve represents the relative refractory period during which the stimulus current required to excite (I) is higher than during diastole and the responses elicited are reduced. In some cell types, there is a short period near the end of repolarization when the stimulus threshold dips below the diastolic level, that is, the supernormal period. On the right are shown the refractory periods of a partially depolarized cell, in which the absolute refractory period outlasts the action potential, and relative refractoriness occurs in diastole.

cylinder and across the resting membrane. The greater the magnitude of this voltage — i.e., the greater the overshoot — the more current will flow and the sooner maximum levels of current will be obtained; 2) the upstroke velocity, which is determined by the quantity of inward current flow in the active region and serves as an indicator of the quantity of excitatory current flowing to the resting (inactive) membrane; and 3) the resistance of the cell interior, which if low allows more excitatory current to flow. Since resistance is related to cross-sectional area, cells with the greatest diameter conduct the most rapidly. In addition, current is divided at sites of branching, so it is less effective for each branch. It appears that conduction is most rapid in regions with the least branching.

The currents generated in the extracellular fluid during conduction are accompanied by gradients of electrical potential which can be recorded. Potentials recorded in the vicinity of the heart are referred to as *electrograms*. Since all the tissues of the body conduct electricity, current generated by the heart flows throughout the body, creating potential gradients at a distance from the heart. Potentials recorded at the body surface are referred to as *electrocardiograms*. Electrocardiograms and electrograms record potentials during repolarization as well as during excitation of cardiac cells.

REFRACTORINESS AND EXCITABILITY

Once excited, the cardiac membrane undergoes a period of total inexcitability (the *absolute refractory period*) and a period of reduced responsiveness immediately following the absolute refractory period (the *relative refractory period*) (Brooks et al., 1955). The relative refractory period has two definitive characteristics: 1) It requires greater current to excite the cell, i.e., the *excitability* is reduced; and 2) the upstroke of the action potential has a reduced overshoot and velocity. Thus, if cardiac tissue is excited during the relative refractory period, conduction is slower than normal.

In normal cardiac cells, refractoriness is primarily a function of the membrane potential during the repolarization of the action potential. The absolute refractory period coincides with the period when the membrane potential is more positive than the threshold potential. The relative refractory period corresponds fairly closely to the phase of repolarization when the membrane potential is between the threshold potential and the resting potential (Fig. 2-7).

In certain cardiac cells, the relative refractory period is followed by a *supernormal* period of enhanced excitability near the termination of repolarization. Action potential upstroke remains reduced. The duration of the refractory period is inversely related to heart rate because the action potential duration varies inversely with rate.

The excitability of cardiac cells, assessed by applied electrical stimuli, has received considerable study (Brooks et al., 1955). The strength, duration, and polarity of the applied current are all important in determining responses. In general, the longer the duration of the stimulus, the less the intensity of current required to excite. The minimal stimulus required to excite is referred to as the *stimulus threshold*. The relationship between current strength and duration for threshold stimuli is approximately hyperbolic (Fig. 2–8).

The influence of stimulus polarity on excitation depends on the time in the cycle when the stimulus is delivered. During diastole, and after the relative refractory period, much less current is required to excite with a cathode (negative electrode) than with an anode (positive electrode). In both anodal and cathodal stimulation, there are dips in the excitability curves during the relative refractory period that coincide with a period of *vulnerability* of the heart to fibrillation (or multiple responses) when very strong anodal stimuli are applied (Fig. 2–8). This vulnerable period occurs near the peak of the T wave of the electrocardiogram. In some types of normal cardiac cells, including cells in the SA or AV nodes, refractoriness is not closely linked to the membrane potential during repolarization. The absolute refractory period outlasts the duration of the action potential, and the relative refractory period occurs entirely in diastole (*post-repolarization refractoriness*).

THE SPECIALIZED CONDUCTION SYSTEM

Generally included in this system are the SA node, some atrial tracts, the AV node, the His bundle, the bundle branches, and the peripheral Purkinje network. There is considerable functional heterogeneity among these com-

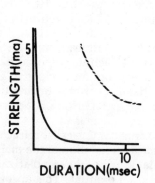
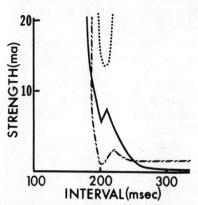

Figure 2–8. The factors that influence the stimulus threshold for excitation. On the left, the strength-duration curve shows the current strength required for stimulation with rectangular pulses of varying duration. The lower curve (solid) was obtained in late diastole. The upper curve (diagonally interrupted) was obtained during the relative refractory period. On the right, the strength-interval curve shows the current strength (duration held constant) required for a stimulus to excite the cardiac cell at any time in the cardiac cycle. The upstroke is designated as time zero. The solid curve was obtained with cathodal stimulation, whereas the diagonally interrupted curve represents anodal stimulation. The upper curve shows the current required to induce ventricular fibrillation. That curve demarcates the vulnerable period.

ponents; however, each has properties of either automaticity and/or conduction that differentiate it from ordinary working myocardial cells.

The SA Node

The dominant pacemaker of the heart is located in the superior portion of the SA node. Its pacemaker cells have the most rapid intrinsic firing rates because of its comparatively rapid rates of diastolic depolarization and less negative maximum diastolic potential. Other automatic cells within the SA node are *latent pacemakers* but may assume the pacemaker function if the primary pacemaker focus is suppressed. The maximum diastolic potential is approximately −60 mV, and the threshold potential is −40 mV.

The action potentials of SA nodal cells have relatively slow upstrokes and low amplitudes. They may result largely from activation of the slow channel, with the fast channel being partially inactivated under normal conditions. Conduction in the SA node is slow and relatively precarious.

Atrial Tracts

Automatic cells exist in the atria outside of the SA node, primarily in the right atrium in the vicinity of the crista terminalis and the ostium of the coronary sinus. However, there is controversy as to the existence of tracts of rapidly conducting fibers connecting the SA and AV nodes and the left and right atria (Janse and Anderson, 1974). Several tracts — the anterior, middle, and posterior internodal tracts and the anterior interatrial tract (Bachmann's bundle) — have been described by some investigators and denied by others.

AV Node

The greatest portion of the delay in impulse conduction occurs in the AV node, a structure specialized for slow conduction (Childers, 1977). The remarkable slowing of conduction in the AV node is the result of a number of anatomic and functional characteristics. The cells are smaller in diameter and arranged in whorls and tangles. Resting potentials are relatively low (−75 mV), and upstrokes of action potentials are slow and diminished in amplitude. In the electrophysiological center of the node, sometimes called the mid-node, the action potentials are slowest and smallest. Proximally, its electrophysiological characteristics are intermediate between those of atrial muscle and mid-nodal cells, and distally they are intermediate between mid-nodal and His bundle cells. Some investigators have given these AV nodal regions the designations AN, N, and, NH, respectively.

The generation of upstrokes by cells in the AV node may, like that in the SA node, depend more on the slow channel (Zipes and Mendez, 1973) than on the rapid channel (in contrast to other cardiac cells). This may have practical clinical importance in therapy, since the slow and rapid channels have different sensitivities to different agents. For example, the slow channel is very sensitive to verapamil, an agent that markedly depresses conduction in the AV node. Conversely, the rapid channel is sensitive to quinidine and procainamide, agents that have little effect on conduction in the AV node.

In addition to delaying transmission of the impulse from atria to ventricles, the AV node serves the important function of limiting the number of atrial impulses that can be transmitted to the ventricles. For example, during atrial fibrillation, only a fraction of the continual barrage of atrial impulses entering the AV node successfully traverse the node to excite the His bundle. The AV node performs this protective function by virtue of its peculiar refractory properties. Because of the substantial and variable conduction delays within the AV node, refractory intervals measured at the input of the AV node differ from those measured at its output.

The *effective refractory period* of the AV node refers to the minimal interval between two atrial impulses that can propagate through it. The *functional refractory period* of the AV node refers to the minimal interval between two impulses exiting the node to excite the His bundle. Because of AV nodal conduction delay, the functional refractory period is longer than the effective refractory period. The determination of effective refractory period and functional refractory period can be made from the relationship between the input intervals (A_1–A_2) and output intervals (H_1–H_2) (Fig. 2–9). The response of AV nodal conduction (A_2–H_2) to different input intervals is also shown in Figure 2–9. While the solid curve was the most common type of relationship observed, occasionally there is an abrupt increase in conduction times at short input intervals. This observation has led to the concept that there may be *dual pathways* in the AV node, one with fast conduction and longer effective refractory periods and the other with slower conduction and lesser effective refractory periods (Moe et al., 1956). The concept of dual pathways is supported by the rare observations of human subjects who spontaneously switch between two different nodal conduction times — that is, different PR intervals on the ECG. It is plausible that dual pathways might make up the elements of re-entry circuit in the AV node if they were presented with an atrial or ventricular impulse that found one pathway refractory but not the other. However, it is likely that the AV node is a fertile field for re-entry even without two distinct pathways because of its intrinsically slow conduction and heterogeneous recovery.

Following an abrupt increase in atrial rate, AV nodal conduction time prolongs progressively over a number of beats to reach a new stable level. If there is marked encroachment on the relative refractory period, AV nodal conduction may prolong progressively over two or more beats until there is complete block of an impulse in the node. Subsequent to the blocked beat, a new cycle will begin with a shorter AV nodal conduction time. Cycles of progressively lenghthening conduction times, culminating in block of an impulse, are referred to as *Wenckebach cycles.* Cellular electrophysiologic correlates and electrocardiographic manifestations of AV nodal Wenckebach cycles are shown in Figure 2–10. Wenckebach cycles are a normal response of the AV node to repetitive excitation early in the relative refractory period. This type of conduction is abnormal in the AV node only if it occurs at relatively slower rates indicating pro-

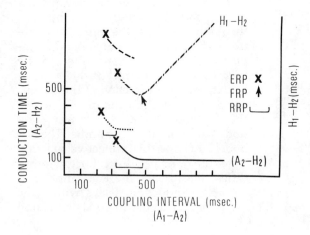

Figure 2–9. A-V nodal conduction time (A_2–H_2) and the interval between His bundle responses (H_1–H_2) following atrial extrasystoles at different coupling intervals (A_1–A_2). The effective refractory period (ERP), the functional refractory period (FRP), and the relative refractory period (RRP) of the A-V node are indicated by the designated symbols. Shorter upper curves of each set show the responses seen in some hearts in which there is an abrupt increase in conduction time at short coupling intervals.

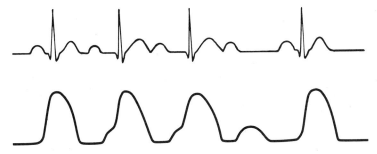

Figure 2–10. Transmembrane potentials of an A-V nodal cell and electrocardiographic characteristics during an A-V nodal Wenckebach sequence.

longation of the relative refractory period. The Wenckebach pattern of conduction is also observed in other types of cardiac cells but almost exclusively under abnormal conditions.

Both conduction and refractoriness of the AV node are quite sensitive to neural, hormonal, and pharmacologic influences (Childers, 1977). Sympathomimetic agents speed conduction and shorten refractoriness. Parasympathomimetic agents and digitalis preparations slow conduction and prolong refractoriness. The effective refractory period lengthens with increasing heart rate, but the functional refractory period shortens.

The His–Purkinje System

Having been slowed in the AV node, the impulse is accelerated in the His bundle. In the transition from the AV node to the His bundle, the cells acquire characteristics that are associated with more rapid conduction: greater resting potentials, more rapid upstrokes, and greater overshoots. These characteristics are even better developed in the bundle branches. At these sites, upstroke velocities and overshoots are the highest found in the heart. If the AV node can be considered as specialized to retard and limit the frequency of conducted impulses, the His–Purkinje system can be viewed as functioning for rapid and widespread dispersal of the impulse to allow subendocardial myocardial cells throughout the heart to be activated nearly simultaneously. In His–Purkinje cells, refractoriness corresponds to the duration of the action potential, except that there is some slight delay after repolarization is complete. Distally, the duration of action potentials and of refractoriness increases progressively.

The refractory period of the right bundle branch is longer than that of the left in most hearts, mainly because the interior septal fibers of the left bundle branch, which originate from the very proximal left bundle branch, have relatively brief refractory periods (Lazzara, 1976). The action potentials of the main right and left bundle grow progressively longer in duration with progression distally (Fig. 2–11). Because of the longer refractory period of the right bundle branch system, early premature beats originating above the His bundle are likely to encounter refractoriness in the right bundle branch at coupling intervals when the left bundle branch block is receptive. Under these circumstances the QRS complex assumes the configuration of a right bundle branch block. The alteration of the QRS complex as a result of conduction block in refractory portions of the ventricular conduction system is termed *"aberrancy"* or *aberrant conduction.*

The border fibers of the left bundle branch appear to be specialized for rapid conduction to the ventricular free

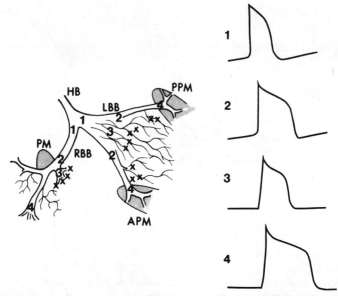

Figure 2–11. Comparison of durations of action potentials at selected sites in the ventricular specialized conduction system. The diagram of the conduction system is shown to the left with the sites designated by numbers. The corresponding numbered transmembrane potentials are shown at right as recorded during antegrade activation. The regions of earliest myocardial excitation (Purkinje-myocardial junctions) are indicated by x's. Note that action potentials become progressively longer distally along the main right bundle branch and the borders of the left bundle branch. However, septal fibers feeding the earliest Purkinje-myocardial junctions have significantly shorter action potentials and refractory periods than fibers at comparable levels on the pathways mentioned above (compare 2 and 3).

walls. Higher values of conduction velocity are attained in the border fibers than in the parallel interior septal fibers. Border fibers are relatively straight and sparsely branched in comparison with interior septal fibers, which are serpentine and rather freely interconnected. Interruption of border fibers appears to delay activation of the corresponding free wall of the left ventricle by 5 to 10 msec in the dog. It is likely that delay in activation of similar magnitude in man, caused by lesions of the border fibers, could account for the axis shifts and electrocardiographic changes referred to as "hemiblock."

The cells of the His–Purkinje system normally manifest gradual diastolic depolarization, the intrinsic rate being highest in the His bundle and proximal bundle branches and least in the peripheral Purkinje fibers. The intrinsic firing rate of the very proximal His–Purkinje system is 35 to 40 beats per minute, but the firing rate of the most peripheral fibers may be less than 10 and irregular (Hope et al., 1976). Some peripheral fibers are quiescent in vitro.

Autonomic influences have little effect on normal conduction and refractoriness in the His–Purkinje system. Sympathomimetic agents increase the automatic firing rate. The influence of the parasympathomimetic agents on automaticity is controversial.

THE ABNORMAL CARDIAC CELL CONDUCTION

A basic response of cardiac cells to various insults is to decrease the absolute magnitude of the resting membrane potential — that is, to partially depolarize. As a result, the rapid sodium channel is partially inactivated, the upstroke velocities and overshoots of action potentials are diminished, and conduction velocity is reduced. In addition, pathologic conditions may depress the rapid sodium channels so that the upstroke is even slower than might be expected at a given membrane potential. It is well known that certain pharmacologic agents depress the responsiveness of the membrane (Fig. 2–12; see also Chapter 23).

Under certain circumstances, greatly depressed upstrokes may occur at low levels of membrane potential where normal cells would be inexcitable because the normal rapid sodium channel is completely inactivated (Cranefield, 1977). Such upstrokes probably result either from calcium flowing through the slow channel or an abnormally functioning rapid sodium channel. The common consequence of depression of the upstroke, whatever the mechanism, is impairment of conduction.

Depression of the upstrokes, especially if coupled with depression of excitability, reduces the safety factor for conduction; that is, the reserve of excitatory current in excess of that required to excite is diminished. At sites where the cells are very depressed, both the direction and configuration of the approaching wavefront of excitation may be important in determining the success of conduction through or across the depressed region. For example, if the wavefront proceeds for relatively long distances through the depressed tissue, it will be more likely to block at a critically depressed site than if it approaches that site over a short distance of depressed tissue. A model of directionally selective or *unidirectional block* based on different spatial gradients of depression is illustrated in Figure 2–13. The configuration of the advancing wavefront may also be an important determinant of the velocity and continuation of conducted impulses. For example, a convergent wavefront may be more effective in excitation of a depressed region than a divergent one (Fig. 2–14). Fragmentation of wavefronts is likely to occur in depressed regions because the pathophysiological conditions are rarely homogeneous.

Refractoriness

Since the action potential duration may be shortened or lengthened under various abnormal circumstances, refractory periods may be shortened or lengthened correspondingly. For example, *hypoxia* characteristically shortens the action potential duration, while *ischemia* lengthens its duration, sometimes to a marked degree. Conditions that primarily alter the action potential plateau would produce changes in absolute refractory period without influencing the duration of the relative refractory period.

Figure 2–12. Membrane responsiveness curves relating maximal upstroke velocities (V̇ max) to the membrane potential (V) at excitation. A normal curve (solid) is compared with a curve (diagonally interrupted) of depressed upstroke velocities generated in a similar range of transmembrane potentials as the normal curve. The lowest curve was obtained from a markedly depressed cell.

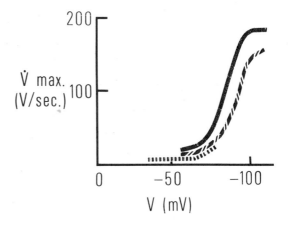

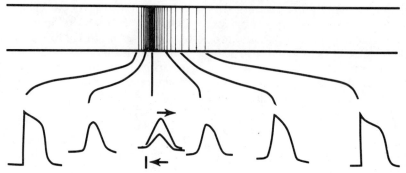

Figure 2–13. Unidirectional block in a fiber with an asymmetrically depressed segment. The degree of depression is indicated by the density of the vertical lines. Samples of transmembrane potentials recorded from different sites are shown below. Conduction from left to right succeeds (note the larger action potential in the most depressed segment) but conduction from right to left fails owing to a more diminished response in the most depressed segment.

Changes in the absolute refractory period operate differently in the generation of arrhythmias than do changes in the relative refractory period. The duration of the absolute refractory period determines the maximum rate at which cells may respond. Thus, the absolute refractory period may provide a limita- tion on the rate of tachyarrhythmias. In this respect, prolongation of the absolute refractory period may be considered advantageous. However, the absolute refractory period may be the basis for a functional "barrier," allowing for the formation of a re-entry circuit (see below). The relative refractory

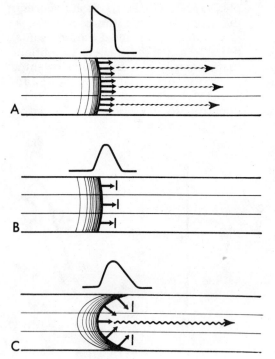

Figure 2–14. The influence of the configuration of the wavefront of propagation on conduction in depressed fibers. In the top diagram (A) the short arrows leading the propagating wavefront signify the density of excitatory current generated by the normal action potential shown above. Each normal segment demarcated by the thinner horizontal lines requires at least one arrow for excitation. In B, the strand is depressed, as indicated by the poor action potential above. The density of excitatory current is reduced (fewer arrows), and the excitability of the fibers is diminished to the extent that *two* arrows are required to excite the segment. Since no segment receives sufficient current, propagation in the strand fails. In C, the strand is equally depressed but the concave wavefront focuses excitatory current on the middle segment (note three arrows) and meets the requirement for excitation (two arrows). Consequently, propagation in the strand succeeds.

period, during which excitability is reduced and upstrokes are depressed, provides a substrate for slow and irregular conduction which is a critical factor in re-entry as well.

Spatial variations in both relative and absolute refractory periods cause irregularity and fragmentation of the wavefronts of propagated impulses which originate during the refractory periods. This factor, which has been called *"dispersion of refractoriness,"* commonly is used to explain *"vulnerability"* — that is, the induction of ventricular fibrillation or multiple ventricular responses by excitation during the T-wave (repolarization phase) of the electrocardiogram (Han and Moe, 1964). Excitation during the T-wave signifies activation during the absolute and relative refractory periods of various cells. Therefore, the progress of this impulse will be irregular, since conduction would be variably slowed or blocked in different regions depending on spatial variations in the duration of absolute and relative refractory periods throughout the ventricular myocardium. It is not difficult to conceive how the propagating wavefront under such conditions might fragment into multiple wavelets proceeding in multiple directions — that is, into *ventricular fibrillation.*

While refractoriness is usually linked closely to repolarization, if *reactivation* of the fast or slow channel is delayed much beyond the completion of repolarization, refractoriness will persist even after the cell is fully repolarized. This type of refractoriness also may be subdivided into absolute and relative refractory periods which operate in the genesis of arrhythmias in the same manner as refractoriness that is linked closely to repolarization. Post-repolarization refractoriness appears to be more prominent when cells are depolarized and depressed and thus is more likely to be significant in markedly abnormal regions that are sources of arrhythmias. It has been observed to last several minutes and may outlast the entire cardiac

cycle, with the result that each basic beat impinges on the refractory period of the abnormal region. This factor may be important in the generation of re-entrant ectopic beats linked to basic beats — for example, in the generation of bigeminal premature ventricular complexes. Moreover, the great variation in these time dependent processes superimposed upon variations in action potential durations amplifies the dispersion of refractory period durations, promoting irregularity and fragmentation of the wavefronts of activation.

Re-entry

Re-entry refers to the repetitive excitation of a site by an impulse propagating continuously around a circuit that includes it. Figure 2–15 illustrates the requisite conditions for re-excitation by means of a re-entrant circuit. First, a barrier must exist in order to form a circuit. In the case of the ring, the barrier is the central hole in the ring, which prevents a short cut from one segment of the ring to the other. Second, the conduction time around the ring must exceed the refractory period of the site that is re-excited by the re-entrant impulse. In the case of normal cardiac muscle, the long refractory period makes re-entry difficult, if not impossible. A locus of abnormally slow conduction helps satisfy the requirement that the transit time exceed the refractory period of the site that is re-excited. (Alternatively, conduction could be slow throughout the ring, or the refractory period of the re-entry site could be short.)

The interrelationship (and sometimes delicate balance!) between transit times and refractory periods in re-entry circuits makes them vulnerable to pre-excitation of an element of the circuit, rendering it inexcitable on arrival of the potential re-entrant impulse. This is the basis for the concept that abolition of a

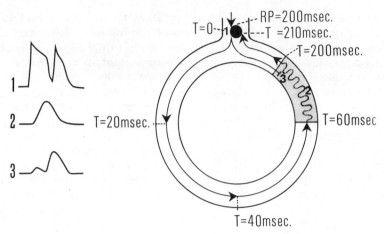

Figure 2–15. Ring model of a re-entry circuit. A segment of slow conduction (shaded) and a site of unidirectional block (3) are shown. The refractory period (RP) of the entry site and the transit times (t) to various points in the circuit are indicated. The transmembrane potentials generated at various sites are on the left.

tachyarrhythmia by means of a relatively premature beat (either induced or spontaneous) strongly suggests a re-entrant mechanism for the tachyarrhythmia.

The third prerequisite for re-entry is that propagation of the impulse must proceed in only one direction around the circuit to avoid collision and extinguishment of the impulse. It is possible that normal anatomic barriers may play a role in re-entry under certain conditions. For instance, the orifices of the venae cavae might be the barrier for a circuit formed in some cases of atrial flutter (see Chapter 7). In abnormal hearts, pathologic and functional barriers may commonly exist in the form of regions of necrosis, scars, or viable but inexcitable myocardium. Undoubtedly, the major deterrent to re-entry in many circumstances is the requirement of conduction in only one direction around the circuit. In the model of Figure 2–15, this requirement is fulfilled by the inclusion of a locus of *unidirectional block*.

Two-dimensional or three-dimensional models can be constructed which are consonant with the multidirectional nature of conduction in the cardiac syncytium. The planar model in Figure 2–16 incorporates the basic features of the ring model: barriers, loci of

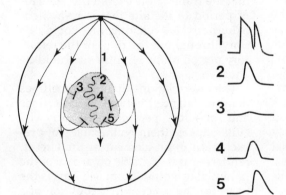

Figure 2–16. Planar surface model of re-entry. The multidirectional spread of activation is indicated by the various arrowheads. There is a depressed region of slow conduction and block (stippled). The impulse blocks at all sites at the margin of this region except one entry site (2) and an exit site (5) of directionally selective conduction. Transmembrane potentials recorded at the various sites are shown to the right.

slow conduction, and *directionally selective* (i.e., unidirectional) block. A "circuit" exists by virtue of barriers to conduction occurring within the abnormal region. Slow conduction occurs along a single pathway in the abnormal region, which has barriers on either side. The impulse exits and circles along normal myocardium around the barriers in the abnormal region to re-excite all the normal myocardium, including the original site of generation of the impulse. Thus, the circuit is complete. As in the linear model, slow conduction is essential to allow time for recovery of the surrounding normal myocardium if the dimensions of the region are relatively small.

It is possible that all the required conditions for re-entry could be fulfilled by changes in refractoriness. The barrier could be a localized region that is absolutely refractory at the time of arrival of the impulse. An adjoining region that is relatively refractory could serve as a slowly conducting pathway. Finally, directionally selective block could occur in a region that was absolutely refractory at the time of initial arrival of the impulse but had recovered by the time of arrival of the slowly conducted impulse from another portion of the circuit.

In tachyarrhythmias in which re-entry has been most strongly implicated in man, refractoriness appears to be the basis for slow conduction and directionally selective block. The tachyarrhythmias of pre-excitation syndromes are illustrative of this point (see Chapter 13). It is felt that re-entry in these tachyarrhythmias is usually initiated by a premature impulse that finds either the AV node or the accessory pathway absolutely refractory and the other relatively refractory. On the first transit, the impulse proceeds slowly along the relatively refractory pathway and blocks at the absolutely refractory pathway. By the time the impulse has crossed the barrier between atria and ventricles (i.e., the AV ring), the absolutely re-

fractory element has become responsive and allows return of the impulse to the chamber of origin. Thus, the three elements of re-entry, slow conduction, directionally-selective block, and a barrier, operate to form a "successful" circuit. Two of the elements, slow conduction and directionally selective block, are dependent on refractoriness. The other element, the barrier, is an anatomic one. There are other examples of tachyarrhythmias — for example, paroxysmal supraventricular tachycardia involving the AV node, and ventricular tachycardia involving the bundle branches in which re-entry has been implicated and the essential elements for re-entry derive from refractoriness.

Abnormal Automaticity

The rate of firing of normally automatic cells is subject to innumerable influences, normal and abnormal. Normal controls acting in excess generally or locally might cause arrhythmias. For example, excess vagal discharge could produce marked *bradyarrhythmia* by depression of SA nodal, atrial, and junctional pacemakers. Conversely, excess sympathetic influence in a local region might accelerate subsidiary pacemakers to the extent that they could usurp control of the heart, producing *ectopic tachycardias*. Abnormal conditions, such as hypoxia or ischemia, may change various factors such as the local distribution of potassium and calcium ions and the concentration of free catecholamines, all of which can affect automaticity. Besides simply increasing the intrinsic firing rate of automatic cells, abnormal conditions may affect the regularity of firing. Ischemic Purkinje fibers have been observed to fire irregularly because of erratic changes in the rate of diastolic depolarization or erratic shifts in threshold potential.

As cells become partially depolarized, the threshold potential tends to shift upward. This might affect the rate, depending on the new relationship between maximum diastolic potential and threshold potential. If cells are depolarized by the passage of depolarizing current, the frequency of firing consistently increases. However, cells depolarized under various abnormal conditions do not always show increased automaticity. Upward shift of the threshold potential would result in slower and smaller upstrokes as well, and consequently slower conduction. This might account for block into and out of some abnormal automatic foci (Singer et al., 1967). If the abnormally automatic focus is in one of the conduction pathways, there might be block not only of automatic beats but also of impulses propagating along the pathway into the abnormal region late in diastole (Cranefield, 1975). Because of diastolic depolarization, and the upward shift of the threshold potential, upstrokes generated late in diastole would arise from low membrane potentials and be slow and diminished. This mechanism may be the basis for *"bradycardia-dependent block"* (Fig. 2–17).

It has been known for many years that automaticity can be induced in non-automatic, ordinary myocardial cells under certain conditions, includ-ing exposure to barium, aconitine, or solutions free of potassium and calcium. Intracellular recordings have revealed that slow diastolic depolarization resembling that of normal automatic cells may appear. Types of automatic firing with distinctive cellular electrophysiological features have also been observed. One type of automatic firing appears as a consequence of transient partial depolarizations that follow action potentials, also called *after-depolarizations* (Cranefield, 1977). After full repolarization, the membrane potential may move positively, much like the usual diastolic depolarization of automatic cells. However, after depolarizing for several hundred milliseconds or more (up to several seconds), the membrane potential returns to a more negative and stable diastolic potential. If the after-depolarization reaches threshold potential, a spontaneous action potential occurs. This, in turn, may be followed by an after-depolarization reaching threshold, and this process can be repetitive.

The magnitude of the after-depolarizations is increased by shorter cycles (higher rate) of the antecedent action potentials. This behavior contrasts with overdrive suppression of diastolic depolarization of normally au-

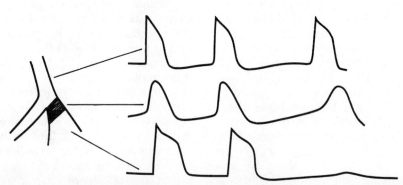

Figure 2–17. Bradycardia-dependent bundle branch block. A diagram of the branching His bundle is shown at the left with an abnormal segment at the origin of the left bundle branch (shaded). Action potentials are depressed at long cycles (bradycardia) because of diastolic depolarization and upward shift of the threshold potential. The action potentials in the abnormal region are adequate for conduction at short cycles. However, after a long cycle, the poor upstroke fails to propagate distally.

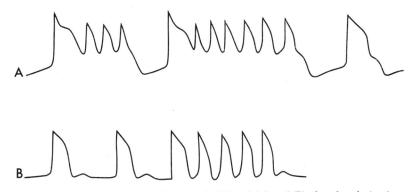

Figure 2–18. Triggerable automaticity due to early (A) and delayed (B) after-depolarizations. In *A*, the after-depolarizations and spikes interrupt repolarization. In *B*, the after-depolarizations occur in the initial portion of diastole. Their amplitude is greater after short cycles. After the third action potential from the left, the after-depolarization attains threshold and fires, initiating a run of tachycardia.

tomatic cells. Tachyarrhythmias due to after-depolarization may be induced (or terminated) by premature beats in a manner reminiscent of re-entrant tachyarrhythmias.

Another type of automatic firing occurs during repolarization of a preceding action potential. One or a series of spikes interrupts the process of repolarization. These spikes sometimes appear after a perceptible short depolarizing drift, which could be called an early after-depolarization (because it appears before the completion of full repolarization) (Fig. 2–18).

These types of automaticity have been termed triggerable automaticity because they are closely linked to repolarization of a previous action potential. The automatic firing will not occur unless an action potential is generated by stimulation or propagation. However, triggerable automaticity has been observed in normally automatic fibers as a phenomenon superimposed upon the slower, normal process of diastolic depolarization. After-depolarizations attracted little attention until the past few years because the circumstances under which they occurred were highly contrived and unphysiologic. Recently, the observation of after-depolarizations in Purkinje fibers exposed to digitalis preparations and in certain fiber types

exposed to catecholamines have given more credence to the possibility that after-depolarizations might be a basis for clinical arrhythmias. As with many phenomena rediscovered during the modern electrophysiological era, after-potentials were postulated as the basis for arrhythmias before they were actually documented in cardiac cells.

REFERENCES

Brooks, C. M., Orias, O., Gilbert, J. L., Siebert, A. A., Hoffman, B., and Suckling, E. E.: Excitability of the Heart. New York, Grune and Stratton, 1955.

Childers, R.: The AV node: Normal and abnormal physiology. Progr. Cardiovasc. Dis. *19*:361, 1977.

Coraboeuf, E., Deroubaix, E., and Hoerter, J.: Control of ionic permeabilities in normal and ischemic heart. Circ. Res. *38*(Supp I):92, 1976.

Cranefield, P. F.: Action potentials, after potentials, and arrhythmias. Circ. Res. *41*:415, 1977.

Cranefield, P. F.: The Conduction of the Cardiac Impulse. The Slow Response and Cardiac Arrhythmias. Mt. Kisco, NY, Future Pub. Co., 1975.

Fozzard, H. A.: Cardiac muscle: Excitability and passive electrical properties. Progr. Cardiovasc. Dis. *19*:343, 1977.

Han, J., and Moe, G. K.: Non-uniform recovery of excitability in ventricular myocardium. Circ. Res. *14*:44, 1964.

Hoffman, B. F., and Cranefield, P. F.: Electrophysiology of the Heart. New York, McGraw Hill, 1960.

Hope, R. R., Scherlag, B. J., El-Sherif, N., and Lazzara, R.: Hierarchy of ventricular pacemakers. Circ. Res. *39*:883, 1976.

Janse, M. J., and Anderson, R. H.: Specialized internodal atrial pathways — fact or fiction. Eur. J. Cardiol. *2*:117, 1974.

Lazzara, R., El-Sherif, N., Befeler, B., and Scherlag, B. J.: Regional refractoriness within the ventricular conduction system. An evaluation of the "gate" hypothesis. Circ. Res. *39*:254, 1976.

Moe, G. K.: Evidence for reentry as a mechanism of cardiac arrhythmias. Rev. Physiol. Biochem. Pharmacol. *72*:56, 1975.

Moe, G. K., Preston, J. B., and Burlington, H.: Physiologic evidence for a dual A-V transmission system. Circ. Res. *4*:322, 1956.

Noble, D.: Applications of Hodgkin-Huxley equations to excitable tissues. Physiol. Rev. *46*:1, 1966.

Reuter, H.: Divalent cations as charge carriers in excitable membranes. Progr. Biophys. Molec. Biol. *26*:1, 1973.

Singer, D. H., Lazzara, R., and Hoffman, B. F.: Interrelationship between automaticity and conduction in Purkinje fibers. Circ. Res. *21*:531, 1967.

Thomas, R. C.: Electrogenic sodium pump in nerve and muscle cells. Physiol. Rev. *52*:563, 1972.

Weidmann, S.: The effect of the cardiac membrane potential on the rapid availability of the sodium carrying system. J. Physiol. *127*:213, 1955.

West, T. C.: Electrophysiology of the sinoatrial node. *In* DeMello, W. C. (ed.): Electrical Phenomena in the Heart. New York, Academic Press, 1972.

Zipes, D. P., and Mendez, C.: Action of manganese ions and tetrodotoxin on AV nodal transmembrane potentials in isolated rabbit hearts. Circ. Res. *32*:447, 1973.

3

GENERAL DISCUSSION OF ARRHYTHMIAS

MONTY M. BODENHEIMER, M.D.,
RICHARD H. HELFANT, M.D.

INTRODUCTION

Normal heart rhythm is generally considered to exist if it originates in the sinus node, is conducted through the normal pathways, and has a regular rate of 60 to 100 beats per minute. Such a definition has the attraction of simplicity; however, it fails to clarify the significance of variations in this rhythm, including those arising from the sinus node. By the standard definition, any sinus rhythm of less than 60 beats per minute is considered abnormal. Yet young adults, particularly those who are athletic, frequently demonstrate resting heart rates of 40 beats per minute or less, often with intermittent junctional escape rhythms and occasionally even with A-V nodal block. Furthermore, children and young adults may manifest grossly irregular heart rates that on closer inspection are seen to constitute a marked sinus arrhythmia that has no pathologic significance. In contrast, these same rhythms in the symptomatic elderly patient are frequently manifestations of serious underlying disease.

The standard definition of sinus tachycardia is equally imprecise. Although a heart rate of more than 100 beats per minute is labeled abnormal, it

may in fact be a normal response to stress. Indeed, a low sinus rate in this situation can be inappropriate enough to suggest an underlying entity such as hypothyroidism. These variations on "normal" make it clear that *a cardiac rhythm must be evaluated in the clinical setting in which it is seen*! This is true of all heart rhythms. Any evaluation of the significance, untoward effects, and treatment of a disorder of the heart beat is inadequate without the relevant clinical information.

The following terms have been used synonymously to describe clinical disorders of the heart beat.

Arrhythmia. This is the most common term and it has become widely accepted, despite the fact that it erroneously suggests an irregularity of the heart beat. On the contrary, many of the arrhythmias have an entirely regular rhythm as, for example, paroxysmal atrial tachycardia, atrial flutter, ventricular tachycardia, complete A-V heart block, and others.

Ectopic Rhythm. Ectopic rhythm implies an abnormal origin of impulse formation outside the S-A node and may therefore refer to a regular or an irregular rhythm. This term may also be misleading, however, since it indicates that a specific mechanism is the cause

TABLE 3–1 ARRHYTHMIAS ON ECG

	Population	Atrial					Ventricular Frequent or			A-V Block		
		Sinus Bradycardia < 60/min	SVC	SVT	Atrial Flutter	A. Fib.	Occas.	Complex	V. Tachy.	1°	2°	3°
Katz and Pick (1956)	50,000	5.8%	6.7%	1.3%	0.5%	11.7%	7.5%	–	0.16%	2.9%	0.79	0.47%
Tecumseh study Ostrander (1965) Chiang (1969)	5129 44% > 40 yrs	–	1.5%	–	0.43%		3.6%	1.7%	–	1.4%	0	2 Persons
Hiss et al. (1962)	122,043 men 17.3% > 40 yrs	23.8%	0.43%	–	5 Persons		0.78%	0.32%	6 Persons	0.65%	8 Persons	3 Persons

SVC = supraventricular complexes; SVT = supraventricular tachycardia; A = atrial.

of the rhythm disorder, which, indeed, may not be the case (see Chapter 2).

Dysrhythmia. This term is applicable not only to cardiac irregularities but also to disturbances of cardiac rhythm in which the rhythm is, nonetheless, regular.

In general, the term arrhythmia will be employed throughout this book because of its widespread usage in referring to disorders of the heart beat. The terms complex, beat, and contraction are used in association with atrial, junctional, and ventricular premature. Some prefer one term to another. For example, since contraction implies that the abnormal beat resulted in ventricular systole, some uses of the terms may be technically inaccurate. However, since these terms are essentially similar, we will use them interchangeably.

ETIOLOGY

The etiology of cardiac arrhythmias can be considered from either of two vantage points. In one situation, the physician is asked to evaluate a rhythm that is a major element in the clinical presentation of the patient and must decide on the specific disease process or processes that may be responsible. In a second situation, the patient may have a known condition (e.g., coronary heart disease) and the clinician must then be aware that different arrhythmias have different prognostic and therapeutic implications, depending on the clinical setting. Thus, the clinician must be prepared to approach arrhythmias either as a primary event without a clear etiology or as a secondary event in a patient with a known disease entity.

Prior to considering specific arrhythmias, a clear understanding of the normal spectrum of rhythm abnormalities in the population at large is useful. For this purpose, we will confine ourselves to examining recordings that were made incidental to the patient's primary condition or are from asymptomatic ambulatory patients as part of prospective studies or studies to clarify the incidence of arrhythmias. These studies have shown that the frequency and type of cardiac arrhythmias vary considerably with the age and medical status of the population examined. The method used to detect arrhythmias — a single ECG comprising less than 1 minute of recording or a long-term monitoring of cardiac rhythm — can also affect the results.

Katz and Pick (1956) reported on the ECG-determined incidence of arrhythmias in 50,000 consecutive in-hospital patients over a 25-year period (Table 3–1). Forty-five per cent of the ECG's showed arrhythmias, including atrial premature complexes (5.6 per cent), ventricular premature complexes (7.5 per cent), atrial fibrillation (11.7 per cent), A-V heart block (4.1 per cent), and A-V dissociation (1.4 per cent). Another 20 per cent demonstrated sinus tachycardia, bradycardia, or irregularities of various other types. Only 35 per cent showed a normal sinus rhythm. In contrast, in a study of electrocardiograms obtained from 5,129 ambulatory adults entered in a longitudinal trial in Tecumseh, Michigan, a significantly lower incidence of arrhythmias was found, including supraventricular contractions in 1.5 per cent and ventricular premature complexes in 3.6 per cent. It is noteworthy, however, that in patients over the age of 40 years the incidence of supraventricular contractions increased to 2.8 per cent and that of ventricular premature contractions to 6.8 per cent (Ostrander et al., 1965; Chiang et al., 1969). In a study involving Air Force men, Hiss and Lamb (1962) found a lower rate of atrial premature complexes of 0.43 per cent and ventricular premature complexes of 0.78 per cent overall. However, as in the Tecumseh study, in subjects over the age of 40 the frequency of ventricular premature complexes was 5.7 per cent.

Few studies are available of long-term monitoring of apparently healthy

TABLE 3–2 ARRHYTHMIAS ON LONG TERM RECORDING

Population	Atrial					Ventricular			A-V Block		
	Sinus Bradycardia <60/min	SVC	SVT	Atrial Flutter	A. Fib.	Occas.	Frequent or Complex	V. Tachy.	1°	2°	3°
Hinkle (1969) 283 Men 55 yrs average	–	76%	0.7%	–	–	62.2%	19.1%	3.2%	0		
Brodsky (1977) 50 Men 23–27 yrs	100%	56%	2%	0	0	50%	12%	2.0%	8%	6%*	–

SVC = supraventricular complexes; SVT = supraventricular tachycardia; A = atrial.
*All Wenckebach.

people. Hinkle and coworkers evaluated 283 active and clinically healthy male telephone workers with an average age of 55 using 6-hour tape recordings. They found that fully 92.6 per cent had some arrhythmia, including 76 per cent with supraventricular beats and 62.2 per cent with ventricular premature complexes (Table 3–1). However, only 19 per cent of the overall population had either definite or suggestive clinical or ECG evidence of heart disease. Interestingly, these patients accounted for only a small percentage of patients with complex ventricular arrhythmia. Thus, only 19 to 29 per cent of patients with bigeminy, trigeminy, or ventricular premature contractions from three of four foci had a clinical picture of definite or probable coronary heart disease. Moreover, of nine with ventricular tachycardia, none had such a clinical picture.

In a series of young nonathletic male volunteers ages 23 to 27, who were clinically normal, including the results of chest x-ray, ECG, and echocardiogram, Brodsky et al. (1977) evaluated 24-hour dynamic ECG recordings and found a high frequency of bradyarrhythmias, including sinus bradycardia of <50 beats per minute in 26 per cent while awake and junctional escape beats in 11 per cent. Premature atrial complexes were seen in 56 per cent and ventricular complexes in 50 per cent. (These findings are not too dissimilar from those of Hinkle in the older age group.) However, complex atrial or ventricular arrhythmias were unusual in this younger population. Only one person demonstrated more than 100 atrial premature complexes in 24 hours, and only one had more than 50 ventricular premature complexes in 24 hours. Moreover, only one subject had a run of ventricular tachycardia, which consisted of five consecutive ventricular premature complexes during sleep with a preceding sinus rate of 45 beats per minute.

These two studies clearly show that ventricular and atrial arrhythmias are common in people of all ages. However, as suggested by early ECG studies, frequent and complex ventricular arrhythmias are unusual in the younger population and become increasingly frequent with age.

Arrhythmia as the Primary Presentation

Etiologies of specific arrhythmias are varied. Sinus tachycardia, although occasionally presenting problems in differential diagnosis (see Chapter 4), usually implies the presence of underlying stress with increased secretion of catecholamines owing to either a direct cardiac or an extracardiac cause. Atrial and junctional tachycardias, frequently grouped as supraventricular tachycardias, are associated with clinically normal hearts in approximately 50 per cent of patients. However, additional etiologies must be considered, including valvular heart disease, pericarditis, drugs, and hyperthyroidism. Furthermore, a very rapid ventricular response of over 250 beats per minute should suggest a preexcitation syndrome as a possible etiology.

Multifocal atrial tachycardia is of interest here (Shine et al., 1968). The clinical setting is often a patient on digitalis therapy, and the drug is thus indicted as the causative agent. Yet several studies have now clearly shown that the most frequent mechanism is pulmonary failure, usually caused by chronic obstructive pulmonary disease. Treatment should be directed primarily toward the lung disease.

Atrial fibrillation and atrial flutter are unusual arrhythmias in clinically normal patients (see Table 3–2). A concerted effort should, therefore, be made to clarify whether the etiology is valvular heart disease (particularly mitral disease), primary myocardial disease or pericardial as opposed to extracardiac causes (e.g., pulmonary parenchymal disease, pulmonary emboli, or hyperthyroidism). Digitalis is only rarely, if ever, responsible for atrial flutter or atrial fibrillation. In contrast, atrial tachycardia with block is caused by an excess of digitalis in the majority of instances, necessitating its discontinuance. (Coronary heart disease, hypokalemia, and rheumatic heart disease should be considered if the patient is not taking digitalis.)

Accelerated rhythms, whether junctional or ventricular, strongly suggest digitalis toxicity. However, such rhythms may also be seen in other conditions, including hypokalemia or acute myocardial infarction. The clinical setting will usually point to both the correct diagnosis and the proper therapy.

Ventricular premature complexes pose a special problem. Although relatively common and apparently benign in younger age groups (see Tables 3–1 and 3–2), their significance is dramatically different in the setting of underlying cardiac disease such as coronary heart disease, cardiomyopathy, or valvular disease (see Chapter 11). Ventricular tachycardia can, based on severity, always be considered abnormal, even though no clear underlying cardiac etiology can be found.

Bradyarrhythmias, wandering atrial pacemakers, and junctional escape rhythms may be normal in some individuals, particularly those who are young and athletic (Tables 3–1 and 3–2). In the elderly, however, these arrhythmias carry a more serious prognosis (Hinkle et al., 1972) and may be a manifestation of the sick sinus syndrome (see Chapter 5). A careful investigation should also be made for drugs such as digitalis and for diseases such as hypertension that are commonly treated with negative chronotropic agents, including reserpine, guanethidine, alpha methyldopa, and propranolol. Other potential causes are hypothyroidism and increased intracranial pressure.

Heart block should always raise the possibility of underlying organic disease. In the elderly, it is frequently attributable to degenerative fibrosis of the conduction system; however, other entities such as coronary heart disease, cardiomyopathy, or aortic valvular disease should be considered. Again, the clinical setting is critical. Young patients who are clinically normal (confirmed, if necessary, by catheterization including electrophysiologic studies) may manifest first degree or Wenckebach type second degree A-V block. These findings should not be cause for alarm. However, viral infections, diphtheria, and even jaundice may at times be responsible. Congenital heart block in the absence of symptoms is usually not an indication for pacemaker treatment, although this has recently been questioned.

Diseases Associated with Cardiac Arrhythmias

Cardiac Factors. These include cardiac abnormalities of coronary, hypertensive, rheumatic, congenital, primary myocardial, infectious, or degenerative origin, as well as the presence of congestive heart failure. Treatment of the primary disorder (such as control of blood pressure or treatment of congestive heart failure) may reduce or eliminate the cardiac arrhythmia. However, specific antiarrhythmic therapy is frequently required.

Extracardiac Factors. These include functional or organic changes originating in organ systems outside the heart as well as drug-induced abnormalities. The primary source may be changes in the autonomic nervous system (including excess of vagal or sympathetic tone), head trauma, or organic brain disease. Psychologic factors such as anxiety and stress may also be responsible. Acute and chronic lung disease, pulmonary embolization, and other conditions that increase right-sided heart strain and decrease ventilation may result in hypoxia and atrial or ventricular arrhythmias. Endocrine disturbances (including hypo- and hyperthyroidism), disturbances in the adrenals (such as hyperaldosteronism), and diabetes can all lead to arrhythmias. Renal disease with secondary hypertension, electrolyte and acid-base disturbances (particularly hyper- and hypopotassemia), and alterations in fluid balance can also be responsible for various arrhythmias. Hyperpotassemia must be remembered as a potential cause of an accelerated rhythm with a wide QRS complex, and this should be actively sought, since correct treatment is life-saving and entirely dependent on recognition (see Chapter 19).

Drug intake is a primary consideration in the evaluation of any patient with an arrhythmia. Not infrequently, cardiac medications (including digitalis, diuretics, and antiarrhythmic drugs) or noncardiac agents (such as major tranquilizers) are responsible for the arrhythmia.

CLASSIFICATION OF ARRHYTHMIAS

Various classifications of arrhythmias are available. The arrhythmias can be classified according to their mechanisms as:

1. disorders of impulse formation (i.e., those caused by abnormal automaticity);

2. disorders of impulse conduction;

3. disorders produced by abnormalities of both impulse formation and impulse conduction. The physiologic concepts underlying these mechanisms have been discussed in detail in Chapter 2, and data pertaining to the mechanism of each arrhythmia are found in the appropriate chapters. The arrhythmias may also be divided into four groups, according to the portion of the heart in which they arise. Subdivisions of these various categories are discussed in detail under each of the arrhythmias.

A. Disturbances of rhythm involving the sinoatrial node
   1. Sinus arrhythmia
   2. Sinus bradycardia
   3. Sinoatrial block
   4. Prolonged sinus pauses (resulting in cardiac standstill or A-V junctional escape)
   5. Wandering pacemaker
   6. Sinus tachycardia

B. Disturbances involving the atria
   1. Atrial premature beats
   2. Atrial paroxysmal tachycardia
   3. Atrial flutter
   4. Atrial fibrillation
   5. Intra-atrial block; intra-atrial dissociation
   6. Atrial standstill
   7. Sinoventricular conduction

C. Disturbances involving the A-V junction
   1. Atrioventricular heart block (prolonged P-R interval, increasing grades of partial block, and complete atrioventricular block)
   2. A-V junctional rhythm
   3. A-V junctional escape, including coronary sinus rhythm
   4. A-V junctional premature beats
   5. Paroxysmal junctional tachycardia
   6. Atrioventricular dissociation (complete or with intermittent capture)
   7. Reciprocal rhythm

D. Disturbances involving the ventricles
   1. Ventricular escape
   2. Idioventricular rhythm
   3. Ventricular premature beats
   4. Ventricular paroxysmal tachycardia
   5. Ventricular flutter and ventricular fibrillation
   6. Cardiac (ventricular) arrest
   7. Heart alternation

SYMPTOMS AND SIGNS

Symptoms

The awareness of one's heart beat is quite variable. A normal person may be exquisitely conscious of either his own normal rhythm or of a benign rhythm disturbance. Often this occurs at night when one is lying on the left side. In contrast, patients with serious cardiac arrhythmias may be totally without awareness of their disorders. Kennedy and coworkers studied 25 asymptomatic patients with arrhythmias on routine ECG's (Kennedy and Underhill, 1976). Only one patient had symptoms referable to cardiac arrhythmias, yet all had more than 30 ventricular premature complexes per hour and 52 per cent had couplets. Similarly, Hinkle and colleagues (1969) found that 92.6 per cent of asymptomatic men had arrhythmias on long-term monitoring. Therefore, symptoms or their absence cannot be taken as evidence of the presence or severity of cardiac arrhythmias. A patient may complain of palpitations which, in reality, are regular sinus rhythm and require only reassurance. In addition, symptoms that are readily attributable to cardiac arrhythmias (such as dizziness, syncope, and faintness) not infrequently are found to be caused by cerebrovascular disease, aortic valvular disease, or diabetes mellitus (with hypoglycemia). Thus, although symptoms may suggest an arrhythmia as the etiology, a major effort should be made to document the presence of the arrhythmia at the time of the symptoms, either by routine ECG or with long-term rhythm monitoring (see Chapter 14).

Manifestations Associated with Rapid Heart Action

The response of the patient to a rapid heart rate depends on the ventricular rate, its duration, and the underlying condition of the heart, as well as on the mental reaction. In general, palpitation, faintness, dizziness, lightheadedness and at times actual fainting, throbbing in the head or neck, shortness of breath, and discomfort in the precordial region may occur. When organic heart disease is present and a rapid rate persists for a sufficiently long period, heart failure, angina, and even myocardial infarction or a shocklike state may ensue. An interesting, although incompletely understood, manifestation often seen after the cessation of a rapid atrial tachycardia is a marked diuresis (Boykin et al., 1975). This may be useful to elicit in order to confirm whether the patient's symptoms are secondary to a paroxysmal tachycardia.

Manifestations Associated with Slow Heart Action

Symptoms associated with a slow heart rate depend on the underlying state of the heart, the age of the patient, the cardiac rate and mechanism (partial or complete A-V block or sinus bradycardia), and the ability of the heart to make circulatory adjustment to the varying requirements of the individual. Moreover, patients with slow heart rates are more susceptible to the development of various other arrhythmias (especially ventricular premature complexes).

Patients with very slow heart rates (below 30 per minute) frequently manifest shortness of breath and fatigue on exertion because of the diminished cardiac output and impaired circulatory adjustments following effort. In addition, many of these subjects have an associated cardiovascular impairment that is aggravated by the slow heart rate. The patient may complain of dizziness and faintness. Symptoms of cerebral insufficiency can be observed if the heart rate is lowered still further for brief periods of time. During periods of ventricular standstill ranging from 3 to 9 seconds, faintness, syncope, and convulsions may occur.

Manifestations Associated with Irregular Action of the Heart

Irregular rhythms usually result from premature beats, marked sinus arrhythmia, S-A heart block, ventricular escapes, partial A-V heart block, or atrial fibrillation. These irregularities may produce few or no subjective symptoms if the ventricular rate is not unduly rapid. Patients often complain of palpitation, periodic thumping of the heart, "the heart appears to turn over," "the heart skips a beat." Generally, the discomfort is moderate but at times it produces considerable anxiety and is interpreted as pain around the heart (simulating the anginal syndrome).

CLINICAL DIAGNOSIS OF CARDIAC ARRHYTHMIAS

Although clinical features may suggest a specific arrhythmia, the ECG is essential in every case to make an accurate diagnosis. Precise delineation of cardiac arrhythmias requires knowledge of the relationship between atrial and ventricular activity. While the history may provide clues as to etiology of the arrhythmia only rarely will it be diagnostic. Some patients are able to feel their pulse accurately and may provide information such as heart rate, regularity, and so forth; however, this at best will only suggest the presence of an arrhythmia and rarely indicates its specific nature.

The physical examination can at times provide specific information regarding the rhythm. This may be accomplished by determining atrial activity, as reflected by the "a" wave in the jugular venous pulse, and ventricular activity, either the arterial pulse, apex beat, or heart sounds. However, this is often difficult, particularly with regard to the "a" wave. Thus, "ectopics" may be palpated; however, their origin (whether atrial or ventricular) cannot be ascertained. Atrial flutter with 2:1 block and paroxysmal atrial tachycardia — both with a ventricular rate of 140 per minute — could be delineated by "a" waves at 300 per minute compared to 150 per minute. Similarly, a palpated

rate of 75 per minute might either be due to sinus at 75 per minute or atrial flutter at 300 per minute with 4:1 block, and again the astute clinician could utilize the frequency of the "a" waves to delineate its nature. This is rarely accurate. Atrial fibrillation, which is diagnosed at the bedside from medical school onward, is frequently said to be characterized by an irregularly irregular pulse and a pulse deficit. However, multifocal atrial tachycardia, numerous ventricular premature complexes, and other rhythm disturbances can easily simulate these conditions. Moreover, a pulse deficit (i.e., a disparity between auscultatory and a peripheral palpated heart rate) simply reflects the presence of ventricular contractions which, primarily because of timing, are insufficient to generate an adequate pulse wave to be palpated.

Similar problems exist with bradycardias. The presence of "Cannon a waves" is considered suggestive of third degree heart block. However, the "a" wave simply reflects atrial contractions against a closed tricuspid valve. Thus, A-V dissociation with a slow ventricular response, junctional escapes, etc., without any true pathologic block may exhibit such waves. It is of historical interest that second degree A-V block of the Wenckebach type was originally described based on the jugular venous pulse, not on the ECG.

In summary, the history and physical examination can provide clues to the presence and etiology of arrhythmias. However, only rarely, if ever, should the clinician assume the diagnosis of a specific arrhythmia without an ECG.

REFERENCES

Boykin, J., Cadnapaphornchai, P., McDonald, K. M., and Schrier, R. W.: Mechanism of diuretic escape response associated with atrial tachycardia. Am. J. Physiol. 299:1486, 1975.
Brodsky, M., Wu, D., Denes, P., Kanakis, C., and Rosen, K. M.: Arrhythmias documented by 24

hour continuous electrocardiographic monitoring in 50 male medical students without apparent disease. Am. J. Cardiol. 39:390, 1977.

Chiang, B. N., Perlman, L. V., Ostrander, L. D., and Epstein, R. H.: Relationship of premature systoles to coronary heart diseease and sudden death in the Tecumseh epidemiologic study. Ann. Intern. Med. 70:1159, 1969.

Hinkle, L. E., Carver, S. T., and Plakun, A.: Slow heart rates and increased risk of cardiac death in middle aged men. Arch. Intern. Med. 129:732, 1972.

Hinkle, L. E., Carver, S. T., and Stevens, M.: The frequency of asymptomatic disturbances of cardiac rhythm and conduction in middle-aged men. Am. J. Cardiol. 24:629, 1969.

Hiss, R. G., and Lamb, L. E.: Electrocardiographic findings in 122,043 individuals. Circulation, 25:947, 1962.

Kennedy, H. L., and Underhill, S. J.: Frequent or complex ventricular ectopy in apparently healthy subjects. Am. J. Cardiol. 38:141, 1976.

Ostrander, L. D., Brandt, R. L., Kjelsberg, M. O., and Epstein, F. H.: Electrocardiographic findings among the adult population of a total natural community, Tecumseh, Michigan. Circulation 31:888, 1965.

Shine, K. I., Kastor, J. A., and Yurchak, P. M.: Multifocal atrial tachycardia. Clinical and electrocardiographic features in 32 patients. N. Engl. J. Med. 279:344, 1968.

SUPPLEMENTAL READING

Brooks, N., Leech, G., and Leatham, A.: Complete RBBB. Echophonocardiographic study of first heart sound and right ventricular contraction times. Brit. Heart J. 41:637–646, 1979.

Opie, L. H., Nathan, D., and Lubbe, W. F.: Biochemical aspects of arrhythmogenesis and ventricular fibrillation. Am. J. Cardiol. 43:131, 1979.

Sutton, R., and Citron, P.: Electrophysiological and hemodynamic basis for application of new pacemaker technology in sick sinus syndrome and AV block. Brit. Heart J. 41:600–612, 1979.

WHO/ISFC Task Force: Classification of cardiac arrhythmias and conduction disturbances. Amer. Heart J. 98:263, 1979.

4

AN APPROACH TO ARRHYTHMIA ANALYSIS

MICHAEL FELDMAN, M.D.,
RICHARD H. HELFANT, M.D.

A systematic approach is critical to establishing the correct diagnosis of a cardiac arrhythmia. This requires an orderly sequence in which atrial activity is intially identified and its rhythm established. Ventricular activity is next evaluated. Lastly, the relationship between the atrial and ventricular activity (if any) is assessed. This simple, orderly method permits the development of a "layered structure" that will allow for an accurate interpretation of even the most complex rhythm disorders.

RHYTHM STRIPS AND SPECIAL LEADS

The first step in evaluating an arrhythmia is to obtain a long rhythm strip. Frequently, recordings must be taken from several ECG leads in order to obtain one in which both atrial and ventricular activity can be clearly identified. The strip must be long enough to allow repeated identification of the various rhythm disorders and should be at least 30 seconds in duration. Leads II and VI are the most commonly utilized, since they generally exhibit the most distinctly visible atrial activity. Unfortunately, however, these conventional leads do not always clearly identify the

atrial mechanisms, and occasionally special leads must be used. These leads include the V3R lead, Lewis lead, esophageal lead and intracardiac electrograms.

V3R Lead. This is a precordial lead taken with the electrodes at the position corresponding to V3 but on the right side of the sternum.

Lewis Lead. This is a chest to right arm lead which is taken with the right arm lead (the positive pole) placed over the left chest wall and the left arm lead (the negative pole) placed either on the right arm or the right chest and recorded from lead I on the ECG machine. This latter lead offers particular advantages in that high voltages are recorded, frequently making atrial activity more distinct.

Esophageal Lead (Fig. 4–1.). This is obtained by using an esophageal electrode attached to a tube or a duodenal catheter. This lead is connected by insulated wire to the arm lead and then to the positive electrogram pole. The ECG machine is set at lead I. The catheter is first passed into the stomach as one would pass a nasogastric tube. Electrocardiograms are then recorded from successive levels in the esophagus as the tube is gradually withdrawn from the subdiaphragmatic to the supracar-

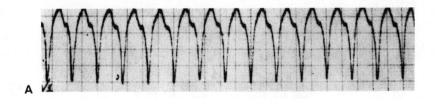

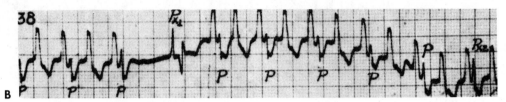

Figure 4–1. Ventricular tachycardia. V_1 and esophageal lead recording. *(A)* (V_1), Note the presence of a regular paroxysmal tachycardia with a ventricular rate of 176 beats per minute. The QRS complexes are widened and notched and no distinct P waves are observed.

   (B) The esophageal lead. The ventricular rate is 176 beats per minute, the P waves are easily seen and occur at the rate of 88 per minute, i.e., exactly half of the ventricular rate. That means that every P wave is related to the preceding QRS in a 2:1 retrograde conduction. The atrial depolarization marked PX1 follows a long pause and represents a sinus escape (note the different shape of the QRS and P wave configuration) followed by another run of ventricular tachycardia. Junctional tachycardia with aberrant conduction and a 2:1 retrograde conduction cannot be ruled out.

diac level. The electrode site is determined from markings on the tube and the presence of the intrinsic deflection of the P wave as long as the tube is contiguous to the atrium. Esophageal electrograms record atrial, transitional, or ventricular deflections according to the position of the electrode. The atrial recordings are generally present at 32 to 47 cm from the anterior nares; the transitional zone is 40 to 50 cm, and the ventricular level is 42 to 52 cm or more.

Intracardiac Electrograms. These are taken from the endocardial surface of the heart via right heart catheterization using a small electrode catheter. The catheter wire is passed from the right brachial or subclavian vein into the right atrium or right ventricle. The characteristic pattern, as obtained from the individual cavities, indicates the exact location of the catheter tip. Progressively larger P waves are recorded as the wire enters the right atrium, and significant ventricular deflections occur as the tricuspid valve is crossed and the right ventricular cavity is entered (Fig.

4–2). Should the catheter bypass the right ventricular cavity and enter the inferior vena cava, the atrial and ventricular complexes would become progressively diminished. The position of the electrode may also be determined by fluoroscopy or (less commonly) by pressure recordings. Although a catheter wire is required, this lead is especially useful for obtaining clear atrial activity and is frequently superior to the esophageal or other special lead systems.

SPECIAL DIAGNOSTIC MANIPULATIONS

Occasionally P waves are buried within the T waves and cannot be visualized despite the use of special leads. Under these circumstances, several diagnostic maneuvers have been helpful. These include: 1) carotid sinus massage, 2) Valsalva maneuver, and 3) exercise. Although carotid sinus massage is frequently a very useful diagnostic (as well as therapeutic) technique, it can be dangerous if not performed properly.

Pressure should be applied over *one* carotid at a time, beginning with the right, and the duration of pressure should *not* exceed five seconds! The patient should be in a Trendelenberg position with the head lower than the feet and the neck extended and rotated to the side opposite the carotid to be mas-

saged. The carotid sinus is located by palpating the strong carotid pulsation above the upper border of the thyroid cartilage and just below the angle of the jaw. The pressure massage is best performed with two or three fingers compressing the artery and sinus posteriorly immediately against the vertebral

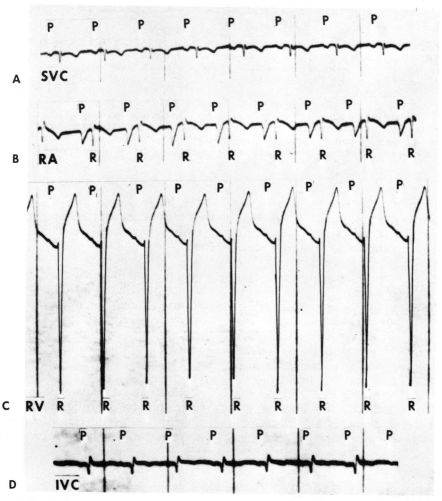

Figure 4–2. Catheter electrode recordings. (A) The complexes obtained as the catheter tip enters the superior vena cava. Note the small initial P wave and the relationship between the size of the atrial and ventricular complexes.

(B) The complexes obtained as the catheter enters the right atrium. Note the significant increase in the P wave amplitude. The atrial complex is now larger than the QRS complex.

(C) The electrode is now in the right ventricle. The P wave is now upright and has been reduced to a small dimension. The QRS is markedly increased in amplitude. Note also the ST segment elevation which is produced as the catheter tip touches the right ventricular wall.

(D) As the catheter tip fails to enter the right ventricle and instead passes into the inferior vena cava, the P wave and QRS complexes progressively diminish in size.

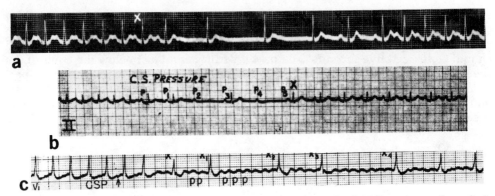

Figure 4–3. (a) The effect of carotid sinus pressure on sinus tachycardia. Initially, a sinus tachycardia is present (rate 150 beats per minute). Carotid sinus pressure is applied at X and results in marked slowing of the sinus rate. With the release of pressure, there is a gradual return to the pre-existing rate.

(b) The conversion of paroxysmal atrial tachycardia to a normal sinus rhythm following carotid sinus pressure. The occurrence of a normal sinus beat at P_1, P_2 and P_4 represents dropped beats with a 2:1 A-V heart block. Note the restoration of normal sinus rhythm in the cycles following X.

(c) The effect of carotid sinus pressure on atrial flutter. The figure shows a rapid arrhythmia, quite regular, at a rate of 160 beats per minute. The exact atrial mechanism cannot be determined at this rapid rate. Following carotid sinus pressure, note that with a slowing of the ventricular rate, the diagnosis of atrial flutter is clearly made. In view of the varying degree of block the P-R interval varies at X, X_3, and X_4.

spine (the artery should not be compressed below the sinus). An ECG rhythm strip should be taken immediately before, during, and following the massage. Carotid massage is often useful in differentiating rhythm disorders with heart rates of 140 and greater (Fig. 4–3): 1) sinus tachycardia will slow gradually; 2) paroxysmal atrial tachycardia or paroxysmal junctional tachycardia either will not change or will "break" to a slower rhythm; 3) atrial flutter will generally not change the flutter rate itself but will usually produce a higher degree of A-V block, and the ventricular response rate will de-crease from 2:1 to 4:1 (allowing better visualization of the basic flutter pattern).

The Valsalva maneuver is another technique that has been useful in evaluating tachyarrhythmias (Fig. 4–4). The response (if any) is similar to that obtained by carotid sinus massage. However, this maneuver is less frequently useful than carotid sinus massage owing to a high incidence of negative responses.

Occasionally, a diagnostic maneuver such as painful pressure over one eyeball with the eyelid closed (involving the oculocardiac reflex) has been advo-

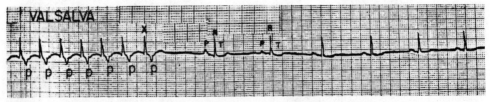

Figure 4–4. The effect of the Valsalva maneuver in terminating supraventricular tachycardia (junctional). Note the tachycardia rate of 140 beats per minute with a QRS followed by an inverted P wave. Following the Valsalva maneuver at X, note the pause and the restoration of normal sinus rhythm.

cated. However, the maneuver is dangerous in that it may result in permanent eye damage, and therefore it is not recommended. Administration of drugs such as atropine or neostigmine has also been advocated in order to alter sinus rate and A-V conduction. However, these drugs are rarely helpful, may cause serious consequences, and are not advised.

ARRHYTHMIA ANALYSIS

Atrial Activity

Once a rhythm strip clearly identifying atrial activity is obtained, a general survey should be made to determine the dominant atrial mechanism. Initially, care should be taken to determine whether the atrial activity is regular or irregular. The rhythms that produce regular atrial activity include sinus rhythm, paroxysmal atrial tachycardia, junctional escape rhythms (also called passive junctional rhythms), nonparoxysmal accelerated junctional rhythms (also called non-paroxysmal junctional tachycardia), paroxysmal junctional tachycardia, atrial flutter, and paroxysmal atrial tachycardia with block. These rhythms are differentiated primarily by their rates and P wave configurations (or vectors).

Sinus rhythm is characterized by a normal P wave configuration with the vector directed from right to left, slightly inferiorly and posteriorly. Thus, the P wave is upright in leads I, II, III and aVF, inverted in lead aVR, and biphasic (initially positive, then negative) in lead VI. The normal sinus rates of adults at rest vary from 60 to 100 beats per minute (those of infants are between 100 and 150 beats per minute). In persons beyond the age of 60, the sinus rate may be slower, often falling between 50 and 75 beats per minute. At any age, a sinus rate below 60 beats per minute is arbitrarily defined as sinus bradycardia and a rate greater than 100 beats per minute as sinus tachycardia. Sinus tachycardia rarely exceeds 160 beats per minute in adults. Interestingly, sinus rhythm is not absolutely regular, in that cycle lengths may vary slightly (Fig. 4–5).

Although there are three types of *junctional rhythms*, all are characterized by abnormal P wave configurations. When discernible atrial activity is present, the P wave vector is oriented precisely opposite the sinus node vector; that is, left to right, slightly anteriorly, and slightly superiorly. Thus, the P

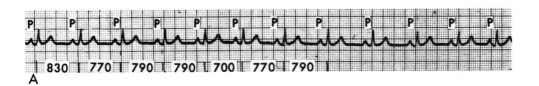

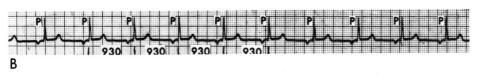

Figure 4–5. *(A)* Sinus rhythm: Note the upright P waves with normal QRS contour and a fixed P-R interval (0.16 seconds). Note also the beat-to-beat variation in the P-P interval. This is a normal feature of sinus node activity.

(B) An example of junctional rhythm (64 beats per minute). Note the inverted P wave, normal QRS and fixed P-R interval (0.16 seconds). The regular P-P interval is a feature of junctional rhythm as opposed to the slight variation in rate seen with sinus node activity.

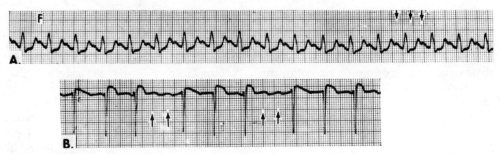

Figure 4–6. Atrial flutter masquerading as sinus tachycardia. *(A)* Note the regular atrial activity preceding each QRS. The ventricular rate is 125 per minute and is suggestive of sinus tachycardia. Note also the wide QRS complexes. The ECG strip is lead II.

   (B) Following carotid massage, a regular "sawtooth" atrial pattern is seen which is readily discernible as atrial flutter (250 per minute). Note also the narrower QRS complexes at this slower conduction rate. The ECG strip is lead V_1.

wave is inverted in leads I, II, III and aVF, upright in lead aVR, and upright in lead V1 (Fig. 4–5). Junctional escape rhythms (also called passive junctional rhythms) have rates of 40 to 70 beats per minute, non-paroxysmal junctional tachycardias have rates between 75 and 130 beats per minute, and paroxysmal junctional tachycardias have rates from 140 to 260 beats per minute.

Paroxysmal atrial tachycardia is also characterized by an abnormal P wave configuration, and both its mechanism and its rate are identical to those of paroxysmal junctional tachycardia. The distinction between the two is made by the lack of discernible atrial activity on the standard ECG in junctional rhythms.

Atrial flutter also produces regular atrial activity. The contour of flutter waves is usually distinctive, exhibiting a "sawtooth" pattern without a flat, isoelectric baseline. The flutter rate ranges between 240 and 360 beats per minute, with the great majority (about 85 per cent) of rates being approximately 300 per minute. Atrial flutter may

present a problem in diagnosis when the ventricular response rate is 2:1, since only every other atrial depolarization may then be seen, the alternate flutter wave being "buried" in the QRS. This can lead to an erroneous diagnosis of atrial or sinus tachycardia (Fig. 4–6). As described previously, carotid sinus massage is useful in differentiating these various rhythm disorders.

Paroxysmal atrial tachycardia with block may be confused with atrial flutter. However, in contrast to flutter, paroxysmal atrial tachycardia with block is characterized by atrial rates from 130 to 240 beats per minute and usually displays a flat isoelectric baseline. Occasionally, however, elderly patients and patients taking quinidine may display a slow atrial flutter rate, making differentiation more difficult.

Several atrial rhythms produce "regularly irregular" atrial activity in which the P waves are not regular but nonetheless have a basic underlying pattern: sinus arrhythmia, sinus arrest, and sinus block. Sinus arrhythmia is merely

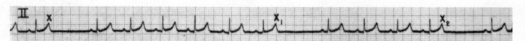

Figure 4–7. S-A Block. Note S-A block in cycle X and cycle X_1. The cycle length is slightly less than that between two normal cycles. The cycles preceding X_2 show a decreasing length, suggesting that this is an example of the Wenckebach type of S-A block.

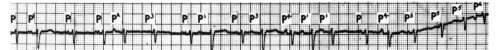

Figure 4–8. Wandering atrial pacemaker with chaotic atrial premature beats. The underlying sinus rate is 92 beats per minute (P). This is interrupted by multiple atrial premature contractions (P_1–P_6) which have abnormal and varying contours and differing P–P' intervals. All of the premature contractions in this strip are conducted (occasionally with aberrancy). The sinus P waves are notched (lead II), suggesting left atrial abnormality.

an exaggeration of the normal tendency of the SA node to beat irregularly. Such arrhythmias are usually related to the respiratory cycle, increasing in rate on inspiration and decreasing with expiration. The less common form of sinus arrhythmia changes rate with no relationship to respiration. These are usually found in older individuals and are associated frequently with bradyrhythms. Sinus arrest results from a pause in sinus activity due to a momentary failure of the sinus node to initiate an impulse. The sinus blocks are usually manifested by a sudden pause during normal sinus rhythm, which is exactly double the P–P interval. Occasionally they may manifest themselves by displaying a gradually shortened P–P interval followed by a pause that is less than twice the normal interval (S-A Wenckebach) (Fig. 4–7).

The arrhythmias that are characterized by "chaotic" atrial activity with no discernible repetitive pattern are atrial fibrillation, sinus or junctional rhythms that are interrupted by frequent multifocal atrial "ectopic" beats and wandering atrial pacemaker (Fig. 4–8). Atrial fibrillation is an arrhythmia characterized by extremely rapid irregular atrial impulses associated with ineffectual atrial contractions. There is no distinct P wave activity and no established baseline.

Ventricular Activity

Once the atrial rhythm is established, attention is directed to ventricular activity, using a similar approach. The normal QRS complex measures 0.04 to 0.10 second in duration (tending to be

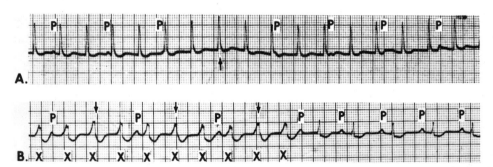

Figure 4–9. A-V dissociation. *(A)* The atrial activity (P) is regular at 64 beats per minute. The ventricular activity is regular at 140 per minute and has a normal configuration. An accelerated nonparoxysmal junctional tachycardia is present. The arrow indicates atrial depolarization buried within the QRS.

(B) The wide and abnormal ventricular complexes (X) are regular (130 per minute) and are independent of the regular sinus activity (P) at 82 beats per minute. Ventricular tachycardia is present. As the P wave moves progressively away from the QRS, atrial capture occurs. Note the normal QRS and regular P-R interval. The initial atrial capture beat has a longer P-R interval because of the concealed retrograde conduction of the ventricular ectopic beat.

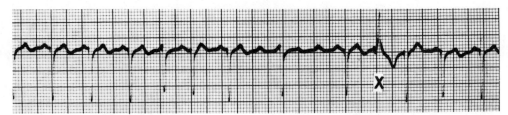

Figure 4–10. Aberrant conduction. Note that the aberrantly conducted beat (X) has a short coupling interval whereas the beat preceding it (which is normal in contour) follows a long pause. The aberrant beat has a right bundle branch block configuration.

shorter in children). The rhythms associated with regular ventricular activity are either supraventricular or ventricular. The supraventricular rhythms are essentially the same as those discussed under atrial activity. Regular rhythms of ventricular origin include slow idioventricular escape rhythms, accelerated idioventricular rhythms (also known as "slow ventricular tachycardia"), and ventricular tachycardia. These rhythms are characterized by wide, "aberrant" ventricular complexes with a duration greater than 0.12 seconds, usually occurring independent of atrial activity (see A-V dissociation under A-V relationships) and are differentiated from each other primarily by rate (Fig. 4–9). The ventricular escape rhythms are usually 50 beats per minute or less, the accelerated idioventricular rhythms are between 90 and 130 beats per minute, and the rapid ventricular tachycardias are between 140 and 250 beats per minute.

The most difficult problem in ventricular rhythm analysis is that of differen-tiating supraventricular tachycardias with rapid ventricular response rates and "aberrant ventricular conduction" from ventricular tachycardia. Aberrant conduction may be defined as a temporarily abnormal intraventricular conduction of a supraventricular impulse (as opposed to a permanent conduction abnormality or bundle branch block). Aberrant conduction is usually caused by a change in the rate at which impulses arrive at the ventricle and is generally associated with a shortening in cycle lengths. Aberrant beats are characterized by: 1) a right bundle branch configuration in greater than 80 per cent of instances (because of the longer repolarization time of the right bundle branch); 2) an initial deflection in the same direction as that of a normally conducted beat; 3) a short cycle followed by a long cycle; 4) a variable "coupling interval" (interval between a normal and abnormal QRS) (Fig. 4–10). Difficulties may also occur in evaluating the site of origin of ventricular complexes (supraventricular or ventricular)

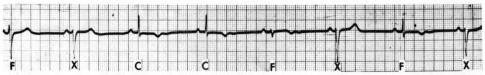

Figure 4–11. Ventricular escape beats with atrial capture and fusion. The ventricular complexes marked C represent atrial capture. The P-R interval is fixed and the QRS contour is normal. The complexes marked X are abnormal in contour and have a variable PR interval. These represent ventricular escape beats. There are several beats (F) which display characteristics of both the ventricular ectopic beats and the atrial capture beats. The degree of aberrancy is determined by the relative contribution of the normal conduction pathway and the abnormal pathway represented by the ectopic beats. The longer the P-R interval, the more normal is the resultant QRS.

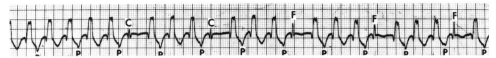

Figure 4–12. Ventricular tachycardia interrupted by atrial capture beats and fusion beats. Note the regular atrial activity (P) at a rate of 68 beats per minute. The dominant ventricular complexes are wide and abnormal in configuration and occur at regular intervals at a rate of 146 beats per minute. There is no relationship between these and the atrial beats. The capture beats (C) occur prematurely, interrupt the ventricular cycle, and have a narrower (more normal) configuration. They are preceded by a P wave and have a fixed P-R interval. These represent atrial capture beats. Occasional beats are also seen with variable configurations (F) which also occur prematurely and interrupt the ventricular tachycardia. These represent fusion beats.

in the presence of persistent bundle branch block.

The major means of differentiating aberrant supraventricular tachycardia from ventricular tachycardia include careful analysis of the A-V relationship and thorough examination of a *long* rhythm strip for capture beats (a QRS complex with normal duration and contour) or fusion beats (a QRS complex with characteristics of both a supraventricular and ventricular beat) (Fig. 4–11). In instances where high grade A-V block is not also present and atrial activity is independent of the ventricular rhythm, ventricular tachycardia may be intermittently interrupted by capture or fusion beats or both (Fig. 4–12). These manifest themseles as intermittent beats with shorter R-R intervals and normal QRS duration (except, of course, in the presence of persistent bundle branch block). These beats occur at irregular intervals and are usually preceded by P waves. A fusion beat results from the simultaneous spread of more than one impulse through the same myocardial territory (either ventricles

or atria). The degree of aberrancy is directly related to the degree of normal conduction as compared to the ectopic activity (see Fig. 4–11). At times, they are the only certain means of recognizing an ectopic ventricular mechanism.

Ventricular premature contractions generally display bizarre QRS complexes. The majority of premature ventricular contractions do not conduct in a retrograde fashion into the atrium and do not reset the sinus pacemaker. The sinus P wave may be buried in a QRS or T wave and not be conducted, although occasionally interpolated premature ventricular contractions are seen (Fig. 4–13). Occasionally (30 per cent), ventricular premature contractions are conducted retrogradely into the atrium, causing atrial depolarization. These may result in echo beats (Fig. 4–14).

Premature atrial complexes may be initiated by an atrial, junctional, or ventricular premature beat (with retrograde activation to the atrium). Atrial ectopic beats are characterized by a premature P wave with an abnormal configuration. Generally this results in a "reset-

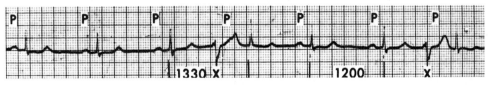

Figure 4–13. A sinus bradycardia is present. The beats marked X are abnormal in contour and represent interpolated premature ventricular contractions. The atrial rate is regular; however, the sinus capture beats following the premature ventricular contractions are conducted with a prolonged P-R interval when compared with the other sinus capture beats. This is due to concealed retrograde conduction resulting in delayed conduction of the subsequent sinus beat through the junction.

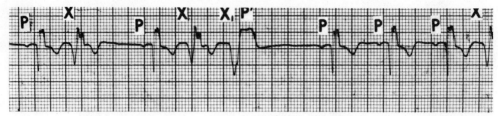

Figure 4–14. Sinus rhythm is present at 82 beats per minute. Premature ventricular contractions are present from two foci (X–X'). The premature ventricular contractions marked X are not conducted in a retrograde fashion to the atrium and do not reset the sinus pacemaker. The premature ventricular contraction marked X', however, is conducted in a retrograde manner to the atrium, resulting in a premature atrial depolarization which subsequently resets the sinus node pacemaker. In this case the premature atrial contraction P' is not conducted back to the ventricle.

ting" of the basic sinus mechanisms with a P-P interval that is greater than that normally expected (Fig. 14–15).

Atrioventricular Relationships

After both atrial and ventricular activity are identified, the relationship between them is examined. The P-R interval (measured from the beginning of the P wave to the beginning of the QRS complex) is evaluated with respect to its constancy and duration. If the P-R relationship is not constant, note is taken as to whether there is a changing relationship; that is, a progressive prolongation of the P-R followed by a nonconducted P wave (second degree block of the Type I or Wenckebach type), an occasional non-conducted P wave with an otherwise constant P-R relationship (second degree block of Type II or Mobitz type), or no relationship between the P waves and the QRS complexes (A-V dissociation) (Fig. 4–16).

When the ventricular response is governed by an accelerated junctional or ventricular mechanism that is faster than the atria, most of the atrial beats will not be conducted to the ventricle because of the retrograde "concealed conduction" within the A-V junction and the subsequent partial refractoriness of the ventricle or junction to the atrial impulses. Similarly, ventricular premature complexes can cause concealed retrograde conduction into the junction and result in delay of the normal antegrade conduction of the subsequent sinus or atrial beat. This results in a longer P-R interval than normal or in a non-conducted atrial beat (see Fig. 4–13). If, however, the P wave falls during an interval in which it is capable of conducting to the ventricle, then capture will occur, resulting in a change in the ventricular rate and rhythm. There

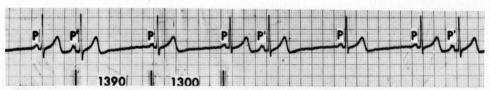

Figure 4–15. Note the difference in contour between the sinus P waves (P) and the premature atrial contraction (P'). The P-R interval for the premature atrial contractions is longer (0.20) than the P-R intervals of the sinus beats (0.16 second). Note also that the sinus rhythm (as represented by the P-P interval) is faster than the sinus node recovery following the premature beat (P'-P), a phenomenon produced by the fact that the sinus node recovery time following premature depolarization is longer than the normal sinus interval.

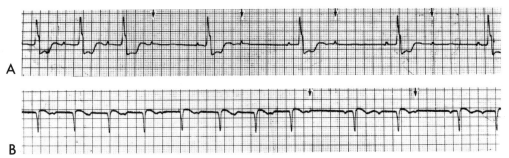

Figure 4–16. Second degree AV block. *(A)* Type II 2° A-V block (Mobitz Type II block). Note the regular P-P interval. The QRS is wide and abnormal in contour. The P-R interval of the first three beats is prolonged (0.38 second) but stable. The shorter P-R interval seen in the conducted beats which follow the blocked sinus beat is due to the longer recovery time in the A-V junction. The arrow points to the non-conducted P waves.

(B) Type 12° A-V block (Wenckebach or Mobitz Type I block). The P-P interval is regular. Note the gradual prolongation of the P-R interval until a sinus beat is finally blocked. The P-R interval for the first beat in each series is identical. Note the normal QRS contour. Pauses engendered by the non-conducted beat are less than twice the sinus rate.

are also occasional situations in which A-V block is present when intermittent capture may occur. In this circumstance, the higher pacemaker fires during a time at which the junction or ventricle is peculiarly prone toward conduction (so-called "supra-normal" conduction).

One of the best methods for analyzing the relationship between atrial, junctional, and ventricular events in a complex arrhythmia involves the construction of a "laddergram" (Figs. 4–17 and 4–18). These may be constructed beneath the ECG rhythm strip with "A" representing atrial activity, "V" representing ventricular activity, and "A-V" representing the events (usually inferred) within the A-V junction. When antegrade conduction is present, the line connecting the preceding atrial activity and subsequent ventricular depolarization represents the duration of the P-R interval. In retrograde conduction,

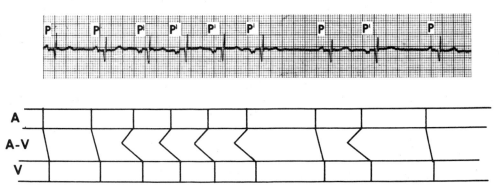

Figure 4–17. Laddergram depicting a junctional rhythm. The sinus beats are characterized by upright P waves (P), which are conducted in an antegrade manner through the A-V junction (A-V) and depolarize the ventricle (V). The junctional beats are preceded by an inverted P wave (P') and a rate that is more rapid than the sinus rhythm. This is represented on the laddergram as originating at a point in the A-V junction (A-V) midway between the atrium (A) and the ventricle (V). Lines drawn in an antegrade and retrograde direction represent conduction to the atrium and ventricle.

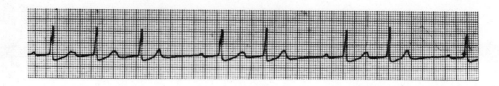

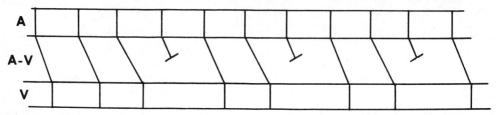

Figure 4–18.   Laddergram depicting type I 2° A-V block (Wenckebach or Mobitz Type I block). Note the regular sinus activity (A) with minor beat-to-beat variations in the sinus rate. Conduction through the A-V node (A-V) is progressively prolonged until finally the last sinus beat in each sequence fails to be conducted to the ventricle (represented by crosshatched lines in the A-V segment). The P-R interval for the first beat in each sequence is identical and the QRS contour is normal. Note also that the pause produced by the non-conducted sinus beat is less than twice the regular P-P interval. 4:3 and 3:2 A-V conduction is present.

the reverse sequence applies. Block of an impulse is shown as a line extending midway through the junction, with a short longitudinal line interrupting it. Impulses arising within the junction are represented by a point midway within the junction with lines extending both antegrade to the ventricle and retrograde to the atrium to indicate ventricular and/or atrial depolarization. This approach, together with accurate identification of atrial and then ventricular activity, allows correct diagnosis of the most complex arrhythmias.

Conditions Simulating Arrhythmias

Certain conditions that do not involve the heart may simulate arrhythmias. The ECG machine may itself produce several types of artifacts, as a result of either malfunction or improper adjustment. Furthermore, a shifting baseline may make interpretation impossible, especially when only a short tracing is available for analysis. Electrocardiographic records may simulate arrhythmia under such conditions as a)

tremors of various types, particularly that of Parkinson's disease (which may disappear from the electrocardiogram during sleep); b) hiccough; c) artifact in the ECG machine; d) poor ECG lead connection to the patient or temporary interruption of connection, either of which will appear as cardiac arrest on the electrocardiogram; e) interference from another electrical apparatus; f) connection through an outside person, as, for example, while holding a precordial lead in place; in these instances, the electrocardiogram of the technician may be superimposed upon that of the patient; and g) diaphragmatic flutter.

Long Term Monitoring (See Chapter 14)

The long term monitoring techniques have provided considerable information about arrhythmias and other electrocardiographic changes occurring during various daily activities (for example, certain stressful situations, either physical or emotional). They can be employed to record the electrocardiograms of patients performing various tasks under various types of chronic and short term stress, including exercise.

The advantages of these techniques over short term resting electrocardiograms are related to the limitations of the "standard" ECG: 1) many rhythm abnormalities are precipitated by activity and are not reproduced on the resting tracings; 2) the standard ECG represents a small sample (60 to 70 beats) of the patient's daily average (greater than 100,000) and most arrhythmias are transient in nature and not detected.

Portable ventricular alarm systems have been produced and serve to alert the patient when ventricular extra systoles have reached a certain frequency or pattern. However, these devices cannot be considered adequate for arrhythmia documentation, since they may not record the arrhythmia that has precipitated the alarm. Some of these systems permit transmission of the ECG via telephone lines to a hospital or physician's office, but many abnormalities are so transient that they are no longer present at the time of telephone transmission, and a false sense of security may result.

Long term monitoring techniques are also useful when assessing the efficacy of antiarrhythmic therapy over the course of a patient's daily activity schedule.

Computer Analysis of Arrhythmias

Computerized systems for analysis of electrocardiograms have been developed that are capable of recognizing P as well as QRS activity and, theoretically at least, of diagnosing complex rhythm disorders. These systems have been available commercially for several years. However, computer system accuracy is extremely important, and the present systems are still not as good as one would like. There are still many difficulties with the electronic interpretation of the electrocardiogram and more particularly in arrhythmia analysis.

Some of the major causes of difficulty in computerized rhythm analysis include: 1) signal noise, which may obscure the baseline and render interpretation of atrial activity impossible; 2) the occasional inability to obtain artifact-free tracings; 3) the inability to interpret some arrhythmias by computer because they require special techniques of electrocardiographic recording; and 4) irregular rhythms (such as atrial fibrillation) with wide QRS complexes secondary to aberrancy or persistent bundle branch block, which make it difficult to detect premature ventricular contractions.

At present, owing to the high number of false positives and false negatives, all tracings should probably be evaluated by trained personnel.

5

ARRHYTHMIAS RELATED TO THE SINUS NODE

VIDYA S. BANKA, M.D.,
RICHARD H. HELFANT, M.D.

GENERAL CONSIDERATIONS

Normal sinus rhythm depends upon the normal functioning of the S-A node, the dominant pacemaker of the heart. Various clinical disorders of the heart beat arise as a consequence of alterations in function of this structure. These include a) sinus tachycardia, b) sinus bradycardia, c) sinus arrhythmia, d) wandering atrial pacemaker, e) sinoatrial block, f) sinus pauses, and others. However, before discussing the arrhythmias related to sinus node dysfunction, it is pertinent to discuss certain features of normal sinus rhythm and the control of the heart rate.

CONFIGURATION OF THE NORMAL ELECTROCARDIOGRAM

The normal electrocardiogram has the following characteristics: 1) The sinus impulses are regular in formation, as demonstrated by P waves. The P waves are upright and smooth in contour in leads I, II, and aVF, and in the precordial leads, except in V_1 and occasionally in V_2, where biphasic (initially positive, then negative); the P waves are normally inverted in aVR. 2) The rate normally ranges from 60 to 100 beats

per minute and usually decreases with age. 3) Every P wave is followed by a ventricular response; that is, by the QRS complex. 4) The P-R interval ranges between 0.12 and 0.21 seconds in duration. In some apparently normal young adults, the P-R interval may be prolonged to the upper limit of normal.

CONTROL OF THE HEART RATE

The heart rate is determined by that of the most rapidly firing pacemaker tissue — normally the S-A node. Its rate is controlled by a balance of two antagonistic forces: cardioinhibitory and cardioaccelerator. The cardioinhibitory forces (vagal) originate from the nucleus ambiguus in the medulla. This center can be affected reflexly or by higher centers. The cardioaccelerator forces (sympathetic) arise in the upper five dorsal segments of the spinal cord and in centers in the hypothalamus and cerebral cortex.

The average heart rate in the adult human subject ranges between 64 and 80 beats per minute. The rate is faster in children and tends to decrease gradually as the individual grows older. At birth, the heart rate ranges from 110 to

58

150 beats per minute; in patients over the age of 60, the heart rate may range from 50 to 75 beats per minute.

In addition to age, several other factors affect the heart rate. Among these are metabolic rate, nutritional state, body temperature, environmental temperatures, body size, posture, exercise, emotional state, sleeping state, and physical conditioning. The adjustments of the heart rate serve an extremely useful purpose in accommodating the heart rate to bodily need for nutrients, for maintaining adequate cardiac output, and for other functions.

RELATION OF S-A NODE AND ATRIA TO ARRHYTHMIAS

Among the automatic tissues of the heart, the sinus node, under normal conditions, possesses the highest spontaneous rate of impulse discharge. However, when the sinus pacemaker slows, when its impulses are carried imperfectly to the remainder of the heart, or when another area of automatic tissue fires more rapidly, an arrhythmia may appear. Other automatic tissues in the region of the atria that might serve as pacemakers are located as follows: 1) at the entrances of the atria, 2) around the atrioventricular valve rings, 3) in the A-V conduction pathway, and 4) about the coronary sinus and in the A-N (atrionodal) region of the A-V junction (Hoffman and Cranefield, 1964).

Disease of the S-A node has been observed in various types of sinoatrial block and atrial arrhythmias. However, pathologic alterations have been studied most frequently in the more serious atrial arrhythmias, such as atrial fibrillation, and more recently in sinoatrial block and the sick sinus syndrome. Ischemic, sclerotic, and inflammatory changes in the S-A node are observed in most patients with the sick sinus syndrome; however, these alterations are seen in only 25 per cent of cases of other atrial arrhythmias (Hudson, 1960; Rubenstein et al., 1972). Isolated causes of muscular dystrophy, amyloid deposition in the atria, cardiomyopathy, systemic lupus erythematosus, and diphtheria have been known to cause atrial bradyarrhythmias. Functionally reversible causes that relate to sinus node dysfunction and arrhythmias include digitalis or quinidine intoxication, hypoxia, hyperkalemia, autonomic imbalance, and endocrine abnormalities (Moss and Davis, 1974).

Sinus Tachycardia

The occurrence of a rapid rate arising from the S-A nodal pacemaker is quite common. Rates greater than 100 beats per minute in adults may be considered sinus tachycardia; occasionally, rates as high as 180 per minute or even higher may be observed. In children, sinus rates as high as 230 per minute have been recorded.

The tachycardia encroaches mainly upon the diastolic period with a resultant decrease in ventricular filling. From the standpoint of work performance, the maximal effective increase in heart rate for the normal adult heart is approximately two and one-half times that of the resting state (that is, from about 70 beats per minute to a level of 160 beats per minute). At faster heart rates, the filling period is curtailed and the stroke volume tends to diminish.

The effect of tachycardia on the electrocardiogram depends upon the underlying clinical state and the precipitating cause of the tachycardia. The P waves are increased in amplitude and the P-R interval is usually shortened, but in occasional instances it is lengthened. The ST-T segments are often depressed; occasionally, they are slightly elevated. ST-T abnormalities may outlast the tachycardia. A previously upright T wave may be flattened and, in rare cases, inverted; occasionally, the

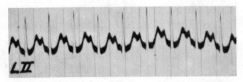

Figure 5–1. Sinus tachycardia with a rate of 186 per minute. (Time intervals measure 0.20 second.) Note the J segment type of ST segment displacement; the P waves follow the peak of the T wave before it has reached the iso-electric line. The P-R interval is relatively short due to the rapid rate.

amplitude of the T wave may be increased. An inconspicuous U wave may become prominent or even inverted (Fig. 5–1).

Following carotid sinus pressure, sinus tachycardia is usually unaffected; occasionally, it is gradually or partially slowed (Fig. 5–2), particularly in the digitalized patients. In paroxysmal atrial tachycardia, the rate either remains unchanged or slows abruptly to about half the original rate.

Sinus Bradycardia

Sinus bradycardia is characterized by a slow sinus rate, usually ranging from 35 to 50 beats per minute (Fig. 5–3). Each atrial impulse is followed by a ventricular beat. The slow rate may persist for relatively short periods of time or for hours, days, or years. It may be associated with or occur independently of a sinus arrhythmia.

Sinus bradycardia frequently occurs in athletes and in normal individuals during sleep. It is also common in the older age group. The following are some of the causative factors: 1) vagal stimulation as a result of Valsalva maneuver, carotid sinus pressure, and ocular pressure results in transient bradycardia; however, vagal reflexes arising from the left ventricle (for example, as a result of posterior myocardial infarction) may produce sinus bradycardia and hypotension. 2) Direct involvement of the sinus node by inflammatory or degenerative processes may cause sinus bradycardia.

Sinus Arrhythmia

Sinus arrhythmia (Fig. 5–4) is caused by a disturbance in the rhythmic production of the impulse at the S-A node. The ventricles and atria participate equally in this irregularity. Each ventricular contraction is preceded by an atrial systole at the usual intervals. Sinus arrhythmia is most frequently encountered in children and young adults and tends to disappear in adult life.

The two types of sinus arrhythmia most commonly observed are: the respiratory form, in which the variations in heart rate are cyclic and related to respiration, and the non-respiratory form, in which the irregularity occurs without correlation to the phases of respiration.

In the more common respiratory form, the irregularity varies with the phases of respiration; the rate tends to increase gradually with inspiration and decrease with expiration. Inspiration

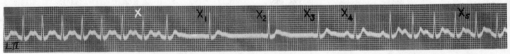

Figure 5–2. Effect of carotid sinus pressure on sinus tachycardia. A sinus tachycardia is present (rate 150 per minute). Carotid sinus pressure applied at X results in marked slowing of the rate. With release of pressure, there is a gradual return to the pre-existing rate. Note the decrease in amplitude and alteration in shape of the P waves and decrease in P-R intervals with the long cycles X_1, X_2, and X_3 (from 0.18 to 0.12 second). This could be the result of shift of the pacemaker within the S-A node as well as improved conduction through the A-V node due to the increased rest period. Note the gradual increase in the P-R interval as the cycle length decreases (X_4) and the return of the P-R interval to 0.18 second as the tachycardia is resumed (X_5).

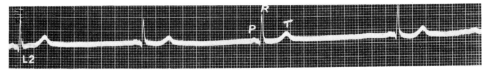

Figure 5–3. Sinus bradycardia, slightly irregular (30 to 34 beats per minute). Both the atrial and ventricular rates are slow (34 per minute) and the P-R interval is normal. With such a slow sinus rate, the possibility of a 2:1 S-A block is to be considered clinically.

tends to diminish vagal tone, while expiration tends to increase it.

In the ventriculophasic type of sinus arrhythmia, the filling of the ventricle mediated through a vagal reflex affects the heart rate. In partial or higher grades of A-V heart block, the ventricle is filled more during those cycles in which the sinus impulse is blocked, and the sinus rate slows (that is, the P-P interval is prolonged) during these periods of increased ventricular filling.

Sinus arrhythmia is observed in normal hearts of children and young adults. By itself, it is not an indication of heart disease; however, its presence does not exclude heart disease, because it often appears in patients with mitral and aortic valvular disease and with various grades of coronary arteriosclerosis in the older age groups.

Other factors include increased intracranial pressure, various types of cerebral dysfunction, and drugs such as digitalis, morphine, and other parasympathomimetic agents.

SINUS NODE DYSFUNCTION:

Sinoatrial Heart Block

Sinoatrial block has been observed in subjects with normal hearts (Averill and Lamb, 1960) and in those with disease processes involving the S-A node or the nodal artery (Greenwood and Finkelstein, 1964). The ratio of males to females is 2:1. The majority of the subjects had associated atrial disease.

Digitalis is the drug most often implicated in the genesis of S-A block. However, quinidine sulfate and potassium salts may occasionally cause human S-A block. Transient or chronic S-A block has often been associated with the following clinical conditions: 1) inflammation, as in acute rheumatic states, other types of myocarditis, and postsurgical trauma; 2) degenerative processes such as postdiphtheric fibrosis and coronary atherosclerosis; and 3) ischemia of myocardial infarction due to occlusion of the coronary artery that supplies the S-A node.

Sinoatrial block is a relatively uncommon condition in which the atria and the ventricles experience a delay or failure of activation by the S-A node for one or more beats. An analogy has been made between the S-A and A-V nodes in grading the degree of block. Theoretically, the block may be divided into first, second, third, or complete S-A block. However, such a differentiation is more difficult to establish with respect to the S-A node.

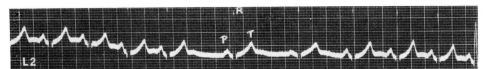

Figure 5–4. Sinus arrhythmia. Note the phasic variation of the R-R interval. The rate increases during inspiration and decreases during expiration. The shorter cycles are associated with a decreased T-P interval. The P-R interval remains constant throughout.

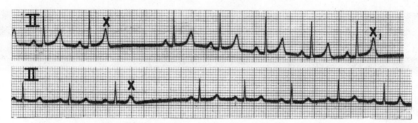

Figure 5–5. Blocked atrial premature beats followed by pauses simulating sinoatrial block. Both tracings represent blocked atrial premature beats occurring superimposed on the T waves marked X and X_1. These represent a superimposition of a P wave on the top of the T wave and are therefore considered as blocked premature atrial beats. The longer cycles are slightly shorter than two P-P intervals. This may be misdiagnosed as S-A heart block.

Theoretically, first degree S-A block may occur, but it cannot be recognized because prolongation of S-A node to atrial muscle conduction time cannot be clinically recognized on a human electrocardiogram, although it may be suspected.

Second degree S-A block consists of the following types:

1. Those manifesting the Wenckebach phenomenon (see Chapter 12).

2. Those in which the long cycle is slightly less than twice that of the usual cycle length. Although the latter type may belong in the Mobitz II category, it is more likely a subdivision of the Wenckebach type; this may be more definitely established if sufficient preceding cycles are studies. Also to be ruled out (when the P-P intervals are longer than the normal sequence) is the presence of a non-conducted atrial premature beat (Fig. 5–5).

3. Those in which the pause is approximately double (or any multiple of) the normal cycle length. Occasionally, the cycle length is less than twice that of the normal R-R interval. There is no evidence of atrial or ventricular activity (no P waves or QRST complexes) during the pause except when a junctional escape occurs during a long pause.

The diagnosis of second degree S-A heart block with Wenckebach phenomenon (analogous to Mobitz type I A-V heart block) is made when the following criteria are fulfilled:

1. The P-P interval, including a blocked S-A impulse, is shorter than double the normal P-P interval.

2. The P-P interval after the dropped S-A impulse is longer than the interval preceding the pause.

3. There is a gradual shortening of the P-P interval preceding the long pause. Thus, every third, fourth, of fifth beat may be dropped in a regular or an irregular sequence (see Figs. 5–6 and 5–7).

Second degree S-A block without Wenckebach phenomenon (analogous to Mobitz type II A-V heart block) is diagnosed when the pause is nearly an exact multiple (two or more) of the basic P-P interval and preceding cycles are constant. The pauses are equal or multiples of a common divisor (Fig. 5–8). Thus, the beats may be regularly or irregularly dropped. Persistent 3:2 S-A block is another type in which short P-P

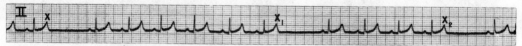

Figure 5–6. S-A block. Note S-A block in cycle X and cycle X_1. The cycle length is slightly less than that between two normal cycles. The cycles preceding X_2 show a decreasing length, suggesting that this is an example of the Wenckebach type of S-A block.

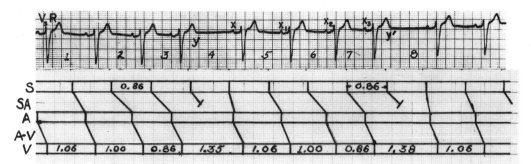

Figure 5–7. Sinoatrial block with Wenckebach phenomenon. A strip of V_3R shows two episodes of 5:4 S-A heart block with Wenckebach phenomenon. The diagram shows theoretical regularly spaced internal sinus node impulses (occurring 0.86 second apart), which are equal to the length of the shortest R-R cycle in each series. The first of these regular internal sinus node impulses is placed 0.08 second before the P wave that starts the cycle; this is the assumed minimal conduction time from the interior of the sinus node to the atrial muscle (X). S marks the theoretic impulses arising from the S-A node. A denotes the interatrial cycle length, and V denotes the interventricular cycle length. The last internal sinus stimulus, Y, is blocked in cycles 4 and 8 and is not conducted to the atrial muscle. Since the increments in time of the prolonged S-A conduction diminished progressively, the P-P intervals become consequently shorter until the last internal sinus stimulus is blocked, thus producing longer P-P and R-P intervals in cycles 4 and 8.

and R-R intervals alternate with long ones; this simulates a sinus bigeminy.

Third degree S-A block is not detectable clinically, because S-A impulses fail to reach the atrial muscle. This type may be suspected in the presence of atrial standstill.

S-A heart block may be acute, intermittent, or chronic. The irregularity may, in fact, be observed for a few cycles only; it may progress gradually or the rate may suddenly be halved (for example, decreased from 75 to 38 beats per minute); this slow rate may persist for several minutes or longer. This type, however, is usually transient. The sudden halving of the heart rate is usually preceded by a slight acceleration, followed by longer cycles, which gradually shorten until the usual cycle length is re-established. The disturbance may

exist for longer periods of time, and it may be the underlying mechanism for long-term bradycardia.

Prolonged Sinus Pauses

Prolonged sinus pauses may occur during S-A heart block (Fig. 5–9). This is probably caused by failure of the impulses to leave the S-A node and inability of the S-A node or any other potential atrial pacemaker to generate impulses. Under these conditions, the A-V junction usually escapes and assumes control of the ventricles for one or more beats (Fig. 5–10). If A-V junctional retrograde conduction occurs, each junctional impulse, by retrograde penetration into the sinus node, continues to discharge the sinus node and

Figure 5–8. Type II second degree S-A heart block. Note that the cycle length, X, is exactly twice that of the normal cycle length.

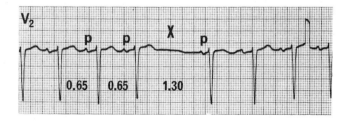

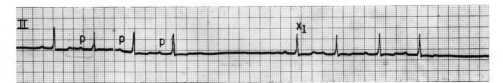

Figure 5–9. Sinoatrial block with prolonged P-R and atrial and ventricular arrest for a duration of three cycles. Following the fourth QRS complex, note the presence of a sinus pause which is equal to that of three cycle lengths. The P-R interval is prolonged; it is shortest after the long pause (0.24 second), and prior to the pause it is 0.28 second. The three complexes following X_1 are similar to those that precede the long pause.

may contribute to the temporary or permanent elimination of the latter from the control of the heart beat.

Prolonged sinus pauses may be caused by increases in vagal tone, which may occur spontaneously or may follow vagal stimulation produced by carotid sinus or ocular pressure, gagging, vomiting, or other conditions. Quinidine and potassium salts particularly tend to produce sinus pauses by slowing the atrial rate; such pauses may lead to atrial standstill. The pauses are extremely dangerous because they may produce syncopal attacks, Stokes-Adams seizures, and cardiac arrest.

It is important to note that the absence of P waves in the electrocardiogram does not exclude a sinus origin of ventricular beats. The P wave is representative of atrial, not S-A nodal, activity. Because of the accumulating evidence of the existence of sinoatrial tracts, recent interest has been aroused concerning the existence of sinoventricular (S-V) conduction, which may transmit the sinus impulse to the A-V junction without atrial contraction (Bel-

let and Jedlicka, 1969). A diagrammatic representation of S-A and S-V conduction is presented in Figure 5–11. Sinoventricular conduction has been noted during experimental hyperpotassemia (DeMello and Hoffman, 1960; Hoffman and Cranefield, 1964; Vassalle and Hoffman, 1965), digitalis intoxication, and hypothermia. Its presence in clinical situations has been proposed.

The pauses observed with S-A block may lead to (a) A-V junctional escape (Fig. 5–10), (b) transient atrial standstill, (c) long periods of bradycardia when 2:1 or higher degrees of S-A conduction occur, and (d) association with A-V block. In about 70 per cent of patients, S-A block is associated with slight grades of A-V heart block. Atrial pacing tends to bring out latent A-V conduction disturbances.

Wandering of Pacemaker from S-A Node to A-V Junction

Occasionally, the sinus pacemaker may shift to another portion of the S-A

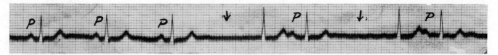

Figure 5–10. Sinoatrial block with junctional escape. At the arrows, a rhythmic atrial beat does not occur, and junctional escape follows. After the escape beat, the P-R interval of the short cycle (fourth and sixth) measures 0.24 second as compared with the normal P-R interval of 0.18 second in the first three beats. This implies concealed retrograde conduction of the preceding beat with antegrade conduction occurring in the relative refractory periods. Note that the P-P interval occurring between the complex preceding the pause and that following the pause are exactly equal to two normal cycles.

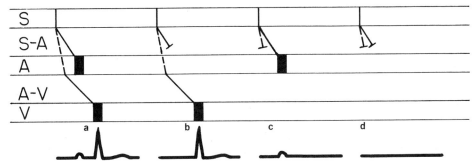

Figure 5–11. (*a*) Normal sequence of P-QRS-T. (*b*) Sinoventricular conduction (without activation of the atrial muscle). Note absence of P wave preceding QRS. (*c*) Sinoventricular block with atrial activation preserved. Note P wave without ventricular activation. (*d*) Sinoventricular block together with the block of the sinus impulse conduction of the atrial muscle. Note absence of both atrial and ventricular activity. (From Bellet, S., and Jedlicka, J.: Amer. J. Cardiol., 24:831, 1969.)

node or to the A-V junction — the so-called "wandering pacemaker." This results in alteration in the configuration of the P waves, the length of the P-R interval, and the heart rate (Fig. 5–12). The P wave changes in size, shape, or direction simultaneously with slowing of the rate and changes in the P-R interval. When the pacemaker returns to the sinus node, these changes are reversed.

Vagal stimulation and various parasympathetic drugs have been demonstrated experimentally to cause a shift of the pacemaker within the S-A node and occasionally to the A-V junction. Wandering of the pacemaker may be initiated by ectopic premature beats or by a run of such beats that transiently suppresses the sinus node. Shift of the

pacemaker may also occur during S-A block (Fig. 5–13).

Atrial Standstill

Atrial standstill may be transient, which is not uncommon, or persistent, which is rare. Transient atrial standstill that lasts from several seconds to hours or days is observed under a variety of conditions. The great majority of cases have been associated with drugs or electrolyte imbalance. Two thirds of cases of temporary standstill are associated with toxic doses of digitalis or the use of quinidine. Transient atrial standstill has been associated with profound sinus bradycardia; S-A block (3:1 or 4:1); responses in A-V junctional

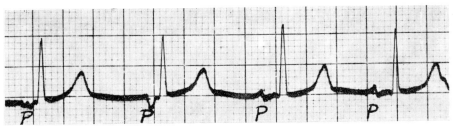

Figure 5–12. Wandering pacemaker. Alteration in configuration of P waves due to a shift in the S-A nodal pacemaker. Note the alterations in configuration of P waves and varying P-R intervals in different cycles. These are due to a shift of the pacemaker to different portions of the A-V node (first two beats) and then to the S-A node (last two beats). The first P wave could be a fusion P (fusion or retrograde and sinus P waves; this is intermediate in type between the second and third P wave).

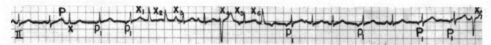

Figure 5–13. Wandering pacemaker with atrial premature beats. (Lead II) Note atrial premature beats at X, X₁, X₂, X₃, X₄, X₆ and X₇; the QRS of X₂, X₄ and X₆ show aberrant conduction. Inverted P waves observed at P₁ are due to a shift of the pacemaker from the S-A toward the A-V node.

rhythm with retrograde conduction to the atria, which render the S-A node refractory; and sinoventricular conduction due to potassium, quinidine, and digitalis.

Persistent atrial standstill may be defined as a condition in which atrial activity is absent for periods of months or years (Allensworth et al., 1960; Bloomfield and Sinclair-Smith, 1965; Lewis et al., 1914).

Atrial standstill may be observed in the terminal phases of many disease states, particularly myocardial infarction. The exact cause of terminal atrial standstill is often difficult to determine; however, in many cases it is the result of hypoxia or hyperpotassemia.

Transient atrial standstill should not be diagnosed merely by the absence of P waves in the routine electrocardiogram but rather by the absence of atrial activity in esophageal or intra-atrial leads (Fig. 5–14) (Bloomfield and

Sinclair-Smith, 1965). Transient standstill must be differentiated from A-V junctional rhythm, sinoatrial block, and sinoventricular conduction. The treatment is that of the underlying etiology: to correct drug toxicity or to treat the underlying cardiac disease.

SICK SINUS SYNDROME

The term "sick sinus syndrome" has been used to describe a group of clinical manifestations that are associated with one or more of the following atrial arrhythmias:

1. Persistent and severe sinus bradycardia;

2. Cessation of sinus rhythm for short intervals (sinus arrest) or for long periods with replacement of this rhythm with atrial and/or junctional escape rhythms;

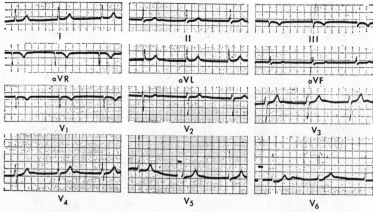

Figure 5–14. Atrial standstill. Electrocardiogram shows a heart rate of 48 beats per minute, QRS duration of 0.08 second and absence of P waves. (From Allensworth, D. C., Rice, G. J., and Lowe, G. W.: Amer. J. Med., 47:775, 1969.)

3. Episodic sinus arrest without a new pacemaker arising, resulting in periods of total cardiac arrest;

4. Chronic atrial fibrillation, often accompanied by an intrinsically slow ventricular rate—that is, not produced by drug therapy;

5. Failure of the heart to assume sinus rhythm after electroversion for atrial fibrillation;

6. Episodes of sinoatrial exit block not related to drug therapy (Ferrer, 1968). Several descriptive terms, such as "sick sinus node," "lazy sinus node," "inadequate sinus mechanism," "sluggish sinus node," and "sino-atrial syncope," have been applied to the impaired sinus mechanism. When an element of tachycardia is associated with the underlying bradycardia, the condition has been called "syndrome of alternating bradycardia and tachycardia" or the "brady-tachy syndrome."

Etiology

The sick sinus syndrome can be caused by ischemic, sclerotic, or inflammatory involvement of the sinus node. Although pathologic studies are meager, the majority of cases appear to occur in patients with coronary heart disease. Of the 56 patients reported by Rubenstein and coworkers (1972), 35 per cent had coronary artery disease. Three patients had evidence of cardiomyopathy and four showed hypertensive heart disease. Rheumatic heart disease, luetic aortic regurgitation, scleroderma, and congenital heart disease were each observed in one patient. No etiologic diagnosis could be made in 42 per cent of the patients. Similarly, in the series of Moss and Davis (1974), 51 per cent of the patients had associated coronary heart disease, while idiopathic cardiac disease accounted for 34 per cent of their patients. Included in the remainder were hypertension, rheumatic heart disease, congenital heart disease, and cardiomyopathy.

Isolated reports of sick have been associated w tomy for calcific tubercu tis, dystrophia myotonia sis, amyloid heart d. diphtheria. A small famili. ...ence of this syndrome has also peen described (Spellberg, 1971; Saracheck and Leonard, 1972).

It should be kept in mind that the electrocardiographic abnormalities consistent with the sick sinus syndrome can be iatrogenic. Digitalis, quinidine, procainamide, and propranolol can all produce an electrocardiogram and clinical picture consistent with the sick sinus syndrome. In some of these patients, determination of the etiology may be almost impossible, as these are the drugs used to control many of the presenting arrhythmias of the syndrome.

Pathogenesis

The sinus node is particularly vulnerable to vascular occlusive disease, since it receives its entire blood supply from a single artery. The sinus node artery originates from the right coronary artery in 60 per cent of the patients and from the left circumflex coronary artery in 40 per cent of the patients, and it supplies the sinus node as well as most of the atria. Occlusion of this vessel will thus affect sinoatrial electrical activity. Indeed, sinus node dysfunction occurs in about 5 per cent of patients with acute myocardial infarctions, and sinus node has frequently been found to be infarcted in patients who develop atrial arrhythmias (Rokseth and Hatte, 1971; James, 1968). Interestingly, however, no significant correlation was found between angiographically documented sinus node artery obstructive disease and sinus node dysfunction assessed electrophysiologically by sinus node recovery time measurements (Engel et al., 1975).

However, idiopathic sclerotic fibrosis

of the sinus node may also be found at necropsy.

Electrophysiology

A reduction in the spontaneous activity of the sinus node may result in sinus bradycardia, sinoatrial exit block of varying degrees, or a complete loss of sinus node function with complete sinoatrial exit block and atrial standstill or sinus arrest. Sinus bradycardia is probably the most common single electrocardiographic manifestation of the sick sinus syndrome, being found in 76 per cent of the patients reported by Radford and Julian (1974) and 22 of the 56 patients reported by Schullman and coworkers (1970). In patients with symptomatic sinus bradycardia, the arrhythmia may have several pathophysiologic causes, which include diminished slope of phase 4 depolarization, increased activation threshold, increased parasympathetic tone, decreased sympathetic tone, or drug and metabolic causes such as propranolol, depressed thyroid function, and hypothermia.

Sinus bradycardia is frequently associated with diffuse disease of the conduction system below the sinus node. Narula (1971), in a study of patients with sinus bradycardia, found that over 60 per cent had conduction disturbances that included abnormalities in the atrial junctional tissue and His-Purkinje system. This would indicate that atrial bradycardias are usually not due to isolated electrical dysfunction of the sinus node independent of other abnormalities in the cardiac conduction system.

The atrial tachyarrhythmias associated with the sick sinus syndrome generally include sinus tachycardia, paroxysmal junctional or atrial tachycardia, atrial flutter, and atrial fibrillation. Sinus tachycardia results from increased slope of phase 4 depolarization, which may be related to changes in parasympathetic and sympathetic tone as well as atrial stretch. Paroxysmal supraventricular tachycardias may result from sustained A-V nodal re-entry or re-entry at the sinus node itself.

Clinical Manifestations

The sick sinus syndrome has similar preponderance in males and females. The peak incidence occurs in the seventh decade, although the syndrome has been recognized in children as well. Table 5-1 shows the clinical presentation of patients with sick sinus syndrome in order of frequency (Moss and Davis, 1974).

The signs and symptoms of sick sinus syndrome are generally related to hypoperfusion of the vital organs, especially the brain and the heart. Cerebral manifestations are the hallmark of symptomatology. These manifestations may include symptoms of fatigue, irritability, and forgetfulness, although more commonly dizziness, near syncope, or true syncope is seen. In the series of Moss and Davis (1974), syncope or near syncope was found in 41 per cent of the patients. Cerebral symptoms may be related either to bradycardia or tachycardia as a manifestation of decreased cardiac output. It is believed that patients with sick sinus syndrome are also greatly at risk for systemic embolism, presumably because of changing atrial rhythms. Cardiac symptoms include palpatation, angina, and manifestations of congestive heart failure. Sudden unexplained episodes of pulmonary edema related to rapid arrhythmias

TABLE 5-1 PRESENTING SYMPTOMS IN SICK SINUS SYNDROME

Syncope or near syncope
Palpitations
Dizziness
Increased congestive heart failure
Increased angina
Cerebral embolism

may also occur. Mild heart failure can occur from persistent or episodic sinus bradycardia.

ELECTROCARDIOGRAPHIC FEATURES

As mentioned previously, the rhythm disturbances seen on the electrocardiogram may include bradyarrhythmias or tachyarrhythmias. In the series of Moss and Davis (1974), sinus bradycardia occurred in 76 per cent of the patients, temporary asystole following tachycardia occurred in 11 per cent, sinus node exit block occurred in 5 per cent, and intermittent sinus arrest occurred in 3 per cent of the patients. The tachyarrhythmias included supraventricular tachycardia and paroxysmal atrial tachycardia in 40 per cent of the patients, atrial flutter and fibrillation in 38 per cent, multifocal supraventricular arrhythmias in 12 per cent, and ventricular tachycardia and/or fibrillation in 10 per cent. Myocardial infarction, bundle branch blocks, and ventricular hypertrophy are often encountered as concomitant findings. A normal electrocardiogram does not exclude the possibility of sick sinus syndrome.

Diagnosis

The diagnosis of sick sinus syndrome often requires a high index of suspicion. It must be considered a possibility in patients with symptoms of syncope, near syncope, light headedness, and palpitations. Syncope and near syncope suggest a much broader differential diagnosis and, unless specific effort is directed toward considering rhythm disturbances, the diagnosis may well be missed. In these patients, a history of drug intake should be reviewed carefully, since the sick sinus syndrome may first appear after cardioactive therapy has been instituted for the control of heart failure, angina, or recurrent tachyarrhythmias.

The physical examintion generally is of limited value in documenting the rhythm disturbance itself. It is useful, however, in ruling out neurological and other cardiac causes for syncope (aortic stenosis, idiopathic hypertrophic subaortic stenosis, and left atrial myxoma). Electrocardiographic documentation of the arrhythmia is, of course, key to the diagnosis of the sick sinus syndrome. A routine electrocardiogram with a long rhythm strip may be all that is necessary to document the rhythm disturbance. However, the arrhythmias characteristic of the sick sinus syndrome are frequently episodic and, therefore, may not be present on a casual rhythm strip. In these circumstances, additional studies are necessary to make the diagnosis.

AMBULATORY ELECTROCARDIOGRAPHIC MONITORING

Long term ambulatory electrocardiographic monitoring has greatly advanced the capability to diagnose episodic cardiac arrhythmias. The brady- and/or tachyarrhythmias of the sick sinus syndrome can be documented with reasonable success using this technique. Occasionally, diagnostic rhythm changes will occur during such monitoring, even in the absence of significant symptoms. Such evidence in a patient with frequent episodes of syncope or near syncope may be all that is necessary to firmly establish the diagnosis and proceed with therapy. More often both symptoms and associated arrhythmias will occur during monitoring.

Provocative Testing

Several provocative tests have been designed to assess sinus node function:

Carotid Sinus Massage and Valsalva Maneuver. Mendell et al. (1972) have suggested that a pause longer than three seconds produced by carotid sinus massage is highly suggestive of inappropriate sinus node responsiveness and thus underlying sinus node disease. Although such a response is not diagnostic in the appropriate clinical context, it should alert the physician and warrants further investigation. Besides a long pause, escape rhythms may supervene. It should be mentioned that carotid sinus massage should be done under direct electrocardiographic monitoring with the usual precautions (see Chapter 4).

The Valsalva maneuver has been used to distinguish the sick sinus syndrome from the physiologic sinus bradycardia of the elderly. In physiologic sinus bradycardia, the expected increase in heart rate during phase 2 of the Valsalva maneuver occurs, as does subsequent slowing of the heart rate during phase 4. In patients with the sick sinus syndrome there is little or no change in the pulse rate. However, this response to the Valsalva maneuver is not diagnostic for sinus node disease.

Atropine Administration and Stress Testing. Administration of intravenous atropine is helpful in ruling out the possibility of increased parasympathetic tone as the cause for sinus bradycardia. Ferrer (1973) has suggested that if intravenous atropine (1 to 2 mg) does not increase the sinus rate to 90 or more per minute and if after atropine sinus node recovery time (see below) remains prolonged, the diagnosis of intrinsic sinus node disease can be made. In the 11 patients with sinus node disease reported by Rosen and coworkers (1971), none developed a heart rate greater than 90 per minute with atropine, although there was a 15 to 125 per cent increase in heart rate in 8 patients. Two patients showed acceleration of the junctional foci prior to an increase in the sinus rate, thus suggesting "sluggishness" of the sinus node.

Treadmill testing has also been used to test the ability of the sinus node to accelerate in an appropriate fashion in response to exercise stress. Established normal values to various stress test protocols are available for this purpose.

Atrial Pacing and Sinus Node Recovery Time. Atrial pacing has been used to determine the recovery time of the sinus node. The "sinus node recovery time" is measured following the rapid atrial pacing (rates between 90 to 150 beats per minute), which temporarily suppresses sinus activity. The interval between the last pacing stimulus and the onset of the next sinus P wave represents the sinus node recovery time. If atrial asystole occurs, the interval from the last pacing stimulus to the junctional escape beat is used. In clinically normal hearts, the interval between the last pacing impulse and the onset of the first intrinsic P wave ranges from 0.8 to 1.1 seconds (mean 0.9 seconds), whereas in patients with clinical evidence of sinoatrial disease, this interval is 1.6 to 7.0 seconds.

Ferrer (1973) feels that the degree of overdrive suppression is best expressed as a percentage of the control heart rate. In her view, at a resting heart rate of 75 to 85 beats per minute, the maximum expected pause should be between 115 and 128 per cent of the control cycle length — that is, a normal sinus node recovery time of 800 to 900 milliseconds. In patients with sinus bradycardia ranging between 45 and 60 per minute, a sinus node recovery time of 1200 to 1600 milliseconds duration should be the normal range, while at control rate of 60 beats per minute, a pause of 125 per cent of control or 1250 milliseconds suggests sick sinus syndrome.

Since the post-pacing suppression or the sinus node recovery time is dependent on the basic sinus rate, Narula et al. (1972) introduced the concept of "corrected sinus node recovery time" as being more indicative of sinus node function. The corrected sinus node recovery time or CSRT is defined as the difference between the recovery interval following cessation of atrial pacing and the average resting P-P interval. In a series of 31 patients reported by Mandel and coworkers (1972), the post pacing CSRT was reported to be 3164 ± 334 milliseconds in 29 patients. The mean CSRT for patients with normal hearts was considered by these authors to be 1073 ± 67 milliseconds. One can also employ sinus to atrial conduction time measurements during these studies. Values greater than 120 milliseconds have been considered abnormal.

Although atrial pacing has been frequently used as a diagnostic aid in patients with suspected sick sinus syndrome, false negatives are frequent. Gupta and coworkers (1974) found that an abnormal CSRT could only be detected in six of their 17 patients with other evidence of the sick sinus syndrome. The insensitivity of CSRT has also been reported by others. The failure of the sinus node recovery time to accurately predict sinus node dysfunction in patients with sick sinus syndrome is related to the fact that the sinus node function depends upon a complex and delicately balanced interaction between intrinsic sinus node electrophysiologic properties, sinoatrial conduction, and factors outside the sinoatrial region, including, importantly, the autonomic nervous system (Chadda et al., 1975; Jordan et al., 1978; Talano et al., 1978). In patients with symptomatic sinus bradycardia, Jordan and coworkers (1978) have been able to differentiate between those who have intrinsic sinus node dysfunction and those with disturbed autonomic regulation by determining the intrinsic heart rate after administration of atropine, 0.04 mg per kg, or propranolol, 0.2 mg per kg.

In summary, although provocative testing using carotid massage, the Valsalva maneuver, atropine administration, or sinus node recovery time studies are helpful in the determination of sinus node dysfunction, the diagnositc hallmark remains documentation of the characteristic rhythm disturbance responsible for the symptoms associated with this syndrome.

Treatment

Current therapy for the treatment of arrhythmias associated with the sick sinus syndrome includes the implantation of a permanent pacemaker, often combined with appropriate pharmacologic agents. According to Moss and Davis (1974), patients with sick sinus syndrome can be divided into two groups: those with major symptoms and those with minor symptoms. The category of patients with major symptoms includes those with symptoms of syncope, near syncope, lightheadedness or dizziness, angina, congestive heart failure, or symptoms of low cardiac output, such as fatigue, activity intolerance, and forgetfulness. The patients in the minor symptoms category are those who may have mild ankle edema easily handled with low dose diuretics or those with subjective palpitations and an uncomfortable awareness of slow, rapid, or irregular heart beat. Additionally, Ajuiss and coworkers (1972) reported a third group of patients with documented bradytachy syndrome who were essentially asymptomatic. Despite atrial bradycardia with a rate of 35 to 40 beats per minute, the cardiac output in these patients was maintained by compensatory augmentation of the stroke volume, and the atrial tachyarrhythmias were not troublesome. Moss and Davis (1974) and Ajuiss et al. (1972) recommend no specific therapy for asymptomatic patients and those with minor symptoms. Patients with major symptoms, however, do require permanent pacing for control of bradyarrhythmias and often an antiarrhythmic drug regimen for suppression of tachyarrhythmias. We are in complete agreement with this approach.

Permanent pacemaker implantation

remains the cornerstone of therapy for the symptomatic patient. Both atrial and ventricular pacing have been used and their efficiency repeatedly demonstrated. Atrial pacing has theoretical advantages over ventricular pacing as long as atrioventricular conduction is preserved, since it allows for maintenance of the atrial transport function. When considering patients for atrial pacing, the integrity of A-V conduction should be determined by atrial pacing and His bundle electrocardiography. Favorable long-term followup studies with atrial pacing electrodes positioned in the coronary vein have substantiated the relative stability, safety, and reliability of this technique. However, these patients not infrequently have A-V conduction abnormalities that preclude atrial pacing. Ventricular pacing, although preventing bradyarrhythmias, may not control the accompanying atrial tachyrhythms. Occasionally, when retrograde ventricular-atrial conduction is present, the atrial depolarization following each paced ventricular beat may suppress ectopic rhythms. In patients with symptoms of low cardiac output, A-V sequential pacing should be considered.

Once a pacemaker system has been implanted, suppressive antiarrhythmic drug therapy can safely be instituted for control of tachyrhythms without concern of further suppressing intrinsic impulse formation. The indications for specific pharmacologic agents are similar to those recommended for management of uncomplicated tachycardias. The ventricular response rate to paroxysmal atrial flutter or fibrillation can be controlled by proper digitalization and may require supplementation with propranolol. Quinidine may prevent the recurrence of paroxysmal atrial tachyarrhythmias but the addition of propranolol to quinidine has been associated with more success than quinidine alone (Fors et al., 1971). Quinidine procainamide, propranolol, or disopyramide can be administered for control of ventricular irritability without the danger of further bradycardia. Digitalis improves myocardial performance and may indirectly inhibit the development of tachyarrhythmias.

Prognosis

The prognosis of patients with sick sinus syndrome manifesting as prolonged periods of sinus standstill, sinoatrial block, or persistent marked bradycardia has improved considerably with improved therapy, especially in the use of artificial pacemakers. In a one to five year followup of 52 patients with sinoatrial disturbances manifesting as syncope, dizzy spells, heart failure, or predisposition to ventricular arrhythmias, permanent pacing was associated with a favorable prognosis. Syncopal episodes were abolished in 32 of 35 patients, congestive heart failure alleviated in seven of 12, and ventricular tachyarrhythmias controlled in two of four patients with pacing and antiarrhythmic drugs (Chokshi et al., 1973).

REFERENCES

Ajuiss, N. S., Rosin, E. Y., Adolph, R. J., et al.: Significance of chronic sinus bradycardia in elderly people. Circulation 46:924, 1972.

Allensworth, D. C., Rice, G. J., and Lowe, G. W.: Persistent atrial standstill in a family with myocardial disease. Am. J. Med. 47:775, 1969.

Averill, K. H., and Lamb, L. E.: Electrocardiographic findings in 67,375 asymptomatic subjects. Am. J. Cardiol. 6:76, 1960.

Bellet, S., and Jedlicka, J.: Sino-ventricular conduction and its relation to sinoatrial conduction. Am. J. Cardio. 24:831, 1969.

Bloomfield, D. A., and Sinclair-Smith, B. C.: Persistent atrial standstill. Am. J. Med. 39:335, 1965.

Chadda, K. D., Banka, V. S., Bodenheimer, M. M., and Helfant, R. H.: Corrected sinus node recovery time: Experimental physiologic and pathologic determinants. Circulation 51:797, 1975.

Chokshi, D. S., Mascarenhas, E., Samet, P., et al. Treatment of sinoatrial rhythm disturbances with permanent cardiac pacing. Am. J. Cardiol. 32:215, 1973.

DeMello, W. C., and Hoffman, B. F.: Potassium ions and electrical activity of specialized cardiac fibers. Am. J. Physiol. 199:1125, 1960.

Engel, T. R., Meister, S. G., Feitosa, G. S., et al.: Appraisal of sinus node artery disease. Circulation 52:286, 1975.

Ferrer, M. I.: The sick sinus node syndrome. Circulation 47:635, 1973.

Ferrer, M. I.: The sick sinus syndrome in atrial disease. J.A.M.A. 206:645, 1968.

Fors, W. J., Vanderark, W. J., and Reynolds, E. W.: Evaluation of propranolol and quinidine in the treatment of quinidine-resistant arrhythmias. Am. J. Cardiol. 27:190, 1971.

Greenwood, R. J., and Finkelstein, D.: Sino-atrial Heart Block. Springfield, IL, Charles C Thomas, 1964.

Gupta, P. K., Lichstein, E., Chadda, K. D., and Badui, E.: Appraisal of sinus node recovery time in patients with sick sinus syndrome. Am. J. Cardiol. 34:265, 1974.

Hoffman, B. F., and Cranefield, P. F.: Physiological basis of cardiac arrhythmias. Am. J. Med. 37:670, 1964.

Hudson, R.: The human pacemaker and its pathology. Brit. Med. J. 22:153, 1960.

James, R. N.: The coronary circulation and conduction in acute myocardial infarction. Prog. Cardiovasc Dis. 10:410, 1968.

Jordan, J. L., Yamaguchi, I., and Mandel, W. J.: Studies on the mechanism of sinus node dysfunction in the sick sinus syndrome. Circulation 57:217, 1978.

Kaplan, B. M., Langendorf, R., Lev, M., and Pick, A.: Tachycardia-bradycardia syndrome (so-called "sick sinus syndrome"). Pathology, mechanisms and treatment. Am. J. Cardiol. 31:497, 1973.

Lewis, T., White, P. D., and Meakins, J.: The susceptible region in A-V conduction. Heart 5:289, 1914.

Mandel, W. J., Hayakawa, H., Allen, H. N., Danzig, R., and Kermaier, A-I.: Assessment of sinus node function in patients with sick sinus node syndrome. Circulation 46:761, 1972.

Moss, A. J., and Davis, R. J.: Brady-tachy syndrome. Progr. Cardiovasc. Dis. 16:439, 1974.

Narula, O. S.: Atrioventricular conduction defects in patients with sinus bradycardia. Circulation 44:1096, 1971.

Narula, O. S., Samet, P., and Javier, R. P.: Significance of the sinus node recovery time. Circulation 45:140, 1972.

Radford, D. J., and Julian D. G.: Sick sinus syndrome: Experience of cardiac pacemaker clinic. Brit. Med. J. 3:504, 1974.

Rokseth, R., and Hatte, L.: Sinus arrest in acute myocardial infarction. Brit. Heart J. 33:639, 1971.

Rosen, K. M., Loeb, H. S., Senno, M. Z., Rahimtoola, S. H., and Gunnar, R. M.: Cardiac conduction in patients with symptomatic sinus node disease. Circulation 43:836, 1971.

Rubinstein, J. J., Schulman, C. L., Yurchak, P. M., and DeSanctis, R. W.: Clinical spectrum of the sick sinus syndrome. Circulation 46:5, 1972.

Saracheck, U. S., and Leonard, J. J.: Familial heart block and sinus bradycardia: Classifications and natural history. Am. J. Cardiol. 29:451. 1972.

Scarpa, W. J.: The sick sinus syndrome. Am. Heart J. 92:648, 1976.

Schullman, C. L., Rubenstein, J. J., Yurchak, P. N., and DeSanctis, R. W.: The "sick sinus syndrome": Clinical spectrum. Circulation 42 (Suppl III) 42, 1970.

Spellberg, R. D.: Familial sinus node disease. Chest 60:246, 1971.

Talano, J. V., Euler, D., Randall, W. C., Eshaghy, B., Loeb, H. S., and Gunnar, R. M.: Sinus node dysfunction: An overview with emphasis on autonomic and pharmacologic consideration. Am. J. Med. 64:773, 1978.

Vassalee, M., and Hoffman, B. F.: The spread of sinus activation during potassium administration. Circ. Res. 17:285, 1965.

SUPPLEMENTAL READING

Ferrer, I. M.: The primary pacemaker: Functions, falterings and false alarms. Chest 75:376–379, 1979.

Rieffel, J., Glöklish, J., Gang, E., Weiss, M., Davis, J., and Bigger, J. T.: Human sinus node electrograms: Transvenous, catheter recorded technique and normal sinoatrial conduction times in adults. Circulation 60(II):63, 1979.

Scheinman, M. M., Strauss, H. C., and Abbott, J. A.: Electrophysiological testing for patients with sinus node dysfunction. J. Electrocardiography 12:211–216, 1979.

6

PAROXYSMAL SUPRAVENTRICULAR TACHYCARDIA

ROBERT I. KATZ, M.D.,
RICHARD H. HELFANT, M.D.

GENERAL CONSIDERATIONS

Although paroxysmal supraventricular tachycardia can include all tachyarrhythmias originating above the His bundle, it generally refers to atrial or A-V nodal tachycardia. Since the significance and treatment of these tachycardias are similar, they can conveniently be discussed together. Both the site of origin of these tachycardias and the electrophysiologic mechanisms causing and sustaining them have been extensively studied over the past several years.

Clinically, paroxysms of atrial tachycardia start and stop suddenly, and last a few seconds, hours, or days. The heart rate during a paroxysm ranges from 160 to 240 (260) per minute. Patients with paroxysmal supraventricular tachycardia often present a history of isolated atrial premature beats which gradually become more numerous and occur more frequently, ultimately eventuating in paroxysms of supraventricular tachycardia. These attacks may occur occasionally (i.e., once per week or month) or quite frequently, with many episodes appearing in a single day.

During the paroxysms the ventricular rate is quite regular. The maximum difference between cycles rarely exceeds 0.01 second. This is in contrast with ventricular tachycardia, in which a slight degree of irregularity is usually present. The rate is not influenced by posture or exercise. Carotid sinus pressure will often stop the paroxysm with resumption of normal sinus rhythm but if ineffective will not even slow the ventricular rate. Relatively few exceptions to this observation have been noted.

ETIOLOGY

Supraventricular tachycardia occurs in approximately 1.1 per cent of hospitalized patients. However, this underestimates the incidence, as most patients who experience the attacks are outpatients, many if not most of whom have otherwise normal hearts. The arrhythmia may be observed in association with many conditions including rheumatic heart disease, coronary heart disease, hypertensive cardiovascular disease and thyrotoxic heart disease, as well as recurrent pulmonary emboli, congenital heart disease (such as atrial-septal defect), mitral valve prolapse, acute myocardial infarction, and acute pericarditis. In addition, the paroxysms in a susceptible individual may be precipitated by hyperventilation, emotional stress, exercise, smoking, caffeine, alcohol intake, and heavy meals. It also occurs commonly as a manifestation of the pre-excitation syndromes (see Chapter 13).

MECHANISMS

Recently, extensive investigation has confirmed that most supraventricular tachycardias result from a "macroreentrant" mechanism (see Chapter 2). This circus movement mechanism or macrore-entrant theory has received substantial report as the electrophysiologic mechanism from several groups. The re-entry pathway usually involves the A-V junction (70%) although the atria and S-A node may also participate. The following findings, characteristic of re-entry, are observed in supraventricular tachycardia: 1) the paroxysm may be initiated or terminated by a premature atrial or ventricular beat. If this is associated with a critical degree of P-R interval prolongation, the re-entrant circuit involves the A-V junction; 2) there is a regular sequence of cycle length that occurs during the establishment of a paroxysm; and 3) once established, the paroxysm has a fixed cycle length. In addition, analysis of the P wave configuration in the initiating atrial premature complex is useful. If the P wave of this atrial premature complex is identical to subsequent P waves, automatic atrial activity is probable, while the initiating P wave will not appear the same as those originating from the re-entrant pathway. In addition, the P wave configuration and is relationship to the QRS during the tachycardia are also important. Thus, absence of a P wave during the tachycardia implies A-V nodal re-entry be-

cause it involves simultaneous atrial and ventricular activation. This is also true if the P wave is inverted. Patients with a P-R interval normal for the underlying rate have either sinus node re-entry or an atrial origin for the arrhythmia (re-entry or an automatic focus). Functional bundle branch block is quite uncommon in supraventricular tachycardia except with tachycardias involving a concealed bypass tract.

Pharmacologic and physiologic maneuvers are helpful in making the diagnosis. Thus, if carotid sinus pressure increases the A-V block while the tachycardia persists, this makes A-V nodal re-entry most unlikely. Conversely, the termination of the tachycardia by these maneuvers suggests that either the S-A node or the A-V node is involved. Automatic ectopic tachycardia may be diagnosed when 1) the tachycardia is spontaneous in onset with the initiating beat being identical to the subsequent beats of the tachycardia; 2) the tachycardia cannot be initiated or terminated with atrioventricular stimulations; 3) electrophysiologic absence of dual pathways is demonstrated. In some patients, the mechanisms of the tachycardia cannot be defined.

PATHOLOGY

Infarction of atrial tissue may be present when paroxysmal supraventricular tachycardia occurs in the patient with acute myocardial infarction. However, in the majority of cases in which there are no underlying clinical abnormalities, no pathologic alteration of the atria or A-V node is observable.

HEMODYNAMICS

The effect of a supraventricular tachycardia on cardiac hemodynamics depends on the rate and duration of the arrhythmia and on the underlying cardiac status. In the normal heart, sinus tachycardia usually causes an increase in cardiac output with rates up to 170 to 180 per minute. At faster rates, the period of ventricular filling is shortened and the stroke volume is reduced. In the previously diseased heart this diminution in cardiac output occurs at slower rates. Similarly, supraventricular tachycardia in the absence of organic heart disease produces little disability initially. However, prolonged episodes can result in progressive hemodynamic impairment. The systemic systolic, diastolic, and pulse pressures decrease, particularly in the upright position, and there is an increase in left atrial pressure and significantly reduced stroke volume (Fig. 6–1). In contrast, during exercise-induced tachycardia, stroke volume is maintained or increased and cardiac output goes up (Befeler et al., 1971).

SYMPTOMS AND SIGNS

Paroxysmal supraventricular tachycardia is characterized by its sudden onset and termination. The symptoms are similar to those observed in the presence of any rapid ectopic rhythm; they depend largely on the state of the heart muscle, its response to an acceleration of the heart beat, the duration of the paroxysm, and the emotional state of the patient. With paroxysms of short duration, the patient may experience relative freedom from symptoms, except for palpitations. In the presence of prolonged paroxysms with rapid ventricular rates, especially in patients with organic heart disease, the symptoms may be quite pronounced and include varying degrees of precordial discomfort or pain, breathlessness, weakness, dizziness, or rarely syncope as well as nausea and vomiting.

The signs of paroxysmal supraventricular tachycardia are those of an accelerated and regular heart rate. The pulse is rapid and weak; the heart sounds are identical. This may be accompanied by a fall in blood pressure, circulatory failure, heart failure, or angina in predisposed patients.

Polyuria, occurring with attacks in all forms of supraventricular tachycardia, is quite typical. Copious diuresis of up to 3 liters begins shortly after the onset

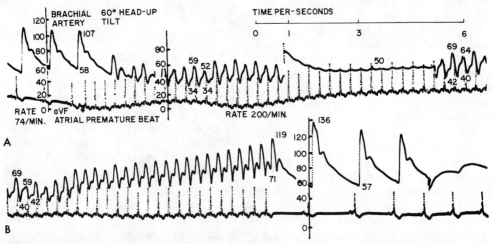

Figure 6–1. Illustrates the drop in brachial artery pressure almost immediately after the onset of paroxysmal supraventricular tachycardia.

(A) Note the brachial artery pressure, which was 107/58, dropped to as low as 52/34. The hypotensive state is the result of inadequate ventricular filling due to shortening of diastole as a consequence of the tachycardia. As a result, there is a drop in stroke volume.

(B) Note the return of blood pressure to normal with the return of normal sinus rhythm at the end of the strip. (From Saunders, D. E., and Ord, J. W.: Amer. J. Cardiol., 9:223, 1962.)

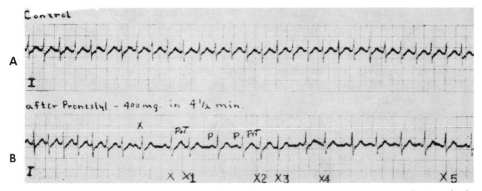

Figure 6–2. Paroxysmal supraventricular tachycardia showing conversion to normal sinus rhythm.
(A) Paroxysmal tachycardia with a rate of 200 per minute is shown. The P wave is superimposed on the preceding T wave. There is no widening of the QRS complex.
(B) Note end of paroxysm at X. The return to a normal sinus rhythm is accompanied by atrial premature beats (P + T) at X_1, X_2, X_3, X_4, and X_5.

of episodes and may last for 30 to 90 minutes in patients with paroxysmal forms of supraventricular tachycardia, atrial fibrillation, or atrial flutter. The mechanism of solute diuresis in these patients is at present believed to be inhibition of ADH secretion.

ELECTROCARDIOGRAM

Paroxysmal Supraventricular Tachycardia

This consists of a rapid, very regular succession of supraventricular premature beats that occur at a rate ranging from approximately 160 to 240 per minute. The P waves seen during the paroxysm vary in configuration (see mechanisms above). They are usually different in contour from those observed in the same patient during sinus rhythm. With very rapid rates, they are often superimposed on the T wave of the preceding beat, making them difficult or impossible to recognize. When this occurs, identification of the disturbance can be made only if one ascertains the beginning or the ending of a paroxysm or employs special methods (such as carotid sinus massage) to determine the atrial mechanism. Alternatively, the P wave may be superimposed on the QRS. This latter form has

also been called paroxysmal nodal (or junctional) tachycardia.

The ventricular complexes are usually normal in paroxysmal supraventricular tachycardia. However, widening may occur as a result of impulses arriving in the conduction system during the relatively refractory period. This may make a definite diagnosis of atrial tachycardia difficult. In the presence of widened QRS complexes the differential diagnosis between atrial and ventricular tachycardia becomes critical because of the marked difference in prognosis and treatment (see Chapter 11).

The following electrocardiographic patterns may be observed during normal sinus rhythm in patients susceptible to the development of paroxysmal supraventricular tachycardia: 1) atrial premature beats, particularly if they are frequent or in groups of two or more or occur coupled to the preceding normal beat; and 2) pre-excitation syndromes.

The transitional period between supraventricular tachycardia and sinus rhythm may be critical because asystole and/or ventricular tachyarrhythmias may transiently occur. The type of transitional arrhythmia observed depends in part upon the methods of conversion (e.g., carotid sinus massage, drugs, countershock) (Fig. 6–2). Conversion to normal sinus rhythm occurs in five general patterns: a) asystole (lasting as long as 6 seconds) followed by normal sinus rhythm; b) slight slowing of the ventricles, followed by sudden conversion; c) precipitous conversion (most common); d) slowing, asystole, and then conversion; and e) ventricular tachycardia, a prefibrillatory ventricular arrhythmia, and premature beats followed by normal sinus rhythm (Hellerstein et al., 1951).

Other Forms of Supraventricular Tachycardias

Multifocal or Chaotic Atrial Tachycardia. Multifocal atrial tachycardia may be defined as a rhythm with an atrial rate of greater than 100 per minute, changing P wave morphology of at least three different types in any rhythm strip, varying P-R intervals, and irregular P-P and R-R intervals. It occurs most commonly in elderly, ill patients with severe underlying pulmonary disease, usually with concomitant heart disease. It may be the forerunner to atrial fibrillation (with which it is often confused). It may be associated with first or second degree block, particularly in the setting of digitalis excess. It is important to differentiate this arrhythmia from atrial fibrillation, as the digitalis which is usually very effective in atrial fibrillation is usually ineffective in controlling ventricular response in chaotic atrial tachycardia.

Its course is usually self-limited and paroxysmal, but it is a difficult rhythm to treat. Vagal maneuvers as well as vagotonic and cholinergic drugs have been uniformly ineffective, as have quinidine, procainamide, phenytoin, and lidocaine. Digitalis is also relatively ineffective in most patients, although occasionally it is of use. However, digitalis toxicity must be considered if A-V block is present. This rhythm is also resistant to cardioversion. One must be careful when using bronchodilators such as aminophyline and isoproteren-

ol in patients with this rhythm and chronic obstructive lung disease, because they may accelerate atrial rhythm. At present the most efficacious means of control (in addition to trying digitalis) is to treat the underlying pulmonary disease.

Repetitive Atrial Tachycardia. The repetitive type of atrial tachycardia consists of brief paroxysms of atrial tachycardia (e.g., three to eight beats), frequently separated by only one or two sinus beats. It is somewhat more resistant to therapy than the continuous type.

DIAGNOSIS AND DIFFERENTIAL DIAGNOSIS

Paroxysmal supraventricular tachycardia should be suspected in a patient who gives a history of a sudden acceleration of the heart beat that lasts for varying periods of time and then suddenly stops. The history of atrial premature beats in the presence of a regular rhythm with a rate ranging from 160 to 240 per minute during the paroxysms should lead one to suspect paroxysmal supraventricular tachycardia. The ECG criteria for diagnosis of paroxysmal supraventricular tachycardia are: 1) P waves usually differ in contour from those of sinus beats, merge with preceding T waves, or are buried in the QRS; 2) the rhythm during the paroxysm is quite regular; 3) the QRS complex is usually normal in contour (but may show aberration); 4) the first normal beat at the end of the paroxysm is usually followed by post-tachycardia pause (Fig. 6–3). Not infrequently, it is difficult to determine the mechanism either because of the rapid rate and consequent poor delineation of the atrial complexes or because of widened QRS complexes. Under these conditions, the following procedures may be utilized: *Carotid sinus pressure* either may be helpful by terminating the tachycardia suddenly or, alternatively,

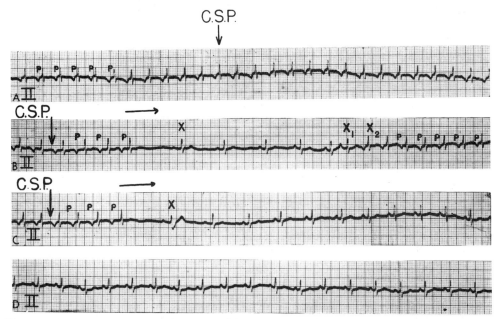

Figure 6–3. Supraventricular tachycardia.

(A) Note the presence of supraventricular tachycardia with a ventricular rate of 150 per minute. The P waves are inverted. The P-R interval measures 0.12 sec.

(B) Ventricular rate 150 per minute; P-R, 0.20 second. Following carotid sinus pressure, note the return to a normal sinus rhythm at X, a premature atrial beat at X_1, followed by a return of the paroxysm at X_2.

(C) Following carotid sinus pressure during another episode, note the return to a normal sinus rhythm at X.

(D) Sinus tachycardia.

has no effect on the rhythm. In contrast, sinus tachycardia will slow with carotid massage, while with atrial fibrillation or flutter the ventricular rate will frequently slow, allowing a better appreciation of the atrial mechanisms. In particularly difficult cases of widened QRS complexes, His bundle electrocardiography can be employed to distinguish between aberrant and ventricular beats (see Chapter 14).

TREATMENT

The principles of therapy of paroxysmal atrial tachycardia involve the use of the following: a) parasympathetic stimulation, primarily by mechanical means (e.g., carotid sinus massage); b) antiarrhythmic drugs; c) electric counter-shock; and d) right atrial pacing in selected cases.

The urgency of therapy depends on the clinical condition of the patient, the presence and severity of underlying heart disease, and the rate, duration, and type of arrhythmia being treated. Carotid massage should be tried initially. If this is unsuccessful, intravenous digitalization may be begun. Alternatively, if the patient is hypotensive, vasopressors such as metaraminol, norepinephrine, or methoxamine may be used in a drip, with monitored blood pressure not to exceed 160 to 180 mm Hg systolic over a period of 5 minutes. Carotid massage may be attempted concomitant with either vasopressor or digitalis administration. Parasympathomimetic drugs are not recommended because of side effects such as bradycardias, asystole, nausea, vomiting, and diarrhea.

If these measures are ineffective, the subsequent approach depends on the status of the patient. In patients without organic heart disease who are tolerating the arrhythmia well, simple sedation may be all that is necessary. However, in patients who are deteriorating, cardioversion should be employed (see Chapter 25).

More recently, cardiac pacing has added a new dimension to the treatment of refractory paroxysmal supraventricular tachycardia. Right atrial or ventricular pacing at varying rates or with single or coupled stimuli has been successful in terminating episodes of supraventricular tachycardia.

If the paroxysms tend to recur frequently, quinidine, procainamide, propranolol, phenytoin and disopyramide may be used. Propranolol in doses of 10 to 20 mg four times a day, alone or with quinidine and digitalis, has been successful in difficult cases. Patients with recurrent attacks frequently can terminate paroxysmal supraventricular tachycardia by 1) applying carotid sinus pressure, 2) performing a Valsalva or Muller maneuver, or 3) forced retching (by putting a finger down the throat).

In the rare situations in which the attacks remain recurrent, refractory, and severe, the possibility of a concealed bypass tract exists and the patient may require electrophysiological study. In patients who are not manageable by drugs but in whom atrial or ventricular stimulation can terminate the tachycardia, permanent pacemakers have been employed to terminate the arrhythmia on demand by the patient.

PROGNOSIS

Prognosis of paroxysmal supraventricular tachycardia is usually good insofar as individual attacks are concerned. Prognosis is less favorable in the following situations: a) in a long-continued paroxysm; b) when severe underlying myocardial damage is present; c) in those infrequent incidences in which the attacks recur repeatedly in spite of therapy; and d) when the attacks are accompanied by precordial pain or cardiac collapse and an association with acute or chronic myocardial infarction.

PAROXYSMAL ATRIAL TACHYCARDIA WITH A-V BLOCK (PAT WITH BLOCK)

General Considerations

Paroxysmal atrial tachycardia with A-V block (PAT with block) is an important arrhythmia. Prompt diagnosis is essential because of its therapeutic and prognostic implications.

Incidence and Etiology

Atrial tachycardia with block is generally considered uncommon, occurring only one sixth to one third as frequently as the common type of PAT (El-Sharif, 1970; Freiermuth and Jick, 1958).

The following etiologic factors are observed: (1) digitalis intoxication (by far the most common cause); (2) hypopotassemia; (3) occasionally, certain drugs other than digitalis (e.g., quinidine and isoproterenol); (4) coronary artery disease or hypertension; and (5) occasionally, A-V junctional disease in elderly persons.

Mechanism

Paroxysmal atrial tachycardia with block is probably caused by a unifocal atrial pacemaker beating at a rapid rate. Intracardiac records have shown that the site of stimulation, at least in some cases, is located in the right atrium near the sinus node and spreads from above downward. The A-V block has been at-

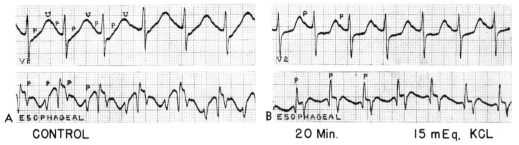

Figure 6–4. Paroxysmal atrial tachycardia with 2:1 A-V heart block due to hypopotassemia (no digitalis medication). Electrocardiogram of a 34-year-old woman with a clinical diagnosis of epilepsy. There was no underlying heart disease or history of digitalis medication, but the patient had intractable vomiting and the serum potassium level was 1.0 mEq./L.

(*A*) The upper strip of the control tracing shows a hypopotassemic pattern and barely visible P waves. In the esophageal lead, the P waves established the diagnosis of an atrial tachycardia with 2:1 A-V block.

(*B*) Following 15 mEq. of potassium, the atrial tachycardia with block has disappeared, although with this amount of potassium the hypopotassemic pattern remains. The administration of a total of 11 gm. of potassium chloride in 48 hours resulted in a return of the electrocardiogram to a normal pattern. (From Bettinger, Surawicz, Bryfogle, Anderson, and Bellet: Amer. J. Med., 21:521, 1956.)

tributed to the following factors: a) the rapid atrial rate; and b) the direct and vagal effects of digitalis on the A-V node, resulting in conduction delay. Hypopotassemia would tend to increase A-V block. The first factor may be the more important, since even in the normal heart an increase in the atrial rate by electrical stimulation predisposes (in the absence of digitalis effects) to the development of A-V heart block (Fig. 6–4).

Symptoms and Signs

Paroxysmal atrial tachycardia with block is usually observed in relatively ill patients. An aggravation of the clinical state characterized by the appearance or worsening of congestive failure and by cardiac or gastrointestinal evidence of digitalis toxically usually occurs following the occurrence of PAT with block. Often, its occurrence may be precipitated by conditions leading to potassium depletion, such as anorexia, vomiting, diarrhea, or administration of powerful potassium-wasting diuretics.

The ventricular rate in PAT usually ranges from 140 to 200 per minute; however, rates of 110 to 230 per minute have been observed. The rhythm may be regular; however, a regular rhythm may be interrupted by varying periods of irregularity due to an increase in or a variation in A-V conduction (Fig. 6–5).

Diagnosis

The diagnosis may be suggested by the presence of the aforementioned symptoms and signs; however, the final diagnosis depends upon the electrocardiogram; in the presence of 1:1 conduction, carotid sinus pressure may occasionally aid in establishing the diagnosis.

This arrhythmia manifests the following characteristics: 1) The P complexes may resemble those of normal S-A origin when the ectopic site is located close to the S-A node; however, it occasionally originates close to the A-V junction, in which case the P waves may be abnormal in morphology. 2) An isoelectric baseline is present between the P waves. 3) The atrial rate is regular and ranges from 110 to 230 per minute; however in 75 per

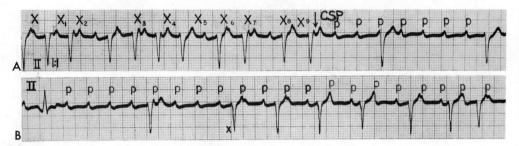

Figure 6–5. Paroxysmal atrial tachycardia with varying degrees of A-V heart block. Complete A-V heart block occurs transiently following carotid sinus pressure.

(A) Paroxysmal atrial tachycardia with block. The atrial rate is 167 per minute; the ventricular rate varies depending upon the degree of A-V heart block. In cycles X and X_1, the ventricular rate is 167 per minute (i.e., 1:1 response); in cycle X_2, 2:1 A-V block is present; cycles X_3, X_4, and X_6 manifest a 1:1 response; X_5 is 2:1; X_7 is 2:1; X_8 is 1:1; and X_9 is 1:1. Following carotid sinus pressure (at arrow), a transient complete A-V heart block can be observed; the atrial rate is unaffected.

(B) Shows paroxysmal atrial tachycardia with varying degrees of A-V block. The first QRS in the record is probably an escape beat.

cent of the episodes it is less than 190 per minute. The lowest reported atrial rate in PAT with block is 106 per minute (Lown et al., 1960). 4) Occasionally, the atrial rhythm may be irregular and an analysis may demonstrate cycle lengths that are multiples of the basic interval, suggesting the presence of an exit block. 5) The degree of block may vary from 2:1 with occasional periods of 1:1 response to a Wenckebach type. 6) The degree of A-V block usually can be increased by carotid sinus pressure (Fig. 6–6).

The differential diagnosis includes the following: 1) Sinus tachycardia may be simulated when the ectopic pacemaker rate is slow (110 to 140 per min-

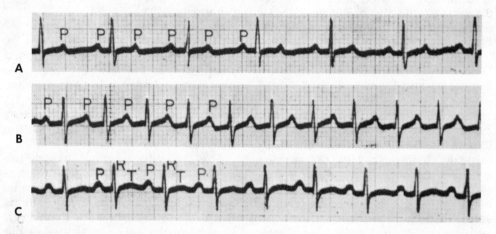

Figure 6–6. Paroxysmal atrial tachycardia with 2:1 A-V block, conversion to normal sinus rhythm.

(A) Shows an atrial rate of 184 per minute and a ventricular rate of 92 per minute (2:1 A-V heart block).

(B) Note that the ventricular rate has increased to 160 per minute. The response is now 1:1 with a prolonged P-R interval, 0.21 second.

(C) Note the return to sinus rhythm with a ventricular rate of 130 per minute; the P-R interval now measures 0.18 second. (From Bettinger, Surawicz, Bryfogle, Anderson, and Bellet: Amer. J. Med., 21:521, 1956.)

ute) or in the presence of a 2:1 A-V heart block when the non-conducted P wave is superimposed on the succeeding T wave. 2) Paroxysmal supraventricular tachycardia of the common type may be diagnosed when the P-R intervals are prolonged. However, the heart rate in PAT usually exceeds 140 per minute; carotid sinus pressure, if successful, converts the tachycardia to a normal sinus rhythm. 3) Atrial flutter is frequently diagnosed in the presence of 2:1 A-V heart block, particularly when the atrial rate ranges from 220 to 250 per minute. However, flutter is almost always greater than 240 (particularly when quinidine has not been present) and a characteristic "saw tooth" pattern is usually seen without an isoelectric baseline (see Chapter 7).

The diagnosis in a puzzling case may often be clarified by the use of the following procedures: carotid sinus pressure, V_3R leads in the third and fourth interspaces, and the esophageal lead.

Treatment

Treatment depends upon the underlying clinical state and, in particular, the underlying cause of the PAT with block. In the presence of digitalis toxicity, administration of the drugs should be stopped. Since diuretic therapy may be an additional factor, this should also be discontinued. Before giving potassium, one should obtain the serum potassium level, since the value may be either low, normal, or elevated. Elevation could be the result of acidosis, dehydration, and a shocklike state. If the serum potassium is low, potassium may be cautiously administered. Hyperkalemia will aggravate the A-V block in the presence of digitalis. If digitalis toxicity is not the cause of the arrhythmia, and hypopotassemia is not present, digitalis may be given as a therapeutic measure (Morgan and Breneman, 1962). Other drugs such as procainamide and quinidine may be used.

Electric countershock has been employed successfully in patients suffering from PAT with block (Mark and Shaw, 1969). However, this is contraindicated if digitalis toxicity is present.

Prognosis

The prognosis generally depends on the etiology, rapid recognition of the arrhythmia, and prompt therapy. Because PAT with block usually occurs with late stage heart disease, the prognosis is often poor. The mortality ranges from 28 to 58 per cent (Freiermuth and Jick, 1958; Lown et al., 1960). The outlook is more favorable in those cases that are associated with transient and correctable types of electrolyte disturbances (e.g., hypopotassemia precipitated by vomiting or diarrhea) and when digitalis toxicity is the chief factor, if these conditions are recognized and the appropriate therapy instituted promptly.

REFERENCES

Barker, P. S., Wilson, F. N., Johnston, F. D., and Wishart, S. W.: Auricular paroxysmal tachycardia with auriculoventricular block. Amer. Heart J. 25:765, 1943.

Barold, S. S., Linhart, J. W., Samet, P., and Lister, J. W.: Supraventricular tachycardia initiated and terminated by a single electrical stimulus. Amer. J. Cardiol. 24:37, 1969.

Barrow, J. G.: Treatment of paroxysmal supraventricular tachycardia with lanatoside C. Ann. Inter. Med. 32:116, 1950.

Befeler, B., Hildner, F. J., Javier, R. P., Cohen, L. S., and Samet, P.: Cardiovascular dynamics during coronary sinus right atrial and right ventricular pacing. Amer. Heart J. 81:372, 1971.

Bellet, S., Zeeman, S. E., and Hirsch, S. A.: Intramuscular use of Pronestyl. Amer. J. Med. 13:145, 1952.

Berry, K., Garlett, E. L., Bellet, S., and Gefter, W. I.: Use of Pronestyl in treatment of ectopic rhythms. Amer. J. Med. 11:431, 1951.

Bjerkelund, C., and Orning, O. M.: An evaluation of DC shock treatment of atrial arrhythmias. Acta Med. Scand. 184:481, 1968.

Bouveret, L.: De la tachycardie essentielle paroxystique. Rev. Med. (Paris) 9:755, 837, 1889.

Denes, P., Delon, W. U., Ramesch, D., Chuqui-mia, R., and Rosen, K.: Demonstration of dual A-V nodal pathways in patients with paroxysmal supraventricular tachycardia. Circulation 48:549, 1973.

Dolara, A., and Possi, L.: Persistent supraventricular tachycardia. Amer. J. Cardiol. 16:449, 1965.

Durrer, D., Schoo, L., Schuilenburg, R. M., and Wellens, H. J. J.: Role of premature beats in the initiation and termination of supraventricular tachycardia in the Wolff-Parkinson-White syndrome. Circulation 35:644, 1967.

El-Sharif, N.: Supraventricular tachycardia with A-V block. Brit. Heart J. 32:46, 1970.

Freiermuth, L. J., and Jick, S.: Paroxysmal tachycardia with atrioventricular block. Amer. J. Cardiol. 1:584, 1958.

Furman, R. H., and Geigen, A. J.: Use of cholinergic drugs in supraventricular tachycardia. J.A.M.A. 149:269, 1952.

Goldreyer, B. N., Bigger, J. T., Jr., and Heissenbuttel, R.: Re-entrant supraventricular tachycardia. Clin. Res. 17:243, 1969.

Han, J.: The mechanism of paroxysmal atrial tachycardia. Amer. J. Cardiol. 26:329, 1970.

Hein, J. J., Wellens, M. D., and Durrer, D.: The role of an accessory atrioventricular pathway in reciprocal tachycardia. Circulation 52:58, 1975.

Hellerstein, H. K., Levine, B., and Feil, H.: Electrocardiographic changes following carotid sinus stimulation in paroxysmal ventricular tachycardia. J. Lab. Clin. Med. 38:820, 1951.

Josephson, M.: PSVT: An electrophysiological approach. A.J.C. 41:1123, 1978.

Lister, J. W., et al.: Rapid atrial stimulation for treatment of supraventricular tachycardia. Circulation 37–38:VI-130, 1968.

Lown, B., Vassaux, C., Hood, W. B., Jr., Fakhro, A. M., Kaplinsky, E., and Roberge, G.: Unresolved problems in coronary care. Amer. J. Cardiol. 20:494, 1967.

Lown, B., Wyatt, N. F., and Levine, H. D.: Paroxysmal atrial tachycardia with block. Circulation 21:129, 1960.

McIntosh, H. D., and Morris, J. J., Jr.: The hemodynamic consequences of arrhythmias. Prog. Cardiov. Dis. 8:330, 1966.

Mark, H., and Shaw, R.: Non-digitalis-induced paroxysmal atrial tachycardia with block. I. Management with cardioversion. J. Electrocardiol. 2:171, 1969.

Meltzer, L. E., and Kitchell, J.: The incidence of arrhythmias associated with acute myocardial infarction. Prog. Cardiov. Dis. 9:50, 1966.

Mendez, C., and Moe, G. K.: Demonstration of a dual A-V nodal conduction system in the isolated rabbit heart. Circ. Res. 19:378, 1966.

Montella, S.: Phasic respiratory paroxysmal atrial tachycardia. Amer. J. Cardiol. 7:613, 1961.

Morgan, W., and Breneman, G.: Atrial tachycardia with block treated with digitalis. Circulation. 25:787, 1962.

Saunders, D. E., Jr., and Ord, J. W.: The hemodynamic effects of paroxysmal supraventricular tachycardia in patients with the Wolff-Parkinson-White syndrome. Amer. J. Cardiol. 9:223, 1962.

Scherlag, B. J., Lazzara, R., and Helfant, R. H.: Differentiation of "A-V Junctional Rhythms." Circulation, 48:304, 1973.

Sowton, E., et al.: Long-term control of intractable supraventricular tachycardia by ventricular pacing. Brit. Heart J. 31:700, 1969.

Ticzon, A. R., and Whalen, R. W.: Refractory supraventricular tachycardias. Circulation 47:647, 1972.

Vassaux, C., and Lown, B.: Cardioversion of supraventricular tachycardias. Circulation, 39:791, 1969.

Wright, J. S., Fabian, J., and Epstein, E. J.: Immediate effect on cardiac output of reversion to sinus rhythm from rapid arrhythmias. Brit. Med. J. 3:315, 1970.

Wu, D., Denes, P., Amat-Y-Leon, F., Dhangia, R., Wyndham, C., Bauernfeind, R., Latif, P., and Rosen, K.: Clinical, electrocardiographic, and electrophysiologic observations in patients with PSVT. A. J. C. 41:1045, 1978.

SUPPLEMENTAL READING

Csapo, G.: Paroxysmal nonreentrant tachycardias due to simultaneous conduction in dual A-V nodal pathways. Am. J. Cardiol. 43:1033, 1979.

Denes, P., Wu, D., Amat-y-Leon, F., Dhingra, R., Wyndham, C., Kehoe, R., Ayres, B. F., and Rosen, K. W.: Paroxysmal supraventricular tachycardia induction in patients with WPW syndrome. Ann. Int. Med. 90:153–157, 1979.

Engle, T. R.: Pacing techniques to guide the therapy of tachycardias. Ann. Int. Med. 90(2):265, 1979.

Rosen, K. W., Barrenfeind, Wyndham, C. R., and Dhingra, R. C.: Retrograde properties of the fast pathway in patients with paroxysmal A-V nodal reentrant tachycardias. Am. J. Cardiol. 43:863, 1979.

7

ATRIAL FLUTTER

ROBERT I. KATZ, M.D.,
RICHARD H. HELFANT, M.D.

GENERAL CONSIDERATIONS

Atrial flutter has been considered somewhat uncommon; however, it probably occurs more frequently than is generally recognized. Since flutter is usually associated with organic heart disease and is amenable to treatment, its recognition is especially important. This can at times be difficult, as flutter comes in many forms and thus must constantly be kept in mind.

Atrial flutter may be observed either as an established disturbance or more commonly as a paroxysmal or transient condition. It is commonly associated with a flutter rate between 250 and 350 beats per minute. In 85 per cent of cases, the flutter rate is 300 per minute with 2:1 block and a ventricular rate of 150 per minute. However, flutter may be observed in conjunction with higher grades of block (i.e., 3:1 and 4:1) and rarely with complete heart block. With the advent of cardioversion and other forms of medical therapy, persistent flutter is rare.

ETIOLOGY AND PRECIPITATING FACTORS

Flutter can occur in association with almost any type of heart disease but most commonly in rheumatic heart disease with mitral valvular involve-ment. It is also found in patients with ischemic, hypertensive, pulmonary, pericardial, and congenital heart disease and cardiomyopathies as well as in patients with such acute conditions as hypoxia, trauma, infection, drug ingestion, acute GI disturbances and pulmonary embolization. In recent years it has also been associated with the "brady-tachy" complication of the sick sinus node syndrome (see Chapter 5) as well as with the prolapsing mitral valve syndrome. There have been reports that flutter may be seen with digitalis intoxication; these cases have been questioned and flutter is probably very rarely if at all due to digitalis toxicity.

MECHANISMS

Atrial flutter is thought to result from either a re-entry or ectopic mechanism. The re-entry or "circus movement" concept postulates an activation front crossing continuously within the atria, mainly around a ring of tissue between the two venae cavae. By definition, the head of this activation front must always encounter responsive (i.e., not refractory) tissue, so that it is continuous (see Chapter 2). The impulse thus travels in one direction through a closed circuit, resulting in a continuous cycle. One can end this movement, theoretically at least, if one of the sites of re-entry becomes refractory to the wave front. This is the postulated mechanism by which quinidine terminates this arrhythmia. There are experimental data in the fish and in the dog to support this mechanism as at least one way in which atrial flutter develops. In addition, recent findings of prolonged atrial conduction intervals in flutter patients with normally sized atria strongly suggest the existence of atrial conduction disease as a major predisposing factor (Leier, 1978).

The second proposed mechanism of flutter is the unifocal hypothesis (a rapid discharge from a unifocal ectopic atrial focus). The only differences between flutter and extrasystolic forms of atrial tachycardia is the rate of discharge. There are as many advocates of this mechanism as there are of the circus movement theory, and the issue remains unsettled. It may be that both forms come into play under different circumstances. It is commonly recognized that atrial flutter is preceded by atrial premature complexes occurring either singly or in couplets and this has been used as evidence to support the unifocal theory (see Fig. 7–1). In a re-

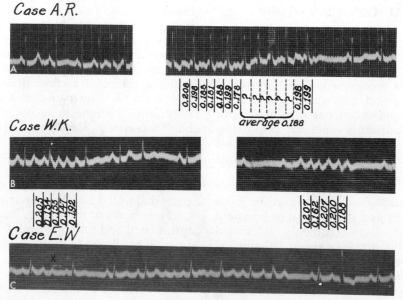

Figure 7–1 Onsets and offsets of atrial flutter (impure). (*A*) In patient A. R., the onsets invariably were precipitated by exercise or by premature atrial beats. Toward the end of the paroxysm illustrated, the atrial waves are fairly regular in time and also in shape except as the irregularity of the ventricular response modifies them. The last two cycles, 0.198 and 0.199 second in duration, while not longer than some individual cycles, are definitely longer than the immediately preceding ones. The preceding seven cycles are impossible to measure accurately; measured *in toto* and averaged, each has an estimated duration of 0.188 second. Such slight and uncertain changes suggest that the termination of flutter was preceded by slowing of the atria.

(*B*) In patient W. K., premature atrial beats were also present and at times initiated paroxysms; at other times, onsets were spontaneous. Both types of onsets are illustrated. The behavior of the atrial rate at the time of offsets was inconstant. In the initial strip of *B*, the last cycle, while not larger than some individual cycles, was longer than the cycle immediately preceding it; in the fourth offset studied the last cycle was definitely shorter than the preceding one. One of each variety of offset is shown.

(*C*) In patient E. W., the flutter was definitely impure. The flutter waves closely approach in shape the P and T waves, and therefore make it difficult to be certain of the exact point of offset. In the first short paroxysm (marked X), the last atrial wave is definitely faster than the preceding wave. The exact point of the other offset illustrated is uncertain. There are numerous premature beats, but we cannot be certain that any of these impulses actually initiated a period of flutter. (From McMillan, T. M., and Bellet, S.: Amer. J. Med. Sci., *184*:33, 1932.)

cent case (Wellens et al., 1971), atrial epicardial excitation mapping was performed during open heart surgery in a patient with atrial flutter. The results obtained in this patient seemed to exclude a circus movement: the possible mechanisms were an ectopic focus located low in the atrium, or a reciprocal rhythm located in a small area low in the atrium or in the upper part of the A–V junction.

Observations with atrial pacing in patients with flutter are also of interest in that there appears to be atrial fusion prior to the interruption of the flutter, suggesting that flutter can be sustained in one part of the atrium even when other parts are being depolarized from a high right atrial site. This suggests that whatever the mechanism, the arrhythmia is generated inferiorly (Waldo, 1977).

SIGNS AND SYMPTOMS

The symptoms and signs of atrial flutter depend critically on 1) the severity and etiology of the underlying heart disease, 2) the ventricular rate associated with the tachyarrhythmia, and 3) the duration of the arrhythmia. Symptoms may vary from minimal palpitations to overt pulmonary edema with hypotension and cardiac collapse. In addition to the severity of the underlying cardiac disease, there are also specific instances in which the loss of the atrial contribution to ventricular filling (which can contribute as much as 20 per cent to the cardiac output) can result in significant deterioration in the clinical state. This is particularly true in patients with left ventricular hypertrophy, a situation which is uniquely dependent on the "atrial kick" for adequate cardiac output (i.e., patients with hypertensive heart disease, valvular or subvalvular aortic stenosis, or hypertrophic cardiomyopathies).

The ventricular rate plays a crucial role in determining the clinical effects of flutter. With ventricular rates higher than 150 per minute, the symptoms are frequently marked; with rates between 100 and 130 they tend to be slight or moderate in severity, and at slower rates they are minimal. Symptoms usually improve when the flutter is converted to atrial fibrillation with a concomitant decrease in the ventricular rate, or more dramatically with return to normal sinus rhythm. Circulatory collapse may occur when the ventricular rate is very rapid, for example, with a 1:1 response (Figs. 7–2 and 7–3).

In some patients with chronic atrial flutter and 3:1 or 4:1 block, although the ventricular rate at rest may be satisfactorily low, the degree of block may abruptly change to 2:1 or rarely to 1:1 with exercise or emotion. When 1:1 conduction does occur under these conditions, a ventricular rate of 240 to 280 per minute suddenly occurs, resulting in severe symptoms. Such cases of flutter should, therefore, be treated with digitalis or converted to sinus rhythm.

PATHOLOGY

The pathology associated with atrial flutter is that of the underlying heart disease. In addition, the atria are frequently dilated with varying degrees of fibrosis present. Some studies have shown that the larger the atria, the slower the flutter rate.

ELECTROCARDIOGRAM

Atrial flutter is characterized by a distinctive "saw-tooth" pattern of atrial activity on the ECG. The vector is inferiorly directed so that it is usually most obvious in leads II, III, and AVF (and often in lead VI). It is characteristically a very regular undulating pattern with no fixed baseline. The atrial rate is usually between 250 and 350 per minute, with certain uncommon exceptions such as very severe heart disease (with huge atria) or in the presence of quinidine or quinidine-like drugs (with de-

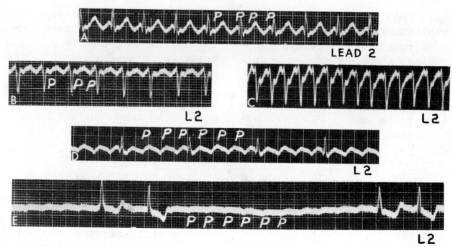

Figure 7-2 Atrial flutter, showing different types of atrial complexes and varying degrees of A-V heart block.

(A) Atrial flutter with a 2:1 heart block. The atrial rate is 250 per minute, the ventricular rate is 125 per minute. Note that the atrial complexes are obscured by the QRS complexes and T waves.

(B) Atrial flutter with a 2:1 heart block.

(C) Atrial flutter with a 1:1 response (atrial and ventricular rate is 250 per minute). The diagnosis of the atrial mechanism was clearly established by other strips that showed higher grades of A-V heart block (Strip B).

(D) Atrial flutter with a 4:1 response.

(E) Atrial flutter with a high degree of A-V heart block and cycle of A-V junctional escapes.

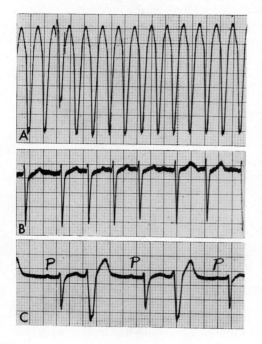

Figure 7-3 Atrial flutter with a 1:1 response showing progressive changes following therapy (all leads V₁). (A) Note rapid ectopic rhythm at rate of 264 per minute. This was considered to be atrial flutter with a 1:1 response. (B) Following digitalis the mechanism was converted to atrial fibrillation, thus confirming the original impression of 1:1 flutter. (C) Digitalis was stopped and conversion to normal sinus rhythm was spontaneous. The P-R interval is slightly elevated (0.22 second). Coupled ventricular premature beats are probably due to digitalis toxicity.

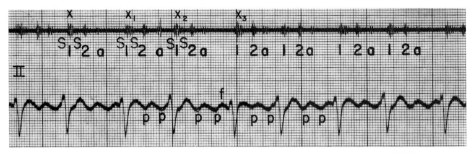

Figure 7–4 Phonocardiogram in atrial flutter with varying degrees of A-V block.

pressed atrial conductivity and prolonged atrial refractory periods). However, 85 per cent of patients in atrial flutter have an atrial rate of 300 per minute and a ventricular rate of 150 per minute (i.e., 2:1 block is present). Therefore, *any electrocardiogram in which the rate of the ventricles is 150 per minute should be examined carefully for flutter!* This is particularly important in cases where a flutter wave is hidden in the previous QRS or T wave (Fig. 7–2A and B).

A-V conduction is often variable in atrial flutter and, therefore, several conduction patterns exist. Although 2:1 A–V conduction is the most common, conduction may alternate between 2:1 and 4:1 A-V block (Fig. 7–4 and 7–5). Odd conduction patterns are unusual (i.e., 3:1, etc.). One can almost always identify a group mechanism if the patient has not been on cardiac medications. The degree of conductivity depends not only on the flutter rate but also on the state of the A-V junctional tissues, the underlying heart disease, and the presence of drugs such as quinidine and digitalis. Thus, as with other supraventricular arrhythmias, one can recognize Wenckebach periods, complete heart block, and A-V dissociation (which is difficult to diagnose because of the presence of concealed conduction associated with this arrhythmia).

Occasionally, flutter with 1:1 conduc-

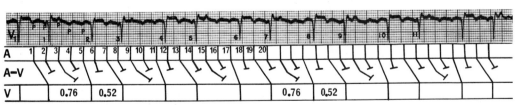

Figure 7–5 Alternating 4:1 and 2:1 flutter, example of "pseudobigeminy." The atrial rate is 280 per minute. Note that *atrial* impulse 5 (see diagram A) is conducted with a short P-R interval. The next impulse (6) is blocked in the A-V node. Impulse 7 is conducted with a longer P-R interval; impulse 8 is again blocked in the A-V node. Impulse 9 has penetrated deeper into the A-V node before being blocked; this shows concealed conduction and represents a dropped beat; impulse 10 is blocked in the node; and 11 is conducted with a short P-R interval. Also note that the longer R-R intervals, measuring 0.76 second, are shorter than four P-P intervals, and the shorter R-R intervals, measuring 0.52 second, are larger than two P-P intervals. This implies that the P-R interval at a 2:1 conduction ratio is longer than the P-R interval at 4:1 conduction ratio.

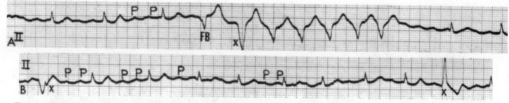

Figure 7–6 Atrial flutter with ventricular tachycardia.

(A) Atrial flutter (rate 216), with 4:1 A-V heart block. Note fusion beat (FB). Starting at X, a 2:1 A-V conduction with aberration of QRS simulating ventricular tachycardia (idioventricular type), 106/minute, is observed.

(B) Note atrial flutter with varying degrees of A-V block. Note abnormal ventricular beats at X.

tion occurs. This is often seen with aberrant conduction because of the very rapid ventricular rate and can be confused with ventricular tachycardia (Fig. 7–3A). Occasionally, the two coexist (Fig. 7–6). It is most often encountered in patients who have been treated with quinidine before being given an A-V nodal blocking agent such as digitalis. In any rhythm in which the ventricular rate is 260 to 300 beats per minute and perfectly regular the possibility of atrial flutter should be part of the differential diagnosis.

The rhythm most often confused with atrial flutter is paroxysmal atrial tachycardia. Several points usually serve to differentiate these two arrhythmias. Paroxysmal atrial tachycardia tends to occur at a lower atrial rate (between 160 and 240 beats per minute) while flutter rates are usually 250 to 350 beats per minute (Chapter 00). One thus must differentiate the P waves of atrial tachycardia from the F waves of atrial flutter — occasionally using esophageal leads (Fig. 7–7). In addition, in contrast to the "saw-tooth" flutter pattern with-

out an isoelectric shelf, paroxysmal atrial tachycardia is characteristically associated with an isoelectric baseline. Exceptions to this, however, not infrequently occur.

Probably the most effective means of differentiating these two arrhythmias is to utilize vagal maneuvers such as carotid sinus stimulation (Figs. 7–8 and 7–9). In atrial flutter, increased vagal activity increases the degree of block in the A-V node and the flutter waves are more easily identified with their characteristic saw-tooth pattern as well as rate. In contrast, with paroxysmal atrial tachycardia, vagal manipulations result in an "all or none" phenomenon; that is, the rate either remains exactly the same or the arrhythmia suddenly "breaks" to normal sinus rhythm. Of less direct value, paroxysmal atrial tachycardia is much more commonly seen in patients with no significant heart disease. Flutter is more common in the elderly while paroxysmal atrial tachycardia occurs primarily in younger individuals.

Paroxysmal atrial tachycardia with A-V

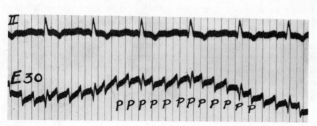

Figure 7–7 Atrial flutter not clearly evident in limb leads, clearly shown by esophageal leads. Limb lead II (*upper strip*) taken simultaneously with esophageal lead (*lower strip*) at atrial level. Upper strip, lead II does not clearly show the atrial complexes. The diagnosis is clearly made by the esophageal lead taken at the atrial level (E_{30}). Note the diphasic atrial complexes occurring at a rate of 310 per minute, which present a characteristic saw-toothed appearance.

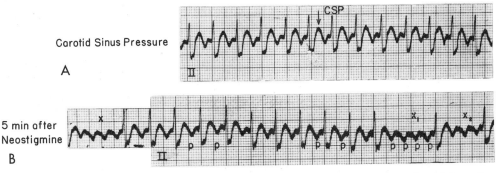

Figure 7–8 The value of carotid sinus pressure (and neostigmine) in the diagnosis of atrial flutter by slowing the ventricular rate.

(*A*) Shows a regular tachycardia with a rate of 155 per minute. Terminal widening of the QRS complex is due to a right bundle branch block. The exact type of arrhythmia is difficult to establish. Carotid sinus pressure was applied at the arrow; however, no slowing was obtained.

(*B*) Five minutes after the administration of neostigmine. Note in cycle marked X, the appearance of typical atrial flutter beats with a rate of 300 per minute. Note the resumption of the rapid rate of 150 per minute with 2:1 A-V heart block until cycle marked X₁ where a 5:1 A-V heart block is seen and atrial flutter beats are observed. At X₂ a 4:1 A-V heart block is present. This varying degree of A-V heart block was maintained 11 hours later after the patient had been digitalized.

block is another important differential diagnostic problem. This arrhythmia is also slower than atrial flutter, the atrial rate being 130 to 220 beats per minute (average, 80 beats per minute). The isoelectric shelf is typically present in PAT with block, and the ventricular response is not nearly as regular as with atrial flutter. However, there are instances in which it is very difficult to differentiate the two arrhythmias, especially in the presence of quinidine therapy. This becomes particularly important if the patient is taking digitalis, since paroxysmal atrial tachycardia with block is usually a manifestation of digitalis intoxication while, as previously mentioned, atrial flutter is rarely, if ever, caused by digitalis excess.

Other arrhythmias, including ventricular tachycardia, easily differentiated from flutter, except in situations in which an intraventricular conduction abnormality occurs or the 1:1 flutter is present (Fig. 7–3). Even in the latter instance, however, if one is suspicious, vagal maneuvers will usually clarify the atrial mechanism as being that of flutter. There are instances in which flutter is accompanied by ventricular tachycardia as a separate arrhythmia with A-V dissociation, but these are rare (Fig. 7–5). In order to elucidate atrial mechanisms of any type in making a diagnosis, one may also, of course, resort to esophageal electrodes (Fig. 7–7) or intra-atrial recordings, but this is usually unnecessary.

DIAGNOSIS

The diagnosis of atrial flutter is usually established by observing dis-

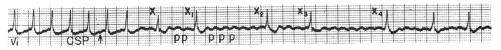

Figure 7–9 Diagnosis of atrial flutter clarified following carotid sinus pressure. The figure shows a rapid arrhythmia, quite regular at a rate of 160 per minute. The exact atrial mechanism cannot be determined at this rapid rate. Following carotid sinus pressure, note that with the slowing of the ventricular rate, the diagnosis of atrial flutter is very clearly made. Note that the P-R interval varies at X, X₃, and X₄.

tinct and characteristic regular flutter waves in leads II, III and AVF as well as in precordial leads VI, V2, and V3R (see Fig. 7–2). These oscillations are very regular and range from 250 to 350, being 300 per minute in 85 per cent of patients. While flutter waves may be buried in the preceding QRS and T complex, carotid sinus massage is often decisive in determining the underlying atrial mechanism in doubtful cases by increasing the A-V block and slowing the ventricular rate. Occasionally, the use of esophageal leads will be necessary to clarify the issue. The relationship between the flutter waves and QRS complexes is often regular and constant, but not invariably so, although the ventricular complexes themselves are very regularly spaced. These variations in the "F-QRS" interval may be due to concealed conduction, A-V dissociation, or depressed A-V conduction, occasionally with Wenckebach type second degree heart block and, less commonly, with complete A-V block.

Flutter with 1:1 Conduction

Atrial flutter with 1:1 conduction occurs when the refractory period of the A-V junction becomes so short that it transmits every atrial impulse. This is accompanied by a very rapid ventricular rate (240 to 280 beats per minute) and usually constitutes a serious cardiac emergency. Its incidence, while small, is probably greater than suggested by the few cases reported in the literature (Sussman et al., 1966). Indeed, this mechanism is often unrecognized and is probably a cause of acute heart failure and sudden death in at least some patients with atrial flutter (Figs. 7–2 and 7–3).

Auscultatory Phenomena

Although auscultation has been emphasized in the past, it is of minor clini-cal value in the diagnosis of atrial flutter.

TREATMENT

The therapeutic approach to atrial flutter can be pharmacological (i.e., digitalis, propranolol, and quinidine) and/or electrical (i.e., cardioversion or, less commonly, right atrial pacing). It has previously been emphasized that the clinical consequences of atrial flutter vary substantially from palpitations to cardiovascular collapse, depending on the severity of the underlying heart disease, the dependence on the "atrial kick," the ventricular rate, and the duration of the arrhythmia. The treatment of flutter is directly related to the patient's clinical state and is not dictated by the arrhythmia per se!

Many cardiologists consider cardioversion to be the treatment of choice in patients with atrial flutter. If the patient is doing poorly, immediate cardioversion is without question the treatment of choice. Certainly, flutter with 1:1 conduction is an emergency requiring immediate cardioversion! It is usually not necessary to use high electrical energy levels to convert atrial flutter to sinus rhythm, and one can start with 10 to 25 watts per second (see Chapter 25). While it may occasionally be necessary to go to higher levels, cardioversion successfully converts flutter to sinus rhythm in more than 90 per cent of cases.

If the patient is clinically stable, one can elect to employ a pharmacologic approach using digitalis as the primary agent. Digitalis is administered to decrease the ventricular rate by increasing the A-V block. It is frequently necessary to use very high doses of digitalis to get appropriate rate slowing, and one should be guided by frequent rhythm strips or telemetric monitoring to assess its effect on the ventricular rate. At the point where satisfactory ventricular rate control is achieved, either atrial fibrillation or normal sinus rhythm may develop spontaneously. If atrial fibrillation occurs, it is treated by continuing digitalis administration with quinidine in hopes of converting the patient to sinus rhythm. It is important to emphasize that quinidine should *not* be used unless the patient has been fully digitalized and the ventricular rate well controlled. Quinidine may increase the refractoriness of the atria, slow the flutter rate, and increase conductivity through the A-V junction, thereby *increasing* the ventricular rate. Under these circumstances, 1:1 atrial flutter can sometimes be precipitated.

Propranolol has become popular in recent years as an adjunct with, or a substitute for, digitalis to slow the ventricular rate in patients with atrial flutter. However, propranolol is a cardiac depressant and can aggravate heart failure, asthma, or chronic obstructive lung disease. If the ventricular rate cannot be well controlled even with high doses of digitalis, one may cautiously add propranolol to attempt more satisfactory rate control; however, its sole use is not recommended except when flutter occurs in patients with a pre-excitation syndrome (see Chapter 13).

Occasionally, atrial flutter is refractory to both pharmacologic interventions and cardioversion. Under these circumstances, rapid right atrial pacing has been proposed to convert the patient to atrial fibrillation or normal sinus rhythm. In this circumstance, a catheter is placed in the right atrium and pacing is performed at high rates to break up the re-entry movement or "entrap" the atria and establish sinus rhythm.

Following conversion to sinus rhythm, digitalis either alone or in combination with quinidine may be used prophylactically to attempt to prevent recurrences of the arrhythmia: the combination of propranolol and quinidine has been found effective, as has triple drug therapy in more refractory cases. There have been reports that atrial pacing on a permanent basis either with an atrial or A-V sequential pacemaker is effective in preventing further bouts of atrial flutter, but in the refractory patient this generally has to be combined with drug therapy.

PROGNOSIS

The prognosis of atrial flutter is that of the underlying heart disease and depends upon the response of the arrhythmia to treatment. It is critical to establish the underlying cause of the disease process (hyperthyroidism, pulmonary embolization, sick sinus node syndrome, drug intake, etc.), since this often yields to specific therapy. It is particularly important to establish the presence of underlying pre-excitation syndromes complicated by atrial flutter, since digitalis is probably contraindicated in this syndrome. When flutter is a complication, it should be treated with propranolol or cardioversion and prophylactically with a combination of quinidine and propranolol (see Chapter 25).

When atrial flutter occurs in patients with severe dysfunction, the prognosis is that of the basic pathologic condition plus the effect of the ventricular rate. However, the prognosis is often favorable in uncomplicated cases and in younger patients. In contrast to atrial fibrillation, and perhaps owing to a somewhat lesser degree of underlying atrial disease, normal sinus rhythm can usually be maintained by utilizing prophylactic digitalis, quinidine, or either of these agents in combination with propranolol.

REFERENCES

Bellet, S., and Kostis, J.: Study of the cardiac arrhythmias by the ultrasonic Doppler method. Circulation 38:721, 1968.
Finkelstein, D., Gold, H., and Bellet, S.: Atrial flutter with 1:1 conduction: Report of six cases. Amer. J. Med. 20:65, 1956.
Korst, D. R., and Wasserberger, R. H.: Atrial flut-

ter associated with complete A-V heart block. Amer. Heart J., *48*:383, 1954.

Leier, C. V., Meacham, J. A., and Schaal, S. F.: Prolonged atrial conduction. Circulation *57*:2, 1978.

Lown, B.: Cardioversion of arrhythmias, II. Mod. Conc. Cardiovasc. Dis. *33*:869, 1964.

Lucchesi, B. R., and Whitsitt, L. S.: The pharmacology of B-adrenergic blocking agents. Prog. Cardiovasc. Dis. *11*:410, 1969.

McMillan, T. M., and Bellet, S.: Auricular flutter: Some of its clinical manifestations and its treatment; based on a study of 65 cases. Amer. J. Med. Sci. *184*:33, 1932.

Rosenbleuth, A., and Garcia Ramos, J.: Estudios sobre el flutter y la fibrilacion. IV. La del musculo auricular aislado. Arch. Inst. Cardiol. Mex. *17*:441, 1947.

Rytand, D. A.: The circus movement (entrapped circuit wave) hypothesis and atrial flutter. Ann. Intern. Med. *65*:125, 1966.

Semerau, M.: Ueber Ruckbildung der Arrhythmia perpetua. Deutsch. Arch. Klin. Med. *126*:161, 1918.

Sussman, H. F., Duqne, D., and Lesser, M. E.: Atrial flutter with 1:1 conduction. Dis. Chest *49*:99, 1966.

Wellens, H. J. J., Janse, M. J., van Dam, R. T., and Durrer, D.: Epicardial excitation of the atria in a patient with atrial flutter. Brit. Heart J. *33*:233, 1971.

Zeft, H. J., Cobb, F. R., Waxman, M. B., Hunt, N. C., and Morris, J. J., Jr.: Right atrial stimulation in the treatment of atrial flutter. Ann. Intern. Med. *70*:447, 1969.

SUPPLEMENTAL READING

Davies, M. J., and Pomerance, A.: Pathology of atrial fibrillation in man. Br. Heart J. *34*:520, 1972.

Greenberg, M. A., Herman, L. S., and Cohen, M. V.: Mitral valve closure in atrial flutter. Circulation *59*:902, 1979.

Haft, J. I.: Treatment of arrhythmias by intracardiac electrical stimulation. Prog. Cardiovasc. Dis. *16*:539, 1974.

Plumb, V. J., MacLedn, W., Cooper, T. B., James, T. N., and Waldo, A. L.: Atrial events during entrainment and interruption of atrial flutter by rapid atrial pacing. Circulation *60*:II-65, 1979.

Scherf, D., and Schott, A.: Extrasystoles and Allied Arrhythmias. London, William Heinemann Medical Books, 1973, pp. 400–419.

Sims, B. A.: Pathogenesis of atrial arrhythmias. Br. Heart J. *34*:336, 1972.

Waldo, A. L., MacLean, W. A. H., Karp, R. B., Kouchoukos, N. T., and James, T. N.: Entrainment and interruption of atrial flutter with atrial pacing. Circulation *56*:5, 1977.

Watson, R., Kastor, J. A., and Josephson, M. E.: Electrophysiologic characteristics of atrial flutter induced by programmed stimulation. Circulation *60*:II-253, 1979.

8

ATRIAL FIBRILLATION

ROBERT I. KATZ, M.D.,
RICHARD H. HELFANT, M.D.

GENERAL CONSIDERATIONS

Atrial fibrillation is one of the most common arrhythmias, and is certainly the rhythm disturbance most frequently associated with organic heart disease and heart failure. It takes one of two forms — paroxysmal or established — and, while both are usually amenable to therapy, the conversion of established atrial fibrillation to normal sinus rhythm usually cannot be maintained on a long-term basis.

INCIDENCE

Of 50,000 consecutive patients, 4316 (8.6%) manifested the chronic variety of atrial fibrillation (Katz and Pick, 1956). It occurs most frequently after the age of 40 but is not uncommon in older children in the presence of rheumatic fever, hyperthyroidism, or certain types of congenital heart disease (i.e., Ebstein's anomaly and atrial septal defect, especially in its late stages).

ETIOLOGY AND PRECIPITATING FACTORS

Atrial fibrillation is almost always observed in the presence of cardiac disease, especially in its advanced forms.

It occurs in about 60 per cent of patients with heart failure. Rheumatic, coronary, and hypertensive heart disease constitute the most common etiologies encountered; less commonly, it is associated with pericardial disease, pre-excitation syndromes, certain types of congenital heart disease, mitral valve prolapse, sinus node disease, and hyperthyroidism. Idiopathic or "lone" atrial fibrillation, however, without evidence of underlying heart disease is not rare.

Patients with the predisposing underlying processes noted tend to develop transient intermittent atrial fibrillation initially which may later progress to the established variety. Established atrial fibrillation is said to be present when it has been present for months or years; whereas in the paroxysmal variety, attacks occur suddenly and last a few seconds, minutes, or days.

Circumstances that affect both sympathetic and parasympathetic tone apparently can lead to the initiation of atrial fibrillation. Precipitating factors include various stress mechanisms, such as nausea, vomiting, acute gastroenteritis, coughing, heavy ingestion of alcohol, hypoglycemia (spontaneous or post-insulin), severe pain or emotional upset, pulmonary embolization, and pancreatitis. Other, less commonly encountered, initiating factors include generalized infections, acute exacerbations of carditis, violent exertion, head or chest trauma, subarachnoid hemorrhage, surgical procedures (particularly open heart surgery), electrolyte disturbances, and sympathomimetic drugs.

PATHOLOGY AND PATHOPHYSIOLOGY

The pathology associated with atrial fibrillation is that of the associated disease state. Hearts of patients with atrial fibrillation often show myocardial changes secondary to hypertensive, coronary, or rheumatic heart disease. In the acute and subacute stages of rheumatic heart disease, the atria are dilated with inflammatory changes which later progress to fibrosis.

No consistent pathology in the S-A node or atria has been found that accounts for the arrhythmia. While Hudson (1960) reported a series of 14 cases of atrial fibrillation in which pathologic findings occurred in the S-A node, in most cases disease of the atrial muscle was also present. The degree of atrial pathology correlates well with the incidence of atrial fibrillation, and this is probably the essential factor in the development of the arrhythmia. In patients with mitral stenosis whose atria are essentially normal, atrial fibrillation occurs rarely. However, moderate to severe fibrosis with disruption of atrial architecture almost always results in fibrillation. The incidence of atrial fibrillation does not correlate as well with the degree of either mitral valvular damage or pulmonary hypertension.

Patients with prolonged atrial fibrillation usually are unable to sustain normal sinus rhythm following correction of the valvular lesions if cardioversion is attempted. This is probably related to the degree of underlying atrial and possibly sinus node pathology. Instead of a normal mechanism, cardioversion may result in chaotic atrial activity (characterized by changing P wave con-

tour), bradycardia, ectopic beats, or the development of atrial re-entrant tachycardia. This has been observed in 5 per cent of patients with atrial fibrillation of less than 1 year's duration and in 45 per cent of cases when the arrhythmia has been present for more than 10 years (Lown et al., 1967).

In patients with previous rheumatic involvement, Aschoff bodies are frequently present in the left atrial appendage, even in the absence of clinical evidence of active rheumatic disease. In the hearts of patients with atrial fibrillation associated with hypertensive or coronary heart disease, there is no definite histologic evidence of a focal change responsible for this arrhythmia, although distention of the atria (especially the left) is usually found. In some patients with atrial fibrillation following a myocardial infarction, occlusion of the sinus node artery causing infarction of the S-A node and atrial muscle has been demonstrated.

ELECTROPHYSIOLOGY

A variety of abnormal mechanisms of impulse formation are operative in atrial fibrillation. Alterations in the diastolic resting potential and markedly inhomogeneous conduction have been demonstrated in atrial tissue obtained at surgery from human subjects with atrial fibrillation. These electrophysiologic abnormalities cause atrial fibrillation by producing diffuse conduction abnormalities which give rise to multiple microre-entry circuits (Harran and Kistler, 1961).

HEMODYNAMICS

Atrial fibrillation is associated with marked hemodynamic alterations which contribute to the symptoms and signs observed as a consequence of this arrhythmia. These hemodynamic changes result from: 1) failure of the atria to contract, 2) the irregular ventricular rhythm, 3) the short cycle lengths associated with a rapid ventricular rate, and 4) the presence of associated valvular abnormalities.

In patients with mitral stenosis and atrial fibrillation, the Starling principle operates on a beat-to-beat basis, since the end diastolic segment length and diastolic pressure are directly related to the length of the cardiac cycle (Braunwald et al., 1960). The preceding cycle length and stroke volume are related not only by the cycle immediately preceding them, but in fact by several preceding cycles.

The increased ventricular rate associated with atrial fibrillation is particularly deleterious in mitral stenosis, because at high rates diastole is abbreviated, resulting in a subsequent decrease in ventricular filling, which has been already compromised both by the absence of atrial systole and by the valvular stenosis. This decrease in ventricular diastolic pressure lessens stroke volume (Starling principle). In addition, left atrial pressure *increases* precipitously under these circumstances, often resulting in pulmonary edema.

Patients with abnormal left ventricular compliance are also particularly susceptible to deleterious hemodynamic abnormalities associated with atrial fibrillation. Thus, patients with hypertension, valvular and subvalvular aortic stenosis, hypertrophic cardiomyopathies, or other diseases associated with left ventricular hypertrophy are particularly dependent on atrial systole ("the atrial kick") to increase ventricular wall tension (manifested by a large "A" wave in the left ventricular pressure tracing) immediately prior to contraction (via the Starling mechanism). The onset of atrial fibrillation in these patients can result in hypotension and/or heart failure with acute clinical deterioration.

The response to exercise, as measured by cardiac output and other parameters of cardiac function, is impaired during atrial fibrillation. This is due to an abnormal heart rate response to the physical effort, which exacerbates the other deleterious effects of atrial fibrillation. In such patients, the increase in the cardiac index with exercise is subnormal and is elicited solely by the increased cardiac rate, since the stroke index is relatively fixed.

Hemodynamic Changes after Conversion to Normal Sinus Rhythm. A great number of studies have been performed to assess the hemodynamic effects of conversion from atrial fibrillation to normal sinus rhythm. The results suggest that conversion leads to little immediate benefit, but when measured after a delay of hours or days, hemodynamics are usually improved. The sequence of improvement following conversion is: 1) at 3 minutes cardiac output is unchanged, but the heart rate is decreased slightly; 2) after three hours the increase in cardiac output is still not significant, but the decrease in heart rate and the increase in stroke volume are both significant; and 3) after three days the cardiac output increases (e.g., 5.1 to 6.5 liters; $p < 0.01$), as does the stroke volume (59 to 93 ml), and the heart rate decreases (88 to 70 beats per minute) (see Chapter 25).

The hemodynamic response to exercise is also improved following conversion. The following changes after conversion were found to be significant: 1) cardiac output increased 8 per cent; 2) stroke volume increased 30 per cent; 3) heart rate decreased 24 per cent; 4) arterial pressure decreased 8 per cent; 5) peripheral resistance decreased 16 per cent; 6) time-tension index increased 103 per cent (Benchimol et al., 1965). Clearly, the efficiency of circulatory adaptations to exercise is markedly improved following conversion to normal sinus rhythm.

The delay in return of atrial function has not been investigated in relation to the duration of the arrhythmia, the characteristics of the fibrillatory state, or the underlying cardiac pathology. Interestingly, no hemodynamic benefit was found in patients classified as "benign fibrillators" after conversion to normal sinus rhythm (Killip and Bear, 1964). This suggests that the underlying cardiac pathology is a vital factor in causing the clinical manifestations.

In summary, the benefit of restoration to normal sinus rhythm depends on a number of factors: 1) if the ventricular rate is lowered, cardiac output will increase; 2) patients with more severe heart disease will benefit more than those with mild impairment in whom the heart is well compensated; 3) the return of normal atrial function may not be fully realized immediately; and 4) the maximal benefits are more fully appreciated with exercise than at rest.

SYMPTOMS AND SIGNS

Relationship Between Ventricular Rate and Clinical Manifestations. The clinical manifestations of atrial fibrillation depend largely on two factors: 1) the ventricular rate and 2) the underlying cardiac status. In most untreated patients, the ventricular rate ranges from 100 to 200 beats per minute or more. Rates over 200 per minute, especially with aberrant conduction, should alert one to the possibility of an underlying pre-excitation syndrome (see Chapter 13) or less commonly hyperthyroidism. Higher rates in susceptible patients may precipitate severe heart failure or hypotension or both. The symptoms are more marked with a rapid rate in association with mitral stenosis or diseases characterized by left ventricular hypertrophy (see above).

Conversely, one may encounter untreated atrial fibrillation in which the ventricular rate (without digitalis) ranges from 40 to 80 beats per minute. These cases are usually observed in older patients and are associated with underlying abnormalities of A-V conduction.

Syncope or other neurological symp-toms occasionally occur. Under these circumstances, the "brady-tachy" syndrome or cerebral embolization (especially with mitral valve disease) must be considered.

Auscultatory Findings. Auscultation reveals the characteristic irregularly irregular ventricular rate. This is most pronounced when rates are below 130 per minute. At rapid rates, the ventricular contraction often fails to lift the aortic valve during a short cardiac cycle. As a result, only one heart sound is heard and the ventricular contraction is too weak to produce a pulse at the wrist. This results in a "pulse deficit" (the difference between the central cardiac rate and peripheral pulse rate). Variations in the intensity of the first heart sound and atrial sounds, although present, are usually of little practical value in the bedside diagnosis of atrial fibrillation.

Systolic murmurs that are audible during normal rhythm are usually preserved during fibrillation. They vary considerably in intensity, depending upon the length of the preceding cycle and the consequent variation in ventricular filling (being louder following the longer cycles and fainter after the shorter cycles). With rapid rates, the murmurs often become inaudible. With the onset of atrial fibrillation and the failure of the atria to contract, the presystolic murmur of mitral stenosis observed during sinus rhythm disappears and only the diastolic rumble is heard. Often left ventricular outflow murmurs can be differentiated from mitral regurgitation murmurs by a variation in intensity with each cycle. Left ventricular outflow murmurs tend to vary in intensity, while the murmur of mitral regurgitation is relatively constant.

ELECTROCARDIOGRAM

The electrocardiographic characteristics of atrial fibrillation are the coarse, rapid fibrillatory waves (in the absence

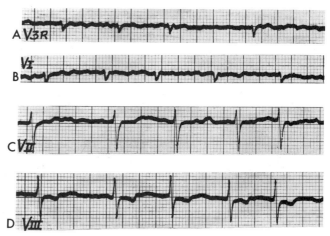

Figure 8–1 Atrial fibrillation showing more marked atrial oscillations in leads from the right side of the precordium. Note that the atrial oscillations are more clearly delineated in the leads V₃R and V₁ (taken from the right side of the precordium). They are less clearly shown in V₂ and V₃ and in leads taken from the left side of the precordium.

of P waves) and the irregularly irregular ventricular complexes. The ECG may thus be divided into a) atrial activity and b) ventricular deflections.

Atrial Activity. The atrial oscillations in the ECG during fibrillation vary from 400 to 700 per minute and thus are much more rapid than in flutter. These oscillations are totally irregular and vary in both size and shape. Although they may be visible in all limb leads, the atrial activity is most marked in leads II, III, and AVF as well as V_1 or locations on the right precordium (Fig. 8–1). In addition, by recording with the right arm electrode placed over the manubrium of the sternum and with the left arm electrode placed parasternally in the fifth intercostal space, various types of atrial oscilla-

tions can also be readily distinguished. Esophageal leads taken at the atrial level occasionally show oscillations which may at times resemble those of atrial flutter but which have rates that usually exceed those of flutter (Fig. 8–2).

The P-R interval is often prolonged prior to the onset and following termination of atrial fibrillation. The prolonged P-R interval probably increases susceptibility to the development of atrial fibrillation.

Ventricular Deflections. The ventricular complexes in atrial fibrillation are usually of normal contour (i.e., "supraventricular") and are irregularly irregular. However, when the ventricular rate is rapid (140 or more/min) various degrees of aberrant conduction of the

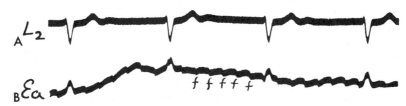

Figure 8–2 The value of esophageal leads in the diagnosis of the atrial mechanism.

(A) Lead II shows a regular ventricular rhythm with a rate of 40 per minute. The atrial mechanism is not clearly shown in this strip. The following possibilities were considered: mid A-V junctional rhythm with hidden P waves, atrial standstill, atrial fibrillation or atrial flutter with a complete A-V block.

(B) An esophageal lead taken simultaneously with A shows the characteristic oscillations of atrial fibrillation.

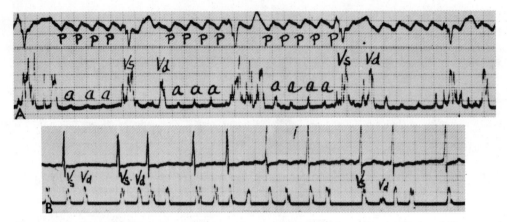

Figure 8–3   (*A*) Atrial flutter. Tracings from a 70-year-old male with arteriosclerotic heart disease and congestive failure. The distance between the thick time lines represents 0.2 second.
   (*B*) Atrial fibrillation. Tracings from patients with hypertensive and arteriosclerotic heart disease and congestive failure.

QRS complex may occur simulating bundle branch block. These aberrantly conducted beats are probably caused by the arrival of an impulse during the relative refractory period of one of the bundle branches, usually the right bundle branch, as a result of the high rate (see Chapter 2). In such cases, the intraventricular conduction often returns to normal following reduction of the ventricular rate (Figs. 8–4 and 8–5).

   The occurrence of conduction block at various levels in the A-V junction causes the irregularly irregular ventricular complexes. This phenomenon can best be explained on the basis of concealed conduction. Following a conducted impulse through the A-V node, the next beat reaches the N region of the node during its absolute refractory period and is blocked. Subsequent impulses are blocked upon reaching refractory tissue that is located progressively closer to the atria. When the N region has recovered its excitability after several impulses have been blocked, the next impulse (when none of the junctional tissue is refractory) can be propagated to the ventricles. In established atrial fibrillation, block occurs primarily between the A-N and N regions of the A-V node.

OTHER ARRHYTHMIAS ASSOCIATED WITH ATRIAL FIBRILLATION

   Atrial fibrillation is often associated with other arrhythmias. Partial A-V block is almost always present with atrial fibrillation (see concealed conduc-

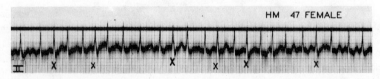

Figure 8–4   Atrial fibrillation with rapid ventricular response (rate 150 per minute). Note aberrant QRS complexes (at X) terminating the shortest cycles.

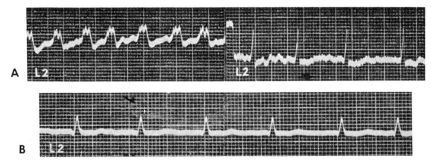

Figure 8–5 Widening of ventricular complexes in association with atrial fibrillation at a rapid ventricular rate. Lead II shows atrial fibrillation with widening of the QRS complexes, and a ventricular rate of 160 per minute. In the second part of *A*, after digitalization, when the ventricular rate had dropped to 80 per minute, the width of the QRS complexes has returned to normal.

(*B*) Atrial fibrillation with an almost regular ventricular rhythm. (From Bellet, S., and McMillan, T. M.: *In* Stroud, W. D., and Stroud, M. W. (eds.): Cardiovascular Diseases. Philadelphia, F. A. Davis Co., 1959.)

tion above), although the degree of block usually varies (Fig. 8–6). However, *complete A-V block* is also occasionally encountered (Fig. 8–6). It may occur as a result of sclerodegenerative changes in the A-V junction and is most often observed in older patients. In this situation, the ventricular rate is slow (40 to 50) and completely *regular*. Most cases of untreated atrial fibrillation with a slow irregular ventricular rate are also due to a high grade of A-V block (Fig. 8–7).

A-V *junctional rhythm* may be present in association with or complicating atrial fibrillation. It is vital to recognize junctional rhythms or high grade A-V block, since they frequently indicate the presence of digitalis toxicity. In A-V junctional rhythms, the ventricles are no longer excited by the irregularly fibrillating atria but are controlled by a pacemaker in the A-V junction per se. Therefore, the R-R intervals are of equal duration (i.e., the QRS complexes are totally regular). The ventricular rate

Figure 8–6 Atrial fibrillation with varying degress of A-V block.

(*A*) Atrial fibrillation with rapid ventricular rate, 160 per minute.

(*B*) Atrial fibrillation with ventricular rate (about 84 per minute), contrôlled by digitalis.

(*C*) Atrial fibrillation with probable complete A-V block. Note the regular ventricular rate, 38 per minute.

(*D*) Atrial fibrillation with a slow ventricular rate and coupled ventricular premature beats due to digitalis toxicity.

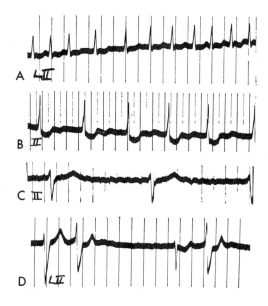

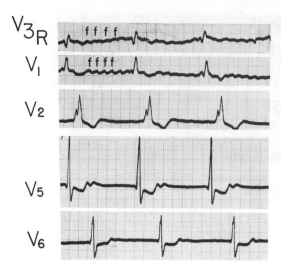

Figure 8–7 Atrial fibrillation with complete AV block. Note the presence of a regular rhythm, rate 40 per minute. The ventricular rate was not altered by moderate exercise or atropine.

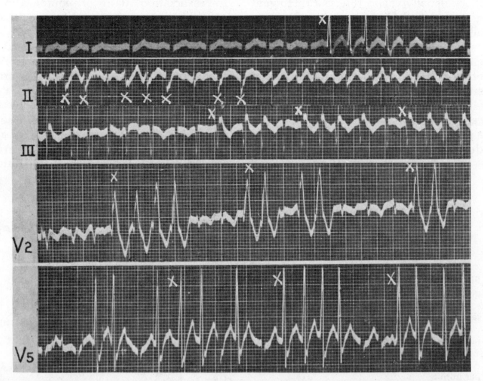

Figure 8–8 Atrial fibrillation accompanied by aberration of the QRS complexes due to delay in the right bundle branch system. These complexes often simulate ventricular beats and ventricular tachycardia. Note the aberration of the ventricular complexes starting at X in lead I. The first beat of the aberrant series is usually following a short pause. The complexes measure 0.10 of a second in width and simulate those of right bundle branch block. Similar episodes are observed at X in leads II, III, V_2 and V_5 (QRS width 0.12 second). Note that the QRS complexes throughout conform to the pattern observed in right bundle branch block.

varies from 40 to 120, but is regular (see Chapter 9 for a description of junctional rhythms).

Ventricular premature complexes are commonly associated with atrial fibrillation. They can occur occasionally or frequently, and are at times coupled or in salvos of three or more. Many of these complexes have a right bundle branch block configuration, suggesting aberrantly conducted beats (Fig. 8–8). *Aberrant conduction* must be differentiated from ventricular premature complexes, since the former are not due to digitalis excess although the latter frequently are, particularly if they occur in a bigeminal or trigeminal pattern (see Chapter 11 for differentiation of aberrant conduction and ventricular premature complexes).

TREATMENT

In addition to the treatment of atrial fibrillation per se, attention must also be directed toward accurately identifying the etiologic and associated precipitating factors predisposing to the previously mentioned arrhythmia. The principles of treating the arrhythmia are sequential, consisting of 1) controlling the ventricular rate (which is best accomplished by the administration of digitalis); 2) treatment of associated congestive heart failure, which is often present; 3) consideration of cardioversion (using quinidine and/or electrical countershock); 4) in cases of paroxysmal atrial fibrillation, prevention of recurrences; and 5) prevention of possible thromboemboli.

Drug Therapy
Digitalis. Digitalis is the drug of choice in treating atrial fibrillation. The primary benefit of digitalis derives from its ability to decrease A-V conduction, thus reducing the ventricular rate. This is accomplished by both a direct and a vagal effect on the A-V junction. The goal of digitalis administration is to decrease the apical rate to about 70

beats per min, with elimination of the pulse deficit. In addition, the ventricular rate should not increase disproportionately with exercise. Digitalis is also helpful in decreasing heart failure by virtue of its positive inotropic effect.

Digitalization should be performed rapidly in patients with severe heart failure, hypotension, or a rapid ventricular rate. It may be accomplished more gradually in those patients in whom the clinical response to the arrhythmia is less severe. Thus each patient must be individualized when determining the dose of digitalis as well as the type and route of digitalis preparation. While any digitalis preparation may be utilized, most clinicians currently prefer digoxin orally or intravenously. It is important to become familiar with at least one type of digitalis preparation for oral and one for intravenous use. The dose of digitalis required to achieve optimal rate control varies widely depending on the etiology of the heart disease, the status of A-V conduction, and the autonomic nervous system. The ventricular rate response is the most important guide to the adequacy of the digitalis therapy. The serum digoxin level is of relatively little value in this regard (Goldman et al., 1975).

The approximate oral digitalizing dose required for a 150 lb person is approximately 2 to 5 mg of digoxin. This dose may be given over a period of days when slow digitalization is desired. When the patient presents a picture of severe congestive heart failure and/or hypotension necessitating rapid digitalization and certainty of absorption, the parenteral route is indicated. Digoxin, 0.5 to 1.0 mg, may be given intravenously followed in 2 to 3 hours by an additional 0.25 to 0.5 mg. This dose may then be repeated every 4 to 6 hours as necessary until adequate ventricular rate control is achieved.

The digitalis preparation, lanatoside C (total digitalizing dose 1.6 mg) intravenously for rapid digitalization has also been used frequently. This should be given in three or four divided doses several hours apart, carefully noting the effects of the preceding dose on rate (preferably with a rhythm strip) before giving an additional dose. Less commonly, ouabain has been utilized, a digitalis preparation with a very rapid onset (even more rapid than lanatoside C). The usual digitalizing dose of ouabain is 0.8 mg given in three or four divided doses over a period of several hours. This very rapidly acting preparation requires experience for clinical use.

Occasionally, digitalis, even in high doses, fails to control the ventricular rate in some patients. Fortunately, such cases are relatively uncommon but when they occur the presence of one or more of the following should be suspected: a) pulmonary embolization, b) cor pulmonale of severe grade, c) toxic factors, d) hyperthyroidism, or e) anemia. In such cases, propranolol administration may be very useful (see below). Conversely, digitalis is usually contraindicated in patients with atrial fibrillation and slow ventricular rates (i.e., below 60 beats/min before therapy), since in such cases further slowing of the ventricular rate may be harmful.

Propranolol. Beta blocking agents such as propranolol have proved efficacious in controlling the ventricular rate when digitalis alone has failed to do so. They are particularly useful when hyperthyroidism or *pre-excitation* is the cause of the arrhythmia. However, in most circumstances, propranolol should be given with care and in small doses to avoid its negative inotropic effect which may either induce or aggravate heart failure.

When atrial fibrillation occurs in patients with a pre-excitation syndrome the ventricular rate is very rapid, and aberrant ventricular conduction is usually present. Digitalis has generally been felt not to be efficacious in this situation, since it tends to decrease normal atrioventricular conduction and therefore rapid conduction over the aberrant pathway may be facilitated (see Chapter 13). Under these circumstances, propranolol is usually the treatment of choice.

Digitalis Toxicity in Atrial Fibrillation. In view of the frequency and chronicity of digitalis therapy in patients with atrial fibrillation, its toxic manifestation complicating this arrhythmia requires particular emphasis. In a digitalized patient, when the ventricular rate becomes completely and persistently *regular* in the presence of atrial fibrillation, the following possibilities should be considered: 1) with rapid rates (80–160), *paroxysmal* or *nonparoxysmal junctional tachycardia;* 2) with slower rates (40–80 beats/min), *A-V junctional rhythm;* and 3) with very slow rates (30–40 beats/min), *complete A-V block* with a pacemaker located in the lower portion of the A-V junction or His-Purkinje system. In this context, digitalis toxicity must always be assumed until proven otherwise.

In addition, the new occurrence of *ventricular premature complexes* especially in bigeminal or trigeminal pattern strongly suggests digitalis excess. This may lead to *ventricular tachycardia* if unrecognized. Other, less common but more potentially ominous, arrhythmias caused by digitalis excess include *paroxysmal atrial tachycardia with A-V block* and *bidirectional tachycardia*.

Indications for Conversion to Normal Sinus Rhythm. There are few current indications for attempting to convert established atrial fibrillation to normal sinus rhythm. It is now clearly established that in the large majority of patients with established atrial fibrillation, conversion to normal sinus rhythm is relatively transient. However, in some patients with recent onset of atrial fibrillation in whom the degree of cardiac damage, cardiac enlargement (particularly of the left atrium), and congestive heart failure is slight, it may be considered. Patients with left ventricular hypertrophy or other abnormalities who tolerate atrial fibrillation particularly poorly even after good control of the ventricular rate would be potential candidates.

Direct current cardioversion has been found to be effective in converting atrial fibrillation to normal sinus rhythm in as many as 90 per cent of patients (Aberg and Cullhed, 1968). This method, as compared to reversion by quinidine, has the advantage of a lower incidence of side effects and a briefer period of hospitalization and is therefore the treatment of choice. The indications, technique, and complications of countershock in the treatment of arrhythmias are discussed in Chapter 25. Unfortunately, the long-term efficacy of direct current cardioversion in maintaining sinus rhythm for 12 months has only been 30 per cent (25% for 24 months). The maintenance of patients in normal sinus rhythm is particularly difficult in those with severe heart disease, particularly associated with mitral valve disease.

The chief complications from the use of direct countershock to convert atrial fibrillation to normal sinus rhythm include: a) the development of ventricular arrhythmias which may be severe at times (more likely if the patient is fully digitalized at the time of conversion); b) the occurrence of occasional instances of cardiac arrest, especially in patients with a history of syncope in whom the "brady-tachy" syndrome may be present; and c) precipitation of thromboemboli (particularly in the presence of mitral valve disease).

Quinidine has also been used either in conjunction with electrical cardioversion or alone in the conversion of atrial fibrillation to normal sinus rhythm. It is successful alone in approximately 60 per cent of patients, although it may vary from 88 per cent (Philips and Levine, 1949) to 58 per cent (Sandoe et al., 1965) depending upon the observer. However, several difficulties are encountered: hospitalization is required; there is a risk of quinidine toxicity (see Chapter 23); and conversion is not real-ized in a large number of patients. As previously noted, quinidine conversion has been indicated less commonly since the advent of countershock, but it still may be of use to convert some patients.

Certainly, quinidine remains the drug of choice for maintenance of normal sinus rhythm after conversion from atrial fibrillation. Following restoration of normal sinus rhythm, maintenance quinidine 0.2 to 0.4 grams four times a day (or a longer acting preparation) is given for several months and continued, depending upon the tendency for recurrence of atrial fibrillation. Most of the patients who revert to normal sinus rhythm have recurrences of atrial fibrillation as a result of many factors including the duration of the arrhythmia prior to therapy, the degree of myocardial damage (Daley et al., 1968) dilatation of the heart beyond the volume of 1000 ml, and especially the presence of mitral regurgitation. The maintenance of adequate plasma levels of quinidine over long periods of time may prove difficult. The use of propranolol in addition to the quinidine has been efficacious in maintaining normal sinus rhythm for a more prolonged period in some instances (Stern, 1971).

Treatment of Paroxysmal Atrial Fibrillation. The treatment of paroxysmal atrial fibrillation is a matter of some controversy. In our experience, digitalis is the drug of choice. Its administration will usually have a salutory effect, particularly in patients with pre-existing heart damage, in those in the older age group, and in the presence of congestive heart failure. It will slow the ventricular rate in paroxysmal atrial fibrillation as effectively as in the established form, and spontaneous reversion to normal sinus rhythm often follows. If this does not occur, other methods of conversion (quinidine and electric countershock) may then be employed.

Anticoagulation and Atrial Fibrillation. In patients with atrial fibrillation there is a definite risk of developing left atrial thrombosis and systemic embolization. This is a particular hazard in patients with atrial fibrillation *and* rheumatic mitral valvular disease. In view of its relative frequency in this situation, long-term anticoagulation therapy is indicated.

PROGNOSIS

The prognosis of patients with atrial fibrillation depends upon the age of the patient, the underlying cardiac condition, the extent of cardiac enlargement or heart failure, and the ease with which the ventricular rate and heart failure are controlled. In general, persistent atrial fibrillation indicates the presence of a rather serious deterioration in the underlying cardiac disease process to which the arrhythmia further contributes. However, with therapy, many patients with atrial fibrillation maintain only moderate decreases in their functional state. Those who exhibit more severe heart failure have a poor prognosis. The outlook is often poor in cases in which there is difficulty in maintaining good ventricular rate control. The sudden appearance of systemic emboli as a complication of the arrhythmia is a serious and at times fatal complication.

The prognosis of atrial fibrillation has been markedly improved in recent years by many advances in therapy, mainly as a result of better treatment of heart failure with high potency diuretics and vasodilators (particularly in mitral regurgitation) and heart surgery. Thus, properly treated atrial fibrillation may reduce life expectancy only moderately in patients without severe diffuse myocardial disease.

REFERENCES

Aberg, H.: Some aspects on atrial fibrillation. Etiology, treatment, complications, and fibrillatory waves using a new technique. Abst. Uppsala Dissertations in Medicine, 63, 1969.

Aberg, H., and Cullhed, I.: Direct current conversion of atrial fibrillation. Longterm results. Acta Med. Scand. *184*:433, 1968.

Arani, D. T., and Carleton, R. A.: The deleterious role of tachycardia in mitral stenosis. Circulation *36*:511, 1967.

Bailey, G. W. H., Braniff, B. A., Hancock, E. W., and Cohn, K. E.: Relation of left atrial pathology to atrial fibrillation in mitral valvular disease. Ann. Intern. Med. *69*:13, 1968.

Bellet, S., Eliamkim, M., and Deliyiannis, S.: The electrocardiogram during electro-convulsive therapy as studied by radio-electro-cardiography. Amer. J. Cardiol. *25*:686, 1962.

Benchimol, A., Lowe, H. M., and Akre, P. R.: Cardiovascular response to exercise during atrial fibrillation and after conversion to sinus rhythm. Amer. J. Cardiol. *16*:31, 1965.

Bjerkelund, C., and Orning, O. M.: The efficacy of anticoagulant therapy in preventing embolism related to DC electrical reversion of atrial fibrillation. Amer. J. Cardiol. *23*:208, 1969.

Braunwald, E., Frye, R. L., Aygen, M. M., and Gilbert, J. W., Jr.: Studies on Starling's Law of the heart. III. Observations in patients with mitral stenosis and atrial fibrillation on the relationships between left ventricular end-diastolic segment length, filling pressure and the characteristics of ventricular contraction. J. Clin. Invest. *39*:1874, 1960.

Cohen, S. I., Lau, S. H., Berkowitz, W. D., and Damato, A. N.: Concealed conduction during atrial fibrillation. Amer. J. Cardiol. *25*:416, 1970.

Corliss, R. J., McKenna, D. H., Crumpton, C. W., and Rowe, G. G.: Hemodynamic effects after conversion of arrhythmias. J. Clin. Invest. *47*:1774, 1978.

Friedberg, H. D.: Atrial fibrillation and digitalis toxicity. Amer. Heart J. *77*:429, 1969.

Horan, L. G., and Kistler, J. C.: Study of ventricular response in atrial fibrillation. Circ. Res. *9*:305, 1961.

Hornstein, T. R., and Bruce, R. A.: Effects of atrial fibrillation on exercise performance in patients with cardiac disease. Circulation *37*:543, 1968.

Hudson, R.: The human pacemaker and its pathology. Brit. Med. J. *22*:153, 1960.

Kastor, J. A., and Yurchas, P. M.: Recognition of digitalis intoxication in the presence of atrial fibrillation. Ann. Intern. Med. *67*:1045, 1967.

Katz, L. N., and Pick, A.: Clinical Electrocardiography. Part I. The Arrhythmias. Philadelphia, Lea & Febiger, 1956.

Killip, T., and Baer, R. A.: Cardiac function before and after electrical reversion from atrial fibrillation to sinus rhythm. Clin. Res. *12*:175, 1964.

Killip, T., and Gault, J. H.: Mode of onset of atrial fibrillation. Amer. Heart J. *70*:172, 1965.

Lau, S. H., Damato, A. N., Berkowitz, W. D., and Patton, R. D.: A study of atrioventricular conduction in atrial fibrillation and flutter in man using His bundle recordings. Circulation 40:71, 1969.

Lown, B., Vassaux, C., Hood, W. B., Jr., Fakhro, A. M., Kaplinsky E., and Roberge, G.: Unresolved problems in coronary care. Amer. J. Cardiol. 20:494, 1967.

Neporent, L. M., and da Silva, J. A.: Heart sounds in atrial flutter-fibrillation. Amer. J. Cardiol. 19:301, 1967.

Phillips, E., and Levine, S. A.: Auricular fibrillation without other evidence of heart disease. Amer. J. Med. 7:478, 1949.

Radford, M. D., and Evans, D. W.: Long-term results of DC reversion of atrial flutter. Brit. Heart J. 30:91, 1968.

Sandøe, E., Hansen, P. F., Aufred, E., and Oleson, K. H.: Defibrilling av Kronisk Atrieflimren. Resultater og Komplikationer. Ugeskr. Laeg. 127:346, 1965.

Shapiro, W., and Klein, G.: Alterations in cardiac function immediately following electrical conversion of atrial fibrillation to normal sinus rhythm. Circulation 38:1074, 1968.

Singer, D. H., Harris, P. D., Malin, J. R., and Hoffman, B. F.: Electrophysiological basis of chronic atrial fibrillation. Circulation 35–36:II–239, 1967.

Stern, S.: Treatment and prevention of cardiac arrhythmias with propranolol and quinidine. Brit. Heart J. 33:522, 1971.

SUPPLEMENTAL READING

Cotoi, S., Georgeseu, C., Kifor, I.: Analysis of human atrial fibrillatory waves using monophasic action potential technique. Am. Heart. J. 98:465, 1979.

Goldman, S., Probat, P., and Seltzer, A.: Inefficiency of "therapeutic" serum levels of digoxin in controlling the ventricular rate in atrial fibrillation. Amer. J. Cardiol. 35:651, 1975.

Greenberg, B., Chatterjee, K., Parmley, W. W., Werner, J. A., Holly, A. N.: The influence of left ventricular filling pressure on atrial contribution to cardiac output. Am. Heart. J. 98:742, 1979.

Morganroth, J., Horowitz, L. N., Josephson, M. E., Kastor, J.: Relationship of atrial fibrillatory wave amplitude to left atrial size and etiology of heart disease. An old generalization re-examined. Am. Heart. J. 97:184, 1979.

Soslinark, T., Jonson, B., and Olsson, A.: Effect of quinidine in maintaining sinus rhythm after conversion of atrial fibrillation or flutter. Brit. Heart J. 37:486, 1975.

9

JUNCTIONAL RHYTHMS

ROBERT I. KATZ, M.D.,
RICHARD H. HELFANT, M.D.

A-V JUNCTIONAL RHYTHM

General Considerations. The major part of the A-V junction is located in the lower portion of the interatrial septum near the fibrous skeleton of the heart, anterior to the ostium of the coronary sinus. The distal portion of the A-V junction includes that portion of the bundle of His proximal to its bifurcation, which extends through the membranous interventricular septum. The term "A-V node" was originally applied by Tawara (1906) to the initial portion of this system; however, the physiology of the A-V junction has recently been reinvestigated. These recent studies have indicated that some of the older concepts are no longer valid; nevertheless, the traditional interpretations can still, in a general way, be utilized clinically.

Until recently, it was held that the "A-V node" possessed a high degree of automaticity and, hence, was considered to be a pacemaker site. Many anatomic and physiologic investigations have modified this view (see Chapters 1 and 2 for a detailed review of this work). Present concepts may be briefly summarized as follows: the traditional "A-V node" of the light microscopist (as most commonly described) corresponds to the N-H region of the electrophysiologist; the "functional A-V

node" of other anatomists, e.g., Truex and Smythe (1964), also includes the electrophysiologic A-N and N regions; the "A-V junction" includes the three regions of the A-V node, in addition to specialized prenodal atrial tissue and bundle of His (DeFelice and Challice, 1969). Automatic fibers have been observed in the A-N and N-H regions, in the coronary sinus region, situated just proximal to the A-V junction, and in the His-Purkinje system (DeFelice and Challice, 1969). If the traditional "A-V node" lacks automaticity, then the A-V rhythms may be explained as originating either somewhat lower down in the nodal-His junction or a little higher up in the coronary sinus area, rather than in the A-V node proper. The possibility that some of the nodal beats may have an origin in the left atrium or in the coronary sinus area has also been considered (DeFelice and Challice, 1969), but this has not been definitely established. Conversely, there is good evidence for His bundle originated rhythms.

Normally the A-V junction serves as a bridge for the transmission of impulses from the atria to the ventricles. This structure may be the site of impulse formation in the following circumstances: (1) when the sinus pacemaker fails; (2) when the automaticity of the S-A node falls below that of the A-V junction; (3) when the rate of impulse formation in the A-V junction is so enhanced that its rate exceeds that of the sinus node; and (4) when conduction fails in the N region due to Wenckebach-type second degree A-V heart block or in certain types of complete A-V heart block.

When, under these conditions, the A-V junction assumes the pacemaker function, an A-V junctional rhythm results, with its various manifestations and modifications. Failure or depression of the S-A node results in unmasking of the natural rate of the A-V junction (approximately 35 to 60 beats per minute); this is termed the *slow* or *passive* type of A-V junctional rhythm. Under certain conditions, the automaticity of the A-V junctional cells may be much greater, producing an A-V junctional tachycardia. Both forms of A-V junctional rhythm are almost always temporary disturbances; in only a few instances have these disturbances approached permanency.

An impulse originating in the A-V junction is usually conducted in both directions: in a forward (antegrade) direction, thus activating the ventricles, and in a retrograde direction, activating the atria. The impulse, however, may be blocked in either one or both directions (Pick and Langendorf, 1968).

The terms "upper," "middle," and "lower" nodal (junctional) rhythms have been used for years. However, one should recognize that these terms represent only rough approximations and, indeed, this classification is without anatomic foundation and may not be applicable under many circumstances (Waldo et al., 1968), particularly in a situation of antegrade or retrograde block.

Scherlag et al., (1973) have pointed out that there are two types of junctional rhythms: (1) true A-V nodal rhythms, which have a rate of 45–60/minute and increase with atropine by 30 to 40 beats; and (2) His bundle rhythms, which have a rate of 30–40/minute and do not increase significantly with atropine.

Incidence and Etiology. A-V junctional rhythm is rare in children; it is noted most frequently in the middle and later decades of life. In a hospital population, 1 per cent (502 of 50,000) manifested A-V junctional rhythm (Katz and Pick, 1956).

Passive A-V junctional rhythms are disorders which usually occur secondary to disturbances of function in the S-A node, to parasympathetic effects, or to the effects of certain drugs such as digitalis. Often, this state is associated with incomplete A-V dissociation. The precipitating factors include: (1) vagal stimulation of various types (e.g., during the phases of respiration or following electric countershock), which may depress S-A nodal functions; (2) injury to the S-A node by toxic or infectious processes, myocarditis (especially rheumatic), and degenerative states; (3) digitalis intoxication; (4) the effect of certain drugs (e.g., potassium, quinidine); (5) atropine during the initial state of its effect; and (6) episodes of sinus bradycardia accompanying acute myocardial infarction; under these circumstances, 7 to 10 per cent of patients manifest A-V junctional rhythm.

Pathology. Relatively few cases present characteristic pathologic findings: the pathology observed is that of the conditions described under etiology. In the persistent type of A-V junctional rhythm, the sinus node may be extensively damaged or entirely destroyed by the disease process. Destruction of the sinus node has been demonstrated by careful pathologic study in several series of patients with chronic atrial fibrillation in whom normal sinus rhythm could not be restored because of damage to this structure. Episodes of A-V junctional rhythm frequently result following countershock in these patients.

Symptoms and Signs. No symptoms or signs are produced by the common type of A-V junctional rhythm it-

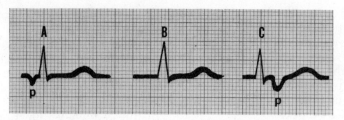

Figure 9–1 Diagrammatic representation of various manifestations of A-V junctional rhythm.
(A) Inverted P wave and the P-R interval measuring 0.12 second.
(B) No P wave is discernible; The P wave is probably hidden in QRS.
(C) The inverted P wave follows the QRS.

self unless it is associated with an extremely slow or rapid heart rate or unless it occurs in subjects with underlying disturbances in circulatory function. Only slight hemodynamic impairment is produced in otherwise healthy individuals by the disruption of the relationship between atrial and ventricular systole in A-V junctional rhythms.

Electrocardiogram. There is one common feature in A-V junctional rhythm: the P waves, if present, often differ in shape from P waves originating in the sinus node. This occurs be-

cause an impulse arising in the A-V junction follows a course through the atria roughly opposite to that of a sinus impulse. The P waves are often inverted in human A-V junctional rhythms, including those instances when the pacemaker is situated in the coronary sinus or bundle of His. However, some instances of A-V junctional rhythms may produce positive P waves. These may include "isorhythmic" A-V dissociation and junctional rhythms in patients with altered cardiac position or derangement of the atrial conduction pathways.

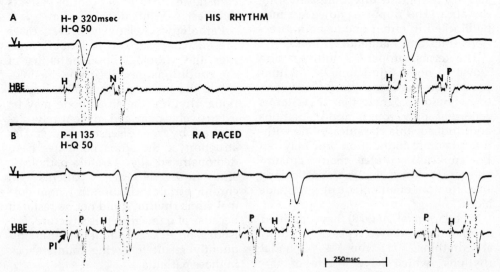

Figure 9–2 A-V junctional rhythm. His bundle recordings. (*Panel A*) His rhythm with retrograde conduction to the atria. Each QRS complex is preceded by a single His deflection (H). (*Panel B*) Antegrade conduction during right atrial pacing. H-V time same as in panel A. (From Damato, A. N., and Lau, S. H.: Circulation, *40*:527, 1969.)

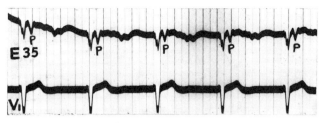

Figure 9–3 A-V junctional rhythm. V_1 taken simultaneously with esophageal lead at atrial level. Note presence of inverted P waves in esophageal lead which follow the QRS complex. This indicates a junctional origin. These P waves are not discernible in V_1.

An A-V rhythm with no visible P wave may occur in the following instances: (a) if the P wave is buried in the QRS or, rarely, in the T wave (Figs. 9–3, 9–4); (b) in the presence of atrial fibrillation; (c) in failure of retrograde conduction to the atrium; or (d) in atrial standstill. This pattern of A-V rhythm may be simulated by sinoventricular rhythm during hyperpotassemia and quinidine intoxication. The diagnosis may be established by careful

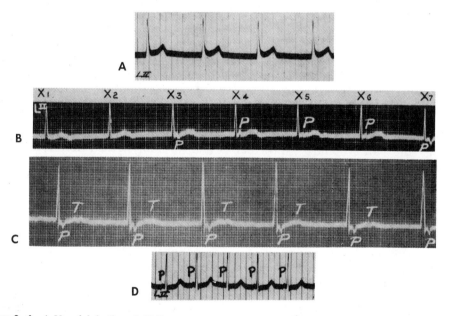

Figure 9–4 A-V nodal rhythm, A-V dissociation, and nonparoxysmal tachycardia.

(*A*) A-V nodal rhythm. No P waves are observed; they either are buried in the QRS complexes or may be absent (atrial standstill).

(*B*) Incomplete and partial A-V dissociation in the presence of sinus bradycardia and nodal rhythm. Regular sequence of ventricular complexes at a rate of 50 per minute. Small positive P waves are buried in the QRS at X_1 (downstroke) and X_2 (upstroke), or follow the QRS complex with practically the same R-P interval but changing amplitude of P at X_4, X_5, and X_6. Negative P waves follow the QRS complex at X_3 and X_7; the latter is deeper than the former. Atrial fusion of sinus and retrograde activation occurred at X_3, X_5, and X_6. P wave at X_4 may be totally of sinus origin, and, at X_7, is probably of nodal origin without fusion.

(*C*) Nodal rhythm. The ventricular rate and atrial rate are both regular at 50 per minute. Note that the P wave follows the QRS at a regular R-P interval of about 0.12 second.

(*D*) Nonparoxysmal tachycardia (rate 115 per minute). The P waves precede the QRS complexes, are diphasic, and the P-R interval is very short (0.08 second).

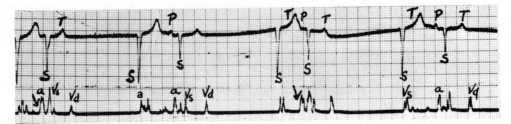

Figure 9–5 A-V nodal escape beats. Tracing from a 43-year-old woman with rheumatic heart disease, mitral insufficiency, and digitalis toxicity. Interval between thick time lines is 0.2 second. Note the relationship of the components of the Doppler tracing to the deflections of the electrocardiogram. The arrow points at a sequence where the P wave is hidden in the T, but the "a" wave is easily recognized in the Doppler tracing.

inspection of a long tracing, since A-V junctional rhythm is generally unstable, and may go in and out of periods of A-V dissociation. In those tracings in which the P waves are continuously buried in the QRS complexes, the atrial mechanism may be difficult to establish.

However, the following procedures may be helpful to demonstrate P waves and the atrial mechanism: (1) Atropine may be administered or the patient exercised; both of these procedures tend to decrease vagal tone, often affecting the two pacemakers unequally and separating the atrial and ventricular rhythms by producing a transient A-V dissociation or a return to normal sinus rhythm. (2) Tracings from a right intra-atrial lead will establish the diagnosis.

Also, transition from sinus to A-V junctional rhythm and back again to sinus rhythm is not infrequent. It may be noted by a gradual change in the P-R interval or the shape of the P wave. This shift in the origin of the impulse may be observed with the "wandering pacemaker" and transient periods of A-V dissociation (Fig. 9–4).

QRS in A-V Junctional Rhythm. Irrespective of the P wave pattern or morphology, the QRS complexes are usually supraventricular in form. They are of normal width and shape, although occasionally one may observe aberration.

Diagnosis. Although an A-V junctional rhythm may be suspected when

the apical rate ranges from 40 to 50 beats per minute, the diagnosis is made only by the electrocardiogram. When the P wave is situated before the QRS complex, the P-R interval is usually short, less than 0.12 second. With a slow (or "passive") A-V junctional rhythm (35 to 60 beats per minute), this can be recognized unmistakably. If the P wave follows the QRS complex, the R-P interval may measure 0.16 to 0.20 second with normal conduction (Scherf and Cohen, 1966). Conduction disturbances may, of course, alter all of these relationships. Inversion of the P wave and variation in the P-R interval should take into consideration variation in antegrade and retrograde conduction times.

The conditions to be differentiated are atrial fibrillation with an almost regular slow ventricular response (A-V junctional rhythm), A-V dissociation, atrial standstill, sinoventricular conduction, and idioventricular rhythm.

Treatment. There is no specific treatment for this condition; therapy should be directed toward the underlying clinical state.

Prognosis. The prognosis in A-V junctional rhythm depends on the underlying clinical state. Persistent A-V junctional rhythm is usually a sign of widespread myocardial damage; however, it may occasionally be the result of a small isolated lesion. The occurrence in the postinfarction period of A-V junctional rhythm (not tachycardia) by itself is not usually associated with a poor prognosis.

CORONARY SINUS AND LEFT ATRIAL RHYTHMS

The terms "coronary" and "left atrial" rhythm should probably no longer be used. This diagnosis, previously based on the P wave vector pattern and P-R interval, has been shown to be inaccurate. Coronary sinus rhythm is a subdivision of A-V junctional rhythm, since the pacemaker arises in the A-V junction or junction–atrial interface. Thus the term can be discarded as an independent rhythm, although it has been used in the past (Waldo, 1967) when the following electrocardiographic criteria were present: (1) P-R interval range from 0.10 to 0.17 second; (2) P wave of low voltage or indiscernible in lead I; (3) the P wave negative in leads II and III; and (4) deviation of the electrical axis of the P wave to the left (Fig. 9–6). This pattern, however, has been produced with pacing from the posterior portion of the left atrium as well as the inferolateral portion of the right atrium.

The diagnosis of left atrial rhythm depends on one or both of the following features: (1) inverted P waves in V_6 with upright, isoelectric, or inverted P waves in lead I; and (2) negative P waves in leads I and V_6 with "dome-and-dart" waves in V_1. These findings are commonly associated with atrial flutter. On the basis of vector analysis, it has been pointed out that the P wave

inversion in V_6 is the most sensitive specific sign of this arrhythmia. However, these P wave vectors have been reproduced by electrical stimulation of several other portions of the right atrium (including the low right atrium), and the term is thus best discarded.

Since the origin cannot be definitely placed in the left atrium, a general term such as "ectopic rhythm" might be used to refer to this rhythm.

A-V JUNCTIONAL TACHYCARDIA

When a sustained junctional rhythm ranges in rate between 60 and 110 beats per minute (the inherent rate, which is unmasked during bradycardia, is 35 to 60 beats per minute), it may be due to what is called *"nonparoxysmal junctional tachycardia" or "accelerated nodal rhythm." This form must be distinguished from "paroxysmal junctional tachycardia,"* which usually has a faster rate (between 140 and 260 beats per minute). The etiologic factors and treatment of paroxysmal A-V junctional tachycardia are similar to those of paroxysmal atrial tachycardia (see Chapter 6).

Paroxysmal Form

Electrocardiogram. The QRS complexes and position of the P waves are similar to those of premature beats of similar origin (Fig. 9–6). Four electrocardiographic patterns of A-V junctional tachycardia, with features similar to the corresponding junctional rhythm, may be recognized. These are (1) P wave preceding the ventricular complex (old classification: "upper nodal");

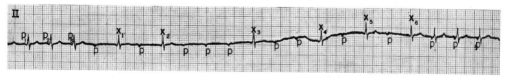

Figure 9–6 Nonparoxysmal junctional tachycardia with varying degrees of A-V heart block. Shows a junctional tachycardia, rate 117 per minute; this is maintained during periods of ventricular standstill. Note the inverted P waves and the short P-R interval at P_2 and P_3. During the ventricular pauses, note the continuance of the inverted atrial beats, which maintain the retrograde conduction and the same heart rate. Note the resumption of the 1:1 response after X_6.

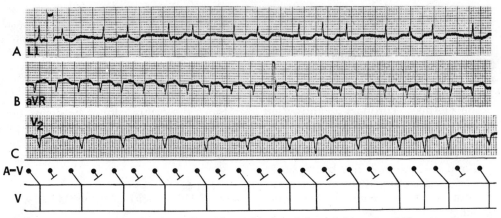

Figure 9–7 A-V junctional tachycardia with exit block and "pseudobigeminy." These tracings were obtained on a 65-year-old female with chronic atrial fibrillation who was in digitalis toxicity. Intermittent second degree A-V block of A-V junctional impulses results in intermittent irregularity or pseudobigeminy of the ventricles.

(A) (Lead I) Atrial fibrillation. At the beginning of this strip, notice regular 3:2 periodicity (pseudobigeminy); at the end of this strip there are 4:3 Wenckebach periods.

(B) (aVR) A-V "junctional" tachycardia with a rate of 160 per minute, probably due to digitalis toxicity. No exit block is present. This pattern could be misinterpreted as supraventricular tachycardia.

(C) (V₂) In lead V₂, repeated 2:1 exit block is manifested as a regular ventricular rate of 80 beats per minute. In the left half of the strip, 2:1 exit block of the A-V junctional tachycardia mimics "A-V junctional tachycardia" with a rate of 80 beats per minute. In the right half of the strip, the following ratios of conduction are present: 3:2, 2:1, 4:3 block (Wenckebach periodicity).

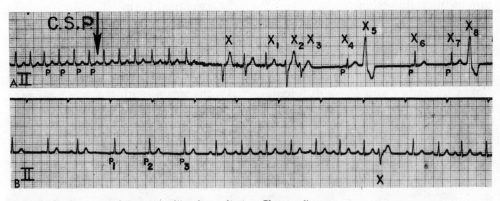

Figure 9–8 Paroxysmal "junctional" tachycardia (see Chapter 6).

(A) The paroxysm manifests a regular rhythm with a rate of 180 per minute. Note that the P waves are inverted and immediately follow the QRS complex. Following carotid sinus pressure, note the presence of a postparoxysmal pause and an escape beat at X, a normally appearing QRS at X_1, followed by premature beats or aberrantly conducted beats at X_2 and X_3. Note the occurrence of a junctional escape beat at X_4 preceded by an inverted P wave and followed by a premature beat, probably ventricular in origin, at X_5. This is followed by a compensatory pause and junctional beats at X_6 and at X_7.

(B) Note the restoration of normal sinus rhythm with a wandering pacemaker from the S-A to the A-V node (inverted P waves at P_1, P_2, and P_3) and the restoration to normal sinus rhythm thereafter, except for a premature beat at X.

(2) P wave concealed by the QRS ("midnodal") (in this case, atrial standstill should be excluded); (3) P wave succeeding the QRS ("lower nodal"); and (4) coronary sinus tachycardia (Scherf and Cohen, 1966).

Therapy. The therapy is that required by the underlying cause. Carotid sinus pressure or other methods for increasing vagal tone result in transient abolition of the complexes of junctional origin, in most cases. If vagal stimulation is not effective, digitalis may be administered, except in those patients in whom the arrhythmia is a manifestation of digitalis intoxication.

Nonparoxysmal (or Accelerated) Form

Etiology and Treatment. In nonparoxysmal junctional tachycardia, the ventricular rate ranges from 70 to 120 (130) beats per minute, in contrast to the more rapid paroxysmal form. The nonparoxysmal type is most often due to excessive digitalis; when digitalis has been given to treat atrial fibrillation, the regularity of the ventricular complexes may simulate conversion to normal sinus rhythm. Such a mechanism may occur as a result of exit block. These episodes may be observed in up to 30 per cent of patients with atrial fibrillation who are receiving digitalis (Urbach et al., 1969). Less frequently this arrhythmia is caused by an acute myocardial infarction, open heart surgery, or rarely acute myocarditis. In about 85 per cent of cases, the atria have an independent mechanism.

A-V JUNCTIONAL ESCAPE RHYTHMS

Following parasympathetic stimulation, the excessive slowing of the S-A node is often interrupted by an A-V junctional impulse or A-V junctional escape beat. This is a very impotant homeostatic mechanism, since sudden death from heart disease would be much more frequent than it actually is if this mechanism were not operative. If escape of the A-V junction does not occur under these conditions, automatic tissue in the region of the bundle of His or below its bifurcation may take over control of the ventricular rhythm. If the latter mechanism also fails, death may result from prolonged cardiac arrest (standstill), or the development of ventricular flutter or fibrillation. Junctional and ventricular escape are secondary either to a higher pacemaker malfunction or to a disturbance of the autonomic nervous system (such as excess vagal stimulation).

Etiology. A-V junctional escape rhythms occur: (1) with spontaneous sinus slowing (Fig. 9–9); (2) with S-A block (see Fig. 5–12); (3) as a result of partial A-V heart block with failure of an atrial impulse to discharge the lower pacemaker; (4) following a premature

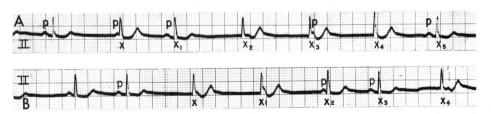

Figure 9–9 Normal sinus beats with periods of A-V junctional escape, and intermittent A-V dissociation.

(A) Note the normal P-R interval, followed by a junctional escape beat at X, the normally conducted beat at X_1, another escape beat at X_2, X_3, and X_4, with a conducted beat at X_5. The sinus rate is 68 per minute with the conducted beats and 58 per minute with the escape beats. Intermittent A-V dissociation occurs at X_2, X_3 and X_4.

(B) Shows periods of A-V junctional escape at cycles marked X, X_1, and X_4. Intermittent A-V dissociation is present at X, X_1, X_2, and X_4.

beat that temporarily suppresses the S-A pacemaker (Fig. 9–8); (5) following carotid sinus pressure during normal sinus rhythm or in the postparoxysmal pause after termination of a supraventricular tachycardia (Fig. 9–8); and (6) when the S-A node is depressed by excessive vagal tone, occurring in a variety of conditions, such as hyperactive carotid sinus reflexes, digitalis intoxication, rheumatic carditis, coronary artery disease, and certain other disease states (see Chapter 5). It is frequently observed in the older age group in association with sinus bradycardia.

Electrocardiogram. A-V junctional escape rhythms are easily recognized in the electrocardiogram by the slow rate (40 to 60 beats per minute). The essential feature of an escaped beat is that it occurs after a long pause. It is usually not preceded by P waves; frequently, when P waves are present, the P-R interval may be short and the P waves may be inverted (Fig. 9–11). The QRS may simulate those of normal beats or aberration may be present. If a series of escape beats appears at a rate slightly in excess of the sinus bradycardia, A-V dissociation may result.

Escape beats may occur singly or in brief runs. Rarely, this same mechanism may initiate persistent junctional rhythm or even junctional tachycardia. If the A-V junctional pacemaker continues to function and does so at a rate greater than that of the re-activated S-A node, the resultant rhythm may be: (a) A-V dissociation, (b) the nonparoxysmal form of junctional tachycardia, or (c) a combination of "a" and "b." This first type has been called "passive junctional rhythm" or the assumption of pacemaker activity by default. The second type occurs when the junctional pacemaker manifests greater automaticity than the sinus node (e.g., due to digitalis effects); this has been regarded as the assumption of pacemaker activity by "usurpation."

Treatment. Treatment depends on the underlying etiology, the hemodyn-

amic consequences, and the presence or absence of other arrhythmias. If A-V junctional escape beats are observed only occasionally, treatment is not necessary. However, in the presence of prolonged periods of junctional escape rhythms, the underlying condition, as previously noted, must be determined and treated. If recurrent episodes occur, treatment may be necessary, particularly if the junctional escape rate is so slow that syncopal attacks occur. Under these conditions, an artificial pacemaker is indicated.

RECIPROCAL RHYTHM

General Considerations. Reciprocal rhythm may be defined as a disturbance of rhythm whereby an impulse arising in the sinus node, atria, A-V junction, or ventricles activates the atrial or ventricular chamber and, during its passage through the A-V junction, enters another A-V pathway, which permits the impulse to return to activate the same chamber once again. Reciprocal rhythm, as it occurs in man, has been associated chiefly with an A-V junctional pacemaker. Two additional types of reciprocal rhythm have been described: reciprocal rhythm with impulses of atrial origin, and reciprocal rhythm with impulses of ventricular origin (Kistin, 1963).

Clinical and experimental evidence suggests that one mechanism for reciprocal rhythm may be the existence of multiple and separate pathways for atrioventricular and ventriculoatrial conduction. (Kistin, 1963; Moe, 1966; Schamroth and Dubb, 1965; Schamroth and Yoshonis, 1969).

The existence of two or more longitudinally dissociated pathways in part or all of the A-V junction has been proposed on indirect physiologic evidence and suggestive anatomic findings (see Chapter 2). Clinical findings have been described which are consistent with the presence of two or more pathways in

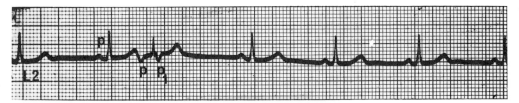

Figure 9–10 Atrial reciprocal beat. (Lead II.) Normal sinus rhythm. The complexes initiated by the inverted P (P-R interval, 0.14 second) probably represent an atrial premature beat. The following inverted P wave represents an atrial reciprocal beat (R-P, 0.08 second).

the upper and middle portions of the A-V junction; these may form a common pathway in the remainder of the junction, or they may be completely separate throughout the length of the A-V junction (Schamroth and Yoshonis, 1969).

Reciprocal rhythm thus represents a form of re-entry. For example, propagation of a junctional impulse proceeds in a forward direction through one portion of the A-V junction to stimulate the ventricles and in a retrograde direction to activate the atria. The impulse from the atria then re-enters another portion of the A-V junction, which is now excitable, and is conducted to activate the ventricles for a second time.

Less commonly, reciprocal beats may arise in the atria or ventricles. Reciprocal rhythm of atrial origin occurs when the sinus or atrial impulse, somewhere in its course toward the ventricles, turns back to activate the atria, thus producing both a QRS complex and a retrograde or reciprocal P wave (Schamroth and Yoshonis, 1969) (see Fig. 9–10). In a reciprocal rhythm of ventricular origin, the impulse arises in the ventricle and is propagated in a retrograde manner through the A-V junction and returns to the ventricle.

Terminology. The term "reciprocating rhythm" is applied to repeated cycles of tachycardia, and "reciprocal beat," to one cycle. The term "return extrasystole" has been used synonymously with "reciprocal beat," but this has the disadvantage that "extrasystole" is used by some writers to mean an accurately coupled ectopic systole or an interpolated systole. The term "echo" is descriptive when the impulse originates in the atrium or ventricle and returns to activate the same chamber a second time but seems less so when the site of origin is in the A-V junction.

Etiology. Reciprocal rhythm ap-

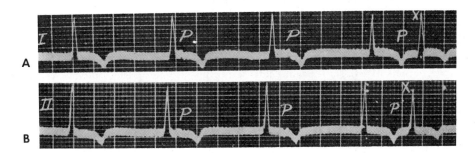

Figure 9–11 Reciprocal beats in a patient with A-V junctional rhythm.
  (A) (Lead I) Shows A-V junctional rhythm in which the QRS is followed by inverted P waves. Note the progressive lengthening of the R-P interval until a critical point is reached (X), when the re-entrant excitation wave finds the antegrade A-V pathway nonrefractory and gives rise to a contraction in the ventricle (reciprocal beat).
  (B) (Lead II) Shows the same phenomenon at X.

pears chiefly in the presence of digitalis toxicity, coronary artery disease, and rheumatic myocarditis, and diseases of the A-V junction.

Diagnosis. The electrocardiographic diagnosis may be made, particularly in the presence of an A-V junctional rhythm, by the presence of an abnormally prolonged R-P interval (over 0.2 second) in which the retrograde P wave is followed by a second ventricular beat (Figs. 9–11, 9–12). This reciprocal beat is separated from the preceding beat by an interval of 0.5 second or less. The R-P interval of successive beats becomes increasingly longer, with the longest R-P interval yielding premature reciprocal beats.

Treatment. The treatment depends on the underlying clinical state and the cause, namely, digitalis toxicity, coronary artery disease, or other factors.

WIDENING OF QRS COMPLEX

The QRS complex may be widened and distorted in the presence of many factors, including (a) ventricular premature beats, (b) supraventricular premature beats and tachycardia (aberration), (c) delayed conduction during bradycardia (e.g., A-V junctional escape), (d) transient or permanent bundle branch block, (e) drugs (quinidine, procaine amide), (f) artificial pacemakers, and (g) hyperkalemia.

Prolongation in the width of the QRS complex depends on a variety of factors, which may be divided into: (a) functional alterations in the physiologic properties of the A-V junction and His-Purkinje system, and (b) organic cardiac changes. The most frequent functional alteration is propagation of an impulse during the partial refractory

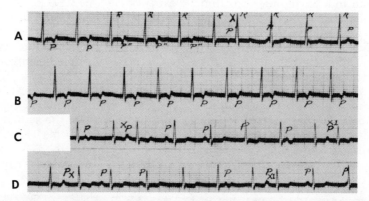

Figure 9–12   A-V junctional rhythm, reciprocal beats, intermittent A-V dissociation and captured beats (lead II).

(A) Note the presence of A-V nodal rhythm in the initial six beats. There is a gradual increase in the R-P interval until in cycle X the R-P interval has increased to 0.32 second and is followed by a premature QRS complex, X (reciprocal beat). The remaining atrial beats in this strip are upright, indicating a sinus origin, the rate of which is slower than that of the ventricular cycles (the ventricular rate is 84 per minute; the atrial rate is 78 per minute). This represents a period of A-V dissociation.

(B) Shows resumption of a regular A-V nodal rhythm with an inverted P wave following the QRS complex at a fixed interval.

(C) A-V dissociation, at X: the P wave captures the ventricle (A-V dissociation with captured beats). Another captured beat is observed at X_1.

(D) A-V dissociation: ventricular capture occurs at X and X_1 and also in the cycle immediately following Px. Note that this cycle length is slightly shorter than that of the A-V nodal beats. Note the difference between reciprocal beats (which have also been considered to be captured beats) and the captured beats of A-V dissociation (so-called pseudoreciprocal beats). In the former, the P wave is inverted, indicating retrograde conduction with a return of the impulse to activate the ventricle; in the latter, the P wave is upright, indicating the usual type of antegrade conduction.

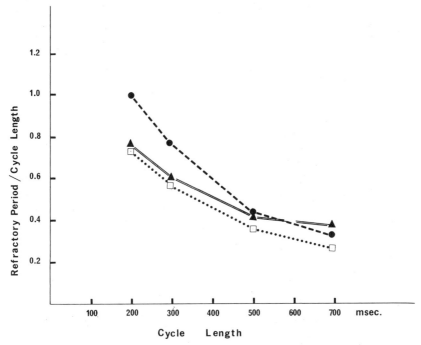

Figure 9–13 The relation of the length of the refractory period in various conduction tissues to cycle length. The circles are the A-V junctional values, the diamonds are the right bundle branch values, and the squares are the bundle of His values. The refractory period length is expressed as a fraction of the total cycle length on the ordinate. Note *that as the cycle length becomes progressively shorter (i.e., as the heart rate increases) the refractory period assumes a greater percentage of the cycle length.* (Compiled from data in Moe *et al.: Circ. Res.*, 16:261, 1965.)

period of the A-V transmission system. Organic factors include: (a) the presence of cardiac hypertrophy or dilatation, (b) disease of the main bundle branches or their smaller subdivisions, and (c) a combination of "a" and "b."

The evidence concerning the modifications of the conducting fibers at rapid rates is complex; several points merit mention here. It has been shown experimentally that the refractory periods of the A-V junction, the bundle of His, and the bundle branches decrease at rapid rates; however, the cycle length decreases percentage-wise more rapidly than does the refractory period (especially in the right bundle branch), with the result that the refractory period of the conduction system may exceed the basic cycle length. Patients who manifest varying grades of myocardial ab-

normality may develop slowed conduction and QRS widening even at relatively slow rates. The factors precipitating deviation from the normal conduction in the presence of arrhythmias may be classified into two groups, depending on whether the QRS widening is due to a derangement that resides primarily in the ventricular part of the conduction system or to a rapid or slow rhythm originating from a supraventricular pacemaker.

Supraventricular impulses may encounter refractoriness or block within the A-V conduction system and cause QRS widening in the presence of (a) atrial or junctional premature beats, (b) A-V junctional escape beats, in which QRS widening following a prolonged pause is due to aberrant transmission of the impulse through one of

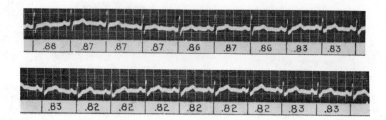

Figure 9–14 Effect of ventricular rate on intraventricular conduction. Note that when the R-R interval is 0.86 second or more, the QRS complex measures 0.08 second. When the R-R interval is 0.83 second or less, the width of the QRS complex increases to 0.12 second.

The critical rate of intraventricular conduction is not a fixed figure for all hearts. It may vary considerably.

the branches of the bundle of His (usually the right bundle branch); (c) the W-P-W syndrome and other pre-excitation syndromes in which fusion of the impulse transmitted through the aberrant pathway and the one propagated through the normal pathway occurs; (d) rapid heart rates (140 to 180 beats per minute), in which the QRS complexes may eventually widen to a level of 0.14 to 0.16 second, similar to that in bundle branch block (Figs. 9–14, 9–15, 9–16). This phenomenon exists because a critical heart rate has been observed above which recovery of the conduction system cannot be completed, thus resulting in aberrant conduction of the impulse; and (e) slow heart rates. In occasional subjects, when the heart rate drops below a critical level,

QRS widening is observed that probably results from diastolic phase 4 depolarization and decremental conduction in the His-Purkinje system (Massumi, 1968).

QRS prolongation may be classified into three types, depending on their relationship to the heart rate: (a) those that occur with either slight or marked acceleration of the heart rate; (b) those that occur at slow heart rates; and (c) those cases in which the widening, which may be either constant or intermittent, occurs independently of the rate.

The term "aberration" has been applied to those instances in which supraventricular impulses occurring at rapid rates or with a short cycle length following a long cycle length produce

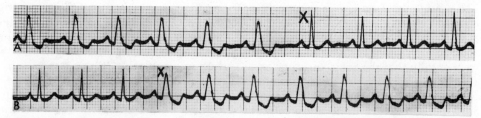

Figure 9–15 Spontaneous transition from bundle branch block to normal intraventricular conduction. (*A* and *B* represent a continuous lead II.) This tracing was taken from a patient with hypertensive heart disease of an advanced degree.

(*A*) Note conversion of bundle branch block to normal intraventricular conduction at X.

(*B*) Note return to bundle branch block at X again. A slight sinus arrhythmia is present.

This type of bundle branch block may be rate-dependent or rate-change-dependent, with two different levels of transition from normal conduction to bundle branch block and from bundle branch block to normal conduction.

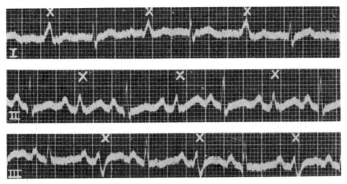

Figure 9-16 Bundle branch block alternating with normal intraventricular conduction. (Leads I, II, and III) Note normal QRS complexes alternating with those of bundle branch block. The interval between the normal and the widened QRS is slightly longer than that between the widened QRS and the following normal beat. P-R times are *constant;* R-R intervals are *constant* as well. This may be called 2:1 bundle branch block.

QRS widening: (1) the QRS widening occurs with only slight increments in rate (e.g., from 70 to 80 or 90 beats per minute); (2) the QRS widening does not depend on the occurrence of a short cycle length following a long one; (3) in general, derangements residing in the ventricular conduction system produce slowed conduction of supraventricular impulses when the heart rate increases; and (4) this pattern frequently progresses to complete bundle branch block. In some instances, especially with intermediate elevations of the heart rate, it is difficult to differentiate "bundle branch block associated with accelerated heart rate" from "aberration."

Mechanisms. The mechanism of QRS widening with acceleration of the heart rate is complicated by several factors: (1) Since the right bundle branch

ordinarily has the longest refractory period in the conduction system, block is most likely to occur there, although it may also occasionally occur in the left bundle branch or in the subdivisions of either bundle branch. (2) The refractory period of each bundle branch is directly proportional to the cycle length of the preceding beat. (3) The refractory period changes relatively slowly after an alteration in the basic cycle length, a phenomenon which has been termed "warming up." (4) The effects of premature beats (and hence, of tachycardia, since both diminish the cycle length) also depend upon their focus of origin, their position in the cardiac cycle, and the presence or absence of organic disease of the conduction system. If the greatest prolongation of refractoriness occurs in the bundle branches or their peripheral ramifica-

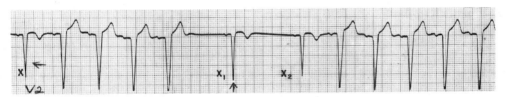

Figure 9-17 Widened QRS complexes, narrowing after long pause. Note the presence of widened QRS complexes, which measure 0.16 second. Note narrowing of the QRS complexes to 0.10 second at X_1 and X_2 following a long pause. This is due to S-A block which was observed in two cycles. X_2 is followed by a resumption of the pre-existent rhythm with widened QRS complexes.

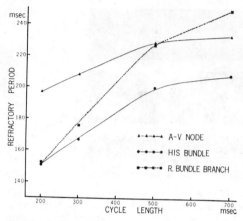

Figure 9–18 Apparent refractory periods of A-V node, His bundle, and right bundle branch as a function of basic cycle length. Open heart preparation. (Moe, G. K., Mendez, C., and Han, J. Circ. Res., *16*:261, 1965.)

tions, QRS widening will result. Such individuals often have normal intraventricular conduction at slow heart rates (i.e., 60 per minute); but they show QRS widening at more elevated rates (see Figs. 7–5, 9–14).

In this light, rate-dependent bundle branch block, manifested by QRS widening and occurring with a slight increase in the heart rate (to 100 beats per minute or less) also may imply the presence of cardiac abnormality due to organic disease, functional alterations, or drug effects.

In occasional cases, 2:1 or 3:1 left bundle branch block may occur with elevation of the heart rate; further acceleration causes complete left bundle branch block.

On occasion, the critical heart rate for normal intraventricular conduction has been observed both clinically and experimentally to be lower for the return of normal conduction than it was for the initiation of abnormal conduction. If, for example, bundle branch block appears whenever the cycle length drops below 0.8 second, the conduction disturbance may persist until the cycle length exceeds 0.90 second. This difference has usually been attributed to the

fact that the refractory period adjusts to rate changes only slowly ("warming up").

QRS Prolongation at Slow Rates. The etiology of bradycardia-dependent bundle branch block is not clearly understood, although most instances reported to date have been in subjects with severe organic heart disease. At present, the most tenable explanation is that during a long diastolic interval phase 4 depolarization of automatic tissues in the bundle branches occurs, altering the excitability in that tissue. Both bundle branches possess automaticity (Hoffman and Cranefield, 1964), and conduction in them may be blocked if diastolic depolarization is sufficiently great.

QRS Prolongation Independent of Rate. Rate-independent QRS widening has considerable clinical significance for several reasons: (a) it frequently precedes the occurrence of complete bundle branch block; (b) sudden death may occur if a ventricular pacemaker does not emerge following the abrupt appearance of complete block; and (c) the same hemodynamic changes that accompany any alteration in intraventricular conduction occur. Block of the bundle branches may occur intermittently, owing to a number of factors other than rapid rates: (a) alteration in autonomic tone, (b) hemodynamic changes, and (c) effect of drugs.

In patients receiving antiarrhythmic drugs, the QRS widening in the electrocardiogram may manifest two patterns: (1) In the initial stages, widening may be present in only occasional ventricular beats, occurring during short intervals with a slight increase in rate, or may appear independent of it. (2) Widened beats may then gradually increase in frequency until all are widened. These complexes usually appear with a rapid rate, and it may be difficult to differentiate them from ventricular premature beats and ventricular tachycardia.

Etiology   and   Clinical   Signifi-

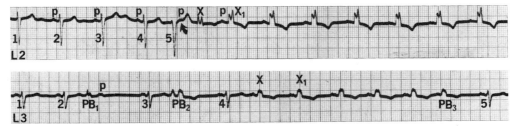

Figure 9–19 Intermittent bundle branch block (not rate-dependent).

(Lead 2) Four sinus beats (1 to 4) are followed by a premature beat, probably A-V junctional or fascicular in origin (X). The next P wave (at arrow) occurs exactly on time and can be seen slightly changing the S-T segment of the premature beat. This P wave is conducted with a P-R time of 0.40 second and the QRS following is that of right bundle branch block (X). Following this, sinus rhythm continues with all QRS complexes exhibiting right bundle branch block. The first QRS after the premature beat represents ventricular aberration (X_1). The morphology of the following QRS — slightly different from the first QRS — may be considered as rate-dependent right bundle branch block after a short cycle. In the remaining QRS complexes, the rate dependency cannot be evoked.

(Lead 3) The first premature beat (PB_1) with QRS aberration does not disturb the sinus rhythm, but the following P is blocked, resulting in a fully compensatory pause. The third sinus QRS is followed by a premature ectopic P wave (PB_2) with aberrant ventricular response. After a nonfully compensatory pause, a normal QRS-T complex appears. The following P wave (X) is premature. The following four beats represent sinus arrhythmia terminated by an ectopic P wave (PB_3). All of these six beats resemble the right bundle branch block pattern.

cance. The etiology of rate-independent bundle branch block is a matter of some question. Many of these patients have hypertension cardiomyopathy, cardiomegaly, or coronary artery disease. However, other individuals have no other clinical evidence of heart disease.

Other Types of Alteration in QRS Width. Paradoxical Narrowing of QRS with Short Cycle. Rarely, a paradoxical effect is observed when the widened QRS complex returns to a normal width following an interval that is shorter than that between the widened complexes (Fig. 9–20). This may be ex-

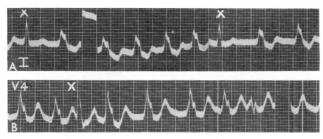

Figure 9–20 Following a run of aberrant, widened QRS complexes, note the occurrence of a QRS of normal width following a short pause.

A and *B* are taken from a patient with atrial fibrillation manifesting a relatively rapid ventricular rate. In cycles marked X, the QRS complexes following the short pause are narrower than the remaining complexes. This may be explained by the concept of supernormal recovery, as applied to the bundle branch fibers; thus, at this critical time, conduction is normal through the bundle branches. This has been described for other conduction tissues, but rarely for the bundle branches. An alternate explanation for the narrowed QRS would be that this is a premature beat arising from the upper midportion of the interventricular septum. Such an origin permits the impulse to travel simultaneously down both branches, thus producing a QRS complex of normal width. Other explanations of paradoxically non-aberrant QRS after a short cycle are longitudinal dissociation within one bundle branch, or the presence in one branch of two consecutive zones with different properties. (See Wellens, H.: Amer. Heart J., 77:158, 1969.)

plained in the following ways: (a) the widened complexes at slower rates may have been due to a bradycardia-dependent bundle branch block; (b) supernormal recovery of the bundle branch fibers could account for it; (c) the narrowed QRS complexes could be the result of a premature beat arising from the upper midportion or the interventricular septum; (d) in the presence of bundle branch block, a premature beat arising in the contralateral ventricle, occurring between P and Q, may bring about a fusion beat resulting in a QRS at normal or almost normal width.

ABERRATION

GENERAL CONSIDERATIONS

Aberrant ventricular conduction is characterized by abnormal spread of the supraventricular impulse in the ventricle brought about by delayed activation of one of the branches of the His bundle (occasionally on the His bundle itself), with resultant widening of the ventricular complex. The right bundle branch is the branch most frequently involved (Fig. 9–21). Such impulses are to be differentiated from those originating in the ventricles, which they very frequently resemble. In the human subject, the effect of atrial pacing in producing aberration depends to some degree upon the control electrocardiogram, the atrial pacing rate, and the cardiac status prior to atrial pacing. For example, Cohen et al. (1968) studied this procedure in normal subjects with a normal electrocardiogram, and in those with left-axis deviation, left ventricular hypertrophy, and delay in the right bundle branch. In 20 of 52 subjects, they observed multiple patterns of aberrant conduction, the most frequent being straightforward RBBB in 31 cases, RBBB with left-axis deviation in 27, left-axis deviation in 14, inferior (rightward) axis deviation in 6, RBBB with inferior axis deviation in 7, and LBBB in 6 (Cohen et al., 1968).

ELECTROCARDIOGRAPHIC CHARACTERISTICS

Gouaux and Ashman (1947) observed the presence of aberration when a su-

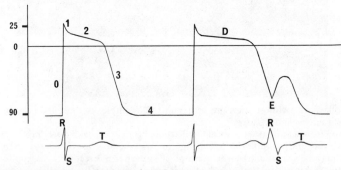

Figure 9–21 Electrophysiologic mechanisms of aberration. The numbers refer to the phase of the transmembrane action potential. The situation in which a premature impulse discharging the ventricular fiber during the repolarization phase and in which phase 4 depolarization causes aberration has been illustrated in Figure 2–8 (p. 23). The long preceding cycle has produced an action potential with a prolonged phase 2 (D). Because of this widening of the action potential, the impulse arriving at (E) discharges the ventricular fiber during the repolarization phase. The resultant aberrant conduction is shown in the simultaneous electrocardiogram.

praventricular beat with a short R-R interval followed a beat of a longer cycle (Ashman phenomenon). In this case, the long cycle predetermines a long refractory period so that the impulse arriving with the succeeding short cycle meets relatively refractory conduction which usually manifests itself in the right branch, thereby exhibiting a picture of RBBB. In fact, 85 per cent of aberrant complexes show an RBBB pattern. Furthermore, 70 per cent of aberrant beats showing the RBBB pattern in V_1 have a triphasic (rsR', rSR', or RsR') pattern, whereas the remaining 30 per cent show a mono- or diphasic pattern. (Sandler and Marriott, 1965). In 44 per cent of aberrant beats manifesting the RBBB pattern, the initial vector of the QRS complex was identical to the sinus beats.

DIFFERENTIAL DIAGNOSIS

The distinction between aberrant complexes and premature beats is often difficult. Certain electrocardiographic characteristics of these two groups may aid in the differentiation. The following favor the diagnosis of ventricular beats: mono- or diphasic complexes in lead V_1; deep S waves in lead V_6; compensatory pauses after a complex; fixed coupling; and the presence of fusion beats, escape beats or parasystole. The following favor the diagnosis of aberration: a triphasic QRS pattern in lead V_1; an initial q wave in lead V_6; variable coupling; and a short cycle preceded by a long cycle. In doubtful cases, His bundle electrocardiography can resolve the issue (see Chapter 14). Supraventricular beats with aberration are characterized by a His spike preceding the QRS complex with an H-V interval equal or greater than the normal beats. In contrast, ventricular beats either have no preceding His spike or an H-V interval shorter than that of the normal complexes.

REFERENCES

Barold, S. S., Linhart, J. W., Hildner, F. J., Narula, O. S., and Samet, P.: Incomplete left bundle branch block. A definite electrocardiographic entity. Circulation, 38:702, 1968.

Berliner, K., and Lewithin, P.: Auricular premature systole. I. Aberration of the ventricular complex in the electrocardiogram. Amer. Heart J., 29:449, 1945.

Bisteni, A., Sodi-Pollares, D., Medrano, G. A., and Pileggi, F.: Nerves Conceptos para el Diagnostico de las Extrasistoles Ventriculores. Arch. Inst. Cardiol. (Mexico), 27:46, 1957.

Bisteni, A., Sodi-Pollares, D., Medrano, G. A., and Pileggi, F.: A new approach for the recognition of ventricular premature beats. Amer. J. Cardiol., 5:358, 1960.

Cohen, S. I., Lau, S. H., Haft, J. I., and Damato, A. N.: Experimental production of aberrant ventricular conduction in man. Circulation, 36:673, 1967.

Cohen, S. I., Lau, S. H., Stein, E., Young, M. W., and Damato, A. N.: Variations of aberrant ventricular conduction in man: Evidence of isolated and combined block within the specialized conduction system. An electrocardiographic and vectorcardiographic study. Circulation, 38:899, 1968.

Damato, A. N., and Lau, S. H.: His bundle rhythm. Circulation, 40:527, 1969.

Damato, A. N., Lau, S. H., Berkowitz, W. D., Rosen, K. M., and Lisi, K. R.: Recording of specialized conducting fibers (A-V nodal, His bundle, and right bundle branch) in man using an electrode catheter technique. Circulation, 39:435, 1969.

DeFelice, L. J., and Challice, C. E.: Anatomical and ultrastructural study of the electrophysiological A-V node of the rabbit. Circ. Res., 24:457, 1969.

Dodge, H. B., and Grant, R.: Mechanism of QRS complex prolongation in man: Right ventricular conduction defects. Amer. J. Med., 21:535, 1956.

Fisch, C., and Knoebel, S. B.: Junctional rhythms. Prog. Cardiov. Dis., 13:141, 1970.

Gardberg, M., and Rosen, I. L.: Observations on conduction in a case of intermittent left bundle branch block. Amer. Heart. J., 55:677, 1958.

Gouaux, J. L., and Ashman, R.: Auricular fibrillation with aberration simulating ventricular paroxysmal tachycardia. Amer. Heart J., 34:366, 1947.

Han, J., and Moe, G. K.: Cumulative effects of cycle length on refractory periods of cardiac tissue. Amer. J. Physiol., 217:106, 1969.

Hoffman, B. F., and Cranefield, P. F.: Physiological basis of cardiac arrhythmia. Amer. J. Med., 37:670, 1964.

Katz, L. N., and Pick, A.: Clinical Electrocardiography. Part I. The Arrhythmias. Philadelphia, Lea & Febiger, 1956.

Kistin, A. D.: Multiple pathways of conduction and reciprocal rhythm with interpolated ventricular premature systoles. Amer. Heart J., 65:162, 1963.

Lisi, K. R., Rosen, K. M., Lau, S. H., and Damato, A. N.: The electrophysiology of coronary sinus rhythm. Circulation, 39–40:III–34, 1969.

MacLean, W. A., Karp, R. B., Kaushoukos, N. T., James, T. N., and Waldo, A. N.: P waves during ectopic atrial rhythms in man. A study utilizing atrial pacing with fixed electrodes. Circulation 52:426, 1975.

Massumi, R.: Bradycardia-dependent bundle-branch block. A critique and proposed criteria. Circulation, 38:1066, 1968.

Mirowski, M.: Left atrial rhythm: diagnostic criteria and differentiation from nodal arrhythmias. Amer. J. Cardiol., 17:203, 1966.

Moe, G. K.: The physiological basis of reciprocal rhythm. Prog. Cardiov. Dis., 8:461, 1966.

Pick, A., and Langendorf, R.: Recent advances in the differential diagnosis of A-V junctional arrhythmias. Amer. Heart J.,76:553, 1968.

Rosenbaum, M. B., Elizari, M. V., and Lazzari, J. O.: The mechanism of bidirectional tachycardia. Amer. Heart J., 78:4, 1969.

Sandler, I. A., and Marriott, H. J. L.: The differential morphology of anomalous ventricular complexes of RBBB-type in lead V_1. Circulation, 31:551, 1965.

Schamroth, L., and Dubb, A.: Escape capture bigeminy. Mechanisms in S-A block, A-V block and reversed reciprocal rhythm. Brit. Heart J., 27:667, 1965.

Schamroth, L., and Yoshonis, K. F.: Mechanisms in reciprocal rhythm. Amer. J. Cardiol., 24:224, 1969.

Scherf, D., and Cohen, J.: Atrioventricular rhythms. Prog. Cardiov. Dis., 9:499, 1966.

Scherf, D., and Harris, R.: Coronary sinus rhythm. Amer. Heart J., 32:443, 1946.

Scherlag, B. J., Lazzarra, R., and Helfant, R. H.: Differentiation of "A-V functional rhythms." Circulation 48:304, 1973.

Tawara, S.: Das Reizleitungsystem des Saugertierherzens. Jena, Gustav Fishcer, 1906.

Truex, R. C., and Smythe, M. Q.: Recent observations on the human cardiac conduction system, with special considerations of the atrioventricular node and bundle. In Taccardi, B., and Marchetti, G. (eds.): Electrophysiology of the Heart. Oxford, Pergamon Press, 1964, pp. 177–198.

Urbach, J. R., Graurnan, J. J., and Strans, S. H.: Quantitative methods for the recognition of atrioventricular junctional rhythms in atrial fibrillation. Circulation, 39:803, 1969.

Waldo, A. L., Vitikainen, K. J., Harris, P. D., Malm, J. R., and Hoffman, B. F.: A new look at the P wave. Circulation 35 (Suppl. 2):260, 1967.

Waldo, A. L., Vitikainen, K. J., Harris, P. D., Malm, J. R., and Hoffman, B. F.: The mechanism of synchronization in isorhythmic A-V dissociation. Some observations on the morphology and polarity of the P wave during retrograde capture of the atria. Circulation, 38:880, 1968.

Wellens, H.: Unusual occurrence of non-aberrant conduction in patients with atrial fibrillation and aberrant conduction. Amer. Heart J., 77:158, 1969.

SUPPLEMENTAL READING

Christopher, R. C., Wyndham, M. B., Dhingra, R. C., Smith, T., Best, D., and Rosen, K. M.: Concealed nonparoxysmal junctional tachycardia. Circulation 60:709, 1979.

Rosen, M., Fisch, C., Hoffman, B., and Knoebel, S.: Delayed afterdepolarization as a mechanism for accelerated junctional escape rhythm. Circulation 60:II–253, 1979.

10

A-V DISSOCIATION

ROBERT I. KATZ, M.D.,
RICHARD H. HELFANT, M.D.

GENERAL CONSIDERATIONS

A-V dissociation is defined as independent beating of the atria and ventricles, each responding to its own pacemaker. Usually, the pacemaker controlling the atria is located in the S-A node, while that controlling the ventricles is located in the A-V junction or in the upper portion of the His-Purkinje system.

An important aspect of A-V dissociation is that it does not occur as a primary disturbance of rhythm but arises secondary to some more fundamental disorder.

DEFINITION OF TERMS

Dissociation. The term "dissociation" refers in a general way to the presence in the same heart of two pacemakers with independent rhythmicity. This may refer to any combination of pacemakers, i.e., atrial, A-V junctional, and ventricular, although the most common type is A-V junctional. The term "A-V dissociation" most often implies that the atria, under the control of the S-A node, and the ventricles, under A-V junctional control, beat independently and that the ventricles usually beat faster than the atria. However, the atria may not necessarily be controlled by the S-A node and the ventricles may

be controlled by a pacemaker other than the A-V junction. Deviations from the common type are discussed later.

The perpetuation of two rhythms depends upon the propagation of the two electrical impulses in such a fashion that each one produces a state of refractoriness to the electrical transmission of the other. It is about this process that most of the disputed terminology has arisen.

Capture (or Interference). The term "capture" or "interference" has been used in a different sense by different authors. (1) The most common use of this term is that in the presence of A-V dissociation the ventricles beat faster than the atria. When the P wave falls far enough beyond the QRS so that the junctional tissues are no longer refractory, the atrial impulse is conducted to (i.e., "captures") the ventricles and the atrial rhythm thus "interferes" with the regular ventricular rhythm by producing an early ventricular beat (capture beat). (2) The term has also been used to mean the mutual extinction of two excitation fronts that meet in any portion of the heart. This form is seen in a "fusion" or summation beat. (3) When the A-V junction discharges its impulse just before the sinus impulse arrives, the latter impulse finds the A-V node refractory. The refractory junctional tissue, therefore, "interferes" with the propagation of the sinus impulse, so

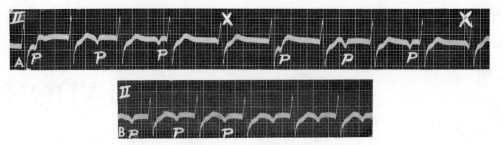

Figure 10-1 A-V dissociation. A and B represent a continuous strip. In A, the atrial rhythm is regular at a rate of 46 per minute and the ventricles beat at a rate of 50 per minute. This is followed by a nodal rhythm seen on strip B.

that the atrial and ventricular rhythms are dissociated.

All three types of "capture" can be observed. Whenever possible, it is preferable to use a more specific term, for example: (1) when one rhythm gains control of the other pacemaker, the terms "ventricular capture" or "atrial capture" are preferable; (2) when two wave fronts meet and extinction results, the term "fusion beat" best describes the result; and (3) when the A-V junction is refractory to the transmission of a sinus impulse, the term "A-V junctional refractory period" is used.

Ventricular Capture. This occurs when, without a significant change in rate of either the atria or the ventricles, the R-P interval approaches a critical level so that the P wave finds the A-V junction nonrefractory and is conducted to the ventricle, producing a ventricular beat after an interval that is shor-

ter than usual (Figs. 10–1, 10–2). With "ventricular capture," restoration to normal atrioventricular and intraventricular conduction may result; however, A-V conduction is frequently prolonged (Fig. 10–1).

Atrial Capture. Occasionally, during periods when the atria are under the control of a junctional or ventricular pacemaker, the sinus impulse may reach the atrial muscle during a nonrefractory phase and result in an atrial beat. This constitutes atrial capture by the S-A node. Conversely, when the atria are under the control of the sinus pacemaker during A-V dissociation, a retrograde impulse arising in the A-V junction or ventricles may reach the atria prior to the sinus impulse. The S-A node may be discharged or depressed by this impulse. This latter situation may result in atrial capture by a junctional or ventricular pacemaker. If

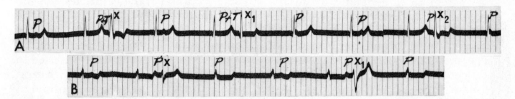

Figure 10-2 Incomplete A-V dissociation with capture beats.

(A) (Lead I) Note the relatively slow regular atrial rate at 48 per minute and the more rapid ventricular rate at 56 per minute. These rhythms are entirely independent of each other; the P waves are upright, indicating a sinus origin. In the cycles marked X, the atrial beat occurs in that phase of the cardiac cycle which finds the A-V conduction system in a nonrefractory state, resulting in a ventricular response (captured beat). Note aberration of the QRS at X and X_2, but none at X_1.

(B) (Lead II) Note that in X and X_1 the QRS of the captured beats is somewhat different in contour from that of the other beats, indicating some alteration in the spread of the impulse through the A-V conduction system (aberration).

the atrial capture is only partial and the two impulses meet in the atrial musculature, a fusion beat results.

MECHANISMS PRODUCING A-V DISSOCIATION

Dissociation may result from three different mechanisms: (1) slowing of the generation of impulse in the primary pacemaker of the heart; (2) acceleration, either paroxysmal or sustained, of impulse formation in the automatic tissue of the A-V junction or ventricles; and (3) permanent or intermittent failure of several successive primary pacemaker impulses, discharging at a normal rate, to reach or to cross the narrow atrioventricular bridge (Pick, 1963). If the failure of conduction is permanent, it is classified as a form of A-V block with concomitant A-V dissociation.

INCIDENCE AND ETIOLOGY

The percentage varies from 0.48 per cent in 10,000 consecutive cases (Marriott et al., 1958) to 1.4 per cent in 50,000 cases (Katz and Pick, 1956). A-V dissociation *always* occurs secondary to some other disturbance in the function of the heart. Sinus slowing may be caused by "sinus arrhythmia," a compensatory pause following a premature atrial impulse, or any factor that decreases automaticity (i.e., decreased catecholamines, increased vagal tone, electrolyte changes, toxic states, or the action of certain drugs, e.g., digitalis). A-V junctional acceleration may be caused by any factor that increases automaticity — digitalis, acute rheumatic fever, acute infections, particularly diphtheria, scarlet fever, pneumonia, and typhus. Quinidine, procaine amide, influences exerted through the autonomic nervous system, and increased intracranial pressure, are causal factors as is inferior myocardial infarction. This rhythm may at times be present in trained athletes with sinus bradycardia. Failure of the impulse to cross the A-V junction may be caused by this tissue being in a refractory state following a previous junctional impulse, depression of conduction by digitalis and other drugs, or various forms of organic heart block. Digitalis toxicity notoriously acts by multiple mechanisms to produce A-V dissociation, including increased automaticity of the A-V junction (Fig. 10–3).

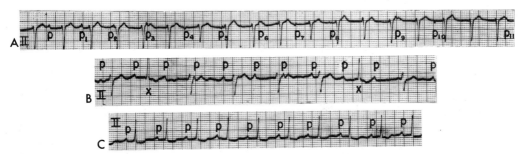

Figure 10–3 Incomplete A-V dissociation with wandering pacemaker caused by digitalis toxicity.

(A) Atrial rate is 79 per minute, ventricular rate, 100 per minute. Note alteration in the configuration of the P waves caused by a wandering pacemaker. The first three cycles (P to P_3) and P_9 and P_{11} show upright P waves and occur at a faster rate than the remaining cycles. P_4 to P_7 and P_{10} are inverted, and P_8 is diphasic. The QRS following P_4 and P_7 probably represent reciprocal beats.

(B) Digitalis is stopped. Atrial rate is 100 per minute; ventricular rate, 56 per minute. Incomplete A-V dissociation with occasional capture beats occur at X. Note the prolonged P-R interval, the slightly narrower QRS width, and the upwardly directed QRS with the conducted beats.

(C) Normal sinus rhythm with slightly prolonged P-R interval (0.24 second). Note the upwardly directed R waves, similar in configuration to the conducted beats in B.

TYPES OF A-V DISSOCIATION AND MODES OF ONSET

The varieties of A-V dissociation may be classified as: (1) complete or incomplete, and (2) persistent or transient. When A-V dissociation without capture of either pacemaker is observed in a long electrocardiographic tracing, "complete dissociation" is said to exist. On the other hand, incomplete dissociation is marked by several types of ventricular capture. An example might be the temporary incomplete A-V dissociation with ventricular capture in a patient with an A-V conduction block due to digitalis intoxication. The common types of A-V dissociation may be classified as follows:

(1) Depression of automaticity of the S-A node allows the impulses from the A-V junction to control the ventricles. Once the "escape beat" of the lower center occurs, it may result in the rhythmic activity of two independent foci, thereby maintaining the dissociation (Fig. 10–4). The dissociation is terminated when a sinus impulse occurs at such a point in the cardiac cycle that it can be propagated through the A-V junction (i.e., when the A-V junction is nonrefractory to impulses from the atrium) and results in a ventricular capture. This may occur, for example, after the disappearance of temporary sinoatrial block. The resumption of S-A nodal activity permits the S-A impulse to reach a position in the cardiac cycle so that it may be conducted (capture beat), with a resultant return to normal sinus rhythm (Fig. 10–5).

(2) Increased automaticity of the A-V junction to a level greater than that of the sinus pacemaker results in "usurpation"; this center then controls the ventricles (Fig. 10–6). This may occur when the junctional rate accelerates, with or without slowing of the sinus rate, or when both pacemakers are slowed or accelerated to an unequal degree (Miller and Sharrett, 1957). In this type, for example, a low junctional premature beat may occur at such a time that it extinguishes the sinus impulse by retrograde conduction or else leaves the A-V node refractory to the passage of a sinus impulse. If the second premature beat occurs early enough to produce the same effect, the resultant refractoriness is perpetuated, resulting in A-V dissociation.

(3) The term *isorhythmic* has been ap-

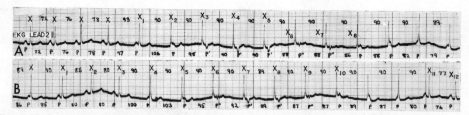

Figure 10–4 Continuous strip of lead II from patient with mitral stenosis. Shows sinus arrhythmia, A-V nodal escape, isorhythmic type of A-V dissociation and nodal rhythm. The numbers above the electrocardiogram denote R-R intervals; those below it denote P-R intervals in msec. P represents the sinus P wave; P', retrograde nodal P_j wave; P", fusion P wave.

(A) Note the first three cycles marked X show the normal sinus rhythm. (P waves are normal). The QRS of X_1 and X_2 represent A-V nodal escape. Note the retrograde P wave in cycles X_3, X_4, and X_5. These are cycles of A-V nodal rhythm. Note the fusion P wave at X_6, X_7, and X_8. Note the variation in the P-P intervals in the initial part of the tracing, indicating the presence of sinus arrhythmia.

(B) Note the occurrence of the isorhythmic type of A-V dissociation in cycles X and X_1, the normal A-V conduction in X_2 and X_3, and an isorhythmic type of A-V dissociation in X_4 and X_5. A fusion P wave occurs at X_6, and retrograde P waves at X_7 and X_8. There is a fusion P wave at X_9, a return to upright P waves at X_{10}, and the restoration of normal sinus rhythm at X_{11} and X_{12}. (From Sackner, Somerson, and Bellet: Amer. J. Cardiol., 4:821, 1959.)

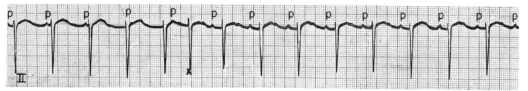

Figure 10–5 A-V dissociation showing transition to normal sinus rhythm.

Note A-V dissociation in the initial four cycles; the atrial rate is 79 per minute and the ventricular rate is 81 per minute. A captured beat occurs at X, following which normal sinus rhythm is restored with a ventricular rate of 79 per minute and a P-R interval of 0.22 second.

plied to A-V dissociation characterized by independent beating of the atria and ventricles at an almost identical rate. The P-R intervals are short, and the P waves often override the QRS complex. Captured beats are observed only rarely (Figs. 10–7, 10–8). This type of dissociation has had various explanations. Segers (1946), on the basis of work with amphibian hearts, proposed that synchronization occurred as a result of contact between two tissues with different rhythms, a process he called "accrochage." He observed that when two separate rhythmic cellular elements are placed in contact without true anatomic continuity, they tend to discharge their impulses at the same rate even though their initial rhythms differ.

A-V Dissociation Presenting Deviations from the Above Types. The following deviations from the above varieties may be frequently observed. Some of these might be easily anticipated. (a) The atria may be controlled, not by the S-A node, but by a lower pacemaker located in the coronary sinus region or in the A-V junction (Fig. 10–9); (b) The ventricles may be controlled not by the A-V junction, but by a ventricular pacemaker. (c) The type of A-V dissociation may change for a series of beats from one in which the rates deviate considerably from each other to one in which they are almost identical. (d) Instances may be observed in which the atria beat slightly faster than the ventricles. This situation may not be due to simple A-V dissociation but to A-V heart block combined with short periods of A-V dissociation. (e) A-V dissociation may be superimposed on a background of 2:1 A-V block. In these tracings the ventricular rate is slower

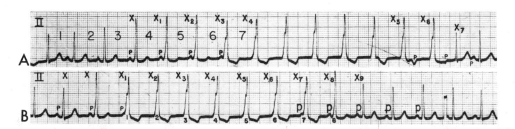

Figure 10–6 Intermittent A-V dissociation showing ventricular tachycardia and fusion beats.

(A) The atrial rate is slightly slower than the ventricular rate (atrial rate, 94 per minute, and ventricular rate, 100 per minute during period of A-V dissociation). The first three beats are normally conducted. From X to X_3, fusion beats with slight aberration of QRS are observed. Thereafter, 6 to the X_6 represent ventricular beats. X_7 represents a fusion beat. The P wave following X_5 is an inverted P wave due to retrograde conduction. A normal upright P wave followed by a normally conducted beat is observed in the last QRS of the strip. It is preceded, following X_6, by an inverted P wave intermediate in form from the preceding one and the one following it. This represents a fusion beat.

(B) The above sequence is repeated in the first part of the strip (X to X_8). Normal sinus rhythm is restored at X_9.

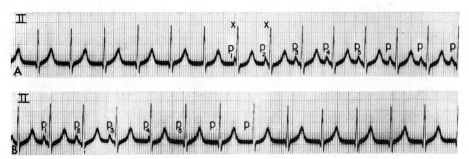

Figure 10–7 A-V junctional rhythm and A-V dissociation (isorhythmic type) observed during right cardiac catheterization.

(A) (Lead II) Note the appearance of A-V junctional beats occurring at a rate of 100 per minute from the beginning of the strip to the cycle marked X. The P waves are apparently buried in the QRS complex; however, at the first cycle marked X, P waves begin to emerge preceding the QRS complexes. The P-R interval gradually increases at P_1, P_2, and P_3. At P_4 and P_5 and in the following cycles, normal rhythm is restored with a P-R interval measuring 0.12 second.

(B) Shows the same process in reverse, namely, a normal P-R interval at P_1, P_2, and P_3, and sudden marked shortening of the P-R interval at P_4 and P_5 as the P wave becomes buried in the QRS complex with the occurrence of an A-V junctional rhythm towards the end of the strip.

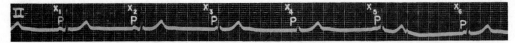

Figure 10–8 A-V dissociation of the isorhythmic type. At the beginning, a sinus bradycardia is present (both atrial and ventricular rates are the same, 38 per minute); at X_3 the atrial rate is slower; at X_5 and X_6, it is faster than the rate of the A-V rhythm. Note the normal P-R interval at X_1 (0.14 second) and X_2. At X_3, the P wave merges into the QRS complex, and at X_4 no P wave can be observed since it is probably buried in the QRS. At X_5, a small P wave is seen to emerge; this becomes larger at X_6.

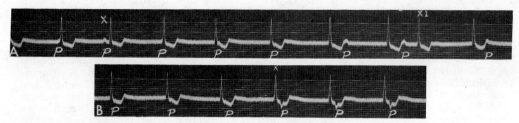

Figure 10–9 A-V dissociation with interference (or capture). Both atrial and ventricular rhythms are slightly irregular. Note capture beat at X_1.

than the atrial rate, but greater than the rate of conducted atrial impulses. (f) Forward conduction is often impaired in the presence of A-V dissociation. This is indicated by the following: the close relationship of the prolonged P-R interval and dissociation in rheumatic fever; and the fact that the P-R interval of the captured beat is often prolonged even when this beat does not occur particularly early in the cardiac cycle as shown by examples of concealed conduction observed in these cases. (g) Retrograde block is not absolute and retrograde conduction to the atria may occasionally occur. (h) Fusion beats may occur in A-V dissociation, in conjunction with any of the types mentioned. These beats represent partial dissociation or, from another point of view, partial capture and occur frequently during the transition between control of the heart by a single pacemaker (e.g., sinus or junctional) and A-V dissociation with two independent pacemakers.

Other Types of Dissociations. Other types of "dissociation" in which two or more pacemakers initiate impulses independent of each other include: (a) atrial dissociation; (b) junctional tachycardia without retrograde conduction, with the maintenance of normal sinus pacemaker activity; (c) two junctional pacemakers beating independently (Fig. 10–9); (d) a rhythm arising from a ventricular focus; (e) complete A-V heart block; (f) two independent ventricular foci; and (g) A-V dissociation with ventricular parasystole.

AUSCULTATORY PHENOMENA

The auscultatory phenomena vary with the type and degree of dissociation. In the presence of A-V dissociation, there is a *variation* in the intensity of the first heart sound due to the difference in the time interval between the P wave and the QRS complex. When the P wave occurs much before the QRS complex, the first heart sound is faint, and when it is close to it, the sound is relatively more intense. This situation is similar to that which occurs in the presence of the A-V dissociation associated with complete A-V heart block.

ELECTROCARDIOGRAM IN A-V DISSOCIATION

There is an inconstant relationship between P waves and the adjacent QRS complexes, while the atrial rate is usually slower than the ventricular rate. In each successive cycle, the P wave moves closer to the ventricular complex to its right and may ultimately coincide with or follow the QRS. When the P wave passes a QRS complex, the following events may occur in subsequent beats: (a) ventricular capture; (b) atrial capture; or (c) synchronization or "accrochage."

Inspection indicates that both atrial and ventricular cycle lengths are constant while bearing no relation to each other (unless a sinus arrhythmia is present). Usually, with a sufficiently long record, there appear to be repetitive "premature" QRS complexes of a supraventricular contour which represent "ventricular capture" beats. With these criteria fulfilled, the diagnosis of A-V dissociation is established. Occasionally, A-V dissociation may transiently develop into an A-V junctional rhythm for a varying number of cycles. This may be apparent from the fusion of the atrial and ventricular beats or by the transient appearance of inverted P waves; when they occur at almost identical rates, they may be superimposed, giving the appearance of an A-V junctional rhythm.

DIFFERENTIAL DIAGNOSIS

The following should be considered in the differential diagnosis of A-V dissociation: (a) First degree A-V heart block with a long P-R interval, with the P wave lying close to the preceding QRS. Tracings of this type closely resemble A-V dissociation with synchronization. However, the response to exercise, emotion, or atropine will alter the relationship of the P wave to the QRS and thus clarify the diagnosis. (b) Complete A-V heart block. Confusion between A-V block and dissociation is not uncommon. Dissociation or independent beating of atria and ventricles may be due to a change in pacemaker rate in one or both of them (without any evidence of A-V block) *or* due to A-V block. When dissociation occurs without block, the lower focus maintains a state of junctional refractoriness interfering with their activation from the atria. However, with appropriate timing, an atrial impulse will arrive in the junctional area when it is not refractory and "interfere" with the regularity of the ventricular depolarization sequence. Thus, the P wave may "march through" the QRS until it is conducted to the ventricles. If, however, under these circumstances the P wave does not conduct to the ventricles, interference and block coexist. (c) 2:1 A-V heart block with dissociation from complete A-V heart block with occasional ventricular captures. These two unusual conditions resemble each other, but careful study of the electrocardiograms will disclose differentiating features (see Fig. 10–3). In complete A-V heart block with occasional transmission of a sinus beat, the ventricular rate usually ranges from 30 to 36 beats per minute with only slight variation of the R-R interval. The QRS complex is often of the idioventricular type and is considerably widened. The atrial rate is frequently 3 to 5 times the ventricular rate and therefore two P-P cycles are shorter than one R-R cycle. When infrequent ventricular capture occurs (this may appear during a supernormal phase) the P-R interval is not fixed because of a varying refractory period of the A-V junction in the transmitted

sinus beats. (d) A-V dissociation between S-A and A-V junctional rhythm with aberrant ventricular conduction. This may sometimes be confused with A-V dissociation between S-A and idioventricular rhythms. (e) Ventricular parasystole may rarely simulate A-V dissociation. The most important distinction is that in parasystole the rhythm of the lower center is slower than that of the upper one. The ventricular center is protected from the higher center by an entrance block; that is, there is unidirectional forward block into the parasystolic center, thereby preventing its capture. The impulses of the parasystolic focus, however, have free exit or egress when the ventricles are not in a refractory phase.

DURATION AND FATE OF A-V DISSOCIATION

Once initiated, A-V dissociation is usually brief or intermittent; it may be observed for a few cycles, a few minutes, hours, or days. It tends to be transient and rarely persists without interruption for any appreciable time.

A-V dissociation may be terminated, transiently or permanently, by one of the following mechanisms: (a) When dissociation is due to an escape mechanism, it will of necessity be short-lived since the S-A pacemaker regains control of the heart after a few beats (Fig. 10–6). (b) Absolute or relative increase in atrial rate or decrease in A-V junctional rate, or a combination of both, may occur spontaneously or may be induced by conditions capable of suppressing or simulating vagal or sympathetic mechanisms (c) Absolute or relative increase in the A-V junctional rate to overcome retrograde A-V block, thereby producing A-V junctional rhythm. This rhythm is usually transient and sinus rhythm usually supervenes. (d) Appearance of an atrial premature contraction, which effects an early discharge of the lower (junctional) pacemaker, thereby creating an opportunity for the sinus node to regain control of the heart (Figs. 10–6, 10–7). (e) Ventricular capture may discharge and depress the A-V junctional pacemaker, thus abolishing the A-V dissociation. Usually a ventricular capture has no effect on the S-A rhythm. (f) A delay in the appearance of the ventricular contraction until the time when it would be expected to appear following a ventricular "captured" beat. This results in a considerably prolonged ventricular cycle (increased R-R interval) and is attributed to the phenomenon of concealed conduction whereby the sinus impulse presumably penetrates the A-V junction, but because of distal refractoriness, cannot activate the ventricles. (g) A-V dissociation may be abolished by various maneuvers or drugs which affect the ectopic focus to a greater degree than the S-A node.

TREATMENT

A-V dissociation itself requires no therapy since it is always a secondary manifestation of an underlying cardiac disorder. Therapy should be directed to the underlying clinical state, drug effects, electrolyte imbalance, or acute rheumatic activity. Cessation of digitalis medication and potassium administration if the serum potassium is low may facilitate reversion to normal sinus rhythm. Often, mere omission of digitalis suffices. Emergency therapy is rarely indicated except with rare types associated with a rapid or very slow ventricular rate.

PROGNOSIS

The prognosis in A-V dissociation per se with or without ventricular capture beats is generally good; much depends on the underlying clinical state and the precipitating cause (e.g., digitalis, infection). Because the heart rate usually does not vary unduly from the normal range, there is no serious concomitant disturbance in the cardiovascular hemodynamics. However, in that type which is accompanied by a rapid ventricular rate, particularly when digitalis-induced paroxysmal atrial tachycardia is associated with incomplete A-V heart block, the mortality is frequently high. A mortality of 58 per cent was reported in a series of 64 patients in whom this occurred (Jacobs et al., 1961). Of the patients with digitalis-induced A-V dissociation, 47 per cent expired as a result of their basic illness shortly after the onset of the arrhythmia (Jacobs et al., 1961). It is interesting that complications are seldom observed as a direct result of this condition. The presence of the A-V dissociation is a warning that there may be a serious derangement in myocardial function due to endogenous or exogenous factors, and if these are not corrected the outcome might be serious or at times fatal.

REFERENCES

Jacobs, D. R., Donoso, E., and Friedberg, C. K.: A-V dissociation — a relatively frequent arrhythmia. Medicine, 40:101, 1961.

Katz, L. N., and Pick, A.: Clinical Electrocardiography. Part I. The Arrhythmias. Philadelphia, Lea & Febiger, 1956.

Levy, M. N., and Edelstein, J.: Mechanism of synchronization in isorhythmic A-V dissociation. Circulation, 41–42: III–99, 1970.

Marriott, H. J. L., and Menendez, M. M.: A-V dissociation revisited. Prog. Cardiov. Dis., 8:522, 1966.

Marriott, H. J. L., Schubart, A. F., and Bradley, S. M.: A-V dissociation: A reappraisal. Amer. J. Cardiol., 2:586, 1958.

Miller, R., and Sharrett, R. H.: Interference dissociation. Circulation, 16:803, 1957.

Pick, A.: A-V dissociation. A proposal for a comprehensive classification and consistent terminology. Amer. Heart J., 66:147, 1963.

Segers, M.: Les phénomènes de synchronisation an nivean du coeur. Arch. Int. Physiol., 54:87, 1946.

Waldo, A. L., Vitikainen, K. J., Harris, P. D., Malm, J. R., and Hoffman, B. F.: The mechanism of synchronization in isorhythmic A-V dissociation. Some observations in the morphology and polarity of the P wave during retrograde capture of the atria. Circulation, 38:880, 1968.

11

VENTRICULAR ARRHYTHMIAS

VIDYA S. BANKA, M.D.,
RICHARD H. HELFANT, M.D.

VENTRICULAR PREMATURE BEATS

General Features

A ventricular premature beat is a complex that originates in the ventricles and results in ventricular depolarization earlier in the cycle than would normally be expected if the ventricles were depolarized by the patient's normal pacemaker. Since the wave of ventricular depolarization is abnormal, the QRS complex is prolonged and bizarre. The coupling interval of the premature complex and the previous normal beat is usually, although not invariably, constant or "fixed." Since ventricular premature beats are conducted retrogradely to the atria in only about 25 per cent of cases, there usually is no interference with the normal sinus mechanism, and therefore the atrial pacemaker is not reset. Under these circumstances, the post extrasystolic pause is "fully compensatory" (Fig. 11–1).

Incidence

Ventricular premature beats compose the most common form of rhythm disturbance observed, both in normal individuals and in those with cardiac abnormalities. Continuous monitoring of patients with acute myocardial infarction has confirmed the presence of ventricular premature beats in the vast majority of these patients (Julian et al., 1964; Meltzer and Kitchell, 1966; Lown et al., 1967; Brown et al., 1965; Stock et al., 1967). Ventricular premature beats were also present in 62 per cent of 300 actively employed and presumably healthy middle-aged men monitored for six hours (Hinkle et al., 1969). Clinically detectable heart disease is observed in only a small percentage of the general population with premature beats; only 26 of 165 (16%) individuals in one series had evidence of coronary heart disease (Chiang et al., 1969). A higher incidence of disease is found when patients are studied for suspected or known heart disease, as in a hospital population. Thus, it should be emphasized that the significance of ventricular premature beats depends primarily upon the presence, type, and severity of the underlying cardiac disorder.

Etiology

Subjects with premature beats may be divided into three groups: 1) those

136

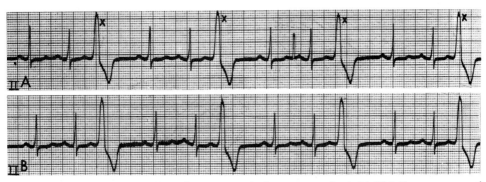

Figure 11–1 The rhythm strip shows frequent ventricular premature beats (x). Note the appearance of a ventricular premature beat every third beat (ventricular trigeminy). These beats do not disturb the normal sinus mechanism, and the post-extrasystolic pauses are fully compensatory (the R-R interval encompassing the ventricular premature beat is double the normal R-R interval). The R-X coupling interval is fixed.

whose hearts are normal; 2) a borderline group in whom underlying heart disease may be suspected because of age or other factors but cannot be demonstrated clinically; and 3) those patients with frank cardiac abnormalities.

In patients with overt heart disease, the most common etiologic disorders are 1) coronary disease, particularly in the acute stage; 2) cardiomyopathies; 3) hypertensive heart disease; 4) rheumatic heart disease; 5) mitral valve prolapse; and 6) congestive heart failure of any etiology.

In patients with normal hearts, as well as those with the above cardiac abnormalities, premature beats may be evoked by a multiplicity of other factors:

1. Autonomic and central nervous system influences. Parasympathetic stimuli may abolish, induce, or have no effect on premature beats. Vagolytic agents, however, generally decrease or abolish premature beats by increasing the heart rate. Sympathetic stimuli are frequently arrhythmogenic.
2. Alterations in certain physiologic states, particularly in pH (both alkalosis and acidosis) and electrolytes (most frequently hypokalemia and hypocalcemia) (Davidson and Surawicz, 1967).
3. Various drugs, including digitalis, sympathomimetic amines, quinidine and other antiarrhythmic agents, calcium, and certain anesthetic agents (particularly cyclopropane).
4. Exercise, which frequently abolishes or decreases premature beats, may elicit ectopic beats, particularly in patients with cardiac abnormalities (notably coronary heart disease — Helfant et al., 1974).
5. Reflexes arising from the gastrointestinal, biliary, and genitourinary tracts, or other viscera.
6. Cigarettes, coffee, or tea.
7. Sudden increases in blood pressure, particularly those produced by isometric exercise, such as heavy lifting.
8. Infections.

Mechanisms (See Chapter 2)

RE-ENTRY

Following a normally conducted impulse, a portion of myocardium may become more refractory than the adjacent area, so that when the next impulse arrives this region is unresponsive and the impulse is of necessity conducted around it. As this area belatedly becomes responsive, the impulse that initially bypassed it may then return and excite it in a retrograde fashion. This late-activated tissue then serves in effect as a potential site of activation for surrounding areas, producing a premature complex.

Automaticity

An ectopic or automatic focus may result in ventricular arrhythmias when its automaticity increases as a result of a change in the slope of diastolic depolarization, in the level of the resting potential, and in the threshold potential.

Ectopic or automatic arrhythmias are frequently manifested as parasystolic rhythms. *Parasystole* may be defined as a persistent and regular ectopic focus coexistent with the dominant pacemaker (usually sinus), located in any part of the conduction system but usually in the ventricles (Fig. 11–2). The inherent rate of the parasystolic focus may range from 20 to 400 beats per minute, having an almost perfect rhythmicity. However, the focus may be only intermittently active.

Normally, the parasystolic focus is not depolarized by impulses from the dominant pacemaker, which arive at a time when it ordinarily would be expected to depolarize the area; this situation is described as "entrance block."

Thus, the parasystolic focus may originate impulses, but impulses traversing the surrounding muscle usually do not affect it. Conversely, "exit block" refers to an inhibition of conduction of the impulse originating from the parasystolic focus to the surrounding tissue.

In a long rhythm strip, premature beats of parasystolic origin can be seen to possess a fixed relationship to each other (although at times beats do not occur when expected). This finding is due to the fact that parasystolic depolarization may occur during the absolute refractory period of the ventricle. When this occurs, the interval between these parasystolic beats may be an exact multiple of those intervals observed between the regularly recurring beats of the ectopic center. The coupling intervals of parasystolic beats are variable. Occasionally the ectopic beat is not seen at an interval where it would be expected to capture the ventricle. At such times, an "exit block" from the parasystolic focus may be present.

Clinical Manifestations

The patient may be subjectively conscious of symptoms that he describes as "palpitations," "the heart turns over," "the heart stops," or "a catch in the throat." If there is a run of premature beats, the subjective sensation may be

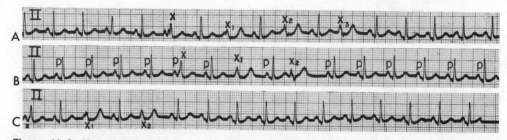

Figure 11–2   Ventricular parasystole. (*A, B,* and *C* represent a continuous strip. The intervals between the ventricular beats are identical.)

(*A*) Note the QRS complexes at X, X_1, X_2, and X_3.

(*B*) Note fusion beat at X indicating that these beats are ventricular in origin. Note also at X_2 that the P wave occurs after the QRS.

(*C*) Note the widened QRS complexes at X, X_1 and X_2.

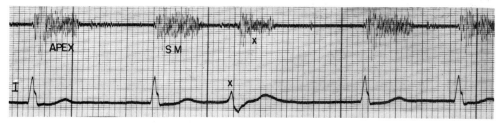

Figure 11-3 Effect of premature beat on character of systolic murmur. Atrial fibrillation. Beat at X represents ventricular premature beat or aberration of a supraventricular beat. The pansystolic murmur recorded at the apex is characteristic of mitral insufficiency. Note that the intensity of the murmur is diminished with the premature ventricular beat at X.

interpreted as "substernal discomfort," "pressure," or "precordial pain." General symptoms such as anxiety, diaphoresis, weakness, and breathlessness may occur. Conversely, many subjects are entirely asymptomatic.

Frequently, the premature beats are not experienced while the individual is working or engaged in an absorbing activity, but are more troublesome while resting, particularly while lying in bed. While the premature beat in itself may be of little or no consequence, the thought of heart disease often causes the individual grave anxiety and he or she may believe that a serious threat to life is imminent. When they occur frequently, these symptoms may cause a profound psychological disturbance with a cardiac fixation and fear of sudden death.

The characteristic auscultatory findings consist of an interruption of the normal rhythm by a premature beat or beats, followed by a pause that is usually but not invariably compensatory. However, the characteristics of the heart sounds vary in different cases. A short, early systolic murmur of low intensity may be present with ventricular premature beats that is not heard with normal beats. Systolic murmurs of the regurgitant type are attenuated, while those of the ejection type may be increased by the premature beats. Ejection murmurs may be increased in the post extrasystolic beats (Fig. 11-3).

Electrocardiogram

Ventricular premature beats may arise from almost any region of the ventricles or the interventricular septum. The resultant abnormal activation produces QRS complexes that are slurred and widened. The T waves following the premature beats are usually large and opposite in direction to the deflection of the QRS complex. However, widening and notching of the premature ventricular complex is not sufficient for the diagnosis, since this may also result from aberrant conduction or may occur in patients with a bundle branch block or an intraventricular conduction defect.

Ventricular premature beats may be isolated or numerous; they may appear to arise from one or several foci; or they may also occur in pairs or runs of three or more beats, thereby constituting ventricular tachycardia (Fig. 11-4).

Ventricular premature beats are usually conducted to the A-V junction, less commonly into the atria. The atrial beats that occur following ventricular premature depolarizations usually arise in the S-A node and, therefore, have a normal configuration. Ventricular premature beats usually do not disturb the normal sequence of atrial depolarization when retrograde atrial activation does not occur. The sinus P wave that occurs during or just after the ventricular premature beat often cannot pro-

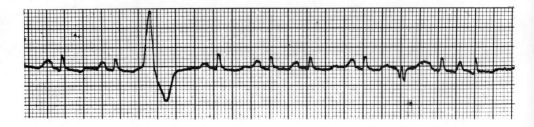

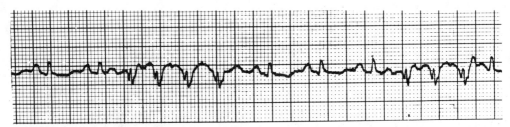

Figure 11–4 Continuous rhythm strip showing ventricular premature beats of different morphology. Note the presence of ventricular premature beats of different QRS configuration (beat 3 and beat 8) in the top part of the strip. Runs of ventricular premature beats (ventricular tachycardia) are noted in the lower part of the strip. These ventricular premature beats are similar to beat #8 (top) in configuration.

duce a ventricular response because it arrives at the A-V junction or ventricle during its refractory period. The first ventricular contraction after the premature beat will then be in response to the subsequent P wave. The interval between the premature beat and the next ventricular beat is, therefore, longer than the usual R-R interval and is referred to as "fully compensatory." The R-R interval between conducted beats under these circumstances is usually twice normal (Fig. 11–5).

If a premature beat occurs early and the heart rate is relatively slow, the A-V junction may be sufficiently recovered from its refractory period so that the next sinus impulse is conducted with a normal ventricular response. No compensatory pause follows. Such a premature beat is referred to as an interpolated extrasystole. The P-R interval following the interpolated beat is often prolonged (Fig. 11–6).

The majority of ventricular premature beats (particularly, although not invariably, those due to re-entry — Michelson et al., 1978) have a constant coupling

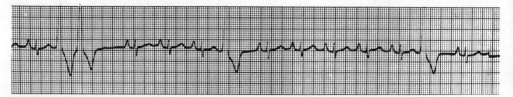

Figure 11–5 Rhythm strip demonstrating the presence of frequent ventricular premature beats. Note that the R-R interval encompassing the single ventricular premature beat is twice the normal R-R interval. This is due to the fact that ventricular premature beats usually do not disturb the normal sequence of atrial depolarization.

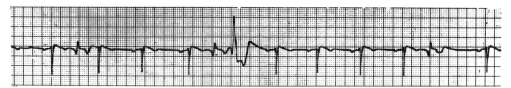

Figure 11–6 Rhythm strip demonstrating frequent ventricular premature beats. Note the presence of an interpolated ventricular premature beat (beat #2). The R-R interval encompassing this ventricular premature beat is the same as the normal R-R interval. Some variation in normal R-R intervals seen in this strip is due to sinus arrhythmia.

interval with the preceding supraventricular beat. Thus, the R-R' interval is similar when the extra beats are of ventricular origin. When present, *"constant"* or *"fixed"* coupling intervals are very useful diagnostically, since aberrant beats and parasystolic beats usually do not have constant coupling intervals (Surawicz and MacDonald, 1964; Moe et al., 1977; Michelson et al., 1978).

Another observation that is of considerable diagnostic importance when present is *ventricular fusion*. Ventricular fusion beats result from the "fusion" of a supraventricular impulse with a ventricular beat. The supraventricular impulse may have its origin in the sinus node, atrium, or A-V junction. (In the

most common form of fusion, a ventricular premature impulse fuses with a sinus impulse.) Fusion beats can be readily identified by the fact that they have a configuration that is intermediate between the ventricular and supraventricular complexes. When analyzing such a complex, it can be seen that the initial portion resembles the beginning of a pure ventricular premature beat and the terminal portion resembles the terminal portion of a ventricular complex from a sinus origin (or vice versa) (Fig. 11–7).

Differential Diagnosis

Ventricular premature beats may be morphologically indistinguishable

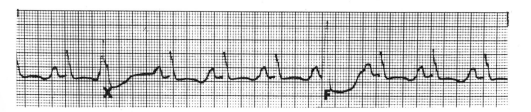

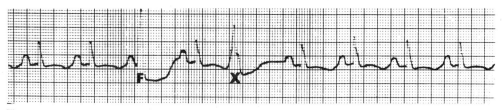

Figure 11–7 Continuous rhythm strip demonstrating ventricular premature beats (X) and fusion beats (F). Note that the QRS of the fusion beats is of intermediate contour between the sinus beat and the ventricular premature beat.

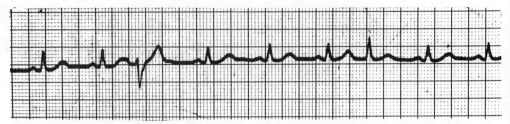

Figure 11–8 Rhythm strip showing the difference in post-extrasystolic compensatory pause between a ventricular premature beat (beat 3) and a premature atrial beat with aberrancy (beat 7). See text.

from supraventricular premature beats with aberrant conduction. There are, however, a number of parameters that may help to distinguish the two: 1) the presence of a preceding P wave early in the cycle suggests the possibility of an atrial premature beat with aberration; 2) premature atrial or junctional beats usually reset the sinus pacemaker, hence the post extrasystolic pause is more often fully compensatory in ventricular beats and less compensatory (the R-R interval for conducted beats is less than twice normal) in supraventricular beats (Fig. 11–8); 3) ventricular premature beats frequently have a constant coupling interval with the preceding beat (in contrast to aberrant beats); 4) the presence of fusion beats indicates the ventricular origin of the premature complexes; 5) the supraventricular beats with aberrancy generally show a right bundle branch type pattern or a triphasic RSR' form in lead V_1, while the ventricular premature beats show a QR or a monophasic R pattern (exceptions, however, not infrequently occur); 6) in the presence of atrial fib-

rillation, a study of cycle sequence may show that the abnormal beat occurs in the sequence of a long pause followed by a short pause. Abnormal ventricular beats in this sequence are more likely to be aberrant than ectopic. Thus, when an anomalous beat ends in a short cycle following a long cycle, the beat is generally supraventricular with aberration (Ashman phenomenon) (Fig. 11–9).

Treatment

The treatment of ventricular premature beats must take into consideration the clinical condition of the patient, particularly the underlying cardiac status and its etiology, the associated symptoms produced, the severity of the arrhythmia, and the patient's reaction to it. In the presence of occasional premature beats, the patient is often unaware of the arrhythmia, and specific treatment is generally unnecessary. In some patients, reduction or elimination of smoking, excessive caffein intake, or

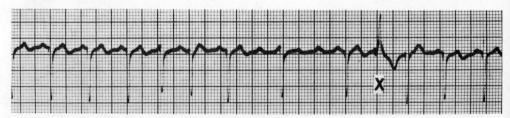

Figure 11–9 *Aberrant conduction.* Note that the aberrantly conducted beat (X) has a short coupling interval whereas the beat preceding it (which is normal in contour) follows a long pause. The aberrant beat has a right bundle branch block configuration.

certain drugs will diminish the frequency of premature beats. The patient who complains of sensations or symptoms due to premature beats is often considerably relieved by a thorough examination. In patients with no evidence of heart disease, reassurance may be all the therapy required. When the premature beats are due to or associated with an underlying cardiac dysfunction, therapy should generally be directed toward the underlying disease. When the premature beats are very frequent or multifocal, or occur in salvos, treatment is usually initiated after a careful search to identify and correct precipitating non-cardiac factors (see Etiology).

The most important antiarrhythmic drugs that may be used to abolish premature beats are lidocaine (in an acute setting), procaine amide, disopyramide, quinidine, diphenylhydantoin, beta blockers (especially if an anxiety factor or excessive sympathetic tone is present), digitalis (when the premature beats are associated with congestive failure and are not caused by digitalis toxicity), and atropine, when ectopic beats are related to an underlying bradycardia. These drugs are discussed in greater detail in Chapter 23. Although each of these agents alone or in combination is known to be effective, the selection of a drug or drugs and their dosages is empirical.

Prognosis

The prognosis of individuals with ventricular premature beats is determined by the presence or absence of heart disease, its etiology and severity, and the severity of the ventricular arrhythmia and its response to therapy.

In individuals with clinically *normal hearts*, if premature beats are infrequent, the condition may be considered relatively benign. However, in one study, the likelihood of sudden death occurring over a 6 year interval in adults was six times as high in the group with documented premature beats as in a group without this arrhythmia (Chiang et al., 1969). A subsequent publication from the same group indicated that the ventricular premature beats were so frequently associated with other factors predisposing to sudden death that the relative contributions of the ventricular premature beats to subsequent cardiac demise could not be determined. The Framingham study also indicated that the presence of a ventricular premature beat on a routine electrocardiogram was of minimal significance relative to sudden death (Weiss, 1969).

In patients with definite *heart disease*, the presence of premature beats may be a cause of concern, especially if the arrhythmia is severe. The appearance of ectopic beats or a significant increase in their frequency may indicate a worsening of the underlying condition. Either may forewarn of ventricular tachycardia, ventricular fibrillation, Stokes-Adams attacks, or sudden death. This is particulary true in the acute coronary heart disease setting, including myocardial infarction, when the danger of sudden death due to a ventricular arrhythmia is particularly high (see Chapter 15).

In an extensive review of the prognostic significance of ventricular premature beats, Moss and Akiyama (1976) indicate that in addition to the underlying heart disease, the severity of the arrhythmia is also important. The parameters that affected the prognosis were 1) the frequency of ventricular premature beats; 2) their prematurity; 3) the presence or absence of bigeminy, trigeminy, pairs, salvos, tachycardia, and multiform appearance; 4) the electrophysiologic mechanisms involved in genesis of ventricular premature beats (i.e., re-entry or automaticity); 5) the location of origin of the ventricular premature beats (i.e., right or left ventricle).

The *frequency* of ventricular beats had

been utilized in determining the prognosis of patients both in epidemiological studies and in patients with myocardial infarction. Ventricular bigeminy, whether induced by digitalis toxicity or myocardial infarction, has frequently been premonitory to the development of ventricular fibrillation. In an ambulatory monitoring study by Hinkle and coworkers (1969), ventricular bigeminy was associated with a tenfold increase in the risk of sudden death from coronary heart disease during a 4 year followup. Repetitive and multiform ventricular premature beats occurring in pairs or salvos also have ominous prognostic significance. The Coronary Drug Project study (Coronary Drug Project Research Group, 1973) demonstrated a twofold increase in 3 year mortality in post-infarction patients with ventricular premature beats in pairs or runs, as opposed to patients with ventricular premature beats without salvos. Similarly, Kotler and associates (1973) found that multiform ventricular premature beats after recovery from myocardial infarction were associated with poor prognosis, being associated with an 18 per cent 2 year mortality. Other studies, however, indicate that no absolute prognostic implications can be derived from the presence or absence of multiform ventricular premature beats (Coronary Drug Project Research Group, 1973).

The *prematurity* of ventricular premature beats can be assessed qualitatively by observing the presence or absence of ventricular premature beats on the T wave of the preceding beat (R on T phenomenon) or using quantitative indices (R-R'/QT ratio). Of the 80 cardiac patients whose electrocardiograms revealed R on T phenomenon, Smirk and Palmer (1960) reported 22 sudden deaths. This observation was later reaffirmed by other investigators (Day, 1963; Brown et al., 1963; Wolff et al., 1968).

To categorize the relative severity of ventricular irritability, several *grading systems* have been used. The more com-

TABLE 11-1 GRADING SYSTEM FOR VENTRICULAR PREMATURE BEATS (LOWN AND WOLF 1971)

Grade	Original	Modified
0	No VPB	No VPB
1	<10 VPB/hour	Occasional isolated VPB
2	>10 VPB/hour	1/min or 30/hour
3	Multiform VPB	Multiform VPB
4	Couplets	Repetitive VPBs a) couplets b) salvos
5	Ventricular tachycardia	Early VPB

monly used have been those of Lown and Wolf (Table 11–1). Utilizing these criteria, Kotler and coworkers (1973) demonstrated that the percentage of deaths following myocardial infarction was much greater in patients who had grade 2 or grade 3 ventricular premature beats than in those with grade 0 or grade 1.

In patients with acute myocardial infarction a frequency of ventricular premature beats greater than five per minute has long been considered to presage ventricular tachycardia and fibrillation (Lown and coworkers, 1967). However, later reports have failed to support the benefit of antiarrhythmic measures in such a setting (Mather et al., 1971; Chopra et al., 1971; Darby et al., 1972). Bennett and Pentecost (1972) found that of the 24 patients experiencing cardiac arrest after admission to the coronary care unit, 19 per cent had no premonitory ventricular beats, 7 per cent had ventricular premature beats recorded for less than 5 minutes before the arrest and 75 per cent had ventricular premature beats for more than 5 minutes. In the latter group, the frequency of ventricular premature beats was less than five per minute. The prematurity of ventricular premature beats in this setting has also long been viewed as a premonitory sign of ventricular tachycardia or fibrillation.

A widespread belief exists that ventricular premature complexes of right ventricular contour (appearing morphologically as an LBBB pattern) have more benign implications than those originating from the left ventricle (appearing as an RBBB pattern). Thus, Lown and associates suggested that the site of origin of a ventricular premature complex may provide pertinent information relative to the risk of sudden death. This is consistent with observations that in persons with a normal heart nearly all ventricular premature complexes arise from the right ventricle. Moreover, when Hiss and coworkers examined the relation between age and the site of origin of ventricular premature complexes, they found that beats of right ventricular origin occurred more frequently than those of left ventricular origin in younger patients, who presumably had more normal hearts. However, the proportion of ventricular premature complexes arising from the right ventricle increased with age, whereas the frequency of those from the left ventricle remained unchanged. Thus, the clinical implications of the site of origin of ventricular premature complexes in patients with a history suggestive of coronary heart disease are unclear. To define more precisely the relationship between the site of origin of ventricular premature complexes and the presence and severity of coronary heart disease in patients with a chest pain syndrome, 39 patients with ventricular premature complexes of right or left ventricular contour who were undergoing cardiac catheterization and coronary arteriography for evaluation of chest discomfort were studied. The findings indicated that in patients with a chest pain syndrome there is no relationship between the site of origin of ventricular premature complexes and either the prevalence or severity of coronary artery disease.

PAROXYSMAL VENTRICULAR TACHYCARDIA

General Features

The diagnosis of ventricular tachycardia is made when three or more ventricular premature beats occur in succession. On routine ECG or more frequently on telemetric or ambulatory monitoring, ventricular tachycardia may evolve as ventricular premature beats that become more numerous and are then followed by a coupled rhythm progressing to sequences of two, three, or more. Not infrequently, however, the paroxysm can occur following a single premature beat. Ventricular tachycardia may last seconds, minutes, or hours, and less commonly days or rarely even weeks. The obvious danger of this arrhythmia lies in its strong predisposition to deteriorate into ventricular fibrillation.

Incidence and Etiology

Ventricular tachycardia is observed more commonly in men (69%) than women (31%). Most cases appear between the ages of 40 and 80 years, with a peak incidence in the sixth decade (MacKenzie and Pascual, 1964).

Paroxysmal ventricular tachycardia usually, although not invariably, occurs in the presence of severe heart disease. By far the most important condition associated with this arrhythmia is coronary heart disease with or without myocardial infarction. Approximately 35 per cent of patients who develop ventricular tachycardia have previously suffered a myocardial infarction, and as many as 60 per cent of patients with acute myocardial infarction may have ventricular tachycardia at some time during their hospital course (Cohn et al., 1966). Patients with ventricular aneurysm resulting from an old myocardial infarction may have a high incidence of ventricular tachycardia. Digitalis toxicity is the causative factor in 25 per cent of cases of ventricular tachycardia, as reported in several series. Severe cardiomyopathic, rheumatic, hypertensive, and infiltrative (i.e., sarcoid or amyloid) heart disease as well as acid-base or electrolyte abnormalities (i.e., hypokalemia or hypocalcemia) may also be causative factors.

More recently, ventricular tachycardia has been reported to occur in 6 per cent of patients with mitral valve prolapse (Swartz et al., 1977). In addition, those factors which predispose patients to ventricular premature beats may also cause ventricular tachycardia.

Occasionally, paroxysmal ventricular tachycardia may be observed in the absence of organic heart disease (Lesch et al., 1967). Some authors have observed 5 to 17 per cent of patients to be in this category (Amburst and Levine, 1962). A psychosomatic etiology has been reported as a precipitating factor, although the precipitation of bouts of paroxysmal ventricular tachycardia with emotional stress is only occasionally encountered.

Mechanism

Ventricular tachycardia may be said to consist of a series of successive ventricular premature beats. Such beats, occurring alone or in various combinations, are usually observed prior to an attack and often follow the paroxysm. The underlying mechanisms are similar to those of ventricular premature beats and include the following: 1) macro- or microre-entry, which is particularly likely to occur around ischemic or infarcted tissue. This mechanism has been emphasized in recent reports, which indicate that sustained ventricular tachycardia can be initiated or terminated in a large number of patients by critically timed test stimuli using programmed single or paired electrical stimulation of the heart (Wellens et al., 1972, 1974, 1976; Josephson et al., 1978) (see Chapter 2). 2) Increased automaticity of an ectopic focus firing at a rapid rate. 3) A parasystolic focus may initiate the paroxysms if the parasystolic pacemaker initiates impulses at a rapid rate. This would presuppose the presence of an exit block, which is normally operative and which tends to prevent the escape of impulses from the parasystolic pacemaker. When this block diminishes or disappears, it allows the ectopic impulses to give rise to premature beats, resulting in a paroxysmal tachycardia.

Hemodynamics

In a study of the hemodynamic alterations caused by atrial and ventricular tachycardia of identical rates, it was found that the cardiac output, coronary blood flow, and mean arterial pressure undergo essentially the same changes in both forms of tachycardia; however, the effects of ventricular tachycardia are more marked (Wegria et al., 1958). Similarly, it has been demonstrated that artificial pacing from a site in one ventricular chamber that results in an abnormal QRS complex is accompanied by a decrease in cardiac output, whereas pacing at the His bundle results in a normal QRS and normal output, provided that the ventricular rate is slow enough to allow for sufficient diastolic filling (Wallace, 1966).

During cardiac catheterization, the occurrence of ventricular tachycardia is usually accompanied by marked hypotension. When the paroxysms persist for a long period, certain circulatory adjustments are made. However, in the presence of coronary disease, this sudden decrease in coronary blood flow adds markedly to the degree of coronary insufficiency and may be fatal. There is usually a marked fall in cardiac output and consequently in cerebral as well as renal blood flow. This is probably due to the fact that ventricular tachycardia usually occurs in patients with myocardial disease, often of a severe grade, and is often associated with profoundly deleterious hemodynamic effects.

Pathology

No distinct pathology is observed; it is that of the underlying conditions already mentioned.

Diagnostic Features

The diagnosis of ventricular tachycardia depends on the electrocardiogram and is often difficult. Heart rate usually ranges from 140 to 200 beats per minute. Patients are usually older, have a history of severe heart disease — e.g., coronary heart disease (usually with a recent myocardial infarction), congestive heart failure, or digitalis toxicity — and usually appear quite ill.

Symptoms and Signs

The symptoms observed during ventricular tachycardia resemble those of any tachyarrhythmia but are usually more marked because of the more severe hemodynamic alterations as compared to supraventricular arrhythmias and its more frequent association with severe ventricular dysfunction. Substernal pain, dyspnea, and syncopal attacks are commonly observed, and occasionally sudden collapse or shock may occur. In patients with either intermittent or persistent paroxysmal ventricular tachycardia not resulting from an acute myocardial infarction, palpitations, weakness, and chest pain are equally apparent; dyspnea appears most often in subjects with persistent ventricular tachycardia. Such patients have a poor prognosis: complications are frequent, and death may be sudden. With the recent improvements in therapy, prolonged attacks are fortunately uncommon. The minor episodes, lasting only seconds or minutes, may present relatively mild or no symptoms, even if repetitive.

The physical signs during ventricular tachycardia are variable and depend upon concomitant atrial activity (Wilson et al., 1964; Harvey and Ronan, 1966) and underlying cardiovascular status. When ventricular tachycardia is accompanied by A-V dissociation, as usually is the case, changing intensity of the first heart sound, beat-to-beat variation in systolic blood pressure (intermittent Korotkov's sounds), and intermittent cannon "a" waves in the jugular pulse may be observed as a result of the changing relationship between atrial and ventricular contractions. If, however, the ventricular tachycardia is associated with 1:1 retrograde conduction, regular cannon waves in the jugular venous pulse and constant intensity of the first heart sound may occur.

Electrocardiogram

The electrocardiographic criteria for ventricular tachycardia include the following: 1) the ventricular complexes are widened (0.12 second or more). 2) The ventricular rate is regular or only slightly irregular at rates of 140 to 250 beats per minute (occasionally as low as 110 to 130). 3) *Atrioventricular dissociation* occurs in the majority of cases, with the atria beating more slowly than the ventricles (Fig. 11–10). However, atrioventricular dissociation does not completely exclude a junctional origin of the tachycardia with aberrant conduction. Conversely, 1:1 ventriculoatrial conduction is not rare in ventricular tachycardia. 4) The QRS complexes frequently have the same morphology as prior or subsequent ventricular premature

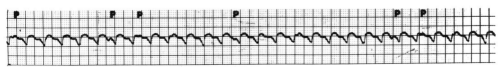

Figure 11–10 Rhythm strip demonstrating ventricular tachycardia. Note that the QRS is wide (0.12 sec.). The ventricular rate is 150 per minute and the P waves can be identified with a rate of 97 per minute, indicating atrioventricular dissociation.

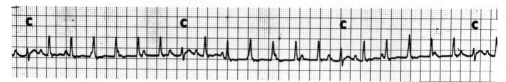

Figure 11–11   Rhythm strip showing ventricular tachycardia (rate 136/min) and occasional capture beats (C) with normal QRS complex. Note that the P wave of the capture beat (C) is conducted with a prolonged P-R interval indicating the presence of first degree A-V block.

beats on the electrocardiogram. 5) The diagnosis is more definitely made when occasional narrow QRS complexes are observed. These are *capture* beats conducted from the atria (Fig. 11–11). They occur when a supraventricular impulse arrives at a time when neither the junction nor the ventricles are refractory, resulting in a normal QRS complex or ventricular *fusion* beats (from combined ventricular and supraventricular impulses). The QRS in this circumstance is intermediate in contour between the normal QRS and that of the ventricular tachycardia. These beats are diagnostic of ventricular tachycardia. In atrial fibrillation, aberrant beats with the configuration of right bundle branch block and, less commonly, of left bundle branch block may be observed; these may simulate ventricular premature beats and paroxysms of ventricular tachycardia. They are usually more grossly irregular than ventricular tachycardia and do not exhibit atrioventricular dissociation, capture, or fusion. Atrial flutter with rapid ventricular responses may also result in aberrantly conducted beats simulating the QRS contour seen in ventricular tachycardias (Fig. 11–12). In doubtful cases, careful study of the initial beat of the paroxysm in all possible leads should be undertaken to determine whether a P wave precedes or is superimposed upon the QRS complex, indicating an atrial or junctional origin (Kistin, 1966). The diagnosis of paroxysmal ventricular tachycardia may be suspected but should not be made unless it meets the aforementioned criteria.

In some cases, the diagnosis cannot be made with absolute certainty unless an esophageal lead or a His bundle electrogram is recorded (see Chapters 4 and 14) during a paroxysm. This may help to determine the origin of the arrhythmia; in the supraventricular beat with aberration, the ventricular activation is preceded by a His spike with a normal or prolonged H-V interval, while with ventricular beats the origin of the impulse is distal to the bundle of His, and thus a His spike does not precede the ventricular activation. In some cases, retrograde activation of the atrium (ventriculoatrial conduction) may take place and the His spike may follow ventricular activation (see Chapter 14).

There are three common types:
1. Those in which the ventricular tachycardia is sustained and all of the ventricular complexes present the same configuration with a rate over 110 and usually 150 to 250 beats per

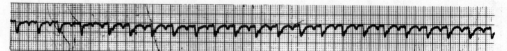

Figure 11–12   Atrial flutter with aberrant QRS complexes and rapid ventricular response simulating ventricular tachycardia. Note that a normal QRS complex can be identified (QRS 4) and flutter waves are seen in cycle 4.

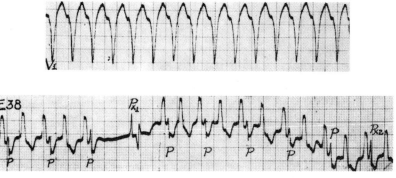

Figure 11-13 Ventricular tachycardia. V₁ and esophageal lead recording.

(A) (V₁) Note the presence of a regular paroxysmal tachycardia with a ventricular rate of 176 per minute. The QRS complexes are widened and notched, and no distinct P waves are observed.

(B) In the esophageal leads, the ventricular rate is 176 per minute, the P waves are easily seen and occur at the rate of 88 per minute.

minute (Fig. 11-13). This sustained ventricular tachycardia is usually associated with serious myocardial derangement and is often premonitory to ventricular flutter or fibrillation.

2. The repetitive type, characterized by short frequent runs of ventricular premature beats occurring in groups of three to six complexes (Fig. 11-14). They may be present for minutes, days, months, or even years.

3. An accelerated *idioventricular tachycardia* ("slow ventricular tachycardia"), which resembles idioventricular rhythm in many respects. The rate is usually 55 to 110 beats per minute, rarely exceeding 100. It usually occurs in association with an acute myocardial infarction and apparently results from an enhancement of latent pacemaker fibers in the Purkinje network.

Often depression of the S-A node during sinus bradycardia or the slow phase of sinus arrhythmia is also present (Fig. 11-15). It is usually observed only for short periods (up to 30 cycles) because of intermittent exit block or sinus capture (Figs. 11-16, 11-17, and 11-18).

Rothfeld et al. (1968) have studied 100 consecutive patients with accelerated idioventricular rhythm by constant electrocardiographic monitoring during the postinfarction period. Thirty-six patients had one or more episodes of accelerated idioventricular rhythm that did not progress to rapid ventricular tachycardia or fibrillation. No apparent deleterious effect on survival was found. More recent studies indicate that the arrhythmia occurs in 9 to 23 per cent of patients with myocardial infarction (Rothfeld et al., 1970; Norris and Mercer, 1974; Lichstein et al., 1975).

Although acute myocardial infarction

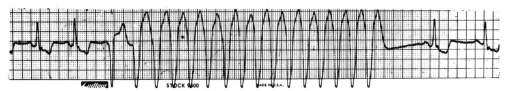

Figure 11-14 Paroxysm of ventricular tachycardia reverting to sinus rhythm.

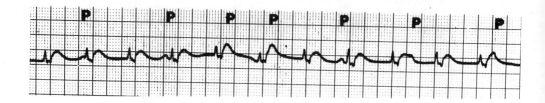

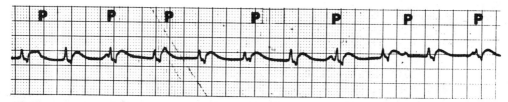

Figure 11–15   Continuous rhythm strip showing slow ventricular tachycardia (ventricular rate 94/min). Note the presence of A-V dissociation and marked sinus arrhythmia. Also called accelerated idioventricular rhythm.

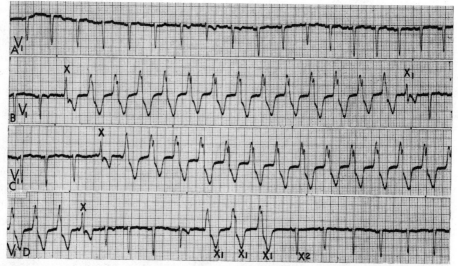

Figure 11–16   (All leads are V_1) Accelerated idioventricular tachycardia, showing fusion beats, and beginning and ending of paroxysm.

(A) Heart rate is 91 per minute in the presence of sinus rhythm.

(B) Note the occurrence of the tachycardia with widened, aberrant QRS complexes and a ventricular rate of 100 per minute. Note the fusion beat (X) at the beginning of the paroxysm and (X_1) at the end of the paroxysm.

(C) Note the recurrence following the fusion beat at X.

(D) Note the end of the paroxysm with a fusion beat at X and the restoration of normal sinus rhythm for four beats ending at X_1, followed by three ventricular beats (X_1); normal sinus beats staring at X_2 are observed at the end of the strip.

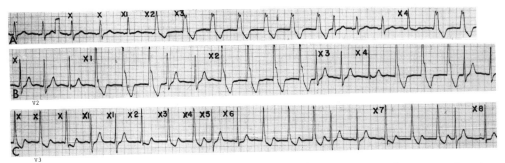

Figure 11–17 Periods of normal sinus rhythm showing beginning and ending of paroxysms of accelerated idioventricular rhythm and fusion beats.

(A) (Lead III) Note normal sinus beats at X. The P waves are diphasic. Note the occurrence of widened QRS complexes with the rate of 75 per minute starting at X_3. X_2 is a beat of intermediate width. Another fusion beat is observed at X_4.

(B) (V_2) Shows two normal sinus beats and one fusion beat at X followed by widened QRS complexes, apparently ventricular in origin, starting at X_1. This is repeated at X_2 for a series of four beats with the resumption of normal sinus beats. A fusion beat is again at X_4.

(C) (V_3) Note the widened QRS complexes starting at X, followed by sinus beats at X_1, a fusion beat at X_2, widened QRS beats at X_3, a normal sinus beat at X_5, and a fusion beat at X_6. Two other fusion beats are observed at X_7 and X_8.

is the most common cause for the occurrence of accelerated idioventricular rhythm, the disorder has also been found in patients with digitalis intoxication (Schamroth, 1968), rheumatic heart disease, primary myocardial disease, and hypertensive heart disease; it has also been found in patients with no evidence of cardiac disease (Massumi and Ali, 1970; Gallagher et al., 1971). Since spontaneous remission is common, this arrhythmia usually requires no therapy. However, it is not necessarily benign because it occurs on the basis of a serious pathophysiologic disturbance and may be associated with or be the forerunner of more serious types of ectopic tachycardias; that is, a more serious type of ventricular tachycardia (Julian et al., 1970; Lichstein et al., 1975; and Sclarovsky et al., 1978). Lichstein et al. (1975) have postulated that in

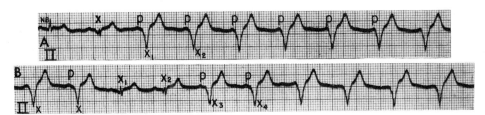

Figure 11–18 Accelerated idioventricular rhythm.

(A) Note normal beat (NB) (rate 68 per minute) ventricular beats starting at X_1 (rate of 79 per minute) and fusion beat at X.

(B) X and X are ventricular beats; X_1 and X_2 are fusion beats, and accelerated idioventricular tachycardia continues at X_3. (The actual rate may be twice the given value due to 2:1 exit block.)

some instances, accelerated ventricular rhythm may represent a true ventricular tachycardia with exit block.

DIFFERENTIAL DIAGNOSIS OF VENTRICULAR TACHYCARDIA

As discussed earlier, the differentiation of tachycardia and supraventricular tachycardia with aberrant conduction is often difficult. Long and multiple electrocardiographic rhythm strips are critical in order to determine the presence or absence of A-V dissociation, fusion, and capture, as well as the initiation or termination of a paroxysm. In addition, the electrocardiographic pattern obtained during normal sinus rhythm are of prime importance. The use of esophageal or intra-atrial leads may at times be helpful in the differential diagnosis by demonstrating the atrial mechanism. Similarly, the availability of His bundle recordings may allow more exact diagnosis of the origin of the tachycardia; however, data derived from this technique are rarely required for therapy. It is axiomatic that when the diagnosis is in doubt, prompt treatment should be instituted for ventricular tachycardia.

SUPRAVENTRICULAR ARRHYTHMIAS SIMULATING VENTRICULAR TACHYCARDIA

Many tachycardias that appear to be ventricular in origin actually arise in the atria or A-V junction. Supraventricular arrhythmias often are associated with abnormal QRS complexes as a result of incomplete recovery of the ventricular conduction fibers prior to the arrival of the next supraventricular impulse. This sequence may lead to an abnormal QRS pattern.

In the presence of widened or abnormal QRS complexes, the following criteria suggest a supraventricular origin (Kistin, 1966):

1. The arrhythmia starts with an ectopic premature P wave which may be confirmed by esophageal or intra-atrial leads.
2. The QRS-to-P interval is too short to be explained by retrograde conduction from a ventricular focus.
3. The configuration of the QRS is the same as that which results from conduction from a known supraventricular site before, during, or after the arrhythmia.
4. The P wave and QRS complex are so related as to suggest that the QRS complexes depend on supraventricular activity (i.e., intermittent block of conduction to the ventricles or Wenckebach phenomenon).
5. The arrhythmia can be terminated by carotid sinus pressure.
6. Clearly establishing the type of atrial mechanism by esophageal leads may definitely rule out atrial tachycardia, junctional tachycardia, or atrial flutter.

An atrial rate slower than the ventricular rate and A-V dissociation does not absolutely establish the diagnosis of ventricular tachycardia, and it is sometimes impossible to differentiate a junctional tachycardia with widened QRS complexes from ventricular tachycardia. However, in our experience, a slower atrial than ventricular rate has, in almost all instances, occurred in a tachycardia of ventricular origin.

VENTRICULAR TACHYCARDIA SIMULATING SUPRAVENTRICULAR TACHYCARDIA

The occurrence of atrial beats with the atrial rate as rapid as that of the ventricles and bearing a constant relationship to the ventricular beat does not rule out a ventricular tachycardia, since these atrial beats may result from retrograde conduction. Indeed, retrograde conduction is not uncommon (Kistin, 1966) (Figs. 11–19 and 11–20). A ventricular origin is difficult to establish in such cases unless associated with fusion and/or capture beats. In view of the

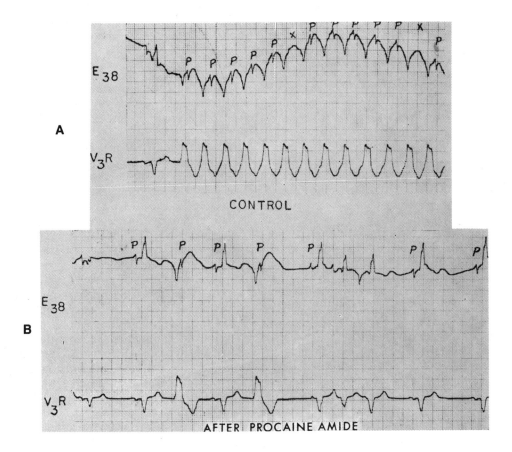

Figure 11–19 Ventricular tachycardia showing retrograde conduction.

(A) The esophageal lead taken at the atrial level is paired with a V_3R lead. Following a normal complex there is a run of ventricular premature beats constituting a paroxysm of ventricular tachycardia. It will be observed in the esophageal lead (E_{38}) that the QRS complex gives rise to a retrograde P wave and that the R-P interval becomes progressively longer until one drops out at X. This sequence is repeated at regular intervals. This represents a V-A Wenckebach phenomenon.

(B) After the administration of procaine amide, there is a return of normal sinus rhythm which is interrupted by frequent ventricular premature beats. Note that the premature beats have the same configuration as the aberrant complexes of the paroxysm and are followed by retrograde P waves in lead E_{38}.

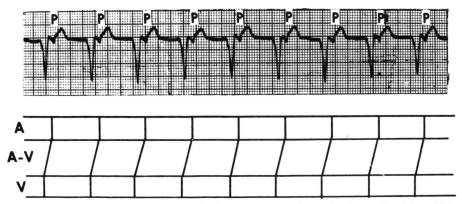

Figure 11–20 Accelerated idioventricular rhythm with retrograde conduction to the atrium. Note the presence of inverted (retrograde) P wave following each QRS complex bearing a constant relationship to the ventricular rate.

153

overriding importance of fusion and capture beats, they should be assiduously searched for with long and repeated rhythm strips.

Treatment

The treatment of ventricular tachycardia depends on the underlying cause (acute myocardial infarction, digitalis toxicity, etc.) and the associated clinical state. These factors will help determine the urgency and intensity of the therapy (Jelinek et al., 1974; Winkle et al., 1976; Denes et al., 1976; Mason et al., 1978; Horowitz et al., 1978). In the treatment of paroxysmal ventricular tachycardia, the methods of choice are the use of 1) drugs, 2) electric countershock, 3) overdrive suppression by artificial pacemaker, and 4) open heart surgery (i.e., ventricular aneurysm resection).

Drugs. Lidocaine is the drug of choice in the therapy of ventricular tachycardia. When lidocaine is ineffective, the drug most commonly employed is intravenous procainamide. If this is ineffective, intravenous diphenylhydantoin may be tried as well as other agents including quinidine, disopyramide, propranolol, potassium, and bretylium. (More detailed indications, dosages, routes of administration, and complications of the agents are discussed in Chapter 23). If the patient is quite ill and the response to drug therapy is not rapid, electric countershock should immediately be instituted if the patient does not respond to an initial or repeated bolus of lidocaine.

Lidocaine, considered to be the therapy of choice, is used prior to electric countershock. It is effective, safe, easy to administer, and rapidly acting. Moreover, when given in therapeutic doses, there is no evidence of myocardial depression of the type commonly observed with other antiarrhythmic drugs. Lidocaine should be administered intravenously in a bolus of 1 mg/kg or 100 mg. It may be effective in as little as 2 minutes and suppresses the arrhythmia for periods up to 20 minutes. An intravenous drip of lidocaine at a rate of 1 to 4 mg per minute is then administered. Recurrences may be treated with a 0.5 to 1 mg/kg lidocaine bolus.

Procainamide is quite effective in the control of ventricular tachycardia. For a rapid effect it should be given intravenously, slowly, in doses of 100 mg every 5 minutes (not exceeding 25 mg/min), to achieve a loading dose of 1000 mg, followed by an intravenous infusion of 1 to 5 mg per minute. The patient may subsequently be placed on an oral maintenance dose.

The use of diphenylhydantoin in therapy of paroxysmal ventricular tachycardia is limited, since other agents are usually more effective. It is particularly useful in ventricular tachycardia due to digitalis toxicity. Occasionally, however, in intravenous doses of 1.0 gram (administered at 25 mg/min) it can be effective. It has been effective in conjunction with procainamide (Helfant, 1968). Bretylium has been shown to be effective in the conversion of ventricular tachycardia to normal sinus rhythm and has recently been released for clinical use in the United States (Becaner, 1968; Holder et al., 1977). It has been useful in some subjects for whom the more traditional agents prove unsatisfactory. Most patients with ventricular tachycardia do not respond to propranolol or potassium but these agents are occasionally of use in cases resistant to other therapeutic agents. Quinidine, used intravenously, has been associated with serious untoward effects, such as severe hypotension, and should be avoided. Disopyramide is currently not available for intravenous use, but clinical trials have shown its therapeutic effectiveness as an intravenous agent for treatment of ventricular tachycardia.

For prevention of recurrence of ventricular tachycardia, maintenance drug therapy is warranted. The more commonly used drugs include procainamide, disopyramide, quinidine, diphenylhydantoin and propranolol. Frequently, combination therapy is required. However, in our experience, the most common cause for "refractory" ventricular tachyarrhythmias is inadequate dosage of the agents employed.

Electric Countershock. Electric countershock is the method of choice in the treatment of drug-resistant ventricular tachycardia not caused by digitalis intoxication. In ventricular tachycardia due to digitalis toxicity, electric countershock should not be used, since it may result in ventricular fibrillation. The vast majority of patients with ventricular tachycardia not caused by digitalis will respond to direct current countershock (Fig. 11–21), which is effective in more than 90 per cent of cases, the majority with low electrical energies. However, ventricular tachycardia is frequently repetitive, requiring multiple cardioversions if other modes of therapy (i.e., drug and/or overdrive) fail to prevent recurrences.

A blow to the precordium ("thumpversion") may terminate episodes of paroxysmal ventricular tachycardia. Pennington et al. (1970) reported termination of 12 episodes of paroxysmal ventricular tachycardia occurring in five patients by using the "thump" method. The sharp thump to the chest provides a low energy depolarizing current to the heart through electromechanical transduction, thereby probably disrupting the re-entry pathway.

Occasionally, one encounters patients with short paroxysms or repetitive continuous paroxysms of ventricular tachycardia who are refractory to the usual types of therapy. Although they may respond to electric countershock, the restoration to normal sinus rhythm is only temporary, and within a few hours the tachycardia recurs. In such cases one must depend on drugs or other therapy to maintain normal rhythm. The results obtained are often unsatisfactory. Many of these cases occur in patients with advanced heart disease, particularly extensive coronary heart disease with healed myocardial infarction(s). In such cases, the following steps should be considered: 1) re-evaluate the myocardial state; 2) rule out the presence of electrolyte imbalance; 3) correct hypoxia or acid-base imbalance; 4) correct congestive heart failure; 5) consider that occasionally these episodes are the result of excessive sympathetic tone (propranolol may be tried in such instances); 6) evaluate cardiac function with particular emphasis on the presence or absence of ventricular aneurysm.

Recently, techniques have been developed to provoke ventricular tachycardia in the laboratory using programmed ventricular stimulation (Wellens, 1974; Mason, 1978; Horowitz, 1978). The ability of an intravenous drug or combination to suppress the tachycardia response to the stimulated beats is used to assess its efficiency (see Chapter 23).

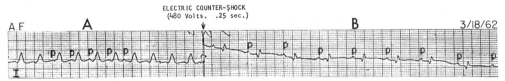

Figure 11–21   Effect of electric countershock in a patient with ventricular tachycardia refractory to drug therapy. (Lead I)

(A) Taken from a patient, age 75, with ventricular tachycardia refractory to the usual methods of therapy. Note the ventricular rate of 145 per minute with markedly widened QRS complexes and P waves occurring at a slower rate independent of the ventricular complexes (complete A-V dissociation).

(B) After the electric countershock (480 volts, 0.25 second). Note the restoration of a normal sinus rhythm with a P-R interval of 0.24 second. (From Medow, A., and Dreifus, L. S.: Amer. J. Cardiol., 11:87, 1963.)

Overdrive Suppression by Artificial Pacemaker. When pharmacologic and D.C. countershock therapy to control recurrent ventricular tachycardia is unsuccessful, ventricular tachyarrhythmias may be terminated with overdrive suppression of the ectopic focus using atrial or ventricular pacing (DeSanctis and Kastor, 1968; Furman and Escher, 1970; Zipes et al., 1968; Haft, 1974; Moss and Rivers, 1974; Hartzler, 1979). This technique is utilized as a temporary or permanent measure in cases of recurrent ventricular tachycardia that are resistant to other forms of therapy. The pacemaker rate to control ventricular tachycardia is usually in the range of 90 to 110 per minute. Frequently, pacing and drug therapy is required for adequate rhythm control. At times, this is a dramatic form of therapy and can be lifesaving.

Surgery for Ventricular Tachycardia. The role of surgery in the management of ventricular tachycardia is still under investigation (Graham et al., 1973). In patients with an old myocardial infarction who develop a ventricular aneurysm, if ventricular tachycardia remains resistant to drugs and overdrive suppression, resection of the aneurysm has given excellent results in some patients (Thind et al., 1971). Nitter-Hauge and Storstein (1973) reported that sympathectomy abolished ventricular tachycardia in two of five patients and ventricular aneurysm resection was accompanied by favorable results in 7 of 12 patients. In our own experience, ventricular aneurysm resection has been helpful in abolishing ventricular tachycardia in about 50 per cent of these patients. Better electrophysiological methods of identifying the site of origin of these arrhythmias may help to enhance the usefulness of surgery in the future.

Prognosis

In general, the prognosis depends on the underlying etiology of the arrhythmia; the severity of the patient's heart disease; the ventricular rate during the paroxysm; the duration of the paroxysm; the hemodynamic response to the tachycardia; and the response to therapy. The overall prognosis has been somewhat improved by the use of cardioversion, overdrive pacing, new developments in drug therapy, and open heart surgery.

Patients may be divided into three groups:

1. Those with apparently normal hearts or with little evidence of heart disease. Such cases are comparatively uncommon, but the prognosis is relatively good, particularly if the attacks can be controlled (although the risk of ventricular fibrillation cannot be minimized).

2. Patients in whom the paroxysms are the result of a severe toxic factor, such as drug toxicity (digitalis, etc.). The paroxysms disappear as the cause is removed and the prognosis then depends mainly on the underlying disease.

3. Patients who have severe heart disease.

Unfortunately the latter constitute the preponderant group. Many of these subjects have sustained a recent myocardial infarction or manifest evidence of severe coronary heart disease. The prognosis is poor in this group. In Strauss' early series of 193 patients, 80 per cent died within a period of only 24 hours. Cooke and White (1943) observed that half of their group died within three weeks of the paroxysm and those who recovered died a few months later, the longest survival being 18 months. The prognosis certainly has improved in recent years with the advent of improved methods of therapy and monitoring. In patients with an acute myocardial infarction, Lown and associates (1967) reported 17 deaths in the coronary care unit among 84 patients (20.2 per cent) who manifested ventricular tachycardia in the immediate postinfarction period, an excess of only two deaths over that expected from the average mortality (17.7 per cent) in their entire series.

In a study by Anderson et al. (1978) of 915 patients who survived the hospital phase of myocardial infarction, 66 showed episodes of ventricular tachycardia (three consecutive ventricular beats or more) during a 4 to 48 month followup period. The mortality rate in patients with ventricular tachycardia was 16 per cent compared to 8 per cent in an age- and sex-matched control group. The 48 month survival rate of ventricular tachycardia patients was 75 per cent compared to 87 per cent in the control group. The causes of death, suddenness of death, and mechanisms of death were similar in the two groups. The ventricular tachycardia patients had more severe cardiac disease and more evidence of ventricular irritability than the matched controls. Within the ventricular tachycardia group, those who died had more severe heart disease than survivors. The prognosis is clearly more grave in patients with more sustained and recurrent episodes that do not respond well to conventional therapy than in those in whom an isolated, short paroxysm is "accidentally" recorded on an ambulatory electrocardiographic tape.

VENTRICULAR FLUTTER AND FIBRILLATION

Ventricular flutter and fibrillation are closely allied to cardiac arrest and standstill, since one mechanism often develops into the other. In fact, the timing of the electrocardiogram after cardiovascular collapse occurs frequently determines which of the two is considered to be present. The exact occurrence of ventricular flutter and fibrillation and its relation to cardiac arrest as well as the clinical manifestations have been studied by continuous electrocardiographic monitoring. In one series (Adgey et al., 1969), when an electrocardiogram was obtained within four minutes of the onset of symptoms, 91 per cent of the patients manifested ventricular fibrillation; after four minutes, 82 per cent manifested cardiac standstill. Therefore, many facets of these two mechanisms may be considered together, since the clinical consequences and immediate treatment (except for defibrillation) are quite similar (see Chapter 26).

Ventricular fibrillation has traditionally been considered a terminal mechanism in an irreversibly damaged heart. However, it is now known that ventricular fibrillation may occur unexpectedly in hearts with relatively little, slight, or moderate degrees of organic damage, resulting from various acute changes caused by ischemia and/or enhanced sympathetic tone with or without myocardial infarction or other factors that tend to cause ventricular electrical instability.

The abolition of ventricular fibrillation with restoration of normal sinus rhythm therefore often results in a resumption of normal function without necessarily decreasing the longevity of the patient. Resuscitation may prove successful in as many as 80 per cent of patients who develop this arrhythmia in a coronary care unit during the course of an otherwise uncomplicated myocardial infarction (Lawrie et al., 1968; Wyman and Hammersmith, 1968; Mogensen, 1971). In these cases, the long-term prognosis is not necessarily affected by the occurrence of ventricular fibrillation during the acute postinfarction period.

Etiology

The causes of ventricular fibrillation in humans are not always clear, and, except under ideal circumstances, there are few opportunities to study the causative factors in the individual patient. Most patients in the hospital who develop ventricular fibrillation suffer from either acute myocardial ischemia or infarction or chronic organic heart disease (especially coronary, hypertensive, rheumatic, or myopathic types). In addition, a severe emotional upset in a predisposed subject may be the immediate cause of increased autonomic tone, which may precipitate ventricular fibrillation (Lown et al., 1976). However, the immediate causes of ventricular fibrillation occurring outside the hospital remain unclear (see Chapter 21).

Ventricular fibrillation may occasionally be initiated by an electrical impulse delivered during repolarization either by an artificial pacemaker, on electric countershock, or a premature beat (R on T phenomenon). It also often occurs during various surgical procedures, especially during cardiac surgery. The primary factor may be anesthesia, hypoxia, surgical trauma, inadequate coronary perfusion, hypokalemia, acid-base disorders, and/or hypothermia. A wide variety of drugs has been implicated in the production of ventricular fibrillation: a) anesthetics (cyclopropane and chloroform), b) sympathomimetic agents, c) quinidine and other antiarrhythmic agents, d) digitalis, e) contrast media used in angiography, and f) tranquilizers. In addition, poor design and improper grounding of common electrical hospital devices may lead to ventricular fibrillation (Briller, 1966).

Relatively rare instances of spontaneous ventricular fibrillation have been documented in human subjects with no indication of myocardial abnormality, drug effects, or trauma (Stern, 1957).

VENTRICULAR FIBRILLATION ASSOCIATED WITH ACUTE MYOCARDIAL INFARCTION

A recent extensive review of the literature indicates that ventricular fibrillation occurs in 1 to 11 per cent of patients with acute myocardial infarction in the coronary care unit (Bigger et al., 1977). However, out-of-hospital ventricular fibrillation is much more common (Cobb et al., 1975) (see Chapter 15). In the setting of acute myocardial infarction,

ventricular fibrillation is defined as *primary* (occurring in patients without left ventricular failure or hypotension) or *secondary* (occurring in patients with left ventricular failure and/or hypotension). It is considered that 80 per cent of the patients with acute myocardial infarction and primary ventricular fibrillation will survive to be discharged from the hospital while only 25 per cent of those with secondary ventricular fibrillation will survive (Lawrie et al., 1968; Wyman et al., 1968; Mogensen, 1971). Although some studies suggest that ventricular fibrillation is more common in patients under the age of 51 (Lawrie et al., 1968; Julian et al., 1964), other studies do not confirm the relationship of age with frequency of ventricular fibrillation (Dhurandhar et al., 1971). The site of infarction (i.e., anterior or inferior) does not seem to affect the incidence of ventricular fibrillation.

There is some evidence that ventricular fibrillation occurs more frequently in patients with large infarcts who develop cardiogenic shock. Although the majority of patients with primary ventricular fibrillation do not exhibit premonitory arrhythmias, some rhythm disturbances and conduction disorders seem to be associated with a higher incidence of ventricular fibrillation: ventricular premature beats, ventricular tachycardia, third degree A-V block, and previous episodes of ventricular fibrillation. Lown and coworkers (1967) suggested that patients having more than five ventricular premature beats per minute, in salvos of two or more, ventricular premature beats of multiform configuration, and ventricular premature beats showing the R on T phenomenon are more liable to develop ventricular fibrillation.

MECHANISMS UNDERLYING VENTRICULAR FIBRILLATION

Ventricular fibrillation is caused by factors that cause electrophysiological inhomogeneity sufficient to result in a severe disorganization of conduction in a critical area of the ventricular myocardium. The presence of areas of myocardium with severely disparate refractory periods leads to disorganized conduction and to the creation of multiple microre-entry circuits. This inhomogeneity then tends to perpetuate itself. These conditions have also been found to occur following one or more premature ventricular beats or an accelerating ventricular tachycardia. Several of the etiologic factors discussed previously cause inhomogeneities in the refractory periods and conduction. Thus, following myocardial infarction, the effects of ischemic injury are not uniform, and varying degrees of circulatory impairment lead to nonuniform depolarization and repolarization.

Clinical Diagnosis

Ventricular fibrillation should be suspected when there is sudden disappearance of a palpable pulse and audible heart sounds and the blood pressure becomes unobtainable. These manifestations are compatible with ventricular fibrillation or cardiac standstill. Since the initial therapeutic approach to these two conditions is essentially the same, a vigorous precordial thump followed by closed chest compression should be done without delay.

Electrocardiogram

The transition from ventricular tachycardia to ventricular flutter and fibrillation is characterized by the QRS complexes of ventricular tachycardia becoming widened and more aberrant until they appear as regular, continuous waves of large amplitude at a rate of 180 to 250 per minute. This stage is called ventricular flutter. Except for the increased amplitude, they bear a striking resemblance to the waves of atrial flutter. The T waves and ST segments cannot be differentiated from the QRS complexes. These complexes become more aberrant and irregular in rhythm and form, resulting in ventricular fibrillation (Figs. 11–22 and 11–23).

Ventricular fibrillation is character-

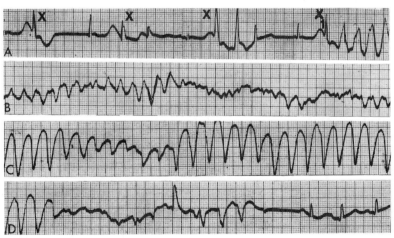

Figure 11–22   Onset and offset of ventricular flutter and ventricular fibrillation.

(A) Note presence of aberrant QRS complex at downstroke of T wave at X and presence of numerous ventricular beats following the cycle with a long Q-T segment at X_1. Note that the premature beats follow close upon the peak of the T waves and that at X they initiate a paroxysm of ventricular flutter.

(B and C) Note changes from ventricular flutter to ventricular fibrillation.

(D) Note the resumption of normal sinus rhythm with normal Q-T length and absent U wave at the end of the strip.

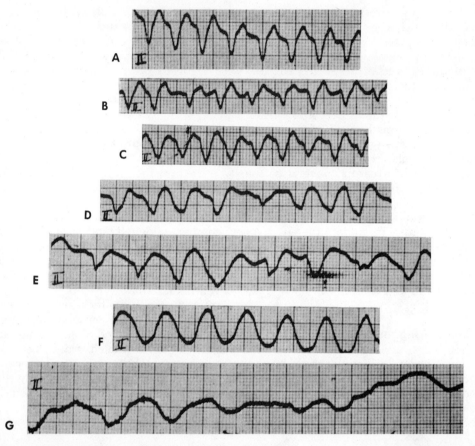

Figure 11–23 Transition of ventricular tachycardia to ventricular flutter and fibrillation following the administration of procaine amide (dying heart). (*A* to *G* represent a continuous strip of Lead II.) Patient, age 70, with arteriosclerotic heart disease was observed to be almost in extremis with a tachycardia (strip *A*) that was considered to be probably ventricular in origin. He was given 400 mg. of procaine amide intravenously in a period of about three to four minutes. This patient was one of the first in which this drug was used in our laboratory.

(*B*) Note the increase in aberration of the ventricular complexes.
(*C*) Increased widening of the ventricular complexes.
(*D*) Increase in abnormality, suggesting beginning of ventricular fibrillation.
(*E*) The irregularity is well marked and the ventricular complexes are more bizarre.
(*F*) This may be considered to be representative of ventricular flutter.
(*G*) A slow and irregular ventricular rate of the dying heart.

ized by bizarre ventricular oscillations without a suggestion of a QRS or T wave; the waves are very coarse and irregular and range from 150 to 300 per minute. The waves are characteristically of varying amplitude, contour, and spacing and, except for the increased amplitude, resemble those of atrial fibrillation. These waves may be divided into several stages: 1) coarse fibrillation; 2) fine fibrillation in which the rate is higher; and 3) a terminal stage, characterized by slow, extremely aberrant complexes.

Treatment

With the increased knowledge of the premonitory and initiating mechanisms and the use of monitoring devices, the *prevention* of ventricular fibrillation assumes crucial importance. The active treatment of ventricular fibrillation depends on the setting in which it occurs, whether inside or outside of the hospital. It consists of cardiopulmonary resuscitation, direct current countershock, and drugs (see Chapter 26).

The result of treatment depends upon several factors: the rapidity with which treatment is begun, the underlying disease state, and the incidence of complications.

Prognosis

The prognosis depends on the underlying disease state and the immediacy and efficacy of treatment of the acute episode. Analysis of mortality rates suggests that the prognosis is poor for patients who had signs of cardiac decompensation prior to the occurrence of ventricular fibrillation. However, among patients without such signs, the expected long-term survival is about 85 per cent. This agrees with the 83 per cent long-term survival in the group studied by Lawrie et al. (1968). Of 23 patients from the working population, 14 have returned to work. These results emphasize that the occurrence of ventricular fibrillation during the *acute* stage of myocardial infarction does not necessarily influence the long-term prognosis, provided cardiac failure is not present.

A recent study from the University of Washington (Cobb et al., 1975) indicates that in the course of 51 months, the Seattle emergency medical system successfully resuscitated 234 patients with out-of-hospital ventricular fibrillation who were hospitalized and later discharged home. Patients surviving ventricular fibrillation unrelated to an acute myocardial infarction showed a two year mortality rate that was three times *higher* than that of patients in whom ventricular fibrillation was associated with acute transmural infarction. Recurrent out-of-hospital ventricular fibrillation was common in these patients, and a pattern of early recurrence was noted, with a median survival of 17 weeks in 34 documented cases.

REFERENCES

Adgey, A. A. J., et al.: Management of ventricular fibrillation outside hospital. Lancet 1:1169, 1969.

Alexander, S., and Ping, W. C.: Fatal ventricular fibrillation during carotid stimulation. Amer. J. Cardiol. 18:289, 1966.

Amburst, C. A., and Levine, S. A.: Paroxysmal ventricular tachycardia: A study of one hundred and seven cases. Circulation 1:28, 1950.

Anderson, K. P., DeCamilla, J., and Moss, A. J.: Clinical significance of ventricular tachycardia (3 beats or longer) detected during ambulatory monitoring after myocardial infarction. Circulation 57:890, 1978.

Bacaner, M.: Bretylium tosylate for suppression of induced ventricular fibrillation. Amer. J. Cardiol. 17:528, 1966.

Bacaner, M.: Quantitative comparison of bretylium with other antifibrillatory drugs. Amer. J. Cardiol. 21:504, 1968.

Baird, W. M.: Prognostic significance of premature beats in acute myocardial infarction. Clin. Res. 17:288, 1969.

Bellet, S., DeGuzman, N. T., Kostis, J. B., Roman, L., and Fleischmann, D.: The effect of cigarette smoke inhalation on VFT in normal dogs and dogs with acute myocardial infarction. Amer. Heart J. 83:67, 1972.

Bellet, S., Horstmann, E., Roman, L. R., et al.: Effect of caffeine on the ventricular fibrillation threshold in normal dogs and dogs with acute myocardial infarction. Am. Heart J. 84:215, 1972.

Bennett, M. A., and Pentecost, B. L.: Warning of cardiac arrest due to ventricular fibrillation and tachycardia. Lancet 1:1351, 1972.

Bigger, T. J., Dresdale, R. J., Heissenbuttel, R. H., Weld, R. M., and Wit, A. L.: Ventricular arrhythmias in ischemic heart disease: Mechanism, prevalence, significance and management. Prog. Cardiovasc. Dis. 19:255, 1977.

Borer, J. S., Kent, K. M., Goldstein, R. E., and Epstein, S. E.: Nitroglycerin induced reduction in the incidence of spontaneous ventricular fibrillation during coronary occlusion in dog. Amer. J. Cardiol. 33:517, 1974.

Briller, S. A.: Electrocution hazards. *In* Dreifus, L., and Likoff, W. (eds.): Mechanisms and Therapy of Cardiac Arrhythmias. New York, Grune & Stratton, 1966, p. 542.

Brown, K. W. G., MacMillan, R. L., Forboth, N.,

Mel'Grano, F., and Scott, J. W.: An intensive care center for acute myocardial infarction. Lancet 2:349, 1965.

Buchner, M., and Effert, S.: Precipitation of tachycardias by extrasystoles. German Med. Monthly 8:3, 1968.

Burgess, M. J., Abildskov, A., and Millar, K.: Early time course of fibrillation threshold in experimental coronary occlusion. Circulation 41–42:III-141, 1970.

Burn, J. H.: The cause of fibrillation. Can. Med. Assoc. J. 84:625, 1961.

Campbell, M.: Inversion of T waves after long paroxysms of tachycardia. Brit. Heart J. 4:49, 1942.

Cass, R. M.: Repetitive tachycardia. A review of 40 cases with no demonstrable heart disease. Amer. J. Cardiol. 19:597, 1967.

Chardack, W. M.: Fibrillation in empty and loaded ventricles. Arch. Surg. 93:795, 1966.

Chiang, B. N., Perlman, L. V., Ostrander, L. D., Jr., and Epstein, F. H.: Relationship of premature systoles to coronary heart disease and sudden death in the Tecumseh epidemiologic study. Ann. Intern. Med. 70:1159, 1969.

Chopra, M. P., Thadani, U., Portal, R. W., and Aber, C. P.: Lignocaine therapy for ventricular ectopic activity after acute myocardial infarction: A double blind trial. Brit. Med. J. 3:668, 1971.

Cobb, L. A., Baum, R. S., Alvarez, H., III, and Schaffer, W. A.: Resuscitation from out-of-hospital ventricular fibrillation: 4 years follow up. Circulation 52(6 Suppl. 3):223, 1975.

Cohen, S. I., Disseroth, A., and Hecht, H. S.: Infra-His bundle origin of bidirectional tachycardia. Circulation 47:1260, 1973.

Cohen, S. I., and Voukydis, P.: Supraventricular origin of bidirectional tachycardia. Circulation 50:634, 1974.

Cohn, L. J., Donoso, E., and Friedberg, C. K.: Ventricular tachycardia. Prog. Cardiovasc. Dis. 9:29, 1966.

Cooke, W. T., and White, P. D.: Paroxysmal ventricular tachycardia. Brit. Heart J. 5:33, 1943.

Corday, E., et al.: Alternating failure of mechanical response to electrical depolarization (the aformed phenomenon) — a new phenomenon in cardiac arrhythmias. Abstr. 18th Annual Scientific Session, Amer. Col. Cardiol., Amer. J. Cardiol. 23:108, 1969.

Coronary Drug Project Research Group: Prognostic importance of premature beats following myocardial infarction. J.A.M.A. 223:1116, 1973.

Danese, C.: Pathogenesis of ventricular fibrillation in coronary occlusion: Perfusion of coronary arteries with serum. J.A.M.A. 179:52, 1962.

Darby, S., Bennett, M. A., Cruickshank, J. C., and Pentecost, B. L.: Trial of combined intramuscular and intravenous lignocaine in pro-

phylaxis of ventricular tachyarrhythmias. Lancet 1:817, 1972.

Davidson, S., and Surawicz, B.: Ectopic beats and atrioventricular conduction disturbances. Arch. Intern. Med. 120:280, 1967.

Day, H. W.: An intensive coronary care area. Dis. Chest 44:423, 1963.

DeSanctis, R. W., and Kastor, J. A.: Rapid intracardiac pacing for treatment of recurrent ventricular tachyarrhythmias in the absence of heart block. Amer. Heart J. 76:168, 1968.

Denes, P., Wu, D., Dhingra, R. C., Amat-y-Leon, F., Wyndham, C., Mautner, R. K., and Rosen, K. M.: Electrophysiologic studies in patients with chronic recurrent ventricular tachycardia. Circulation 54:229, 1976.

Dhurandhar, R. W., MacMillan, R. L., and Brown, W. G.: Primary ventricular fibrillation complicating acute myocardial infarction. Am. J. Cardiol. 27:347, 1971.

Easley, R. M., Jr., and Goldstein, S.: Differentiation of ventricular tachycardia from junctional tachycardia with aberrant conduction. Circulation 37:1015, 1968.

Fisher, F. D., and Tyroler, H. A.: Relationship between ventricular premature contractions on routine electrocardiography and subsequent sudden death from coronary heart disease. Circulation 47:712, 1973.

Furman, S., and Escher, D. J.: Temporary transvenous pacing. In Furman, S., and Escher, D. J.: Principles and Techniques of Cardiac Pacing. New York, Harper & Row, 1970.

Gallagher, J. J., Damato, A. N., and Lau, S. H.: Electrophysiologic studies during accelerated idioventricular rhythms. Circulation 44:671, 1971.

Gerst, P. H., Fleming, W. H., and Malm, J. R.: Increased susceptibility of the heart to ventricular fibrillation during metabolic acidosis. Circ. Res. 19:63, 1966.

Graham, A. F., Miller, D. C., Stinson, E. B., Daily, P. O., Fogarty, T. J., and Harrison, D. C.: Surgical treatment of refractory life-threatening ventricular tachycardia. Am. J. Cardiol. 32:909, 1973.

Haft, J. I.: Treatment of arrhythmias by intracardiac electrical stimulation. Prog. Cardiovasc. Dis. 16:539, 1974.

Han, J.: Ventricular vulnerability during acute coronary occlusion. Amer. J. Cardiol. 24:857, 1969.

Han, J., DeTraglia, J., and Moe, G. K.: Incidence of ectopic beats as a function of basic rate in the ventricle. Amer. Heart J. 72:632, 1966.

Han, J., Garcia de Jalon, P. D., and Moe, G. K.: Adrenergic effects on ventricular vulnerability. Circ. Res. 14:516, 1964.

Han, J., Malozzi, A. M., and Lyons, C.: Ventricular vulnerability to paired-pulse stimulation during acute coronary occlusion. Amer. Heart J. 73:79, 1967.

Harris, A. S., Estandia, A., and Tillotson, R. F.:

Ventricular ectopic rhythm and ventricular fibrillation following cardiac sympathectomy and coronary occlusion. Amer. J. Physiol. 165:505, 1951.

Hartzler, G. O.: Treatment of recurrent ventricular tachycardia by patient activated radiofrequency ventricular stimulation. Mayo Clin. Proc. 54:75, 1979.

Harvey, W. P., and Ronan, J. A.: Bedside diagnosis of arrhythmias. Prog. Cardiovasc. Dis. 8:419, 1966.

Helfant, R. H., Pine, R., Kabde, V., and Banka, V. S.: Exercise-related ventricular premature complexes in coronary heart disease: Correlations with ischemia and angiographic severity. Ann. Intern. Med. 80:489, 1974.

Hinkle, L. E., Jr., Carver, S. T., and Stevens, M.: The frequency of asymptomatic disturbances of cardiac rhythm and conduction in middle-aged men. Amer. J. Cardiol. 24:629, 1969.

Hiss, R. G., and Lamb, L. E.: Electrocardiographic findings in 122,043 individuals. Circulation 25:947, 1962.

Holder, A. A., Sniderman, A. D., Fraser, G., and Fallen, E. L.: Experience with bretylium tosylate by cardiac arrest team. Circulation 55:541, 1977.

Horowitz, L. N., Josephson, M. E., Farshidi, A., Spielman, S. R., Michelson, E. L., and Greenspan, A. M.: Recurrent sustained ventricular tachycardia. 3, Role of electrophysiologic study in selection of antiarrhythmic regimens. Circulation 58:986, 1978.

Huppert, V. F., and Berliner, K.: The intraventricular conduction time (QRS duration) of ventricular premature systoles. Cardiologia 27:87, 1955.

Jelinek, M. V., Lohrbauer, L., and Lown, B.: Antiarrhythmic drug therapy for sporadic ventricular ectopic arrhythmias. Circulation 49:659, 1974.

Josephson, M. E., Horowitz, L. N., Farshidi, A., and Kastor, J. A.: Recurrent sustained ventricular tachycardia: I. Mechanisms. Circulation 57:431, 1978.

Julian, D. T., Valentine, P. A., and Miller, G. G.: Disturbances of rate, rhythm and conduction in acute myocardial infarction. A prospective study of 100 consecutive unselected patients with the aid of electrocardiographic monitoring. Am. J. Med. 37:915, 1964.

Julian, D. G., Vellani, C. W., Godman, M. J., and Terry, G.: Prolongation of QRS duration in acute myocardial infarction. Prog. Cardiovasc. Dis. 13:56, 1970.

Kastor, J. A., and Goldreyer, B. N.: Ventricular origin of bidirectional tachycardia. Case report of a patient not toxic from digitalis. Circulation 48:897, 1973.

Katz, M. J., and Zitnik, R. S.: Direct current shock and lidocaine in treatment of digitalis-induced ventricular tachycardia. Amer. J. Cardiol. 18:552, 1966.

Kent, D. M., Smith, E. R., Redwood, D. R., and Epstein, S. E.: Beneficial electrophysiologic effects of nitroglycerin during acute myocardial infarction. Am. J. Cardiol. 33:513, 1974.

Kistin, A. D.: Problems in the differentiation of ventricular arrhythmias from supraventricular arrhythmias with abnormal QRS. Prog. Cardiovasc. Dis. 9:1, 1966.

Kotler, M. N., Tabatznik, B., Mower, M. M., and Tominaga, S.: Prognostic significance of ventricular ectopic beats with respect to sudden death in the late postinfarction period. Circulation 67:959, 1973.

Lawrie, D. M., et al.: Ventricular fibrillation complicating acute myocardial infarction. Lancet 2:523, 1968.

Lesch, M., Lewis, E., Humphries, J. D., and Ross, R. S.: Paroxysmal ventricular tachycardia in the absence of organic heart disease: Report of a case and review of the literature. Ann. Intern. Med. 66:950, 1967.

Lichstein, E., Ribas-Meneclier, C., Gupta, P. K., and Chadda, K. D.: Incidence and description of accelerated ventricular rhythm complicating acute myocardial infarction. Am. J. Med. 58:192, 1975.

Lown, B., Temte, J. V., Reich, P., Gaughan, C., Regestein, O., and Hamid, H.: Basis for recurring ventricular fibrillation in the absence of coronary heart disease and its management. New Engl. J. Med. 294:623, 1976.

Lown, B., et al.: Unresolved problems in coronary care. Amer. J. Cardiol. 20:494, 1967.

Lown, B., Fakhro, A. M., Hood, W. B., et al.: The coronary care unit. New perspective and directions. J.A.M.A. 199:188, 1967.

Lown, B., Kleiger, R., and Williams, J.: Cardioversion and digitalis drugs. Changed threshold to electric shock in digitalized animals. Circ. Res. 17:519, 1965.

Lown, B., Vassaux, C., Hood, W. B., Fakhro, A. M., Kaplinsky, E., and Roberge, G.: Unresolved problems in coronary care. Am. J. Cardiol. 20:494, 1967.

Lown, B., and Wolf, M.: Approaches to sudden death from coronary heart disease. Circulation 44:130, 1971.

MacKenzie, G. J., and Pascual, S.: Paroxysmal ventricular tachycardia. Brit. Heart J. 26:441, 1964.

Maling, H. M., and Moran, N. C.: Ventricular arrhythmias induced by sympathomimetic amines in unanesthetized dogs following coronary artery occlusion. Circ. Res. 5:409, 1957.

Mason, J. W., and Winkle, R. A.: Electrode-catheter arrhythmia induction in the selection and assessment of antiarrhythmic drug therapy for recurrent ventricular tachycardia. Circulation 58:971, 1978.

Massumi, R. A., and Ali, N.: Accelerated isorhythmic ventricular rhythms. Am. J. Cardiol. 26:170, 1970.

Mather, H. G., Pearson, N. G., Read, K. L. Q.,

Sharo, D. B., Steed, G. R., Thorne, M. G., Jones, S., Guerrier, C. J., Eraut, C. D., McHugh, P. M., Chowdhury, N. R., Jafary, M. H., and Wallace, T. J.: Acute myocardial infarction: Home and hospital treatment. Brit. Med. J. 3:334, 1971.

Meltzer, L. E., and Kitcheel, J. B.: The incidence of arrhythmias associated with acute myocardial infarction. Prog. Cardiovasc. Dis. 9:50, 1966.

Michelson, E. L., Morganroth, J., Spear, J. F., Kastor, J. A., and Josephson, M. E.: Fixed coupling: different mechanisms revealed by exercise induced changes in cycle length. Circulation 58:1002, 1978.

Moe, G. K., Jaliffe, J., Mueller, W. J., and Moe, B.: A mathematical model of parasystole and its application to clinical arrhythmias. Circulation 56:968, 1977.

Mogensen, L.: A controlled trial of lignocaine prophylaxis in prevention of ventricular tachyarrhythmias in acute myocardial infarction. Acta Med. Scand. 513:1, 1971.

Moss, A. J., and Akiyama, T.: Prognostic significance of ventricular premature beats. Cardiovascular Clinics 6:274, 1976.

Moss, A. J., and Rivers, A. J.: Termination and inhibition of recurrent tachycardias by implanted pervenous pacemakers. Circulation 50:942, 1974.

Muller, O. F., Cardenas, M., Bellet, S.: QRS alterations produced by auricular and ventricular paroxysmal tachycardia in the presence of bundle branch block pattern: An experimental study in dogs. Amer. J. Cardiol. 7:697, 1961.

Nitter-Hauge, S., and Storstein, O.: Surgical treatment of ventricular tachycardia. Brit. Heart J. 35:1132, 1973.

Norris, R. M., and Mercer, C. J.: Significance of idioventricular rhythms in acute myocardial infarction. Prog. Cardiovasc. Dis. 16:455–468, 1974.

Palmer, D. G.: Interruption of T waves by premature QRS complexes and the relationship of this phenomenon to ventricular fibrillation. Amer. Heart J. 63:367, 1962.

Pantridge, J. F., and Adgey, A. A. J.: Pre-hospital coronary care. The mobile coronary care unit. Amer. J. Cardiol. 24:666, 1969.

Pennington, J. E., Taylor, J., and Lown, B.: Chest thump for reverting ventricular tachycardia. New Engl. J. Med. 283:1192, 1970.

Robinson, G. C., and Hermann, G. R.: Paroxysmal tachycardia of ventricular origin and its relation to coronary occlusion. Heart 8:59, 1921.

Rothfeld, E., Zucker, R., Leff, W. A., et al.: Idioventricular rhythm in acute myocardial infarction: A reappraisal. Circulation 42(Suppl. 3):111, 1970.

Rothfeld, E. L., Zucker, I. R., Parsonnet, V., and Alinsonorin, C. A.: Idioventricular rhythm in acute myocardial infarction. Circulation 37:203, 1968.

Schaal, S. F., Wallace, A. G., and Sealy, W. C.:

Protective influence of cardiac denervation against arrhythmias of myocardial infarction. Cardiovasc. Res. 3:241, 1969.

Schamroth, L.: Idioventricular tachycardia. J. Electrocardiol. 1:205, 1968.

Scherf, D.: The mechanism of flutter and fibrillation. Heart Bull. 16:88, 1967.

Scherlag, B. J., Samet, P., and Helfant, R. H.: The His electrogram: A critical appraisal of its uses and limitations. Circulation 44:601, 1972.

Sclarovsky, S., Strasberg, B., Martonovich, G., and Agmon, J.: Ventricular rhythms with intermediate rates in acute myocardial infarction. Chest 74:180, 1978.

Smirk, F. H., and Palmer, D. G.: A myocardial syndrome. With particular reference to the occurrence of sudden death and of premature systoles interrupting antecedent T waves. Amer. J. Cardiol. 6:620, 1960.

Spurrell, R. A. J., Yates, A. K., Thorburn, C. W., Sowton, G. E., and Deuchar, D. C.: Surgical treatment of ventricular tachycardia following epicardial mapping studies. Brit. Heart J. 37:115, 1975.

Stern, T. N.: Paroxysmal ventricular fibrillation in the absence of other disease. Ann. Intern. Med. 47:552, 1957.

Stock, E., Goble, A., and Sloman, G.: Assessment of arrhythmias in myocardial infarction. Brit. Med. J. 1:719, 1967.

Stock, J. P. P.: Repetitive paroxysmal ventricular tachycardia. Brit. Heart J. 24:297, 1962.

Strauss, M. B.: Paroxysmal ventricular tachycardia. Amer. J. Med. Sci. 79:337, 1930.

Surawicz, B., and MacDonald, M. G.: Ventricular ectopic beats with fixed and variable coupling: Incidence, clinical significance and factors influencing the coupling interval. Am. J. Cardiol. 13:198, 1964.

Swartz, M. H., Teichholz, L. E., and Donoso, E.: Mitral valve prolapse: A review of associated arrhythmias. Am. J. Med. 62:377, 1977.

Thin, G. S., Blakemore, W. S., and Zinsser, H. F.: Ventricular aneurysmectomy for the treatment of recurrent ventricular tachyarrhythmias. Am. J. Cardiol. 27:690, 1971.

Wallace, A. G.: Personal communication cited in McIntosh, H. D., and Morris, J. J., Jr.: The hemodynamic consequences of arrhythmias. Prog. Cardiovasc. Dis. 8:330, 1966.

Wallace, A. G., et al.: The electrophysiologic effects of beta-adrenergic blockade and cardiac denervation. Bull. N.Y. Acad. Med. 43:119, 1967.

Wegria, R., Frank, C. W., Wang, H. H., and Lammerent, J.: Effect of atrial and ventricular tachycardia on cardiac output, coronary blood flow and blood pressure. Circ. Res. 6:624, 1958.

Weiss, A. N., Jobe, C. L., Gordon, T., Lange, P. H., and Frommer, P. L.: Relationship of premature ventricular contractions and left ventricular hypertrophy to sudden cardiac death. Circulation 39, 40 (Suppl. III): III–213, 1969.

Wellens, H. J. J., Durrer, D. R., and Lie, K. I.:

Observations on mechanism of ventricular tachycardia in man. Circulation 54:237, 1976.

Wellens, H. J. J., Lie, K. I., and Durrer, D.: Further observations on ventricular tachycardia as studied by electrical stimulation of the heart. Chronic recurrent ventricular tachycardia and ventricular tachycardia during acute myocardial infarction. Circulation 49:647, 1974.

Wellens, H. J. J., Schuilenburg, R. M., and Durrer, D.: Electrical stimulation of the heart in patients with ventricular tachycardia. Circulation 46:216, 1972.

Wilson, W. S., Judge, R. D., and Siegel, J. H.: A simple diagnostic sign in ventricular tachycardia. New Engl. J. Med. 270:446, 1964.

Winkle, R. A., Alderman, E. L., Fitzgerald, J. W., and Harrison, D. C.: Treatment of recurrent symptomatic ventricular tachycardia. Ann. Intern. Med. 85:1, 1976.

Winkle, R. A., Derrington, D. C., and Schroeder, J. S.: Characteristics of ventricular tachycardia in ambulatory patients. Am. J. Cardiol. 39:487, 1977.

Wolff, G. A., Veith, F., and Lown, B.: A vulnerable period of ventricular tachycardia following myocardial infarction. Cardiovasc. Res. 2:111, 1968.

Wyman, M. G., and Hammersmith, L.: Coronary care in a small community hospital. Dis. Chest 53:584, 1968.

Zipes, D. P., et al.: Treatment of ventricular arrhythmia by permanent atrial pacemaker and cardiac sympathectomy. Ann. Intern. Med. 68:591, 1968.

SUPPLEMENTAL READING

Jalife, J., and Moe, J. K.: A biologic model of parasystole. Am. J. Cardiol. 43:761, 1979.

Josephson, M. E., and Horowitz, L. N.: Electrophysiologic approaches to therapy of recurrent sustained ventricular tachycardias. Am. J. Cardiol. 43:631, 1979.

Pederson, D. H., Zipes, D. P., Foster, P. R., and Troup, P. J.: Ventricular tachycardia and ventricular fibrillation in a young population. Circulation 60:988, 1979.

Resnekov, L., and Das Gupta, D. S.: Prevention of ventricular rhythm disturbances in patients with acute myocardial infarction. Am. Heart J. 98:653, 1979.

Zipes, D. P.: Diagnosis of ventricular tachycardia. Drug Therapy p. 83–87, April 1979.

12

A-V HEART BLOCK

RICHARD H. HELFANT, M.D.,
BENJAMIN J. SCHERLAG, Ph.D.

GENERAL CONSIDERATIONS

A-V block refers to conduction disturbances occurring between atrial and ventricular activation, i.e., in the A-V conduction system. This includes the A-V node, the bundle of His, and the bundle branches. The conducted impulse may either be delayed or fail completely to reach the ventricles.

The heart is composed of two types of cardiac muscle: the regular or working myocardium (which makes up the walls of the atria and ventricles) and the specialized conducting tissue (S-A node, A-V node, and the His-Purkinje system) (see Chapter 2). Activation of the working myocardium results in the inscription of the P wave and QRS on the electrocardiogram. However, activation of the specialized conduction tissue (Fig. 12–1) is not seen as positive or negative waves in conventional electrocardiograms owing in part to the small total tissue mass of these structures. Its activation is represented instead by the isoelectric interval just prior to the P wave (S-A node) and during the P-R segment (A-V node, bundle of His, and bundle branches) of the standard electrocardiogram. However, the method of recording from one of these sites — the His bundle — has allowed for considerable increases in our understanding of atrioventricular conduction and heart block, particularly in enabling a more

166

precise localization of the site or sites as well as the degree of cardiac conduction abnormalities (Fig. 12–2).

ETIOLOGY OF A-V HEART BLOCK

Several pathologic processes can result in A-V heart block. These include: sclerodegenerative disease; coronary heart disease; drugs such as digitalis, propranolol, and antiarrhythmics; in-

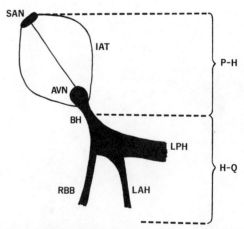

Figure 12–1 Diagrammatic representation of the cardiac conduction system illustrating the intervals measured in the His bundle electrogram. SAN = sinoatrial node; IAT = intra-atrial tracts; AVN = atrioventricular node; BH = bundle of His; LPH = left posterior hemibranch; LAH = left anterior hemibranch; RBB = right bundle branch.

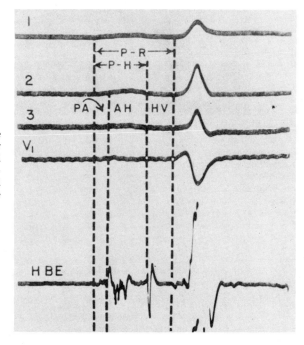

Figure 12–2 Recording of a His bundle electrogram (HBE) and simultaneously recorded electrograms, leads I, II, III and V_1. The P-R interval is divided into intra-atrial conduction time (PA); A-V nodal conduction time (AH) and His-Purkinje time (HV).

flammatory conditions such as rheumatic fever and myocarditis; and congenital abnormalities. The first three represent the most frequently seen etiologies, and they will be discussed extensively, since much interest (and some controversy) has arisen in the diagnosis, treatment, and prognosis of patients with A-V heart block resulting from these causes.

Sclerodegenerative disease is characterized by the progressive replacement of the specialized muscle cells of the conduction system by fibrotic tissue. The histopathologic studies of Lenegre and his associates in 1964 and Davies and Harris (1969) established peripheral bundle branch fibrosis as a primary disease entity leading to A-V heart block. The work of Yater (1935) and Lev (1964) revealed similar sclerodegenerative changes in the proximal His-Purkinje system. In its pure form, primary conduction system disease does not affect the working cardiac muscle nor the coronary arteries in these hearts. The course of this disease process is chronic and complete A-V heart block is, therefore, manifested most frequently in old age.

Coronary heart disease causes A-V heart block as a result of impaired blood flow to the specialized conduction tissue. Since the A-V node is supplied with blood primarily by the A-V nodal artery, decreased blood flow through the vessel may lead to A-V nodal conduction disturbances. The His-bundle and proximal portion of the left and right bundle branch systems are supplied primarily by the first major septal perforator artery. Thus, decreased flow through this vessel may result in conduction abnormalities in these areas.

Drugs such as digitalis and propranolol decrease conduction through the A-V node. In excessive doses, therefore, nodal conduction abnormalities or block may occur (see Chapter 23).

FORMS OF A-V HEART BLOCK

Atrioventricular block is classified according to both its location and severity. Thus, *type I* block refers to an

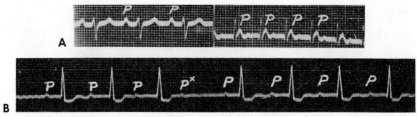

Figure 12–3   Various types of partial A-V heart block. (A) Initial strip shows prolongation of the P-R interval which measures 0.22 second. Second strip: note the P-R interval prolongation with the tachycardia (ventricular rate, 150 per minute). Note that the P wave of the prolonged P-R interval is situated immediately following the preceding QRS complex between the QRS and T wave. This P wave controls the following QRS complex. (B) Shows progressive prolongation of the P-R interval until a dropped beat is observed at P^x (Wenckebach phenomenon). The same sequence is repeated in the latter part of the tracing.

abnormality in the A-V node whereas *type II* is "infranodal" (i.e., below the A-V node). The severity of the block is 1°, 2°, or 3° (complete heart block).

First degree A-V block is manifested on the electrocardiogram as a prolonged P-R interval (greater than 0.21 seconds, Fig. 12–3A). By itself (that is, without associated bundle branch block or higher degrees of block), first degree A-V block is usually benign, representing some degree of delay greater than normal in impulse transmission through the A-V node.

Second degree A-V block is characterized by the failure of some, but not all, atrial impulses to reach the ventricles. This form of block is seen on the electrocardiogram as two relatively distinct

patterns: (1) *Wenckebach* or *Mobitz type I* block, in which the P-R interval progressively prolongs prior to the blocked P wave (Figure 12–3B), and (2) *Wenckebach type II* or *Mobitz type II* block, in which the blocked P wave is preceded by P-R intervals which are relatively constant and the same as the P-R interval of the first conducted beat after the block (Figure 12–4). (Recent studies suggest that both forms represent different degrees of slowed conduction prior to the blocked beat [El-Sherif et al., 1975].) However, type II block carries a higher risk of 3° A-V heart block — i.e., complete heart block — than the type I form. Thus, pacemaker therapy is indicated when type II block is seen.

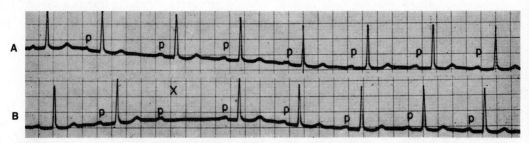

Figure 12–4   Partial A-V heart block: Mobitz type II. A and B represent a continuous record. Note the presence of a partial A-V heart block with a constant degree of P-R interval prolongation measuring 0.28 second. Slight irregularity in the ventricular rate is due to a sinus arrhythmia. Note the sudden appearance of a 2:1 A-V heart block in cycle X of strip B, without any change in the length of the preceding P-R intervals. The P-R after the A-V block is slightly shorter (0.24 second) than that observed in previous short cycles and this is followed by cycles of P-R prolongation similar to those that preceded the 2:1 A-V heart block.

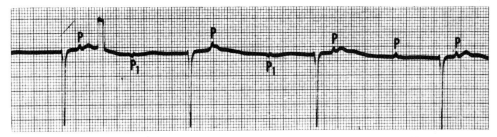

Figure 12–5 Complete A-V heart block with narrow QRS complexes (0.08 second) in an 80-year-old male with arteriosclerotic heart disease. The ventricular rate is 33 per minute; the atrial rate is 75 per minute; there is no relationship between the atrial and ventricular contractions. The atrial beats vary in configuration. The narrow QRS complexes suggest that the ventricular pacemaker is located in the bundle of His.

Third degree A-V block or *complete heart block* is seen on the electrocardiogram as completely independent activity of the atria and ventricles, the former at a rate of 60–80 per minute, the latter at a rate of 30–50 per minute (Fig. 12–5). Permanent complete heart block may occasionally be interrupted by the return of sinus rhythm with 1:1 A-V conduction. Sudden onset of A-V block can often result in a prolonged period of ventricular asystole prior to the "warmup" of a subsidiary ventricular escape pacemaker. Such paroxysmal episodes, known as Stokes-Adams attacks, represent the greatest danger to the patients since they are associated with dizziness, syncope, and sudden death. The patient may suffer severe traumatic damage as a result of syncope, or ventricular fibrillaton may occur during this period of cardiac instability.

HARBINGERS OF IMPENDING A-V BLOCK

Fascicular Block or Bilateral Bundle Branch Block

With the increased acceptance and use of electronic pacemakers, attention has been focused on the detection of individuals at risk for the development of paroxysmal, complete A-V block. Two major advances in the detection of impending Stokes-Adams attack have been the establishment of the trifascicular concept of the His-Purkinje system and the development of the His bundle recording technique.

Figure 12–6 Diagrammatic representations of the A-V conduction system illustrating the various types of complete A-V heart block (top row) and the individual fascicular blocks (bottom row). RBBB = right bundle branch block; LAH = left anterior hemiblock; LPH = left posterior hemiblock.

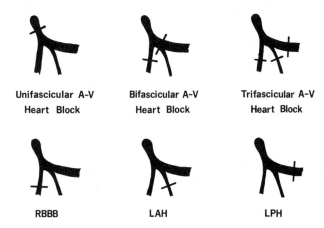

Unifascicular A-V Heart Block   Bifascicular A-V Heart Block   Trifascicular A-V Heart Block

RBBB   LAH   LPH

The trifascicular concept of Rosen-baum et al. (1970), based on prior ex-perimental (Rothberger and Winter-berg, 1917; Watt and Pruitt, 1965) and clinical studies (Wilson and Hermann, 1920; Grant, 1959), envisions a His-Purkinje system composed of the main or common bundle — i.e., His bun-dle — which has three branches or fas-cicles: the right bundle branch; and two divisions of the left bundle branch, the anterior-superior division and the posterior-inferior division (see Fig. 12–6). Various forms of partial infranodal or fascicular block can occur. Thus, when two fascicles are blocked, this ab-normality (referred to as bifascicular block or bilateral bundle branch block) may precede complete A-V heart block. The most common types of bifascicular or bilateral bundle branch block seen clinically are right bundle branch block with left axis deviation (frontal plane axis greater than −45°), referred to by Rosenbaum et al. as left anterior hemi-block (LAH). Less commonly seen is right bundle branch block with right axis deviation (frontal plane axis +80° to +120°) or left posterior hemiblock (LPH).

The electrocardiographic pattern of right bundle branch block and left an-terior hemiblock is shown in Figure 12–7. It is characterized by a wide QRS (greater than 0.10 sec), predominant R waves in V1, and primarily negative deflections in leads II, III and aVF. Right bundle branch block and left pos-terior hemiblock (Figure 12–8) also shows the widened QRS and predomi-nant R wave in V1 characteristic of right bundle branch block. In addition, there is the S1 Q3 pattern characteristic of right axis deviation (or left posterior he-miblock).

The association between bifascicular block or bilateral bundle branch block, particularly the electrocardiographic pattern of right bundle branch block and left anterior hemiblock, and im-pending complete A-V block was ini-tially established by the retrospective

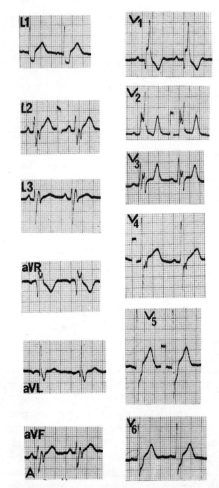

Figure 12–7   Right bundle branch block with left anterior hemiblock shows right bundle branch block with left-axis deviation. Note the terminal widening of the QRS complexes in leads I, II, and III and the tall R waves in the right precordial leads. This is due to the combination of right bundle branch block and left anterior hemiblock.

studies of Lasser et al. in 1968. By ex-amining patients with documented complete heart block, they found that almost 60 per cent showed the pattern of right bundle branch block and left anterior hemiblock on electrocardio-grams prior to the complete block. It is equally important that the prospective portion of the study showed that only 10 per cent of patients with the electro-cardiographic pattern of right bundle

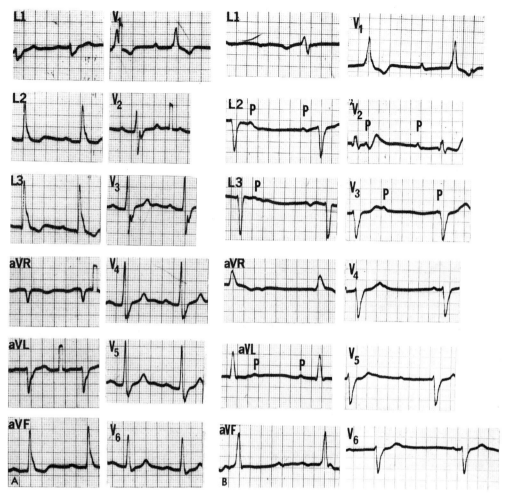

Figure 12-8 (A) Right bundle branch block with left posterior hemiblock. Note the right axis deviation, widened QRS, and prolonged P-R interval (0.28 second). Tall R waves are observed in the right precordial leads. (B) One year later, patient has developed complete A-V heart block.

branch block and left anterior hemiblock went on to complete A-V block. The reason for the differences in the retrospective and prospective studies probably relates to the inclusion of many more patients with myocardial infarction in the former group. In these patients the time between the infarction which induces the electrocardiographic pattern of right bundle branch block and left anterior hemiblock is short — i.e., hours (Lie et al., 1974) — whereas in patients with this bifascicular block pattern due to primary conduction system disease, the end-stage, complete heart block, usually occurs after many years. The long course of primary conduction disease may account for the marked variability found by several investigators for the incidence of complete heart block in patients with bifascicular block.

HIS BUNDLE RECORDINGS

The technique for recording the His bundle electrogram was introduced by

Scherlag et al. (1969). It requires the positioning of an electrode catheter, usually inserted through a femoral vein, against the lower right atrial septum in the area of the A-V node and His bundle. In conjunction with several standard electrocardiographic leads, the His bundle electrogram allows a more precise determination of the site and degree of delay or block in the cardiac conduction system. Using the His bundle electrogram and the electrocardiogram (His bundle-electrocardiography), the P-R interval can be subdivided into specific conduction compartments (Fig. 12–2). The P-A interval represents intra-atrial conduction from the beginning of the P wave (the area of the sinus node) to the beginning of atrial activation (A) near the A-V node. It ranges from 10 to 55 msec in the normal heart. A-V nodal conduction can be quantitated by measuring the interval from the beginning of the A wave to the onset of the His bundle deflection, the A-H interval. This varies from 50 to 120 msec in the normal heart. His-Purkinje conduction time can be measured from the onset of the His bundle potential to the earliest activation of the ventricles in any of the electrocardiographic leads recorded. The H-V interval ranges from 35 to 55 msec in the normal heart.

Atrial pacing and programmed stimulation (see Chapter 14) are commonly used in conjunction with His bundle-electrocardiography. In normal hearts atrial pacing at progressively increasing rates results in prolongation of A-V nodal conduction until A-V nodal Wenckebach periodicity ensues at heart rates above 130 per minute. Block of the atrial impulses is normally localized proximal to the His bundle deflection. An A-H interval greater than 120 msec during sinus rhythm and normal heart rate or a Wenckebach type pattern of A-H intervals at rates below 130/minute (Rosen 1971) are considered to be indications of abnormal A-V nodal function.

In the normal heart at all paced rates the H-V interval remains constant. Abnormal H-V intervals can be seen when conduction is delayed at both the right and left bundle branches or in the His bundle itself. If a delay occurs in only one bundle branch the ventricles will be activated at the normal time but not in normal sequence by the other bundle branch. The ability to localize the site of H-V delay is limited unless split His bundle potentials — i.e., intra-His bundle block — or electrocardiographic patterns of right or left bundle branch block are seen in conjunction with normal H-V intervals.

When the His bundle recording technique was introduced, clinical investigators realized an opportunity to utilize this technique in patients with electrocardiographic patterns of bifascicular block in order to more definitively identify those at risk for impending complete heart block. In the series of Narula et al. (1975), of 131 patients with right bundle branch block and left axis deviation or left anterior hemiblock, 72 per cent showed H-V prolongation. Thus, conduction delay existed not only in the right bundle branch and left anterior division of the left bundle branch but also in the posterior division of the left bundle as well.*

Recent studies by Narula et al. (1975), Scheinman et al. (1973), Ranganathan et al. (1972), and Vera et al. (1976) have shown that H-V prolongation is observed in a high percentage of patients with a suspicious electrocardiographic pattern; i.e., right bundle branch block plus left anterior hemiblock. These patients are symptomatic and exhibit diz-

---

*Of interest is the high percentage of H-V prolongation, 79 per cent in the 123 patients with left bundle branch block pattern on the electrocardiogram. In these cases there must be right bundle branch block to a lesser degree or intra-His bundle block coexisting with the left bundle branch block. The H-V prolongations for other forms of intraventricular conduction defects indicate that the electrocardiogram was not a specific indicator of the degree and site(s) of lesion in the ventricular conduction system.

ziness and syncope not related to neurological disorders. In the study of Narula et al., 24 symptomatic patients with right bundle branch block and left axis deviation or left anterior hemiblock had prolonged H-V intervals and were treated by pacemaker implantation. These patients were followed for a period up to six years. The average annual mortality was 13 per cent. Of the 34 who were asymptomatic (without pacemakers) the average yearly mortality was almost three times as great, 36 per cent. These findings have been confirmed in a recent prospective study by Altschuler et al. (1977). Thus, these investigators found that the H-V interval has considerable prognostic significance in terms of mortality, supposedly from A-V block, and thus, in determining the method of management, i.e., whether or not to implant a permanent pacemaker.

On the other hand, another study of 119 asymptomatic patients with right bundle branch block and left anterior hemiblock, followed for up to two years by Denes et al. (1975) did not show the marked increases in the incidence of A-V block or mortality. The differences between the studies may be explained by two important factors regarding the etiology of A-V block. Firstly, the average age of the patients in the Narula study was 72 and in the study by Altschuler et al., 69. On the other hand, the average age in the study by Denes et al. was 62. Thus, it would be expected that the older patients would represent a population showing a higher incidence of primary conduction system disease and a greater tendency, owing to age, for the conduction system disease to go on to complete heart block. Indeed, in the study by Narula et al. it was noted that almost 30 per cent of the patients studied were diagnosed as exhibiting primary conduction system disease as the major if not the sole disease entity. Moreover, in the population study by Denes et al., the majority of patients showed moderate to severe coronary artery disease as reflected by a high incidence of cardiomegaly, functional class III and class IV status, and presence of third heart sound gallop and other indications of severe hemodynamic impairment. Thus, even in those cases with prolonged H-V intervals, the severe coronary heart disease may be overriding, with a lethal factor preventing them from reaching an age at which the primary conduction system disease would progress to complete A-V heart block. In fact, the annual mortality of 10 per cent in the 33 asymptomatic patients would preclude the large majority of them reaching the average age represented in the studies by Narula et al. (1975) and Altschuler et al. (1977). The differences in patient population can also be seen in recent studies of patients with electrocardiographic patterns of right bundle branch block and left anterior hemiblock induced by acute myocardial infarction. Lie et al. (1974) found that prolongation of H-V intervals in these patients was associated with a high mortality and that permanent pacemaker implantation in a comparable group significantly decreased mortality. Similar findings were reported by Lichstein et al. (1977).

On the other hand, Ginks et al. (1977) followed 25 patients who survived acute myocardial infarction and transient A-V block for an average of 49 months. The majority, 14, had bifascicular block on the electrocardiogram. At the end of the follow-up period, 10 of the 14 were alive. Of four in whom permanent pacing was established, two died. These authors concluded that "long term pacing is not justified in patients, otherwise asymptomatic, with (bifascicular) block persisting after . . . anterior myocardial infarction." Unfortunately, only eight patients were studied using His bundle-electrocardiography and no apparent relationship between the H-V interval and outcome was evidenced. Further studies are required to determine the long term prognostic value of H-V intervals in patients with bifascicular block resulting from acute anterior wall myocardial infarction. It is highly probable, however, that the high mortality associated with the development of bundle branch block in acute anterior wall myocardial infarction (Norris et al., 1972; Godman et al., 1970) is mainly the result of pump failure and much less attributable to cardiac conduction disorders.

NEW APPROACHES TO DETECTION OF IMPENDING OR INTERMITTENT COMPLETE HEART BLOCK

Both the electrocardiographic patterns and measurements of H-V intervals in patients with partial A-V heart block are limited in determining impending complete heart block. The limitations are based on the chronic course of primary conduction system disease generally and the variable nature of the disease process in any given individual (Ranganathan et al., 1972; Vera et al., 1976). It is controversial whether a single determination of an abnormal H-V interval in a patient with right bundle branch block and left anterior hemiblock is indicative of impending complete heart block even if the value is greater than 65 msec (Narula, 1975a; Vera, 1976; Dreifus, 1977). Similarly, problems exist in patients with disease in the His bundle itself, since His potentials may or may not be recorded in this situation (see Chapter 14).

Recently, non-invasive means of recording His-Purkinje system activation has been reported by several groups (Berbari et al., 1973; Hishimoto and Sawayama, 1975), based on signal averaging of an amplified rapid sweep speed standard electrocardiogram. This may allow for serial studies to be performed in patients with conduction system disorders in the future. At the present time, this remains in the investigative sphere.

Long Term Ambulatory ECG Monitoring

In patients who are suspected of having episodes of complete heart block, long term electrocardiographic monitoring has become an important mode of obtaining clinical information (see Chapter 14). These monitoring techniques, originated by Holter, consist of outfitting patients with a portable, self-contained tape-recording unit which the patient then carries with him for up to 24 hours in the course of his daily activities. Analysis of these tape recordings is then made using a scanning device which allows rapid data reduction and graphing. To date, most of the experience has been gained with the Holter-Avionics system (see Chapter 14). In patients with suspected evidence of episodic severe heart block, paroxysmal symptoms such as lightheadedness, faintness, disorientation, or syncope can then be correlated by simultaneously determined patient diary entry and electrocardiographic reading at the time of symptoms. Arrhythmias of some type have been found in 25 to 40 per cent of patients who have symptoms of syncope, dizziness, or other transient neurological symptoms, including evidence of sinus node dysfunction (see Chapter 5), A-V block with long periods of non-conduction, and occasionally other ectopic arrhythmias as well. Thus, this technique is a most valuable adjunct in the detection of patients with suspected A-V block.

Stress Testing

Stress testing is another means by which conduction defects involving the atrioventricular junction and bundle branches may be unmasked. The increased adrenergic drive evoked during exercise usually shortens atrioventricular conduction. Thus, a lengthening of the PR interval or more importantly the development of higher degrees of A-V block with exercise are considered abnormal responses indicative of underlying conduction system disease. While the development of intraventricular conduction disturbances — i.e., right or left bundle branch blocks — can be observed during exercise in patients without pathologic disease of the conduction system, the usual "tachycardia dependent bundle branch block" involves the right bundle branch. Abnormalities resulting in a left bundle branch with left anterior hemiblock type patterns are more suspicious of underlying conduction system disease. Similarly, the development of tachyarrhythmias of atrial or ventricular origin with exercise and accompanying symptoms relative to the central nervous system is strong incrimination of this being the etiology of the patient's problem and lessens the possibility of conduction system disease as a primary underlying etiology.

CLINICAL FEATURES

The symptoms of *incomplete or partial A-V block* are largely influenced by the underlying clinical state. However, unless the heart rate is slow, there are few symptoms due to the incomplete heart block itself. The clinical manifestations of *complete heart block* depend upon the type and duration of the cardiac disturbance as well as the state of the cerebral circulation. The manifestations of cerebral origin may range from lightheadedness and dizziness, which may be relatively transient, to loss of consciousness with or without convulsive episodes. This will generally correlate with either ventricular standstill or very low rates, i.e., 20 beats per minute or less. Occasionally, ventricular fibrillation is noted. These arrhythmias may occur singly or in various combinations. However, in the presence of varying degrees of cerebral atherosclerosis, heart rates below 40 may result in cerebrovascular insufficiency of a generalized or localized nature. Symptoms associated with myocardial dysfunction

also may occur, such as easy fatigability and/or shortness of breath.

On physical examination, the cardinal sign of complete heart block (aside from the slow heart rate) is a change of intensity in the first heart sound which is best heard at the apex, due to the variation in relationship between atrial and ventricular contractions. Frequently, faint atrial sounds may be heard. The venous pressure is elevated and cervical venous pulsations are unrelated to ventricular activations with characteristic "cannon waves" observed in the neck occurring when the P wave falls between the QRS and T wave (i.e., when the right atrium contracts against a closed tricuspid valve).

ELECTROCARDIOGRAM

First Degree A-V Block

The ECG clearly shows regularly recurring normal P waves with P-R intervals which are prolonged beyond 0.21 second in adults (0.18 second in children). Dropped beats are not encountered.

Second Degree A-V block

Wenckebach Type (Mobitz Type I). This pattern of A-V block is characterized by progressive lengthening of the P-R interval until a point is reached at which no ventricular complex follows the P wave. The increment of delay, however, is progressively less with each cycle. There is, therefore, the appearance of progressively shorter R-R cycles (despite the progressive lengthening of the P-R interval), separated by a long cycle with the long cycle being less than the sum of the two short cycles preceding it.

Mobitz Type II. In this situation, the P-R interval is fixed although it may be less than, equal to, or greater than 0.21 second. At intervals, a single ventricular beat is dropped. Frequently associated with Mobitz type II block, the QRS complex is widened to 0.12 second or longer. This widening is indicative of the conduction disturbance in the His-Purkinje system discussed previously.

Complete A-V Block

Complete block is characterized by ventricular complexes which occur regularly at a rate usually between 20 and 40 beats per minute while the atria are usually beating independently at a more normal rate. In cases of congenital complete heart block, however, the ventricular rate may be higher. Occasionally, complete heart block may occur in the presence of atrial fibrillation or other atrial arrhythmias.

The ventricular complexes in complete heart block are usually characterized by prolonged interventricular conduction with notched and slurred QRS complexes. This type of pattern occurs in 85 per cent of the adult cases of complete A-V heart block. In the second type, the QRS is characterized by normal width and duration and is most commonly seen in the congenital variety, although it may occasionally occur in the acquired type of A-V block. The conduction abnormality in the latter circumstance is usually due to block within the His bundle itself. Widened ventricular complexes in complete heart block may be due to unusual pacemaker location as well as different combinations of bundle branch block. Not infrequently, widened ventricular complexes may occur intermittently or change their contour, presumably due to shifts in pacemaker location and/or conduction pathway.

The ventricular rate in patients with A-V block characterized by wide QRS complexes is generally between 20 and 40 beats per minute. These beats tend to be irregular at times and patients are prone to episodes of unexplained cardiac arrest. Occasional irregularities may occur when the pacemaker site itself is slightly irregular, when the pacemaker site shifts from one focus to another, when ventricular premature complexes are present, when occasional normally conducted beats occur, when two or more lower pacemakers compete, or in the presence of atrial fibrillation when a supraventricular beat emerges, also after emergence from a Stokes-Adams attack when the ventricular rate may initially be rapid (100 or more beats per minute), then gradually slowing to the original rate.

The A-V conduction system has a bi-directional capacity and thus retrograde conduction from the ventricles to atrium may occur during ventricular tachycardia or premature beats as well as in the presence of complete antegrade atrioventricular block. The ECG under these circumstances exhibits complete antegrade block with ventriculoatrial conduction and the atrial component represented by inverted P waves.

It has frequently been observed that in cases of A-V block (partial or complete) the P-R intervals that contain a ventricular complex are shorter than those that do not. The best explanation for this effect is that the ventricular contraction produces traction on the right atrium and this mechanical stretch increases sinus node automaticity.

Fascicular Blocks and Bilateral Bundle Branch Block

Right Bundle Branch Block. The electrocardiographic criteria for the diagnosis of right bundle branch block are (1) QRS duration of more than 0.12 second; (2) delayed onset of the intrinsicoid deflection (R') in the right ventricular leads; (3) increased amplitude of the R' deflection in the right precordial leads; (4) secondary ST and T wave changes; and (5) often a QR or SR' pattern in lead aVR.

Left Anterior Hemiblock (block of the anterior-superior division of the

left bundle branch). The electrocardiographic criteria for pure left anterior hemiblock are (1) electrical axis equal to or more than 60°; (2) main QRS forces oriented superiorly and to the left; (3) Q1,S3 pattern or an apparent counterclockwise rotation of the heart on the longitudinal axis; and (4) a QRS complex of normal width or not prolonged by more than 0.02 second.

Left Posterior Hemiblock (block of the posterior inferior division of the left bundle branch). The electrocardiographic criteria are (1) electrical axis between +80 and +120 degrees, (2) S1, Q3 pattern with prolongation of the QRS pattern. A simple vertical heart and right ventricular hypertrophy must be ruled out. Clinically pure left posterior hemiblock is very uncommon and is rarely seen unless diffuse conduction system abnormalities are present. In these cases it is usually accompanied by right bundle branch block or intermittent left anterior hemiblock.

TREATMENT OF A-V HEART BLOCK

The treatment of A-V block depends on its location, degree, etiology, and clinical manifestations. In general, first degree block does not require treatment. Heart block can be divided into acute and chronic settings.

Acute Heart Block

The most common causes of acute heart block are a fresh myocardial infarction and drug excess, notably digitalis toxicity. In acute myocardial infarction, type I block usually occurs in the context of an inferior infarct affecting the A-V nodal artery. In this setting, Wenckebach block and complete heart block usually do not require therapy. Since the heart block is of type I variety in this setting, the ventricular rate is usually 50 or more with a stable

pacemaker and no significant hemodynamic impairment. Under circumstances in which the rate is slower or unstable or if hemodynamic impairment is evident, temporary ventricular pacing is indicated. Type I block due to digitalis toxicity is approached in the same general manner with the obvious primary treatment being cessation of digitalis.

Patients with anterior myocardial infarction can be complicated by A-V block of the type II variety. In this circumstance, complete block is unpredictable in its occurrence. It is frequently accompanied by a slow, unstable ventricular rate and severe hemodynamic abnormalities. Occasionally, infarcts of this type, involving the first septal perforator of the left anterior descending coronary artery result in fascicular and bundle branch blocks. Thus, the development of Mobitz II block, complete block, or a new bundle branch block (or more particularly bifascicular block) in this setting is an absolute indication for temporary pacemaker implantation.

Chronic Heart Block

In chronic A-V block, those of the type I variety are usually drug related, less commonly being due to infections or a congenital etiology. Specific therapy is usually not necessary.

Type II block in a more chronic setting is usually due to either primary sclerodegenerative conduction system disease or less commonly chronic coronary heart disease or primary myocardial disease. Most authorities recommend permanent pacemaker therapy for patients with complete heart block of the type II variety or Mobitz type II block even in the absence of symptoms.

In patients with bifascicular block (i.e., bilateral bundle branch block), the indications for pacemaker therapy are somewhat less clear. In the absence of neurological abnormalities, patients with strongly suggestive symptoms (see above) and evidence of bilateral bundle branch block should, in our judgment, be strongly considered for pacemaker therapy, particularly when episodes of higher degrees of block can be demonstrated either with long term ECG monitoring or stress testing or if His bundle studies reveal severe prolongation, i.e., ≥70 milliseconds H-V time. However, it is also our view that the symptoms, not the H-V time should be the decisive index for pacemaker consideration in this circumstance.

Patients who are totally asymptomatic with evidence of bifascicular or bilateral bundle branch block should be followed carefully for the exhibition of classic neurological symptoms relating to higher degrees of block. However, unless Mobitz type II or complete heart block is demonstrated, it is our view that pacemaker therapy is not warranted.

DRUG THERAPY

The therapy of choice for symptomatic heart block is clearly temporary or permanent pacing, depending on the clinical context in which the block occurs. This is because drugs are rarely effective in abolishing A-V block. However, certain drug preparations will act temporarily to improve the situation and allow a more optimal circumstance for pacemaker implantation. *Atropine* is used for the drug treatment of patients with type I block because of its low incidence of serious side effects. By reducing vagal tone, it often will augment A-V block of the Type I variety (although its effect may be transitory) and has little effect on infranodal or type II block.

Isoproterenol is at times a life saving agent in the emergency treatment of severe heart block complicated by very slow ventricular rates or ventricular standstill. It acts to increase the automaticity of cardiac pacemakers as well as to temporarily increase cardiac output due to the increased ventricular rate. In patients with recurrent Stokes-Adams attacks complicated by exceedingly low ventricular rates (i.e., 20 or less or ventricular standstill), intravenous isoproterenol is utilized to stabilize the rhythm while a temporary pacemaker is inserted.

A complete description of the indications, uses, types, and follow-ups of patients with pacemakers is presented in Chapter 24.

PROGNOSIS

The prognosis for patients with complete A-V block is not clear since the incidence and natural history are only available in those who have been symptomatic. Prior to the availability of pacemaker therapy, 50 to 60 per cent of patients who suffered Stokes-Adams attacks died within a year, most often from a subsequent attack. In many series, artificial pacing has been found to markedly improve long term survival rates. The life expectancy of patients with pacemakers is now within 10 per cent of that of a normal population comparable in age and sex (see Chapter 24).

Death frequently occurs during a Stokes-Adams attack and this is the most common cause of death in untreated complete A-V block. In the series of Penton et al. (1956) the average duration of life after the first sign of A-V block was 26.2 months. With the advent of reliable pacemaker therapy, the prognosis of patients with Stokes-Adams seizures thus has become much improved.

Chardack (1969) has found that 25 of 48 (52%) are alive 5 to 8 years after surgical implantation of myocardial electrodes in an early experience with pacemakers. Other authors have reported similar results (Johanson, 1966; Siddons and Sowton, 1967). At present, the principal limitations on longevity are 1) the age of the patient; 2) the severity of underlying cardiac disorder; 3) the occurrence of a rhythm in competition with the pacemaker leading to ventricular fibrillation; 4) the various forms of failure and other complicating factors of the pacemakers themselves. However, with further improvement in the reliability and longevity of pacemakers and their batteries, there has been continued improvement in the prognosis of these patients.

REFERENCES

Adolph, R. J.: Diagnosis and medical management of complete atrioventricular block. Heart Bull. 17:16, 1968.

Alanis, J., and Benitez, D.: Transitional potentials and the prolongation of impulses through different cardiac cells. In Santo, T., Mizukira, V., and Matsuda, K. (eds.): Electrophysiology and Ultrastructure of the Heart. New York, Grune and Stratton, 1967, pp. 153–175.

Altschuler, H., Fisher, J. D., and Furman, S.: Prolonged H-V interval. Preventable early mortality in symptomatic patients without documented heart block. Clin. Res. 25:203A, 1977 (Abst).

Bazett, H. C.: Analysis of time relations of electrocardiogram. Heart 7:353, 1920.

Bellet, S., and Wasserman, F.: Indications and contraindications for the use of molar sodium lactate. Circulation 15:591, 1957.

Bellet, S., Wasserman, F., and Brody, J. I.: Molar sodium lactate; its effect in complete A-V heart block and cardiac arrest occurring during Stokes-Adams seizures and in terminal state. New Engl. J. Med. 253:891, 1955.

Bellet, S., Wasserman, F., and Brody, J. I.: Effect of molar sodium lactate in increasing cardiac rhythmicity: Clinical and experimental study of its use in the treatment of patients with slow heart rates, Stokes-Adams syndrome and episodes of cardiac arrest. J.A.M.A. 160:1293, 1956.

Benchimol, A., Evandro, E. G., and Dimond, E. G.: Stroke volume and peripheral resistance during infusion of isoproterenol at a constant fixed heart rate. Circulation 31:417, 1965a.

Benchimol, A., Palmero, H. A., Liggett, M. S., and Dimond, E. G.: Influence of digitalization on the contribution of atrial systole to the cardiac dynamics at a fixed ventricular rate. Circulation 31:417, 1965b.

Benchimol, A., Wu, T., and Liggett, M. S.: Effect of exercise and isoproterenol on the cardiovascular dynamics in complete heart block at various heart rates. Amer. Heart J. 70:337, 1965c.

Berbari, E. J., Lazzara, R., Samet, P., and Scherlag B. J.: Noninvasive technique for detection of electrical activity during the P-R segment. Circulation 48:1005, 1973.

Bevegard, S., et al.: Effect of changes in ventricular rate on cardiac output and central venous pressure at rest and during exercise in patients with artificial pacemakers. Cardiovasc. Res. 1:21, 1967.

Chardack W. M.: Cardiac pacemakers and heart block. In Gibbon, J. H., Sabiston, D. C., and Spencer, F. C.(eds.): Surgery of the Chest. Philadelphia, W. B. Saunders Co., 1969, pp. 824–865.

Chatterjee, K., et al.: The electrocardiogram in chronic heart block. A histological correlation with ECG changes in 42 patients. Amer. Heart J. 80:47, 1970.

Damato, A. N., Lau, S. H., Helfant, R. H., Stein, E., Berkowitz, W. D., and Cohen S. I.: Study of atrioventricular conduction in man using electrode catheter recordings of His bundle activity. Circulation 39:287, 1969.

Davies, M., and Harris, A.: Pathological basis of primary heart block. Brit. Heart J. 31:219, 1969.

DeLeon, A. C., Bellet, S., and Muller, O. F.: The effect of acidosis and of hyperpotassemia on the idioventricular rate in complete A-V heart block (unpublished data, 1961).

Denes, P., Dhingra, R. G., Wu, D., Chaquima, R., Amat-y-Leon, F., Wyndham, C., and Rosen, K. M.: H-V interval in patients with bifascicular block (right bundle branch block and left anterior hemiblock). Amer. J. Cardiol. 35:23, 1975.

Dreifus, L. S.: Clinical judgement is sufficient for the management of conduction defects. In Corday E, (ed.): Controversies in Cardiology. Philadelphia, F. A. Davis Co., pp. 195–201, 1977.

El-Sherif, N., Scherlag, B. J., and Lazzara, R.: Pathophysiology of second degree atrioventricular block: A unified hypothesis. Amer. J. Cardiol. 35:421, 1975.

Fisch, C., and Knoebel, S. B.: Junctional rhythms. Prog. Cardiov. Dis. 13:141, 1970.

Friedberg, H. D., and Schamroth, L.: The Wenckebach phenomenon in left bundle branch block. Amer. J. Cardiol. 24:591, 1969.

Ginks, W. R., Sutton, R., Winston, O. H., and Leatham, A.: Long-term prognosis after acute anterior infarction with atrioventricular block. Brit. Heart J. 39:186, 1977.

Godman, M. J., Lasser, W. D., and Julian, D. J.: Complete bundle branch block complicating acute myocardial infarction. New Engl. J. Med. 282:237, 1970.

Grant, R. P.: Peri-infarction block. Prog. Cardiovasc. Dis. 2:237, 1956.

Hanssen, P.: Incidence of auricular flutter and auricular fibrillation associated with complete auriculoventricular dissociation. Acta Med. Scand. 136:113, 1949.

Hishimoto, Y., and Sawayama, T.: Non-invasive

recording of His bundle potential in man. Brit. Heart J. *37*:635, 1975.

Johansson, B. W.: Complete heart block. A clinical, hemodynamic, and pharmacological study in patients with or without an artificial pacemaker. Acta Med. Scand. *180*: Suppl. 451, 1966.

Johnsson, R. A., Averill, K. H., and Lamb, L. E.: Non-specific T wave changes. In Lamb, L. E. (ed.): First International Symposium in Cardiology in Aviation. Texas, Brooks Air Force Base, 1969.

Kastor, J. A., Sanders, C. A., Leinbach, R. C., and Hawthorne, J. W.: Factors influencing retrograde conduction. A study of 30 patients during cardiac catheterization. Brit. Heart J. *31*:580, 1969.

Katz, L. N., and Pick, A.: Clinical Electrocardiography, Part I. The Arrhythmias. Philadelphia, Lea & Febiger, 1956.

Kaufman, J. G., Wachtel, F. W., Rothfield, E., and Bernstein, A.: The association of complete heart block and Adams-Stokes syndrome in two cases of Mobitz type II block: Case reports. Circulation *23*:253, 1961.

Korst, D. R., and Wasserberger, R. H.: Atrial flutter associated with complete heart block. Amer. Heart J. *48*:383, 1954.

Kulbertus, H.: The magnitude of risk of developing complete heart block in patients with left axis deviation-right bundle branch block. Amer. Heart J. *86*:278, 1973.

Kulbertus, H., and Collignon, P.: Association of right bundle branch block with left superior or inferior intraventricular block. Its relation to complete heart block and Adams-Stokes syndrome. Brit. Heart J. *31*:435, 1969.

Langendorf, R., and Mehlman, J. S.: Blocked (non-conducted) A-V nodal premature systoles imitating first and second degree A-V block. Amer. Heart J. *34*:500, 1947.

Langendorf, R., and Pick, A.: Approach to the interpretation of complex arrhythmias. Prog. Cardiovasc. Dis. *2*:706, 1960.

Langendorf, R., Pick, A., Edelist, A., and Katz, L. N.: Experimental demonstration of concealed A-V conduction in the human heart. Circulation *32*:386, 1965.

Lasser, R. P., Haft, J. I., and Friedberg, C. K.: Relationship of right bundle branch block and marked left axis deviation to complete heart block and syncope. Circulation *37*:429, 1968.

Lenegre, J.: Etiology and pathology of bilateral bundle branch block in relation to complete heart block. Prog. Cardiovasc. Dis. *6*:409, 1964.

Lev, M.: Anatomic basis for atrioventricular block. Amer. J. Med. *37*:742, 1964.

Lev, M., Kinare, S. G., and Pick, A.: The pathogenesis of atrioventricular block in coronary disease. Circulation *42*:409, 1970.

Lev, M., and McMillan, J. B.: A semi-quantitative histopathologic method for the study of the en-tire heart for clinical and electrocardiographic correlations. Amer. Heart J. *58*:140, 1959.

Lichstein, E., Gupta, K. D., Chadda, H., Liu, H., and Sayeed, M.: Findings of prognostic value in patients with incomplete bilateral bundle branch block complicating acute myocardial infarction. Amer. J. Cardiol. *32*:913, 1977.

Lie, K. I., Wellens, H. J., Schuilenberg, R. M., Becker, A. E., and Durrer, D.: Factors influencing prognosis of bundle branch block complicating acute anteroseptal infarction. Circulation *50*:935, 1974.

Logue, R. B., and Hanson, J. F.: Heart block. Amer. J. Med. Sci. *207*:765, 1944.

Lopez, J. F.: Electrocardiographic findings in patients with complete atrioventricular block. Brit. Heart J. *30*:20, 1968.

McNally, E. M., and Benchimol, A.: Medical and physiological considerations in the use of artificial cardiac pacing. Parts I and II. Amer. Heart J. *75*:380, 864, 1968.

Moe, G. K., Childers, R. W., and Merideth, J.: An appraisal of "supernormal" A-V conduction. Circulation *38*:5, 1968.

Narula, O. S.: Intraventricular conduction defects. In Narula, O. S. (ed.): His Bundle Electrocardiography and Clinical Electrophysiology. Philadelphia, F. A. Davis Co., 1975, Chapter 10.

Narula, O. S., Gann, D., and Samet, P.: Prognostic value of H-V intervals. In Narula, O. S. (ed.): His Bundle Electrocardiography and Clinical Electrophysiology. Philadelphia, F. A. Davis Co., 1975, Chapter 20.

Narula, O. S., and Samet, P.: Wenckebach and Mobitz type II A-V heart block within the His bundle and bundle branches. Circulation *41*:947, 1970.

Narula, O. S., Scherlag, B. J., Samet, P., and Javier, R. P.: Atrioventricular block: Localization and classification by His bundle recordings. Amer. J. Med. *50*:146, 1971.

Norris, R. M., Mercer, C. J., and Croxson, M. S.: Conduction disturbances due to anteroseptal myocardial infarction and their treatment by endocardial pacing. Amer. Heart J.: *81*:560, 1972.

Penton, G. B., Miller, H., and Levine, S.: Some clinical features of complete heart block. Circulation, *13*:801, 1956.

Ranganathan, N., Dhurandhar, R., Phillips, J. H., and Wigle, E. D.: His bundle electrogram in bundle branch block. Circulation *48*:282, 1972.

Rosen, K. M.: The contribution of His bundle recordings to the understanding of cardiac conduction in man. Circulation *43*:961, 1971.

Rosenbaum, M. B., Elizari, M. V., and Lazzari, J.: Los Hemibloqueos. Buenos Aires, Ed. Paidos, 1967.

Rosenbaum, M. B., Elizari, M. V., and Lazzari, J. L.: The hemiblock. Oldsmar, Florida, Tampa Tracings, 1970.

Rosenbaum, M. B., et al.: Intraventricular trifascicular blocks. The syndrome of right bundle branch block with intermittent left anterior and posterior hemiblock. Amer. Heart J. *78*:306, 1969.

Rosenbaum, M. B., and Lepeschkin, E.: The effect of ventricular systole on auricular rhythm in atrioventricular block. Circulation *11*:240, 1955.

Rothberger, C. J., and Winterberg, H.: Experimentelle beitrage zur kenntnis der reizleitungsstorungen in den kammern des saugetierherzens. Zeitschr. f.d. ges. exper. Med. *5*:264, 1917.

Scanlon, P. J., Pryor, R., and Blount, S. G.: Right bundle branch block associated with left superior or inferior intraventricular block: Clinical setting, prognosis and relation to complete heart block. Circulation *42*:1123, 1970.

Scheinman, M., Weiss, A., and Kunkel, F.: His bundle recording in patients with bundle branch block and transient neurological symptoms. Circulation *48*:322, 1973.

Scherlag, B. J., Lau, S. H., Helfant, R. H., Berkowitz, W. D., Stein, E., and Damato, A. N.: Catheter technique for recording His bundle activity in man. Circulation *39*:13, 1969.

Siddons, H., and Sowton, E.: Cardiac Pacemakers, Springfield, Ill. Charles C Thomas, 1967.

Stock, R. J., and Macken, D. L.: Observations on heart block during continuous electrocardiographic monitoring in myocardial infarction. Circulation *38*:993, 1968.

Vera, Z., Mason, D. T., Fletcher, R. D., Awan, N. A., and Massumi, R. A.: Prolonged His-Q interval in chronic bifascicular block: Relation to impending complete heart block. Circulation *53*:46, 1976.

Watanabe, Y., and Dreifus, L. S.: Second degree atrioventricular block. Cardiovasc. Res. *1*:150, 1967.

Watanabe, Y., and Dreifus, L. S.: Newer concepts in the genesis of cardiac arrhythmias. Amer. Heart J. *76*:114, 1968.

Watt, T. B., Murao, S., and Pruitt, R. D.: Left axis deviation induced experimentally in a primate heart. Amer. Heart J. *70*:381, 1965.

Watt, T. B. Jr, and Pruitt, R. D.: Character, cause and consequence of combined left axis deviation and right bundle branch block in human electrocardiograms. Amer. Heart J. *77*:460, 1969.

Wenckebach, K. F., and Winterberg, H.: Irregular Heart Action. Leipzig, Wilhelm Engelmann, 1927.

Wilson, F. N., and Hermann, G. R.: Bundle branch block and arborization block. Arch. Intern. Med. *26*:153, 1920.

Wilson, F. N., Johnston, F. D., and Barker, P. S.: Electrocardiogram of an unusual type in right bundle branch block. Amer. Heart J. *9*:472, 1934.

Yater, W. M., and Cornell, V. H.: Heart block due to calcareous lesions of the bundle of His. Review and report of a case with detailed histopathologic study. Ann. Intern. Med. *8*:777, 1935.

Zoll, P. M., et al.: Intravenous drug therapy of Stokes-Adams disease: Effect of sympathomimetic amines on ventricular rhythmicity and atrioventricular conduction. Circulation *17*:325, 1958.

SUPPLEMENTAL READING

Dhingra, R. C., Wyndham, C., Amat-y-Leon, F., Denes, P., Wu, D., Sridhar, S., Bustin, A. S., and Rosen, K. W.: Incidence and site of A-V block in patients with chronic bifascicular block. Circulation *59*:238–246, 1979.

Ginks, W., Leatham, A., and Siddons, H.: Prognosis of patients paced for chronic A-V block. Brit. Heart J. *41*:633–636, 1979.

Schneider, J. F., Thomas, H. E., Kreger, B. E., McNamara, P. M., and Kannel, W. B.: Newly acquired left bundle branch block: The Framingham Study. Ann. Int. Med. *90*:303–310, 1979.

13

ANOMALOUS ATRIOVENTRICULAR CONDUCTION AND THE PRE-EXCITATION SYNDROMES

RALPH LAZZARA, M.D.

In normal hearts, the A-V node, His bundle, and bundle branches constitute the sole pathway for the conduction of the impulses between the atria and the ventricles. Normally, this pathway links the atrial myocardium at its proximal end (the A-V node) with the ventricular myocardium at its distal end (the Purkinje ramifications of the bundle branches) and there are no other connections with ordinary myocardial cells. However, anatomists for many years have found tracts of fibers in occasional human hearts which bypassed parts or all of this normal pathway, connecting the atria and ventricles by "accessory" routes (Kent, 1893; Mahaim, 1947; James, 1961). These tracts, termed "bypass tracts," "accessory pathways," or "accessory bundles" were brought to the attention of clinicians and electrocardiographers after the report of Wolff, Parkinson, and White (1930) of subjects whose ECGs exhibited short P-R intervals, prolonged QRS complexes, and paroxysmal arrhythmias. This report resurrected the original findings by Kent, and later by others, of accessory

tracts of fibers crossing one or the other of the atrioventricular rings in certain human hearts. It was postulated that such accessory bundles would transmit the impulse relatively rapidly from atria to ventricles, since the normal A-V nodal delay would be circumvented. This would explain the short P-R interval. Prolonged duration of ventricular activation could be accounted for by entry of the impulse into the ventricles in their superior portions out of the reaches of the Purkinje network.

Despite the attractiveness of this hypothesis, it has been under continual and vigorous siege. However, in the past decade, the utilization of electrophysiological techniques and the results of surgical interruption of accessory bundles have validated the original hypothesis of the existence of functional accessory bundles in subjects with the Wolff-Parkinson-White syndrome (Durrer and Roos, 1967; Burchell et al., 1967; Cobb et al., 1968).

Although the Wolff-Parkinson-White syndrome and Kent bundles have generated the most interest, other forms of anomalous atrioventricular conduction have been postulated on the basis of anatomic, electrophysiologic, and clinical observations. Subjects with abnormally rapid atrioventricular conduction (i.e., short P-R intervals but normal ventricular activation, i.e., normal duration and configuration of the QRS complex) have been identified by Lown, Ganong, and Levine (1952) as a group also especially susceptible to supraventricular tachyarrhythmias. In this group, it has been hypothesized that all or part of the A-V node may be bypassed by fibers which have electrophysiological properties more like ordinary myocardial cells than A-V nodal fibers, viz., they conduct more rapidly and have shorter refractory periods than the A-V nodal fibers. Fibers connecting atrial myocardium with distal portions of the A-V node and the His bundle have been described anatomically. It was emphasized by James (1961) that these fibers might functionally bypass the A-V nodal delay and participate with the A-V node in re-entry circuits.

In addition to Kent bundles, which bypass the entire normal atrioventricular conduction system, and James fibers, which may bypass the proximal portions of the system, fibers have also been described by Mahaim (1947) and others, that bypass the distal portion of the normal atrioventricular conduction system, connecting the distal A-V node, His bundle, or proximal bundle branches to the myocardial fibers of the upper septum. Mahaim fibers have been observed in hearts of subjects who had no electrocardiographic abnormalities or arrhythmias (Becker and Anderson, 1976). There are rare descriptions of subjects who had the predictable electrocardiographic and electrophysiological consequences of functioning Mahaim fibers: Normal P-R intervals, short H-V intervals, and a slow initial inscription of the QRS (delta wave). In Figure 13–1 are depicted the basic anatomic, electrocardiographic, and electrophysiologic features of Kent, James, and Mahaim tracts. It is useful to refer to Kent bundles as complete bypass tracts, James fibers as partial proximal bypass tracts, and Mahaim fibers as partial distal bypass tracts.

In addition to these anatomic bypass tracts, a type of anomalous atrioventricular conduction that does not involve bypass of the atrioventricular conduction system has been identified electrophysiologically but not yet anatomically (Denes et al., 1973). This entity of "dual A-V nodal pathways" consists functionally of two pathways, one with relatively rapid conduction and longer refractoriness, the other with slower conduction and shorter refractoriness.

Figure 13–1 Anatomic relationships, electrocardiographic features, and characteristic atrioventricular conduction intervals in complete and partial bypass tracts. At the top are diagrammatic sketches showing the major elements of the normal conduction system and the various types of bypass tracts in bolder block superimposed on the outline of the atria and ventricles. In the middle are typical electrocardiographic patterns for each type of bypass tract. At the bottom are typical electrocardiograms, and recordings of atrial, His bundle, and ventricular electrograms, with measured A-V nodal (AH) and His-Purkinje (HU) conduction times in msec.

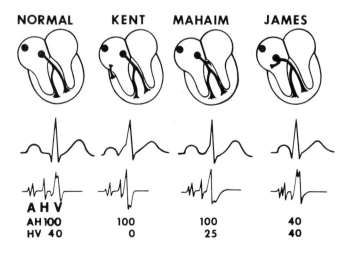

NORMAL	KENT	MAHAIM	JAMES

AHV
AH 100 ...... 100 ...... 100 40
HV 40 ...... 0 ...... 25 40

Both are contained within the A-V node. The two pathways can form limbs of a re-entry circuit within the A-V node generating supraventricular tachyarrhythmias.

WOLFF-PARKINSON-WHITE SYNDROME

The characteristic electrocardiographic features of Wolff-Parkinson-White (WPW) syndrome are a short P-R interval (less than 0.12 second), prolonged QRS (greater than 0.12 second) but normal P-J interval, and initially slow inscription of the QRS (delta wave). The incidence of this combination in otherwise normal subjects has been estimated to be between 1:10,000 and 3:1000 in different studies (Averill et al., 1960; Chung et al., 1965; Sears and Manning, 1964). However, the true incidence is probably underestimated. Some accessory bundles conduct only in a retrograde direction, so that the conventional electrocardiogram is not altered. In addition, spontaneous changes in the properties of accessory bundles may make them intermittently latent or manifest. Thus, the standard electrocardiogram at times is normal and at other times typical of WPW during the life of such an individual. Sometimes normal and WPW beats can be seen on the same ECG. Although it was considered by some that WPW syndrome could be acquired, it is more plausible that congenital accessory bundles can become manifest later in life either as a result of slowing of conduction in the normal pathway or of the institution of antegrade conduction in a previously blocked accessory pathway.

Wolff-Parkinson-White syndrome appears with greater frequency in association with certain congenital anomalies such as Ebstein's anomaly and idiopathic hypertrophic subaortic stenosis (Gallagher et al., 1975). However, it occurs most commonly in subjects otherwise free of organic heart disease.

The tachyarrhythmias which often accompany the anomaly are usually benign. However, it has recently been documented that tachyarrhythmias sometimes may be hazardous and occasionally fatal (Kaplan and Cohen, 1969; Dreifus et al., 1971).

Diagnosis

The electrocardiogram continues to be the mainstay of diagnosis. The findings of short P-R interval, prolonged QRS duration, normal P-J interval, and slow initial inscription of the QRS are secure evidence of an accessory atrioventricular bundle. Diagnostic problems arise when one or more of the findings are absent or borderline. All of the electrocardiographic abnormalities depend on "pre-excitation" of some portion of the ventricles by the accessory pathway(s). In most cases, the ventricles are activated by way of both the accessory pathway and the normal pathway, and the resultant QRS complex represents fusion of both sequences of activation. The early portion of the QRS is usually a reflection of activation of some region in the superior aspect of the ventricle close to the site of insertion of the accessory bundle. Since the superior regions of the ventricles are sparse in Purkinje fibers, conduction is relatively slow. Normal activation occurs in the middle and inferior regions of the septum where the Purkinje network connects initially with ventricular myocardium. Then activation is rapidly disseminated over wide areas of the free wall by the Purkinje network. As a consequence of this Purkinje-facilitated rapid spread of ventricular activation, the normal QRS is more rapidly inscribed (higher frequency components) than the initial delta wave of the QRS in the WPW syndrome.

Early excitation of ventricular myocardium by the accessory bundle occurs because the ordinary myocardial cells of the accessory bundles conduct more rapidly than A-V nodal cells. However, if the accessory bundle is itself activated late relative to the A-V node, the ventricles may be "pre-excited" to a lesser degree or not at all. In general, the ventricles are pre-excited to a lesser degree when the accessory bundle is on the left side, rather than the right (Gallagher et al., 1975), because the left atrium is activated later than the right atrium. In cases in which the presence of a delta wave is equivocal and the P-R interval is borderline, slow changes in the early vectors may be more apparent on the vectorcardiogram than on the electrocardiogram. However, slow inscription of the electrocardiogram or vectorcardiogram can be produced by other pathologic processes which alter normal activation, such as disease in the bundle branches or septal myocardium. If such pathologic processes were combined with a fortuitously short P-R interval, the electrocardiogram might resemble the WPW syndrome. Generally such clinical mimics present borderline findings but not the full-blown picture of WPW syndrome. The vectorcardiogram is not especially helpful in differentiating these clinical conditions from WPW syndrome, since initial slow change in QRS vectors from any cause would be reflected on the vectorcardiogram as well as on the electrocardiogram. In equivocal cases, therefore, the most precise diagnosis is obtained by electrophysiological studies.

Electrophysiological Characteristics of Accessory Bundles

The introduction of His bundle electrocardiography has allowed several electrophysiological features of the WPW syndrome to be clarified. In the WPW syndrome, the His bundle electrogram either follows the onset of the QRS complex or precedes it by an abnormally brief interval (less than 35 msec) (Castellanos et al., 1970; Wallace et al., 1971). Indeed, detection of His bundle activation after the onset of the QRS can be considered the definitive electrophysiological characteristic of complete bypass tracts. Premature atrial stimulation or rapid atrial pacing will slow conduction in the A-V node so that His bundle activation is further delayed in relation to the onset of QRS. The QRS, therefore, is more reflective of conduction through the accessory pathway. The relationship of the His bundle electrogram to the QRS during sinus rhythm and atrial pacing is shown in Figure 13–2. The technique of atrial stimulation can be used to unmask complete bypass tracts which are not obvious during sinus rhythm because the normal atrioventricular conduction pathway is more rapid than the tract. The use of atrial pacing to unmask the bypass tract depends on the fact that the refractory period of the accessory bundle is shorter than the relative refractory period of the A-V node. As a result, premature atrial impulses will delay in the A-V node but not in the accessory bundle. In some subjects, accessory bundles have long refractory periods. The frequency distribution of refractory periods in one series of subjects (Gallagher et al., 1975) is shown in Figure 13–3. Accessory bundles with very brief refractory periods are of great clinical significance because in the event of atrial fibrillation the ventricles could respond at a very rapid rate. This is believed to be a mechanism for sudden death in some cases of WPW syndrome.

Accessory bundles differ from ordinary myocardium in that their refractory periods often depend upon the direction of conduction. Most commonly, the refractory period during antegrade conduction is longer than during retrograde conduction (Wellens, 1976). In fact, it has become apparent in recent years that accessory bundles may conduct poorly or not at all antegrade but perfectly well retrograde (Wellens,

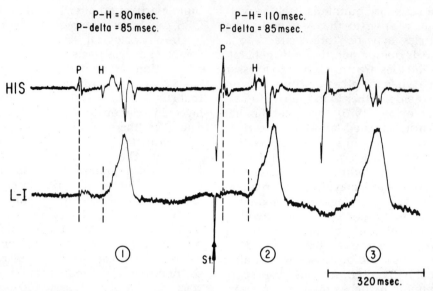

Figure 13–2   The effect of atrial pacing on atrioventricular conduction intervals in Wolff-Parkinson-White syndrome. At the left (1), is the intracardiac recording of atrial (P) and His bundle (H) electrograms and lead I of the electrocardiogram. Note that the QRS onset precedes the His deflection. The onset of atrial pacing in the first beat shows further delay of the His bundle electrogram, even later than the onset of the QRS complex. However, the interval between the atrial electrogram and the onset of the QRS remains the same because bypass conduction is not delayed. With the second atrial beat, there is still further delay, so that the His bundle electrogram is lost in the QRS. The QRS is even more deformed, indicating relatively pure accessory pathway conduction. (From Wallace, A. G., et al.: Wolff-Parkinson-White syndrome. A new look. Am. J. Cardiol. *28*:509, 1971.)

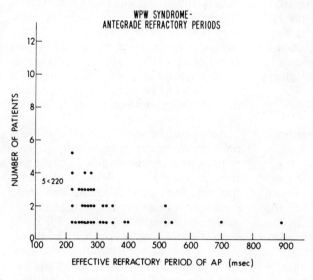

Figure 13–3   Distribution of refractory periods in a group of patients with Wolff-Parkinson-White syndrome. (Reproduced by permission of the American Heart Association, Inc. From Gallagher, J. J. et al.: Wolff-Parkinson-White syndrome: The problem, evaluation, and surgical correction. Circulation *51*:767, 1975.)

1976). Such bypass tracts are "concealed" because they do not affect the electrocardiogram. However, concealed bypass tracts may form critical links in re-entrant circuits.

There are several ways to localize bypass tracts. The simplest and oldest method employs the electrocardiogram. The anterior and rightward direction of the initial forces (delta wave) in type A WPW (lead V1 mainly positive) suggests a posterior and leftward location of the bundle with a connection between the left atrium and left ventricle; the posterior and leftward direction of the delta wave vector (V1 mainly negative) in type B WPW indicates that the accessory bundle bridges the right atrium and right ventricle anteriorly (Rosenbaum et al., 1945). Examples of each of these electrocardiographic types are shown in Figure 13–4. In typical cases, these deductions from the electrocardiogram generally have been verified with more precise methods. However, careful analysis of subjects with WPW syndrome reveals that the initial vectors are quite variable in direction among subjects (Gallagher et al., 1975). This is not surprising in view of the findings of bypass tracts in many locations throughout the A-V rings, including septal sites.

Stimulation of the atria or ventricles may aid in localizing the tracts. With right-sided tracts, stimulation of the right atrium results in greater prominence of the pre-excitation pattern as compared with stimulation of the left atrium. The converse applies with left-sided tracts. Similarly, stimulation of either ventricle can alter atrial activation to a greater or lesser degree, depending on the location of the tract. In the case of atrial activation, it is usually not feasible to use the P-wave as a guide in the same manner that the QRS is used as a guide to ventricular activation. Usually atrial activation is crudely mapped by recording atrial electrograms from several crucial sites, including the right atrium, the atrial septum (His bundle recording catheter), and the left atrium (coronary sinus catheter). For example, if the accessory bundle is left-sided, the earliest atrial electrogram will be recorded in the left atrium, especially if the left ventricle is stimulated.

Finally, the most precise method of localizing bypass tracts has been mapping of epicardial activation in the exposed heart (Gallagher et al., 1975). Normally during sinus rhythm the earliest epicardial electrograms are recorded over the trabecular zone of the right

Figure 13–4   The initial vectors (delta wave) in WPW syndrome. At top are shown examples of the two types of electrocardiograms according to the most common classification of WPW syndrome, i.e., type A, with initial vectors directed anteriorly, and type B, with initial vectors directed posteriorly. The actual distribution of initial vectors among a group of subjects with WPW syndrome is shown superimposed upon sketches of the torso in frontal and horizontal planes below. It is apparent that the simple classification is inadequate. (Reproduced by permission of the American Heart Association, Inc. From Gallagher, J. J. et al.: Wolff-Parkinson-White syndrome: The problem, evaluation, and surgical correction. Circulation *51*: 767, 1975.)

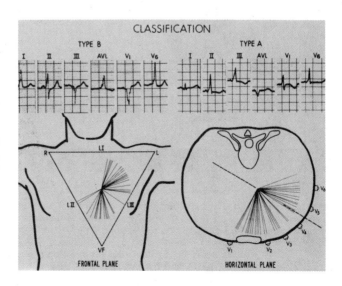

ventricle. With conduction over accessory bundles, the earliest electrograms occur in the superior aspect of the ventricles adjacent to the site of insertion of the tract. With ventricular stimulation, the site of earliest atrial activation is adjacent to the site of earliest ventricular activation. Septal tracts cannot be precisely localized unless the endocardial surfaces are explored. An example of the results of the intraoperative mapping in WPW syndrome is shown in Figure 13–5.

By means of electrophysiological studies, the effects of many pharmacologic agents on the refractory periods of bypass tracts and of the normal conducting system have been determined. In general, agents which prolong refractoriness in either the bypass tract or the A-V node have been therapeutically efficacious. The effects of a number of agents as compiled by Wellens (1976) are summarized in Table 13–1.

Incidence and Mechanisms of Arrhythmias

Various studies have estimated that the incidence of supraventricular tachyarrhythmias is between 40 and 80 per cent of all cases of WPW syndrome (Newman, Donoso, and Friedberg, 1966). Since electrocardiographic features of WPW syndrome may not be apparent at certain times in a subject's lifetime, and since tachyarrhythmias may appear or disappear at different stages of life, the true incidence is uncertain. It is generally considered that the majority of tachyarrhythmias are supraventricular, predominantly paroxysmal junctional tachycardia and less commonly, atrial fibrillation. There are reports of ventricular tachyarrhythmias (Newman, Donoso, and Friedberg, 1966), but some or all of these may have been cases of aberrant ventricular activation due to atrioventricular conduc-

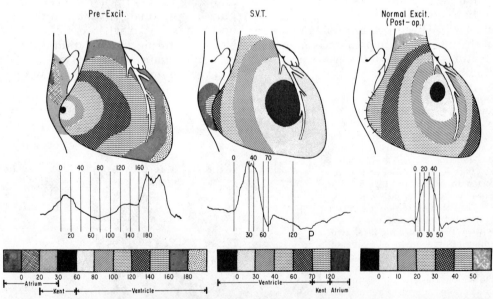

Figure 13–5 Epicardial activation sequence before (left) and after (right) interruption of a right-sided accessory pathway. Note the locus of early activation of the right ventricle adjacent to the A-V groove on the left map. On the right, the point of breakthrough in the right ventricle is the trabecular zone of the free wall, a normal pattern. (Reproduced by permission of the American Heart Association, Inc. From Boineau, J. P., and Moore, E. N.: Evidence for propagation of activation across an accessory atrial ventricular connection in types A and B pre-excitation. Circulation 41:375, 1970.)

TABLE 13–1

| | | Length of Effective Refractory Period | | | |
	Atr.	AV node	His-Purkinje	Ventr.	Acc. P.
Digitalis	±	+	?	±	−
Procaine amide	+	0	+	+	+
Quinidine	+	±	+	+	+
Ajmaline	+	0	+	+	+
Phenytoin	±	−	−	±	±
Atropine	0	−	?	0	0
Propranolol	±	+	?	±	0
Lidocaine	±	0	?	+	+
Verapamil	±	+	?	±	±
Amiodarone	+	+	+	+	+

+ = lengthened, − = shortened, 0 = no change, ± = inconsistent, ? = not known.

tion exclusively by way of the accessory bundle.

Tachyarrhythmias usually can be induced during electrophysiological studies by premature stimulation of either the atria or the ventricles (Durrer and Roos, 1967). The re-entry circuit is created by the inequality of refractory periods of the bypass tract and the A-V node. This inequality of refractory periods allows appropriately timed premature beats to cross between atria and ventricles by one route, to find the other route refractory, then to return via the second pathway. Four basic possibilities for re-entry circuits generated by premature beats in atria or ventricles are shown in Figure 13–6. If the route from atria to ventricles is by way of the normal conducting system, the QRS will usually be narrow and normal, but sometimes it will reflect bundle branch block due to rate-dependent aberrancy. If the path from atria to ventricles is through the bypass tract, the QRS will be prolonged and deformed, reflecting

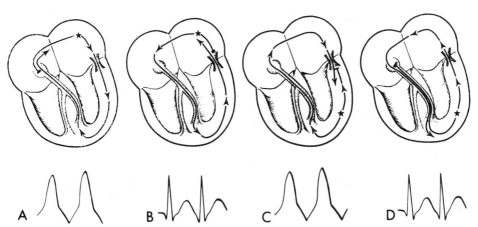

Figure 13–6 Re-entry circuits and electrocardiographic patterns in tachyarrhythmias in WPW syndrome. The site of origin of the initiating premature impulse is designated by a star. The initial passage of the impulse, including the site of block and the pathways of conduction, is shown by the arrows. The elements of the normal conduction system and the accessory pathway are included in the outline of the cardiac chambers. Note that a normal QRS can result from a site of origin in the atrium with initial block in the accessory pathway (B) or a site of origin in the ventricles with initial block in the AV node (D). When the impulse conducts antegradely down the accessory pathway, the QRS assumes a completely aberrant pattern.

a pure pattern of pre-excitation. In tach-ycardias with a regular rate the QRS is usually narrow because the refractory period of the bypass tract is longer than the effective refractory period of the A-V node in the antegrade direction and shorter than the effective refractory period of the A-V node in the retro-grade direction. These conditions are reflected in Figure 13–6B and D. Atrial fibrillation occurs relatively frequently because the relatively brief refractory period of the bypass tract in the retro-grade direction allows return of the im-pulse to the atria during their vulnera-ble period.

Spontaneous tachyarrhythmias may not always originate with premature beats. For example, with increasing sinus rate, the sinus beat might en-counter refractoriness antegrade in the bypass tract but not in the A-V node, setting the stage for re-entry into the atria retrograde by way of the bypass tract. In cases of bypass tracts which conduct only retrograde (concealed by-pass tracts), the situation is somewhat different. In such cases, the antegrade pathway down the A-V conduction sys-tem and the retrograde pathway up the bypass tract supply an ever-present cir-cuit for potential re-entry with each sinus beat. It appears that the major obstacle to the consummation of re-entry is atrial refractoriness, which usually outlasts the time spent in trans-mission of the sinus impulse down the conduction system, through the ventri-cles, and retrogradely up the bypass tract. Re-entry can therefore be con-summated by factors shortening atrial refractoriness — e.g., increased rate — or by factors lengthening the transit time of the impulse — e.g., A-V nodal delay or bundle branch block ipsilateral to the bypass tract. The resultant tachyarrhythmia would take the form of a regular supraventricular tachy-cardia. With modern methods of detec-tion, concealed bypass tracts are being found more frequently in studies of

subjects with recurrent supraven-tricular tachycardia (Gillette, 1977).

Pharmacologic agents that prolong refractoriness in either the A-V node or the bypass tract, or reduce the frequen-cy of premature beats, would be expect-ed to suppress tachyarrhythmias. In general, the agents that have been found empirically to be therapeutically effective have one of these properties. The most effective agents have been digitalis preparations and propranolol, which prolong refractoriness in the A-V node, and procainamide and quini-dine, which prolong refractoriness in the bypass tract and suppress prema-ture beats. Certain newer agents show great therapeutic promise because of their striking effects on refractoriness in the bypass tract (see Chapter 23). Some investigators have cautioned against the use of digitalis preparations alone because of their tendency to *shorten* re-fractoriness in the bypass tracts (Table 13–1), an effect which could be danger-ous in the event of atrial fibrillation. In difficult cases, it may be necessary to employ combinations of agents direct-ed at the normal conducting system, the bypass tracts, and the premature beats.

Occasionally, in cases refractory to medical therapy, the bypass tracts can be interrupted surgically (Gallagher et al., 1975). This requires detailed elec-trophysiological studies to localize the tracts approximately, and epicardial mapping during operation for more precise localization. Occasionally, mul-tiple tracts are encountered. Septal tracts present particular problems for surgical interruption. However, in cases where the accessory bundles can-not be interrupted, interruption of the normal atrioventricular pathway also will eliminate the problem of the re-entrant tachyarrhythmias.

Since attacks of tachycardia can be both initiated and terminated by pre-mature stimuli, pacemakers have also been employed as therapy. The rationale for this therapy is that the introduction of a premature depolarization can render a portion of the re-entrant circuit refractory, thus terminating the arrhythmia.

LOWN-GANONG-LEVINE SYNDROME

Since it was observed that subjects with a short P-R interval (less than 0.12 msec) have a higher incidence of supraventricular tachyarrhythmias (approximately 10 per cent) than matched subjects with a normal P-R interval (Lown, Ganong, and Levine, 1952), speculation concerning the basis for the abnormally rapid atrioventricular conduction and susceptibility to tachyarrhythmias has focused on the so-called James fibers (James, 1961). These are tracts of myocardial fibers that connect atrial myocardium with the inferior margin of the A-V node. James observed that in some subjects these fibers appear anatomically to insert into the distal part of the node or into the

upper His bundle (see Figure 13–1). It is presumed that these fibers have electrophysiological properties similar to ordinary myocardium. Consequently, the slow conduction and long refractoriness of the A-V node could be partially or completely bypassed by these fibers if they inserted at a distal site in the node. Also the James fibers, the A-V node, and the atrial myocardium could form a potential circuit, which could produce re-entry if an impulse was unidirectionally blocked in one limb of the circuit but conducted in the return direction. One possible sequence leading to re-entry is diagrammed in Figure 13–7, which shows a premature atrial impulse conducting antegrade down the bypass tract but blocked at the atrial margin of the A-V node because of refractoriness, then returning retrograde through the node to the atrium. It is possible to postulate other possible re-entrant sequences depending on the site of origin of the impulses, whether in the atria or the ventricles, and depending on the relative refractory periods of the bypass tract and the A-V

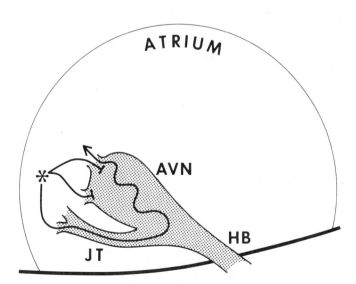

Figure 13–7 Diagram of a James tract (JT) inserting at the junction of the A-V node (AVN) and His bundle (HB). An impulse originating in the atrium is shown to follow a re-entrant circuit by blocking initially at the input to the A-V node and conducting down the bypass tract and retrogradely up the node.

node. A re-entrant circuit in this location should lead to regular supraventricular tachyarrhythmias which, indeed, are prevalent in these subjects.

Although this hypothesis is attractive, it has not been universally accepted. Some investigators have pointed out that tracts which anatomically appear to bypass much or all of the A-V node are common (Becker and Anderson, 1976). It is possible that a site of insertion which appears anatomically to be distal in the A-V node may not be functionally distal. There is evidence from experimental studies that impulses may take circuitous routes through the node, depending on sites of entry (Janse et al., 1976). In other words, there does not seem to be a simple axial spread of activation through the node.

The LGL syndrome is defined by one electrocardiographic feature (the short P-R interval) which represents a quantitative, not qualitative, deviation from normal. The definition of "normal" is arbitrarily based on statistical prevalence of measured values of P-R intervals in the population. One might surmise that many subjects with short P-R intervals may not have A-V nodal bypass tracts. They may have nothing more than unusually rapid A-V nodal conduction, a condition which is not of itself arrhythmogenic. In short, the electrocardiographic marker for proximal partial bypass tracts is not as reliable as the electrocardiographic markers of complete bypass tracts.

ELECTROPHYSIOLOGICAL STUDIES

In most subjects, His bundle electrocardiographic studies (Castellanos et al., 1971) have shown that a short P-R interval results mainly from rapid conduction between the atrium and the His bundle, i.e., an abbreviated A-H interval (see Figure 13–1). Assessment of the refractory properties of the atrio-His conduction pathway by means of atrial pacing or atrial extrastimuli has disclosed two different types of responses (Bissette et al., 1973). In one type, the A-H interval remains constant when the interval between the atrial impulses is shortened. This type of "flat" response is suggestive of complete bypass of the A-V node. The other type of response is qualitatively similar to that of the A-V node itself in that A-H intervals prolong with closer coupling of the atrial impulses but the prolongation is not as great as normal. The two types of response are shown in Figure 13–8 in comparison with the normal relationship between A-H intervals and A-A intervals. The second type of "blunted" response could result from a partial bypass of the A-V node, or from A-V nodal fibers which conduct and recover

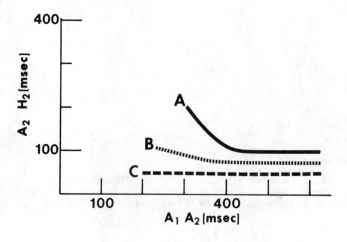

Figure 13–8 The relationship of A-V nodal conduction time (A_2H_2) to the coupling interval between atrial beats (A_1A_2) in normal subjects (A) and subjects with short P-R intervals (B and C).

excitability more rapidly than usual. In short, electrophysiological studies leave open the possibility that many subjects with short P-R intervals simply represent extremes of normal function. Occasional subjects with short P-R intervals present electrophysiological characteristics other than those described, including recovery curves suggestive of dual pathways which will be described below.

THERAPY

There have been relatively few studies of subjects with James fibers in which the pharmacological properties of atrioventricular conduction have been characterized. It is presumed that partial proximal bypass tracts, when present, have the same pharmacologic sensitivities as complete bypass tracts in the WPW syndrome. Since the re-entry circuit includes both the bypass tract and the A-V node, it is likely that the same principles apply to drug therapy. One would anticipate that agents prolonging refractoriness and depressing conduction in the A-V node — i.e., propranolol and digitalis preparations — and agents prolonging refractoriness and depressing conduction in the bypass tracts — i.e., quinidine or procainamide — would be effective in the prevention and therapy of the supraventricular tachyarrhythmias. In general, this appears to be so.

Surgical interruption of James fibers is not feasible. The creation of heart block by interruption of the normal A-V conduction pathway would prevent the participation of the ventricles in the tachyarrhythmia. This radical approach rarely, if ever, should be necessary.

MAHAIM FIBERS

There have been few reports of subjects that present the expected electrocardiographic and electrophysiologic effects of functioning Mahaim fibers. The electrocardiogram would be expected to show a P-R interval that is normal or borderline short, and a QRS complex with initial slow inscription (delta wave). The A-V nodal delay, as indicated by the A-H time, should be in the normal range and should show the normal prolongation with premature atrial beats or with rapid atrial pacing. The interval from His bundle activation to ventricular activation (H-V interval) should be short. These features are illustrated in Figure 13–1. The Mahaim fibers, the ventricular myocardium, and the His-Purkinje system form a potential re-entry circuit. However, since this re-entry circuit does not contain a slowly conducting element such as the A-V node, it could be anticipated that re-entrant tachyarrhythmias would not be as common in these subjects as in subjects with the types of anomalous atrioventricular conduction described above. In the other types of accessory pathways, the potential re-entry circuits contain the A-V node, which normally can retard conduction to the degree necessary to consummate re-entry with ease.

The incidence of functioning Mahaim fibers and re-entrant tachyarrhythmias attributable to them has not been accurately assessed, but case reports have been sparse (Tonkin et al., 1975). The tachyarrhythmias would be expected to respond to agents that slow conduction in ordinary myocardial cells or the His-Purkinje system, such as procainamide or quinidine, but not to agents which predominantly affect conduction in the A-V node, such as propranolol or digoxin.

DUAL PATHWAYS

Some time ago, physiologists observed that the relationship between atrioventricular conduction times and coupling intervals between atrial beats was discontinuous in some experimen-

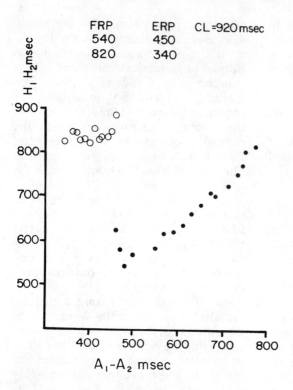

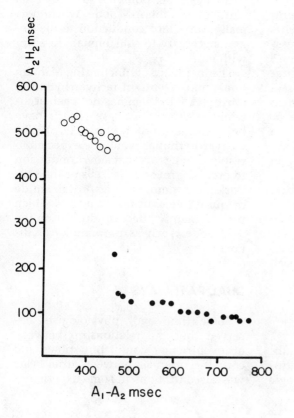

Figure 13–9   A-V nodal conduction characteristics in subjects with dual A-V nodal pathways. On the top, the intervals between His bundle electrograms ($H_1 H_2$) are plotted against the intervals between atrial beats ($A_1 A_2$) as the atrial coupling interval is shortened with atrial extrastimuli. The coupling intervals, represented by open circles, are associated with echo beats. On the bottom, A-V nodal conduction time ($A_2 H_2$) is plotted against the coupling interval between atrial beats. (Reproduced by permission of the American Heart Association, Inc. (From Denes, P., et al.: Demonstration of dual A-V nodal pathways in patients with paroxysmal supraventricular tachycardia. Circulation *48*:549, 1973.)

tal animals (Mendez and Moe, 1966). The same type of discontinuity could be found with retrograde as well as antegrade conduction. Recently, it has been confirmed that similar discontinuous curves can be demonstrated in man (Denes et al., 1973). An example of this discontinuous relationship is shown in Figure 13–9.

When the curves are discontinuous, both segments of the curve are affected similarly by autonomic influences. These observations have led to the hypothesis that the discontinuity is due to the existence *within the A-V node* of two parallel pathways, one with more rapid conduction and longer refractoriness, the other with slower conduction but shorter refractoriness. At closer A-V intervals, the rapid pathway is refractory, and the impulse is conducted solely by way of the slower pathway. The break in the curve corresponds to the effective refractory period of the rapid pathway. A diagram of the postulated pathways is shown in Figure 13–10. It would be

expected that these parallel pathways along with the proximal and distal common pathways could form a re-entry circuit when activated by an appropriately timed premature impulse. Clinical surveys confirmed that subjects with electrophysiologically demonstrable dual pathways have a greater incidence of supraventricular tachyarrhythmias than normals. This condition rarely has electrocardiographic markers except for the rare occurrence of spontaneous vacillation between two different P-R intervals in the same subject (Rosen, Mehta, and Miller, 1974).

Since its detection requires electrophysiological studies, the true incidence is unknown. It would be expected that agents which depress conduction in the A-V node would be most useful in treating the tachyarrhythmias associated with this syndrome.

REFERENCES

Averill, K. H., Fosmoe, R. J., and Lamb, L. E.: Electrocardiographic findings in 67,375 asymptomatic subjects. IV Wolff-Parkinson-White syndrome. Am. J. Cardiol. 6:108, 1960.

Becker, A. E., and Anderson, R. H.: Morphology of the human atrioventricular junctional area. *In* Wellens, H. J. J., Lie, K. I., and Janse, M. J. (eds): The Conduction System of the Heart. Philadelphia, Lea and Febiger, 1976, p. 264.

Bissette, J. K., Thompson, A. J., deSoyza, M., and Murphy, M. L.: Atrioventricular conduction in patients with short PR intervals and normal QRS complexes. British Heart J. 35:123, 1973.

Burchell, H. B., Frye, R. L., Anderson, M. W., and McGoon, D. C.: Atrioventricular and ventriculoatrial excitation in Wolff-Parkinson-White syndrome (Type B): Transitory ablation at surgery. Circulation 36:663, 1967.

Castellanos, A., Castillo, C. A., Agha, A. S., and Tessler, M.: His bundle electrograms in patients with short PR intervals, narrow QRS complexes, and paroxysmal tachycardias. Circulation 43:667, 1971.

Castellanos, A., Chapunoff, E., Castillo, C., Maytin, O., and Lemberg, L.: His bundle electrograms in two cases of Wolff-Parkinson-White (pre-excitation) syndrome. Circulation 41:399, 1970.

Chung, K. Y., Walsh, T. J., and Massie, E.: Wolff-Parkinson-White syndrome. Am. Heart J. 69:116, 1965.

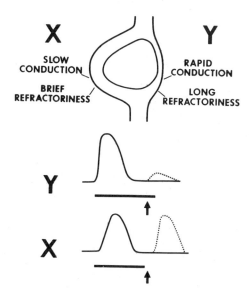

Figure 13–10 Diagram of hypothesized dual pathways within the A-V node. Below are shown postulated action potentials from each pathway and the response to a close-coupled beat which interrupts the refractory period (denoted by horizontal bar below the action potential) of pathway Y.

Cobb, F. R., Blumenschien, S. D., Seally, W. C., Boineau, J. P., Wagner, G. S., and Wallace, A. G.: Successful surgical interruption of the bundle of Kent in a patient with Wolff-Parkinson-White syndrome. Circulation 38:1018, 1968.

Denes, P., Wu, D., Dhingra, R. C., Chuquimia, R., and Rosen, K. M.: Demonstration of dual A-V nodal pathways in patients with paroxysmal supraventricular tachycardia. Circulation 48:549, 1973.

Dreifus, L. S., Haiat, R., Watanabe, Y., Arriaga, J., and Reitman, N.: Ventricular fibrillation. A possible mechanism of sudden death in patients with Wolff-Parkinson-White syndrome. Circulation 43:520, 1971.

Durrer, D., and Roos, J. P.: Epicardial excitation of the ventricles in a patient with Wolff-Parkinson-White Syndrome (type B). Circulation 35:15, 1967.

Durrer, D., and Roos, J. P.: The role of premature beats in the initiation and the termination of supraventricular tachycardia in the Wolff-Parkinson-White syndrome. Circulation 36:644, 1967.

Gallagher, J. J., Gilbert, M., Svenson, R. H., Seally, W. C., Kasell, J., and Wallace, A. G.: Wolff-Parkinson-White syndrome. The problem evaluation, and surgical correction. Circulation 51:767, 1975.

Gillette, P. G.: Concealed anomalous cardiac conduction pathways: A frequent cause of supraventricular tachycardia. Am. J. Cardiol. 40:848, 1977.

James, T. N.: Morphology of the human atrioventricular node, with remarks pertinent to its electrophysiology. Am. Heart J. 62:756, 1961.

Janse, M. J., van Capelle, F. J. L., Anderson, R. H., Touboul, P., and Billette, J.: Electrophysiology and structure of the atrioventricular node of the isolated rabbit heart. In Wellens, H. J. J., Lie, K. I., and Janse, M. J. (eds.): The Conduction System of the Heart. Philadelphia, Lea and Febiger, 1976.

Kaplan, M. A., and Cohen, K. L.: Ventricular fibrillation in the Wolff-Parkinson-White syndrome. Am. J. Cardiol. 24:259, 1969.

Kent, A. F. S.: Researches on the structure and function of the mammalian heart. J. Physiol. 14:233, 1893.

Lev, M., Fox, S. M., Bharati, S., Rosen, K. M., Langendorf, R., and Pick, A.: Mahaim fibers as a basis for a unique variety of pre-excitation. Am. J. Cardiol. 35:152, 1975.

Lown, B., Ganong W. F., and Levine, S. A.: Syndrome of short PR interval, normal QRS complex and paroxysmal heart action. Circulation 5:693, 1952.

Mahaim, I.: Kent's fibers and the AV paraspecific conduction through the upper connection of the bundle of His-Tawara. Am. Heart J. 33:651, 1947.

Mendez, C. and Moe, G. K.: Demonstration of dual AV nodal conduction system in the isolated rabbit heart. Circ. Res. 19:378, 1966.

Newman, B. J., Donoso, E., and Friedberg, K.: Arrhythmias in the Wolff-Parkinson-White syndrome. Prog. Cardiovasc. Dis. 9:147, 1966.

Rosen, K., Mehta, A., and Miller, R. A.: Demonstration of dual atrioventricular nodal pathways in man. Am. J. Cardiol. 33:291, 1974.

Rosenbaum, F. F., Hecht, H. H., Wilson, F. N., and Johnston, F. D.: The potential variations of the thorax and the esophagus in anomalous atrioventricular excitation (Wolff-Parkinson-White syndrome). Am. Heart J. 29:281, 1945.

Sears, G. A., and Manning, G. W.: The Wolff-Parkinson-White pattern in routine electrocardiography. Can. Med. Assoc. J. 87:1213, 1964.

Tonkin, A. M., Dugan, F. A., Swenson, R. J., Seally, W. C., Wallace, A. G., and Gallagher, J. J.: Coexistence of functional Kent and Mahaim-type tracts in the pre-excitation syndrome. Circulation 52:193, 1975.

Wallace, A. G., Boineau, J. P., Davidson, R. M., and Seally, W. C.: Wolff-Parkinson-White syndrome. A new look. Am. J. Cardiol. 282:509, 1971.

Wellens, H. J. J.: The electrophysiological properties of the accessory pathway in the Wolff-Parkinson-White syndrome. In Wellens, H. J. J., Lie, K. I., and Janse, M. J. (eds.): The Conduction System of the Heart, Philadelphia, Lea and Febiger, 1976, 567.

Wolff, L., Parkinson, J., White, P. D.: Bundle branch block with short P-R interval in healthy young people prone to paroxysmal tachycardia. Am. Heart J. 5:685, 1930.

SUPPLEMENTAL READING

Denes, P., Wu, D., Amat-y-Leon, F., Dhingra, R., Wyndham, C., Kehoe, R., Ayers, B. F., and Rosen, K. M.: Paroxysmal supraventricular tachycardia induction in patients with Wolff-Parkinson-White Syndrome. Ann. Intern. Med. 90:153, 1979.

Engle, T. R.: Pacing techniques to guide the therapy of tachycardias. Ann. Intern. Med. 90(2):265, 1979.

14

STRESS TESTING, AMBULATORY MONITORING, AND ELECTROPHYSIOLOGICAL TESTING: CLINICAL USES AND LIMITATIONS

RICHARD H. HELFANT, M.D.

INTRODUCTION

The electrocardiogram is the principal means of diagnosis when a cardiac arrhythmia is continuously present. However, many patients with symptoms of palpitations or syncopal episodes exhibit normal sinus rhythm at the time of initial examination and routine electrocardiogram. Under these circumstances, an occult, transient arrhythmia which is responsible for the patient's symptoms may remain undetected. Transient rhythm disturbances may be innocuous; they can also constitute the basis for severe and life threatening tachycardias or bradycardias.

In patients with coronary heart disease, ventricular arrhythmias may be rare and sporadic and yet may be harbingers of sudden death. Similarly, patients with disease of the atrioventricular conduction system may only sporadically exhibit evidence of heart block, which may result in transient syncopal episodes or other Stokes-Adams symptoms (including sudden death). In addition, patients with paroxysmal supraventricular tachycardia characteristically manifest these rhythm disturbances on an intermittent and transient basis, making diagnosis and treatment difficult.

In recent years important advances have been made in developing methods for exposing and elucidating cardiac rhythm disturbances which are not seen on the routine electrocardiogram. These include stress testing, long term ambulatory electrocardiographic monitoring, and electrophysiological testing (including His bundle electrocardiography). In this chapter the uses, limitations and clinical indications for these procedures in clinical practice will be discussed.

STRESS TESTING

The relationship between exercise and arrhythmias depends on many factors, including the state of the heart (normal or diseased), the patient's age and physical condition, the type of exercise, the rapidity with which it is performed, and its duration. The effects of exercise on the heart involve the central nervous system, endocrine system, and biochemical alterations. Thus, exercise manifests the following effects: 1) decreased vagal tone; 2) increased circulating catecholamines and sympathetic tone; and 3) increased plasma cortisol and growth hormone levels. These factors tend to increase cardiac rate and output. In addition, the effects of exercise may result in ischemia if myocardial oxygen requirements exceed oxygen supply. During physical exercise these physiologic changes that occur may result in the development of a cardiac arrhythmia.

The increase in adrenergic drive and the concomitant decrease in parasympathetic tone are related to the level of work performed. Changes in autonomic background activity may reflect themselves as effects on the action potential increasing the rate of phase 4 depolarization, resulting in increased normal as well as ectopic cardiac automaticity. The increased sinus rate that occurs during exercise may protect against the development of ectopic cardiac rhythms by the mechanism of overdrive suppression. However, conversely, the rapid rate may impinge upon the relative refractory period of some fibers with abnormal action potentials, resulting in re-entrant arrhythmias (see Chapter 2). This is particularly important when exercise causes myocardial ischemia, since this may result in regional abnormalities of depolarization, repolarization, automaticity, and conduction, allowing for both automaticity and re-entrant arrhythmias. In many individuals, arrhythmias do not become manifest until immediately following cessation of exercise when rapid deceleration of heart rate occurs but the systemic effects of the exercise stress are still manifest.

Tachyarrhythmias. Almost all known supraventricular arrhythmias have occurred during exercise testing, although the prevalence of these rhythm disturbances is small. In particular, paroxysmal atrial flutter and fibrillation are infrequent and usually terminate spontaneously. Conversely, paroxysms of supraventricular tachycardia are more common. Ventricular arrhythmias are by far the most common rhythm disorders observed during exercise. These vary from isolated ventricular premature complexes to bouts of ventricular tachycardia, and rarely ventricular fibrillation. Depending on the population studied and type of stress performed, ventricular arrhythmias occur in 20 to 50 per cent of patients. These arrhythmias are observed most commonly in the post-exercise period. Most bouts of ventricular tachycardia have been reported to occur in patients who previously exhibited isolated ventricular premature complexes. However, this is not invariably the case.

Considerable interest has also focused on whether or not the ventricular premature complexes are induced, increased, or actually decreased by exercise. The relationship between the development of premature beats during exercise and the presence of coronary heart disease was first made in 1927 (Bourne, 1927), and in 1948 it was reported that the premature beats induced by exercise occurring concomitantly with angina pectoris probably indicated a grave prognosis (Porter, 1948). An additional study indicated that unless exercise-related premature beats were accompanied by S-T segment abnormalities indicating ischemia, they were probably of no significance (Rozzak, 1963). In the study of Helfant et al., ventricular premature complexes that were either precipitated or increased by exercise were associated with coronary heart disease in 22 of 38 patients; 18 of these 22 coronary patients showed extensive disease with significant two- or three-vessel obstruction. However, 16 of these 38 patients either showed a cardiomyopathy or were normal by catheterization. In contrast, only 6 of the 22 patients with ventricular premature complexes that decreased with exercise showed coronary heart disease angiographically, and four of these six patients had one-vessel coronary disease only. Most workers have concluded that ventricular premature complexes which occurred with exercise were of no significance unless accompanied by clinical evidence of cardiac disease.

Premature beats that are precipitated following moderate or severe exertion in normal subjects usually occur in young subjects and may be the result of increased reactivity to catecholamines, recent infections, or excessive amounts of nicotine or caffeine. In the experience of Bellet, in normal subjects aged 17 to 25, moderately severe exercise resulted in the production of a tachycardia with the heart rate increasing to as much as 160 to 180 per minute. However, arrhythmias are quite rare in this group. Unless associated with unusual circumstances, such as strenuous exercise, physical exhaustion, toxic states, drugs, or excessive intake of caffeine, the precipitation of numerous premature beats or a tachyarrhythmia by exercise in Bellet's opinion constituted evidence of some degree of deviation from the normal.

Conduction Defects. Conduction abnormalities involving the sinoatrial node, atrial ventricular junction, and bundle branches may also occur during exercise. However, it is very uncommon for sinus node dysfunction to be induced during exercise. The increased adrenergic drive during exercise normally shortens the P-R interval. Thus, when a patient exhibits P-R lengthening or actual A-V block during exercise, this is considered an abnormal response implying underlying A-V conduction system disease. Intraventricular conduction disturbances, including right or left bundle branch and unspecified conduction abnormalities, have also been occasionally observed during exercise stress. Usually the bundle branch block disappears with the cessation of exercise when the heart rate declines. These changes are usually indicative of tachycardia-dependent bundle branch block. With the increase in sinus rate associated with exercise, higher grades of block may occasionally be elicited. The clinical and prognostic significance of exercise-related arrhythmias has been controversial.

Arrhythmias Induced by Isometric Exercise

Isometric exercise has been observed to have a significant immediate effect on left ventricular function (Helfant et al., 1971), acting primarily to markedly and precipitously increase afterload. However, in our experience handgrip isometric stress evoked considerably fewer arrhythmias than the isotonic stress of either bicycle ergometry or treadmill exercise testing. These observations have been confirmed by several other groups.

Psychological Stress Testing

Both neural and psychological factors have been implicated as risk factors in the production of arrhythmias, including ventricular tachyarrhythmias and sudden death in man. Lown and coworkers (Lown, 1978) have recently examined the effect of psychological stress testing in patients with advanced grades of ventricular arrhythmias. Psychological stress consisted of mental arithmetic, reading from color to cards, and recounting emotionally charged experiences. Such testing induced a significant increase in the frequency of ventricular premature beats in 11 of 19 patients. Thus, subjective psychological stress testing may become a useful means of precipitating ventricular arrhythmias in suitably susceptible patients (Bellet and Roman, 1970; Bellet et al., 1968).

LONG-TERM AMBULATORY ELECTROCARDIOGRAPHIC MONITORING

During the past 15 years, small recorders have been developed which allow for continuous taping of the electrocardiograms of individuals performing normal daily activity. High speed playback displays and, more recently, newer computer techniques allow this electrocardiographic information to be analyzed relatively rapidly. These long-term monitoring techniques have allowed an opportunity to correlate patients' symptoms with the concomitantly recorded rhythm. In addition, the increasing emphasis on arrhythmias in the context of predisposing to sudden death (see Chapter 15) has led to the progressively widespread use of these ambulatory arrhythmia monitoring techniques.

Originally developed by Holter and associates, several ambulatory electrocardiographic recording systems are now available. Their common denominator consists of a small electrocardiographic amplifier and precision amplitude and frequency modulation tape recorders capable of recording 24 or more hours of electrocardiogram readings from electrodes attached to the patient's chest. Many new recording systems now allow two ECG channels to be recorded simultaneously as well as having "event markers" to more precisely correlate the time of a patient's symptoms with the rhythm present on the recording.

Recorder

Holter recorders are small, battery operated instruments utilizing exceptionally slow tape transport speeds. In ambulatory patients, the recorder may be carried over the shoulder like a camera case. The two basic lead systems that are employed are a modified bipolar V4 and modified V1.

The patient is instructed to keep a diary during the recording period, entering all symptoms and pertinent activities. This permits subsequent correlation of symptoms and activities with electrocardiographic changes. During the recording, the patient may engage in all his usual activities, particularly encouraged activities are those that are known to cause symptoms.

The data are analyzed using either a high-speed, technician-operated playback system or computer techniques. The high-speed playback retrieval systems are all potentially limited by operator fatigue; thus, the newer computer systems appear to provide more consistent arrhythmia analysis.

EXPERIENCE WITH AMBULATORY ELECTROCARDIOGRAM

Experience with long-term ambulatory ECG recordings has led to several observations of particular note. For example, if the clinician has a preconceived clinical judgment as to the type of arrhythmia causing the paroxysmal symptoms (e.g., paroxysmal supraventricular tachycardia) he is likely to be right in only a small minority of cases. In situations in which paroxysmal supraventricular tachycardia was suspected to be the cause of palpitations studies have found that only 25 percent of patients have documentation of supraventricular tachycardia (the remainder having sinus tachycardia). When patients report palpitations in their diary, by far the most common rhythm found is sinus tachycardia. The most common Holter diagnosis found in cases where paroxysmal supraventricular tachycardia was suspected was frequent premature ventricular complexes. Other diagnoses included incomplete A-V dissociation, runs of ventricular tachycardia, and frequent, occasional, and rare atrial premature complexes. Similarly, when the cause of symptoms was suspected to be ventricular tachycardia, this is documented in less than 20 per cent of cases, each time terminating spontaneously.

When monitoring was performed because of syncope, transient dizziness, or transient neurological symptoms, a relatively high number of cases yield objective evidence of a probable cause for symptoms. In approximately 40 per cent of cases a probable cause is found, including evidence of sinoatrial block or arrest with an adequate escape mechanism, Mobitz II A-V block, runs of ventricular tachycardia, variable A-V block, atrial fibrillation with long pauses, extreme sinus bradycardia, and malfunctioning pacemaker. Thus, the general experience has been that in 20 to 25 per cent of cases presenting with these types of symptoms, long-term electrocardiographic monitoring will significantly clarify the underlying problem.

Clinical Uses of Ambulatory Electrocardiographic Monitoring

Ambulatory electrocardiographic monitoring is potentially useful for any patient in whom arrhythmias are considered to be important from a symptomatic or prognostic standpoint. Even when patients are already known to have an arrhythmia, ambulatory monitoring frequently provides additional information concerning its frequency, relationship to symptoms, and physical (as well as other) activity. It can also be useful in assessing the efficiency of antiarrhythmic therapy. A patient diary for recording activities and symptoms allows correlation of symptoms with heart rhythm. Studies utilizing ambulatory monitoring have determined that a large number of cardiac arrhythmias

produce no symptoms. Conversely, a large number of symptoms experienced by patients with and without heart disease which are suggestive of cardiac arrhythmias occur at times when no arrhythmias are present.

Arrhythmias detected on ambulatory monitoring must also be evaluated from a prognostic standpoint. It is well to emphasize that 1) arrhythmias can be present in apparently healthy subjects; 2) the prognostic significance of many of the rhythm disturbances detected on ambulatory electrocardiograms is not known; and 3) conversely, an arrhythmia may be the first manifestation of heart disease.

Ambulatory electrocardiographic monitoring may also be useful in judging the efficacy of treatment for a cardiac rhythm disturbance. It may also be useful in determining the type of treatment. For example, rhythm disturbances that are aggravated by physical activity may be controlled by its avoidance; those occurring during emotional stress may respond to tranquilization; and those occurring at more rapid heart rates may be treated efficaciously with propranolol.

Indications for Ambulatory Electrocardiographic Monitoring

Ambulatory electrocardiographic monitoring should be considered for any patient whose symptoms suggest an underlying cardiac arrhythmia as the cause. Before considering therapy, the relationship, if any, between symptoms and the presence or absence of an underlying heart rhythm disturbance must be determined. Thus, patients with palpitations should undergo monitoring to determine whether an arrhythmia is responsible for these symptoms. If an arrhythmia is determined to be the cause of palpitations, the exact type of arrhythmia can be identified and appropriate therapy instituted. If no arrhythmia is found, the cost, inconvenience and possibly toxic side effects of antiarrhythmic therapy can be avoided. Patients with unexplained syncope or syncope-like episodes should also undergo ambulatory electrocardiographic monitoring to determine whether an underlying brady- or tachyarrhythmia is detectable that can explain these symptoms. Caution must be urged when interpreting asymptomatic arrhythmias exhibited on the ambulatory electrocardiogram in a patient with intermittent symptoms. To be certain of cause and effect, the symptoms and arrhythmias should be observed simultaneously.

Another major use for ambulatory electrocardiograms is in patients with coronary heart disease. In this situation, the frequency and severity of ventricular premature complexes can be determined as a possible harbinger of sudden death. Although specific criteria still are controversial, there seems to be an increasing recognition that the presence of ventricular premature complexes that are frequent or complex in patients with coronary heart disease or previous myocardial infarction defines an increased risk of subsequent sudden death (see Chapter 15).

Thus, long-term electrocardiographic rhythm monitoring has rapidly assumed an important role in the diagnosis and management of disorders of the heart beat. The technique has been most useful in uncovering transient arrhythmias and in clarifying the relationship between symptoms and the presence or absence of concomitant rhythm disturbances. It has also yielded important information concerning underlying severe and otherwise unsuspected rhythm disturbances in addition to allowing improved evaluation of the efficacy of therapy.

CLINICAL ELECTROPHYSIOLOGICAL STUDIES

HIS BUNDLE ELECTROCARDIOGRAPHY

Although the standard electrocardiogram has been of invaluable clinical use to physicians for more than 50 years, it only partly records the electrical activity that takes place during each cardiac cycle. This is particularly important when one attempts to evaluate conduction through the A-V node, the His bundle, the bundle branches, and Purkinje fibers, since an impulse traversing these areas is depicted on the standard electrocardiogram by the isoelectric period of the P-R interval. The advent of a simple clinical method of recording the His bundle potential has enabled a more precise localization of the site of cardiac conduction abnormalities and blocks to be made. This technique has also been a useful aid in arrhythmia analysis.

Technique. The technique for recording a His bundle electrogram consists simply of inserting a standard bipolar (or multipolar) pacing electrode catheter with tip electrodes 1 cm apart percutaneously into a femoral vein and advancing it under fluoroscopic and electrocardiographic control into the right ventricle. The catheter is then slowly withdrawn to the A-V junctional area so that the electrodes lie in close proximity to the midportion of the base of the tricuspid valve. The bipolar electrode leads are connected to the AC input of an electrocardiogram amplifier (filtered from 40 to 200 Hz.) to display

TABLE 14–1   USES OF HIS BUNDLE RECORDINGS

Heart block
   Site
   Degree
   Prognosis
   Indications for Pacemaker

Arrhythmia-analysis
   Aberrant conduction
   Ventricular premature complexes

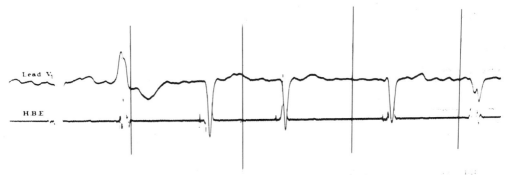

Figure 14–1   The second and sixth beat of the surface ECG are "abnormal." The second beat exhibits a right bundle branch block pattern. However, both beats are not preceded by a His bundle spike, while the "normal" complexes are; therefore, these two beats are of ventricular origin. (From Helfant, R. H., and Scherlag, B. J.: His Bundle Electrocardiography. New York, MEDCOM Press, 1974, pg. 35.)

and record the His bundle electrogram. The electrical potential from the sensing pacemaker electrode is monitored oscilloscopically as the catheter is slowly withdrawn or advanced through the region in which atrial and ventricular deflections are both apparent until a clear His bundle potential appears.

P-A, A-H, H-V Intervals and Normal Values.   Figure 14–1 illustrates the intervals defined by the His bundle electrogram (Hb), showing leads I (L-1), II (L-2), AVR, and an electrode (BE), demonstrating sinus activity (SA) in addition to the His bundle (Hb). The first deflection represents atrial activation (A wave) in the area of the low atrial septum at the A-V junction. The second deflection represents His bundle activation (H) and is usually a rapid bi- or triphasic deflection occurring during the isoelectric portion of the P-R segment seen on the standard electrocardiographic leads. The third deflection of the His bundle electrogram represents activation of the ventricles (V); this potential coincides with the QRS complex. Thus, the His bundle electrogram, in conjunction with the simultaneously recorded surface electrocardiogram, allows a division of the P-R interval into three components (see broken lines of Figure):

1.   The *P-A interval*, measured from the earliest onset of the P wave in any of the surface electrocardiograms to the beginning of the A wave, corresponds to a representative portion of intra-atrial conduction between the area of the sinus node and the area of the A-V junction.

2.   The *A-H interval*, measured from the onset of the A wave to the initial deflection of His bundle activation in the bipolar recording, is a relatively accurate measure of conduction through the A-V node.

3.   The *H-V interval*, taken from the onset of the His bundle deflection to the earliest appearing ventricular activity seen in the bipolar His bundle electrogram or in any of the standard electrocardiographic leads, measures conduction through the specialized conduction system of the ventricles; i.e., the His bundle, the bundle branches and their major fascicles, and the Purkinje fibers.

A conduction delay in the *A-V node* will be manifested by a prolongation of the A-H interval. A beat that is blocked at the level of the A-V node will be seen as an A wave with no accompanying His spike, since it is blocked proximal to the His bundle. A delay of conduction in the *His-Purkinje system* will be reflected on the electrogram as a prolongation of the H-V interval. With beats

TABLE 14–2 NORMAL VALUES OF CONDUCTION INTERVALS IN MAN*
(Mean and standard deviation)

P-A	A-H	H-V
43 ± 14	88 ± 21	41 ± 4
37 ± 11	78 ± 18	37 ± 5

*Conduction time in milliseconds of the three conduction intervals within the P-R interval of the standard ECG as measured in two laboratories by the His bundle electrogram. The P-A interval corresponds to intra-atrial conduction, A-H to conduction through the A-V node, and H-V to conduction through the specialized fibers of the ventricle.

that are blocked below the A-V node in the distal His bundle, fascicles below will be seen as an A wave accompanied by a His spike.

The normal values for the conduction times composing the P-R interval are summarized in Table 14–2

Location of Heart Block. The use of His bundle electrocardiography has allowed a more precise understanding of the localization and quantification of conduction defects in man. Table 14–3 summarizes these findings. The results of these clinical studies have closely correlated with earlier experimental findings in animals as well as with the ingenious deductive reasoning of many clinical investigators using the electrocardiogram alone.

TABLE 14–3 LIMITATIONS OF HIS BUNDLE RECORDINGS

Validation of His spike
  Nonuniformity of criteria
  Technically difficult (especially His pacing)
Definition of normal values
Split or fragmented His spikes
  Incidence unknown
  Can lead to misinterpretation of H-V or
    localization
Prognosis and indications for pacemaker
  Patients with complete heart block with
    normal H-V correlation of H-V with severity
    of heart disease

In the great majority of patients with *first-degree heart block* of the acquired or congenital type, prolongation of the A-H interval has been found to be the major determinant of the prolonged P-R interval. Although in most patients the H-V times have fallen within the range of normal values, some patients with acquired first-degree heart block have the major site of delay in the His-Purkinje system.

Mobitz I or Wenckebach type second-degree A-V block is characterized on the surface electrocardiogram by a progressive prolongation of the P-R interval until there is a blocked or nonconducted P wave. This "Wenckebach period" is repetitive in whatever ratio (4:3, 3:2, etc.) may be present. His bundle electrocardiography has demonstrated that the site of progressive delay, as the P-R interval prolongs, is usually in the A-H portion of the cycle. In addition, the blocked P wave is characterized by an A deflection that is blocked proximal to the bundle of His. These findings indicate that this type of second degree heart block usually occurs proximal to the His bundle or in the A-V node. Although Mobitz I block has also been shown to be due to a focal lesion within the His bundle itself, this is quite infrequent.

Mobitz II second-degree block is less common than the type I variety. The P-R interval is constant and may be within the normal range, but isolated P waves are unexpectedly not followed by a QRS. Varying ratios of block occur (8:7, 5:4, etc.). In contrast to type I, the site of block in patients with this conduction abnormality is usually below the A-V node. This has been shown by the fact that the blocked P waves have a His bundle spike that follows the atrial deflection on the electrogram. Thus, the site of block is "infranodal" (i.e., below the A-V node). However, occasional exceptions have been reported, particularly in patients in whom His bundle lesions accounted for the sudden failure of A-V conduction and in those in whom true or simulated Mobitz type II block have been shown to occur above the recorded His bundle deflection (probably in the A-V node).

In most patients with *complete heart block* who have been studied with the His bundle method, the site of block has been found to be below the level of the A-V node. This has been shown by the fact that the nonconducted P waves are blocked distal to the bundle of His and that the ventricular electrogram is not preceded by a His deflection. This finding is almost invariable in patients with a widened QRS complex (0.12 second or greater) and a slow idioventricular rate (below 40 beats per minute). However, in patients with complete heart block of the congenital variety (in whom the QRS complex is of normal or "supraventricular" morphology), the His bundle potential is temporally associated with ventricular activity and not with activity of the atria. This indicates that the site of block in these patients is in the A-V node. In some patients, however, the site of the lesion can be localized within the His bundle itself.

Bundle Branch Block and Hemiblocks. In the presence of right or left bundle branch block, His bundle electrocardiography allows an assessment to be made of the contralateral bundle branch system. This is based on the concept that the propagation of electrical impulses to nonspecialized cardiac muscle occurs virtually simultaneously from the three fascicular pathways of the specialized conduction system. Therefore, the "H-V time" in a patient with bundle branch block represents activation of the contralateral bundle-branch system. It follows that significant prolongation of the H-V time indicates at least a partial abnormality of conduction of *all* functioning portions of the specialized conduction system — i.e., the common bundle branches and their fascicles or Purkinje system. It should also be pointed out that lesions occurring at the origins of the bundle branches may also affect the bundle of His. This situation may reveal itself as a right or left bundle branch block with a prolonged H-V time. Therefore, in the presence of bundle branch blocks of the right or left types, or *bifascicular blocks* (RBBB with left or right anterior hemiblock) (see Chapter 12), the H-V time can be used to assess the conduction status of the remaining fascicle, fascicles, or distal common bundle. This differentiation cannot be made on the basis of the electrocardiogram alone. Although the significance of the H-V times in these patients may potentially be of prognostic importance, this still remains controversial (see below).

Analysis of Arrhythmias. His bundle electrocardiography can be of considerable value in the analysis of some complex arrhythmias. Its primary clinical use in arrhythmia analysis has been in differentiating ventricular ectopic beats from supraventricular beats with aberrant conduction. The differentiation of ventricular premature beats from supraventricular beats with aberrant ventricular conduction is often difficult on the basis of the surface electrocardiogram (see Chapter 8). This difficulty usually arises in a patient with underlying atrial fibrillation. The diagnosis of aberrant conduction has been based largely on the presence of 1) a right bundle branch block pattern, 2) a cycle revealing an abnormal ventricular complex in the sequence of a long pause, followed by a short pause and, 3) a variable coupling time.

This differentiation is often inexact, and in many instances the differentiation cannot be definitively made on the basis of the surface electrocardiogram. Use of His bundle electrocardiography allows precise differentiation of these two phenomena. This is based on the temporal relationship of the His bundle deflection to the subsequent ventricular complex. In a patient with atrial fibrillation in which the "abnormal" beat is preceded by a His bundle deflection with an H-V time equal to or longer than the normally conducted ventricular beats, this is diagnostic of aberrant ventricular conduction. However, if no His bundle spike precedes the abnormal QRS complex or if the His bundle spike precedes the QRS in question with an H-V time shorter than the supraventricular complexes, the site of origin of the beat in question is ventricular.

In Figure 14–2 the surface electrocardiogram demonstrates an abnormal ventricular beat in a right bundle branch block pattern in the sequence of a long and short pause. This would therefore meet the majority criteria for aberrant ventricular conduction. Note, however, that in this His bundle electrogram (HBE), although clear-cut His bundle spikes precede the "supraventricular" beats, the normal beat is not preceded by a His bundle spike, indicating that this is of ventricular origin.

Limitations of His Bundle Recordings. There are several important limitations of His bundle recordings which have important implications for the clinical use of this technique. Validation that the spike seen between the atrial and ventricular depolarizations represents the His depolarization has been a particular problem. There has in general been no uniform criterion for validating whether or not a spike originates from the bundle of His or one of the other portions of the specialized conduction system, or is an artifact. At times, validation of the His bundle spike is technically difficult, particularly when one attempts pacing from the His bundle itself (unfortunately the most precise means of validation). In addition, the definitions of normal values of P-A, A-H, and A-V have often not been uniformly agreed to.

Another major difficulty relates to "split" or fragmented His bundle spikes. The incidence of conduction abnormalities involving the bundle of His itself (which result in either split or fragmented His bundle activation on the catheter recording) is unknown but has profound implications in interpreting His bundle recordings. Since even with the most careful catheter search for a split His bundle spike may be unrewarding, it is almost impossible to be certain that a split His bundle spike exists except by actually recording it. If indeed a split or fragmented His bundle spike is missed, this can result in gross

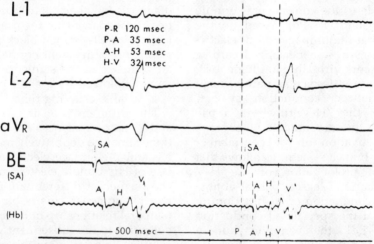

Figure 14–2   Recording of His bundle bipolar electrogram (Hb) and simultaneously recorded bipolar electrogram from the sinus node area (BE, SA) with three standard ECG leads (L-1, L-2, and aVR). The P-R interval (120 msec) is divided into intra-atrial conduction time (P-A = 35 msec), A-V nodal conduction (A-H = 53 msec); and His-Purkinje system conduction time (H-V = 32 msec) (Scherlag, et al: Circulation 46:601, 1972).

misinterpretation of either the location of conduction abnormalities or of the H-V interval.

Lastly, the use of the H-V interval as a prognostic guide and a determinant for cardiac pacemaker implantation has not been determined and remains controversial to the present time (see Chapter 12). Narula et al. (1978) have presented strong evidence for using the H-V interval as *the* major indication for pacemaker implantation in patients with bilateral bundle branch block. However, this has been disputed by many authorities (see Chapter 12). Patients have been reported with documented complete heart block and a normal H-V interval (Haft, 1977). In addition, correlations have been made between the degree of H-V prolongation and the underlying severity of heart disease overall (i.e., the severity of congestive heart failure, heart size, functional classification of the patient, etc.) (Rosen, 1975). Additional studies are needed with patient subsets relating to the etiology of heart disease, perhaps with serial electrophysiologic observations to clarify this issue. Until then, the prognosis of the H-V interval remains controversial and probably should not, in our view, be used as a major parameter in clinical decisions regarding pacemaker implantation.

Clinical Indications for His Bundle Electrograms

Heart Block. Most patients with chronic complete heart block or with well documented intermittent complete heart block not associated with acute myocardial infarction, digitalis intoxication, or other transient clinical conditions should have permanent pacemakers implanted. Similarly, most patients with a history of documented syncope, seizures, or associated neurological symptoms without a neurological cause who have right bundle branch block with either anterior or posterior hemiblock or left bundle branch block should have a permanent pacemaker implanted. In addition, patients with documented Mobitz type II block and a prolonged QRS complex are candidates for permanent pacemakers. Occasionally, patients with fixed-ratio heart block will require a His bundle electrogram to determine the site of block if the decision for pacemaker cannot be made on the basis of the clinical findings, such as the ventricular rate, symptoms, or underlying heart disease.

In patients with first degree heart block associated with bifascicular block without symptoms, a pacemaker is probably not indicated. A His bundle electrogram can be performed to determine whether the P-R prolongation is due to block in the distal conduction system and the H-V interval since it *may* have some prognostic value. However, while in some centers it is felt that all patients with bifascicular block should have a His bundle electrogram performed regardless of symptomatology, this currently is not our view for the reasons previously indicated.

Arrhythmia Analysis. As discussed previously, when it is difficult to deduce from the surface electrocardiogram whether a tachycardia originates from the ventricles or is supraventricular with aberrant conduction, a His bundle study will usually clarify the origin of the arrhythmia in question. In addition, an exceedingly rare arrhythmia has been diagnosed with a His bundle electrogram: an arrhythmia which looks like Mobitz type II block on the standard electrocardiogram but which has blocked His bundle premature beats.

Pre-excitation Syndromes. His bundle electrocardiography has been employed in patients with pre-excitation syndromes to allow a determination to be made of the type and function of the bypass tract (see Chapter 13). However, clinically it is rarely necessary to employ His bundle electrocardiography in patients with pre-excitation syndromes except in severe and refractory cases or under other special circumstances (see Chapter 13).

SINUS NODE RECOVERY TIME

Following termination of rapid atrial pacing, spontaneous sinus rhythm normally resumes with the first post-pacing cycle length being longer than the spontaneous cycle length. This phenomenon, the sinus node recovery time, has been used to evaluate patients with the *sick sinus syndrome* (see Chapter 5), characterized by sinus bradycardia, sino-atrial arrest, sino-atrial block and "brady-tachy" syndrome (see Chapter 5). However, the sinus node recovery time measurement has several problems that limit its clinical usefulness (see Table 14–4). It is reportedly abnormal in from 35 to 93 per cent of patients (depending on the report) with classic clinical and electrocardiographic evidence of the sick sinus syndrome and thus is insensitive, since many patients with marked sinus bradycardia may have a normal sinus node recovery time measurement. This relative insensitivity may be due to sino-atrial conduction disturbances, sinus node entry block, a shift in the sinus node pacemaker, or changes in the autonomic nervous system. For example, experimental and clinical studies have indicated that changes in the autonomic nervous system can have profound effects on sinus node recovery time. Thus, while this measurement may at times be helpful in confirming the diagnosis of sinus node dysfunction, prolonged electrocardiographic ambulatory monitoring is usually more valuable in diagnosis (see Chapter 5).

TABLE 14–4   LIMITATIONS OF SINUS NODE RECOVERY TIME

Abnormal in 35 to 93% of patients with sick sinus syndrome
Patients with marked bradycardia may have normal SNRT
Relative insensitivity may be due to:
  S-A conduction disturbances
  Sinus node entry block
  Shift in sinus node pacemaker
  Changes in autonomic nervous system

ATRIAL AND VENTRICULAR PACING AND PROGRAMMED STIMULATION

The techniques of atrial and ventricular pacing and programmed stimulation in conjunction with intracardiac recordings from the His bundle and other areas of the heart have greatly expanded our understanding of the mechanisms of supraventricular and ventricular tachyarrhythmias and have resulted in a reclassification of several of these arrhythmias based on their electrophysiological characteristics (Wellens, 1972). These studies have also been used to measure the sino-atrial conduction times in patients with the suspected sick sinus node syndrome as well as to determine the site and electrophysiologic characteristics of bypass tracts in patients with pre-excitation syndromes.

Pacing techniques to provoke ventricular (and supraventricular) tachycardia have also been used to evaluate drug treatment regimens (Denes, 1976; Mason, 1978; Horowitz, 1978). This technique involves induction of ventricular tachycardia with programmed ventricular stimulation using an intravenous pacemaker and then testing the ability of a given drug or combination to suppress the tachycardia response to the stimulated beats. This approach is currently in the investigative stages and several important questions will have to be answered before it becomes accepted for undisputed clinical use (Scheinman, 1978): 1) What is the risk of the procedure? In the experience of Mason and Winkle (1978), fully 52 per cent of patients required emergency cardioversion because of hemodynamic instability. It seems clear that this technique has serious potential risks. 2) How predictable can this technique induce the ventricular tachycardia? This has varied widely depending at least in part on the particular technique used (which varies considerably in different laboratories). 3) What is the precise relationship between the ability of an intravenous drug to suppress pacing stimulated ventricular tachycardia in the laboratory and its long-term clinical efficacy? Conversely, how certain is it that a drug which fails to suppress stimulated ventricular tachycardia is clinically ineffective? (The need for intravenous drug trials with this method currently limits the number of antiarrhythmic agents that can be tested, i.e., those that are only available for oral use). 4) What are the advantages of this technique compared with the use of ambulatory and/or telemetric monitoring to assess the efficacy of oral drug trials?

REFERENCES

Altschuler, H., Fisher, J. D., and Furman, S.: Prolonged H-V interval. Preventable early mortality in symptomatic patients without documented heart block. Clin. Res. 25:203A, 1977 (Abst).

Bellet, S., Roman, L., Kostes, J., et al.: Continuous ECG monitoring during automobile driving. Am. J. Cardiol. 22:856, 1968.

Bleifer, S. B., Bleifer, D. J., Hansmann, D. R., et al.: Diagnosis of occult arrhythmias by Holter electrocardiography. Prog. Cardiovasc. Dis. 16:569, 1974.

Crook, B. R. M., Cashman, P. M. M., Stott, R. D., et al.: Tape monitoring of electrocardiogram in ambulant patients with sinoatrial disease. Br. Heart J. 35:867, 1973.

Damato, A. N., Lau, S. H., Helfant, R. H., et al.: A study of heart block in man using His bundle recordings. Circulation 39:297, 1969.

Damato, A. N., Lau, S. H., Helfant, R. H., Stein, E., Berkowitz, W. D., and Cohen, S. I.: Study of atrioventricular conduction in man using electrode catheter recordings of His bundle activity. Circulation 39:287, 1969.

Denes, P., Dhingra, R. G., Wu, D., Chaquima, R., Amat-y-Leon, F., Wyndham, C., and Rosen, K. M.: H-V interval in patients with bifascicular block (right bundle branch block and left anterior hemiblock). Am. J. Cardiol. 35:23, 1975.

Denes, P., Wu, D., Amat-y-Leon, F., Dhingra, R., Wyndham, C., Kehoe, R., Ayers, B. F., and Rosen, K. M.: Paroxysmal supraventricular tachycardia induction in patients with Wolff-Parkinson-White Syndrome. Ann. Intern. Med. 90:153, 1979.

Dhingra, R. C., Wyndham, C., Amat-y-Leon, F., Denes, P., Wu, D., Sridhar, S., Bustin, A. S., and Rosen, K. W.: Incidence and site of AV block in patients with chronic bifascicular block. Circulation 59:238–246, 1979.

Dreifus, L. S.: Clinical judgement is sufficient for the management of conduction defects. In Corday, E. (ed.): Controversies in Cardiology, Philadelphia, F. A. Davis Co., 1975, pp. 195–201.

Engle, T. R. (Editorial): Pacing techniques to guide the therapy of tachycardias. Ann. Intern. Med. 90(2):265, 1979.

Fitzgerald, J. W., and DeBusk, R. F.: Early postinfarction ambulatory monitoring and exercise testing in detection of arrhythmias. Am. J. Cardiol. 35:136, 1975.

Gilson, J. S., Holter, N. J., and Glasscock, W. R.: Clinical observations using the electrocardiocorder-AVSEP continuous electrocardiographic system: Tentative standards and typical patterns. Am. J. Cardiol. 14:204, 1964.

Goldberg, A. N.: Exercise stress testing in the uncovering of dysrhythmias. Med. Clin. of North. Amer. 60:315, 1976.

Goldschlager, N., Coke, D., and Cohn, K.: Exercise induced ventricular arrhythmias in patients with coronary artery disease. Am. J. Cardiol. 31:434, 1973.

Haft, J. I.: Clinical indication for the His bundle electrogram. Cardiovasc. Med. 449, 1977.

Harrison, D. C., Fitzgerald, J. W., and Winkle, R. A.: Ambulatory electrocardiography for diagnosis and treatment of cardiac arrhythmias. N. Engl. J. Med. 294:373, 1976.

Helfant, R. H., Meister, S. G., and DeVilla, M. A.: The effect of sustained isometric handgrip exercise on left ventricular performance. Circulation 44:982, 1971.

Helfant, R. H., Pine, R., Kabde, V., Banka, V. S.: Exercise-related ventricular premature complexes in coronary heart disease. Ann. Intern. Med. 80:589, 1974.

Helfant, R. H., and Scherlag, B. J.: His bundle electrocardiography. MEDCOM Press New York, New York, 1974.

Hinkle, L. E., Jr., Carver, S. T., and Stevens, M.: The frequency of asymptomatic disturbances of cardiac rhythm and conduction in middle-aged men. Am. J. Cardiol. 24:629, 1969.

Hinkle, L. E., Meyer, J., Stevens, M., et al.: Tape recordings of the ECG of active men: Limitations and advantages of the Holter-Avionics instruments. Circulation 36:752, 1967.

Holter, N. J.: New method for heart studies: Continuous electrocardiography of active subjects over long periods is now practical. Science 134:1214, 1961.

Horowitz, L. N., Josephson, M. E., Farshidi, A., Spielman, R., Michelson, E. L., and Greenspan, A. M.: Recurrent sustained ventricular tachycardia. 3. Role of the electrophysiologic study in selection of antiarrhythmic regimens. Circulation 58:986, 1978.

Jelinek, M. V., and Lown, B.: Exercise testing for exposure of cardiac arrhythmias. Prog. Cardiovasc. Dis. 16:497, 1974.

Josephson, M. E., Horowitz, L. N., Farshidi, A., and Kastor, J. A.: Recurrent sustained ventricular tachycardia. I. Mechanisms. Circulation 57:431, 1978.

Kosowsky, B. D., Lown, B., Whiting, R., et al.: Occurrence of ventricular arrhythmias with exercise as compared to monitoring. Circulation 44:826, 1971.

Lamb, L. E., and Hiss, R. G.: Influence of exercise on premature contractions. Am. J. Cardiol. 10:209, 1962.

Mann, R. H., and Burchell, H. B.: Premature ventricular contractions and exercise. Mayo Clin. Proc. 27:383, 1952.

McHenry, P. L., Fisch, C., Jordan, J. W., and Corya, B. R.: Cardiac arrhythmias observed during maximal treadmill exercise testing in clinical normal men. Am. J. Cardiol. 29:331, 1972.

Mason, J. W., and Winkle, R. A.: Electrode-catheter arrhythmia induction in the selection and assessment of angiarrhythmic drug therapy in recurrent ventricular tachycardia. Circulation 58:971, 1978.

Michelson, E. L., and Josephson, M. E.: Uses and limitations of the ambulatory ECG. Cardiovasc. Med. 4:533, 1979.

Michelson, E. L., Morganroth, J., Spear, J. F., Kastor, J. A., and Josephson, M. E.: Fixed coupling: Different mechanisms revealed by exercise-induced changes in cycle length. Circulation 58:1002, 1978.

Morganroth, J., Michelson, E. L., Horowitz, L. N., Josephson, M. E., Pearlman, A. S., and Durkman, W. B.: Limitations of routine long term ambulatory ECG monitoring to assess ventricular ectopic activity. Circulation 58:408, 1978.

Narula, O., Quazi, N., Samet, P., et al.: Ten year prospective observations based on H-V interval in patients with right bundle branch block and left axis deviation. Circulation II-197, 1978.

Narula, O. S., and Samet, P.: Wenckebach and Mobitz type II A-V heart block within the His bundle and bundle branches. Circulation 41:947, 1970.

Narula, O. S., Scherlag, B. J., Samet, P., and Javier, R. P.: Atrioventricular block: Localization and classification by His bundle recordings. Am. J. Med. 50:146, 1971.

Porter, W. B.: The probably grave significance of premature beats occurring in angina pectoris induced by effort. Am. J. Med. Sci. 216:509, 1948.

Ranganathan, N., Dhurandhar, R., Phillips, J. H., and Wigle, E. D.: His bundle electrogram in bundle branch block. Circulation 48:282, 1972.

Razzak, M. A.: Bigeminy on exertion. Circulation 28:32, 1963.

Rosen, K. M.: The contribution of His bundle recordings to the understanding of cardiac conduction in man. Circulation 43:961, 1971.

Rosenbaum, M. B., et al: Intraventricular trifascicular blocks. The syndrome of right bundle branch block with intermittent left anterior and posterior hemiblock. Am. Heart. J. 78:306, 1969.

Ryan, M., Lown, B., and Horn, H.: Comparison of ventricular ectopic activity during 24 hour monitoring and exercise testing in patients with coronary heart disease. N. Engl. J. Med. 292:224, 1975.

Sandberg, L.: Studies on electrocardiographic changes during exercise tests. Acta Med. Scand. 169(suppl): 1–117, 1961.

Scheinman, M., Weiss, A., and Kunkel, F.: His bundle recordings in patients with bundle branch block and transient neurological symptoms. Circulation 48:322, 1973.

Scheinman, M. M., Peters, R. W., Modin, G., et al.: Prognostic value of infranodal conduction time in patients with chronic bundle branch block. Circulation 56:240, 1977.

Scherlag, B. J., Lau, S. H., Helfant, R. H., Berkowitz, W. D., Stein, E., and Damato, A. N.: Catheter technique for recording His bundle activity in man. Circulation 39:13, 1969.

Scherlag, B. J., Samet, P., and Helfant, R. H.: The His electrogram: A critical appraisal of its uses and limitations. Circulation 44:601, 1972.

Tzivoni, D., and Stern, S.: Pacemaker implantation based on ambulatory ECG monitoring in patients with cerebral symptoms. Chest 67:274, 1975.

Vera, Z., Mason, D. T., Fletcher, R. D., Awan, N. A., and Massumi, R. A.: Prolonged His-Q interval in chronic bifascicular block: Relation to impending complete heart block. Circulation 53:46, 1976.

Wellens, H. J. J., Duren, R. D., and Lie, K. I.: Observations on mechanisms of ventricular tachycardia in man. Circulation 54:237, 1976.

Wellens, H. J. J., Lie, K. I., and Durrer, D.: Further observations on ventricular tachycardia as studied by electrical stimulation of the heart. Circulation 49:647, 1974.

Wellens, H. J. J., Schuilenburg, R. M., and Durrer, D.: Electrical stimulation of the heart in patients with ventricular tachycardia. Circulation 46:216, 1972.

Wu, D., Amat-y-Leon, F., Simpson, R. J., Jr., Latif, P., Wyndham, C. R. C., Denes, P., and Rosen, K. M.: Electrophysiologic studies with multiple drugs in patients with atrioventricular re-entrant tachycardia utilizing an extranodal pathway. Circulation 56:727, 1977.

15

CORONARY HEART DISEASE AND SUDDEN DEATH

Coronary Disease

MONTY M. BODENHEIMER, M.D.
RICHARD H. HELFANT, M.D.

GENERAL CONSIDERATIONS

Coronary heart disease is one of the major public health problems today, being associated with 600,000 to 700,000 deaths per year in the United States. Its major manifestations include myocardial infarction, angina, congestive heart failure, arrhythmias (both tachycardias and bradycardias) and sudden death—each of which may be the presenting feature. With the advent of the coronary care unit and its widespread utilization in the 1960's, it soon became evident that arrhythmias were very common in acute myocardial infarction. More recently, it has also become clear that the majority of patients dying from coronary heart disease succumbed before reaching the hospital, presumably of a sudden catastrophic arrhythmia. In addition, many unexpected sudden deaths were occurring both after discharge from the coronary care unit and after discharge from the hospital in the healing stage of the disease process.

In the past decade, there has been a massive effort directed at better understanding as well as reduction of high incidence of out-of-hospital mortality due to lethal cardiac arrhythmias. Several epidemiologic and experimental studies have defined risk factors for coronary artery disease as well as those factors which predispose to arrhythmias. Emphasis on pre- and post-Cardiac Care Unit management of the patient has led to the development of rapid response teams, including mobile coronary care units and fire rescue squads for immediate cardiopulmonary resuscitation in the pre-hospital phase, and the establishment of intermediate coronary care units to monitor patients after discharge from the intensive care unit.

PATHOGENESIS OF CORONARY HEART DISEASE

Coronary heart disease is caused by atherosclerotic lesions, which are usually confined to the proximal extramural coronary arteries. The earliest

211

lesions, detectable in males in the late teens and early 20's, are fatty streaks, deposits consisting mainly of cholesterol in the intima. Over the ensuing years, these slowly evolve into the mature lesions of atherosclerosis: obstructive intimal plaques consisting of fibrosis, lipids (mainly cholesterol), calcium, and necrotic material. These lesions usually do not produce clinical consequences until reduction of the luminal cross section of the coronary artery reaches 75 per cent or more.

Other mechanisms proposed as playing a role in arterial obstructive disease include hemorrhage into a cholesterol plaque, platelet aggregation, thrombosis, coronary spasm, and neuropsychiatric mechanisms. Any or all of these processes could result in a critical reduction in coronary blood flow, with resultant myocardial ischemia, infarction, or a catastrophic arrhythmia. Yet, some patients who have clearly had a myocardial infarction are subsequently found to have no evidence of coronary obstruction on arteriography. The mechanism(s) in these cases is speculative.

Risk Factors

Although the basic etiologic factors and mechanisms involved in the atherosclerotic process remain uncertain, several have been identified that statistically correlate with a higher incidence, more rapid progression, or greater severity of coronary heart disease. Studies have established a significant association for age, sex, familial history of coronary heart disease, cigarette smoking, hypercholesterolemia, hypertension, and diabetes mellitus. Other factors not as clearly involved include a sedentary life style and a compulsive hard-driving perfectionistic personality (type A).

Unfortunately, despite these statistical epidemiologic correlations, the cause and effect relationship between these factors and the atherosclerotic process remains obscure. This is best illustrated by the Coronary Drug Project, in which an attempt was made to prevent or retard the development of atherosclerotic heart disease by reducing hyperlipidemia in patients who survived a myocardial infarction. While the ability to control or reduce blood cholesterol was good, no effect on mortality was observed.

ELECTROPHYSIOLOGIC CORRELATES OF MYOCARDIAL ISCHEMIA

Considerable experimental data are available which describe the effects of ischemia on the myocardium. Reduced coronary blood flow causes myocardial ischemia, which results in the accumulation of metabolites within the affected zone. Electrophysiologically, hypoxia results in a small decrease in the amplitude and duration of the action potential with little effect on threshold potential. In contrast, ischemia results in more marked changes in the amplitude and duration of the action potential, with a marked loss of resting membrane potential as well. Presumably, these differences relate to the accumulation of potassium and other metabolites as well as acidosis (although the relative importance of these changes is unclear). It has also become apparent that within the zone of infarction, cells are present that show slow channel activity (see Chapter 2). It has been proposed that these latter changes are responsible for many of the arrhythmias seen, particularly since catecholamines and high extracellular potassium (both present in the setting of acute myocardial infarction) can result in these conditions (Cranefield, 1975). However, within the same infarct, areas of fast channel activity also exist. The relative importance or interrelationship between these two electrophysiological abnormalities in arrhythmogenesis is unclear.

The QRS complex, which reflects ventricular depolarization, shows a decrease in amplitude, fractionation, increase in duration, and delayed activation compared to the QRS complex of nonischemic myocardium. An increase in excitability occurs within 5 minutes of coronary occlusion. In addition, the ventricular fibrillation threshold (which, according to some authors, measures the propensity of the ventricle to fibrillate) decreases dramatically within the first few minutes after coronary occlusion.

Myocardial ischemia also results both in conduction delays and changes in refractoriness. Han and Moe (1964) and Durrer et al. (1964) have found evidence of slowed conduction in ischemic myocardium, while Williams et al. (1974) observed a delay in conduction in the ischemic zone that progressively increased from the time of coronary occlusion. In addition, Williams et al. noted persistence of electrical activity during diastole. The progressive delay in conduction coincided with appearance of ventricular arrhythmias. Levites et al. (1975) demonstrated that coronary occlusion resulted in a decrease in the refractory period of 28 per cent without a change in the nonischemic zone, resulting in a dispersion of refractoriness. These changes in conduction, as reflected by prolongation of electrical activity throughout the cardiac cycle and refractoriness, also predispose to re-entrant arrhythmias (see Chapter 2).

Lethal arrhythmias may not invariably be associated with an actual myocardial infarction (see Sudden Death). This has raised the question of whether arrhythmias in the setting of acute coronary heart disease (myocardial ischemia or infarction) are a consequence of the coronary occlusion per se as opposed to being due to "reperfusion" of the ischemic area, at least in some cases. Experimental studies, beginning with Tennant and Wiggers in the 1930's and more recently confirmed by several groups, have shown that coronary re-

perfusion is accompanied by marked ventricular irritability including ventricular tachycardia and fibrillation. Restoration of coronary flow into a previously ischemic area results in a rapid washout of metabolites including lactate and potassium and it is conceivable that the rapid alteration in the extracellular milieu may be responsible for these arrhythmic changes.

It is of interest that the electrophysiologic changes seen after reperfusion differ considerably from those of coronary occlusion. Levites et al. (1975) showed that the refractory period immediately after reperfusion increases markedly compared to the shortening seen after coronary occlusion. Battle et al. (1974), as demonstrated by others, showed that the ventricular fibrillation threshold decreased markedly after coronary occlusion, but the ventricular fibrillation threshold then gradually returned to baseline. However, after reperfusion no change was seen in the ventricular fibrillation threshold.

EXPERIMENTAL MYOCARDIAL ISCHEMIA AND INFARCTION

Experimentally, there are two phases of ventricular arrhythmias after coronary ligation. The first stage occurs within 15 to 30 minutes and is characterized by re-entrant VPC's, ventricular tachycardia, and a high incidence of ventricular fibrillation. Lidocaine and procainamide are relatively ineffective in altering the appearance of re-entry arrhythmias in this phase. (This is consistent with the clinical experience of some authors that these agents are relatively ineffective in the very early phase of myocardial infarction — Adgey et al., 1971).

Harris and coworkers also described a second phase of experimental arrhythmias 24 to 48 hours after coronary artery ligation characterized by multifocal ectopic beats and repetitive ventricular premature depolarizations. These arrhythmias, thought to be due to enhanced automaticity, were associated with much lower mortality than in the early phase. This experimental phase has several similarities to the coronary care unit phase in patients.

Recent animal studies have also shown that there is a third, subacute phase of ventricular arrhythmias 3 to 10 days after coronary artery ligation in which ventricular arrhythmias occur spontaneously or can be readily induced (Scherlag et al., 1974). These ventricular arrhythmias occur after the phase of enhanced automaticity has subsided. Fractionation and delay in conduction could be induced by pacing during this phase, again suggesting reentry as the mechanism. Temporally, there is a similarity between these ventricular arrhythmias in the experimental animal and those seen in patients after discharge from the coronary care unit.

In patients with acute myocardial infarction, tachyarrhythmias cause hemodynamic changes that range from a momentary change in stroke volume due to a ventricular premature beat to complete cessation of circulation due to ventricular fibrillation. Rapid but coordinated contraction of the atria (supraventricular tachycardia) with a rapid ventricular rate usually causes a decrease in cardiac output because the rapid rate is unable to compensate for the decrease in stroke volume. Ventricular tachycardia impairs stroke volume even further. Occasionally, patients with acute myocardial infarction may tolerate episodes of tachyarrhythmias rather well for brief periods; in others, the arrhythmia encroaches upon the remaining cardiac reserve, leading to rapid deterioration, shock, and eventual death.

Complete A-V heart block occurring during acute myocardial infarction has an especially deleterious effect on the circulation, because the myocardial impairment limits the maximal stroke volume. The infarction often causes acute pump dysfunction and failure, and, as a result, arterial pressure may fall markedly when complete A-V heart block occurs. Temporary cardiac pacing is often a mandatory emergency measure (see Chapter 24).

SINUS BRADYARRHYTHMIAS

Several centers have found that a significant number of patients manifest bradyarrhythmias within one hour of onset of acute myocardial infarction (Fig. 15–1). Adgey et al. (1971), in a study of 284 patients, found that 26 per cent had sinus bradycardia or junctional rhythm, with the incidence in posterior myocardial infarction being 36 per cent compared to 18 per cent in

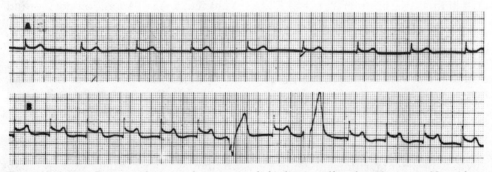

Figure 15–1 (A) Patient with acute inferior myocardial infarction of less than 30 minutes. No evidence of atrial activity could be detected and a junctional rhythm at 58 per minute is present. (B) One hour later, patient was given 0.6 mg atropine, which increased heart rate to 85 beats per minute. Multifocal VPC's appeared. Again no atrial activity was seen.

anterior myocardial infarction. The same group (Webb et al., 1972), in a selected series of 74 patients seen within the first 30 minutes, found brad-yarrhythmias in 20 patients (27 per cent), of whom 12 required atropine either for marked bradycardia or for hypotension. This high incidence decreased markedly, such that only 7 per cent had bradyarrhythmia after 4 hours.

Different mechanisms for these brad-yarrhythmias have been proposed. Involvement of the sinus nodal artery with secondary ischemia could result in bradyarrhythmia. The sinus node artery arises from the right coronary artery at the crux (posterior junction of the atrioventricular and interventricular grooves) in 55 per cent of patients and from the proximal portion of the left circumflex artery in 45 per cent. Its origin from the vessel supplying the inferior wall of the left ventricle would explain the higher incidence of such arrhythmias in posterior infarction. However, the excellent response frequently observed after atropine administration suggests that vagotonia is responsible. There are known to exist a large number of cholinergic ganglia and nerve endings in the lower posterior portion of the interatrial septum between the ostium of the coronary sinus and the posterior margin of the A-V node. Ischemia of this region could result in a vagotonia response which would be expected to improve with atropine.

Bradyarrhythmias acquire significance in the setting of acute myocardial infarction if hypotension or ventricular arrhythmias appear concomitantly. While some experimental studies have indicated that bradycardia may have beneficial electrophysiologic effects (Epstein, 1973), others have shown that bradyarrhythmias predispose to ventricular arrhythmias and that an optimal heart rate reduces the propensity to arrhythmias (Chadda, 1974). Chadda et al. used atropine to treat patients with bradyarrhythmias and hypotension in the early phase of acute myocardial infarction. Sinus bradycardia was relieved in 32 of 32 patients, hypotension was relieved in 61 of 68 patients, and the incidence of VPC's was decreased in all 26 patients in whom they appeared. No patient manifested an increase in VPC's. Although the course of such patients without treatment is speculative, it is clear that if a patient manifests brad-yarrhythmia with hypotension sufficient to either impair perfusion or result in ventricular arrhythmias, careful use of intravenous atropine, begun with 0.4 mg, is beneficial. However, rapid atropine administration may induce potentially dangerous arrhythmias (Fig. 15–1) (Mussumi, 1972).

ATRIOVENTRICULAR CONDUCTION DISTURBANCES

In an extensive review of the literature, Bigger et al. (1977) found the incidence of first degree atrioventricular block to range from 5.8 to 19.5 per cent, second degree block from 2 to 10 per cent and complete heart block from 1.8 to 8 per cent. It is clear, however, that the significance of block depends not only on its presence and severity but also on the site of myocardial infarction. Thus, the mortality of patients with complete heart block in inferior myocardial infarction is approximately 30 per cent, whereas in anterior myocardial infarction it is over 80 per cent.

MECHANISMS OF HEART BLOCK

The A-V node is supplied by an A-V nodal artery of the right coronary artery branch, which arises from the right coronary artery in 90 per cent of patients (the remainder arises from the left circumflex artery). Coronary occlusion involving this vessel is generally manifested as an inferior or posterior myocardial infarction on electrocardiogram and not infrequently is associated with A-V block, usually first degree block or type I (Wenckebach) second degree A-V block. (Fig. 15–2). Necropsy studies in such patients have shown typical pathologic evidence of myocardial infarction. Yet the A-V node itself is rarely involved. This explains the observation that in the vast majority of patients the block completely disappears after several days.

Infranodal tissues, including the major fascicles of the right and left bundles, are supplied by penetrating branches of the left anterior descending artery. The appearance of bundle branch block or heart block in the presence of anterior myocardial infarction is associated with extensive irreversible damage to the interventricular septum, and a high incidence of cardiogenic shock. The prognosis in such patients is generally determined by the associated failure. Thus, although a transvenous pacemaker is required to maintain an adequate heart rate, the patient often succumbs to pump failure.

CLINICAL FEATURES

Norris and Mercer (1974), in a series of 503 patients with inferior myocardial infarction, found first degree block in 21 per cent, second degree in 16.5 per cent, and 3rd degree in 10.5 per cent. Of the 103 patients with first degree A-V block, 70 per cent progressed to second degree block and 39 per cent progressed to complete heart block. Similar results were reported by Adgey et al. (1971) and Stock and Macken (1968). The usual sequence of events is a gradual increase in the P-R interval, followed by Wenckebach type second degree A-V block and, in the minority of patients, progression to third degree A-V block. In addition to the usual electrocardiogram finding of inferior myocardial infarction and the gradual progression, heart block in this setting is characterized by a ventricular rate of 50 to 60 per minute and a narrow QRS. The natural history of such block is almost always of gradual improvement following a similar reversed sequence to complete recovery over a period of hours to several days.

Major differences are seen in the setting of anterior wall infarction (Fig. 15–3). In such patients, type II second degree A-V block, bundle branch block, and asystole are the usual manifestations, with complete heart block appearing suddenly in some cases without any premonitory evidence of lesser degrees of block. Stock and Macken

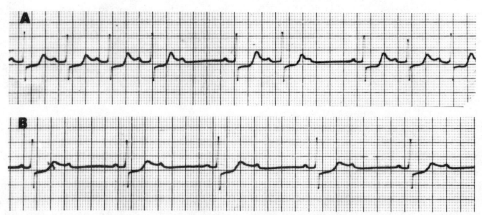

Figure 15–2 (A) Intermittent Mobitz type I (Wenckebach) 3:2 block approximately 48 hours after admission in a patient with an inferior myocardial infarction. (B) Progression to 2:1 A-V block. Patient reverted to normal sinus rhythm over the subsequent 48 hours. Neither hemodynamic deterioration nor tachyarrhythmias appeared and patient returned to normal sinus rhythm without evidence of A-V block over the subsequent 48 hours.

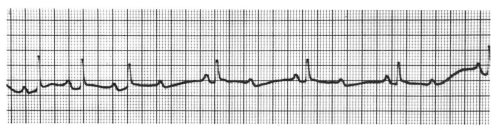

Figure 15–3   Mobitz type II block. Note absence of P-R prolongation prior to appearance of A-V block.

(1968) found that of eight patients who developed complete heart block, five had no warning and three had Mobitz II preceding. No patient exhibited first degree or Wenckebach phenomenon. Norris and Mercer (1974) found that second or third degree A-V block developed in 35 of 658 cases of anterior myocardial infarction (5.3%) and ventricular asystole occurred in 28 of the 35. Escape rhythms, in contrast to those seen with inferior myocardial infarctions, are generally slower, averaging less than 50 beats per minute, and have a wide QRS. These workers found that right bundle branch block almost always preceded complete heart block. Godman et al. (1970) also found that bundle branch block, usually bilateral, preceded the appearance of complete heart block.

SUPRAVENTRICULAR ARRHYTHMIAS

Supraventricular arrhythmias are relatively uncommon. Adgey et al. (1971) found that 4 per cent of patients seen within one hour showed atrial fibrillation or flutter and only 0.4 per cent showed supraventricular tachycardia. After four hours, the incidence of these two arrhythmias was only 5 per cent and 3.5 per cent. Liberthson et al. (1976) found atrial arrhythmias in 109 of 862 patients (12.6%), including atrial fibrillation in 7.8 per cent, atrial flutter in 3.4 per cent, and paroxysmal atrial tachycardia in 3.8 per cent. In 57 patients, atrial tachycardia was preceded by atrial premature contractions. Cristal et al. (1975) reported an even higher fre-

quency, with supraventricular arrhythmias in 44 per cent of 318 patients with acute myocardial infarction, including atrial flutter or fibrillation in 11 per cent, which was associated with supraventricular contractions in 87 per cent.

Lown et al. (1969) have emphasized the frequent association between atrial arrhythmias (including sinus tachycardia) and left ventricular pump failure. Cristal et al. (1975) found that supraventricular arrhythmias were more likely to be associated with a poor prognosis. Atrial flutter or fibrillation followed the onset of pump failure in 65 per cent, and atrial fibrillation was associated with a 41 per cent mortality. They also noted that the site of infarction was important, with anterior infarcts being significantly worse prognostically than those located inferiorly. In contrast, Liberthson et al. (1976) could not find an association between supraventricular arrhythmias and either a worse prognosis or a higher incidence of pump failure. These authors emphasized other etiologies which are associated with atrial tachyarrhythmia (in 23.6% of cases), particularly pericarditis and atrial infarction. It is of interest that no difference in prevalence of atrial arrhythmias was found in either study between anterior and inferior myocardial infarction.

Sinus tachycardia, although not an arrhythmia in the usual sense, deserves special attention. Lown et al. (1969) found that of 300 patients with acute myocardial infarction, mortality was 4.4 per cent in patients with sinus bradycardia and 33.9 per cent in patients with sinus tachycardia. This higher mortali-

TABLE 15–1   VENTRICULAR ARRHYTHMIAS WITHIN ONE HOUR OF ACUTE MYOCARDIAL INFARCTION

	Ventricular Premature Contractions	Ventricular Tachycardia	Ventricular Fibrillation
Adgey (1971)	25%	3.5%	10%
Grace (1970)	10%	2%	4%
Rose (1974)	93.6%	–	36%
Moss (1972)	–	–	6%

ty reflects the association of persistent sinus tachycardia with pump failure. Other factors to be considered include persistent or recurrent chest pain, fever, and pericarditis. In view of its adverse affect on oxygen consumption and resultant potential worsening of the ischemia, active treatment of the underlying cause is important. It should be noted, however, that direct slowing of the sinus rate, such as with beta blockers, is not indicated.

VENTRICULAR ARRHYTHMIA

Pre-Hospital

Several studies (Table 15–1) that have observed patients during the pre-hospital phase of acute myocardial infarction have found a high incidence of ventricular arrhythmias. Adgey et al. noted ventricular fibrillation in 10 per cent of a series of 284 patients within one hour and 19 per cent over the first 48 hours. Ventricular tachycardia was seen in 3.5 per cent of patients within one hour and in 31 per cent within 48 hours. Similar observations have been made by others (Table 15–1, Fig. 15–4).

In-Hospital

Numerous factors affect the detection of arrhythmias once the patient arrives in the coronary care unit: these include the patient population, the type of monitoring (observer or taped for re-review), the time of arrival, the drug therapy, and the clinical status of the patient (Table 15–2). The major thrust and raison d'être of both intensive monitoring of cardiac rhythm and active treatment has been the realization that aggressive treatment of serious ventricular arrhythmias markedly reduces mortality (Fig. 15–5).

WARNING OR PREMONITORY ARRHYTHMIAS

Lown (1969) has been instrumental in developing the concept that prior to the onset of lethal arrhythmias the majority of patients with acute myocardial infarction will manifest warning arrhythmias sufficiently early to permit institution of prophylactic therapy. These arrhythmias include frequent ventricular premature contractions (>5 per minute), bigeminy, couplets, multiform

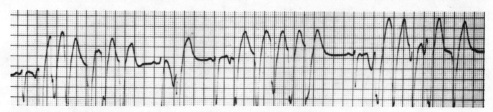

Figure 15–4   Recurrent runs of ventricular tachycardia, unifocal in origin. Atrial activity is clearly delineated and is seen to be unrelated to the ventricular tachycardia.

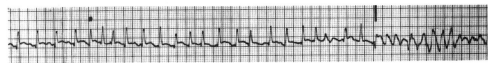

Figure 15–5   Patient 24 hours after acute inferior wall myocardial infarction with a sinus tachycardia at 135 per minute (far left of strip). An APC (*) is followed by a rapid irregular supraventricular tachycardia which is interrupted by a VPC (|) and ventricular fibrillation.

short coupling interval, and R on T phenomenon (i.e., a ventricular premature contraction on the T wave of the preceding beat). However, others have questioned this concept. Lawrie et al. (1968) found that even if the patients had been monitored for sufficient time prior to ventricular fibrillation, five of 15 with primary ventricular fibrillation (defined as the appearance of ventricular fibrillation without evidence of clinical left ventricular failure) had no warning arrhythmias. It is of interest that late ventricular fibrillations (those episodes occurring more than 48 hours after onset of symptoms) were preceded by warning arrhythmias in seven of 10 patients. Dhurandhar et al. (1971) found no warning arrhythmias in two of 20 and in an additional three patients, warning arrhythmias were seen for only seconds prior to fibrillation. Lie et al. (1975) performed continuous taping on 262 consecutive patients without antiarrhythmic therapy within six hours of onset of chest pain. Of 20 patients who developed primary ventricular fibrillation, 12 demonstrated warning arrhythmias while eight had none. Conversely, 59 per cent of the 252 patients demonstrated warning arrhythmias. Thus, although warning arrhythmias may be a useful premonitory feature of ventricular fibrillation in some patients, the majority of patients do not deteriorate to ventricular fibrillation. Moreover, the absence of warning arrhythmias cannot be taken as indicating the absence of risk of ventricular fibrillation in such patients.

It is commonly stated that ventricular premature contraction with a short coupling interval or a ventricular premature contraction occurring during the vulnerable period (R on T phenomenon) is particularly dangerous. It is true that ventricular fibrillation or runs of ventricular tachycardia, in retrospect, can often be demonstrated to have started with a ventricular premature contraction during this phase. Dhurandhar et al. (1971) found that the R on T phenomenon was an invariable finding in primary ventricular fibrillation except where ventricular tachycardia preceded the fibrillation. However, Lie et al. (1975) found that only nine of 20 patients with primary ventricular fibrillation were initiated by early cycle ventricular premature contractions. Conversely, only nine of 27 with R on T ventricular premature contractions deteriorated to ventricular fibrillation. Thus, the presence or absence of such warning arrhythmias provides no absolute guidelines.

ACCELERATED IDIOVENTRICULAR RHYTHM

Recognition of this arrhythmia is important with regard to both prognosis and treatment in the patient with acute myocardial infarction. Although variably defined (see Chapter 11), most authors consider it an accelerated ventricular rhythm at a rate of approximately 70 to 110 beats per minute, usually occurring in the setting of a sinus bradycardia or A-V block. Its incidence in acute myocardial infarction varies widely from 8 to 46 per cent. It is not associated with either an increased incidence of ventricular fibrillation or hospital mortality and usually does not require treatment. If associated with a

TABLE 15–2 IN-HOSPITAL FREQUENCY OF VENTRICULAR ARRHYTHMIAS

	Ventricular Premature Contractions	Ventricular Tachycardia	Ventricular Fibrillation
Julian (1964)	67%	6%	10%
Jewitt (1967)	34%	6.3%	9.4%
Lown (1969)	80%	28%	–
Lie (1975)	–	5%	7.5%

decrease in blood pressure, atropine administration usually increases the sinus rate and is usually all that is required therapeutically. However, many of these patients may also manifest associated rapid (more than 150 beats per minute) ventricular tachycardia. This association between the two arrhythmias has suggested a common electrophysiologic basis (such as ventricular tachycardia with intermittent 2:1 exit block).

It is thus clear that ventricular arrhythmias, including complex forms, are very common in the early phase of myocardial infarction and that as many as 10 per cent of patients will manifest primary ventricular fibrillation during the early hospital course (Table 15–2). It is equally apparent that anywhere from a third to a half of the patients with lethal arrhythmias will *not* manifest warning arrhythmias, while, conversely, the majority of patients with "warning arrhythmias" will not progress to ventricular fibrillation.

CORRELATION BETWEEN SIZE OF INFARCTION, ARRHYTHMIA, AND PROGNOSIS

At present, the major prognostic factor related to patient survival during the acute phase is the status of the left ventricle. Thus, involvement of increasingly large portions of the left ventricle results in progressively more severe left ventricular dysfunction manifesting as left ventricular failure or cardiogenic shock, and if more than 40 per cent of

the left ventricle is involved, death of the patient. Although left ventricular dysfunction is associated with a high incidence of both atrial and ventricular arrhythmias, it is important to note that patient outcome in this setting is determined primarily by the degree of left ventricular dysfunction itself. Lawrie et al. (1968) found that 72 per cent of patients with "secondary" ventricular fibrillation (i.e., secondary to left ventricular failure) died in the hospital. In contrast, in the patient without evidence of left ventricular failure who developed "primary" ventricular fibrillation, only 17 per cent died in hospital. Thus, the immediate short-time prognosis in patients with primary ventricular fibrillation is good, provided treatment is rapid. Such patients may show continued ventricular irritability, but generally these arrhythmias decrease over two to four days and the patient then tends to follow an uncomplicated in-hospital course.

It is of interest that the frequency of ventricular arrhythmias is similar in patients with transmural myocardial infarction characterized by new Q waves and enzyme elevation and nontransmural myocardial infarction characterized by ST and T wave and enzyme abnormalities without Q waves (Scheinman and Abbott, 1973). Thus, the absence of Q waves suggesting a lesser extent of myocardial infarction should *not* be taken as indicating a reduced risk of serious ventricular arrhythmias and such patients require as close observation as patients who develop Q waves.

MANAGEMENT OF PATIENTS WITH ACUTE MYOCARDIAL INFARCTION

Pre-Hospital

Optimal pre-hospital care for the patient who has suffered acute myocardial infarction depends on several strategies. Patients must be educated to recognize and respond to the early symptoms of infarction, since many go unrecognized for the crucial minutes (or hours) of the immediate post-infarction period (Schroeder, 1978). A tentative diagnosis must be made promptly by self-referral to nearby medical facilities so that treatment can be instituted at the first signs of significant arrhythmias or cardiac decompensation.

In addition, large scale education in cardiopulmonary resuscitation has increasingly become recognized as an important adjunct to the total care system of these patients. The Seattle Heart Watch Program has demonstrated the value of this type of approach.

MOBILE CORONARY CARE UNITS

In view of the large number of deaths that occur prior to hospitalization, considerable effort has recently been devoted to developing better medical systems of pre-hospital care. Chief among these is the mobile coronary care unit. A special ambulance equipped and staffed to cope with arrhythmias and to provide immediate on-site therapy was introduced by Pantridge and Geddes (1967) and has now been instituted in several cities in the United States. The ambulance is usually staffed with highly trained paramedics and equipped with a battery-operated electrocardiogram monitor and direct writer, a D.C. defibrillator, antiarrhythmic medications, and a pacemaker. In addition, the ambulance is often in voice and electrocardiogram communication with a central facility or emergency room staffed by a physician who can direct more complicated treatment prior to arrival at the hospital. The patient is monitored with no attempt to transfer him to the ambulance until ventricular irritability has been treated. Of 312 patients encountered over a 15-month period when this mobile unit was in use, no deaths occurred in transit, as compared to a one-year study of coronary deaths at the same hospital in which 102 of 414 patients were dead on arrival.

Problems faced by such mobile units include traffic congestion, false alarms, cancelled calls, and other problems, many of which are peculiar to a metropolitan area. In addition, the initial investment in personnel and equipment required to establish the unit is high, as are operating and upkeep costs. Despite the problems in organization, communication, staffing, and financing posed by the mobile coronary care unit, its usefulness appears beyond question as a life-preserving extension of the hospital intensive care concept. Several centers have shown that 50 to 87 per cent of patients resuscitated outside the hospital eventually leave the hospital alive and many return to productive lives.

In-Hospital

CORONARY CARE UNIT

The coronary care unit is by far the best location for patients with an acute myocardial infarction. Its effectiveness is based on constant observation by a team of physicians and nurses well trained in the diagnosis and treatment of the complications of myocardial infarction. The unit contains electronic equipment for constant monitoring of the electrocardiogram, heart rate and rhythm, and physiological parameters and provides immediate availability of resuscitative equipment, including defibrillator, pacemaker, and respirators. Modern electronic equipment can be

used most effectively in specific diagnoses and treatment to support the patient through the first few critical days.
Complications can be quickly detected
and appropriate therapy immediately
instituted. In addition, a constantly
available, highly trained nursing service is reassuring to the patient and
contributes substantially to his recovery.

The prevention of cardiac arrest requires highly trained nursing personnel, competent in recognizing electrocardiographic patterns and capable of
knowing when significant changes
occur in the clinical state of the patient
and in the electrocardiogram.

Computer assisted arrhythmia detection, although potentially useful, is limited in its ability to differentiate complex and, at times, even simple
arrhythmias. Thus, such systems
should be considered supplementary to
the trained cardiac nurse, who must be
a specialist in the management of myocardial infarction, prepared to institute
life-sustaining measures, including administering intravenous drugs, closed-
chest heart massage, artificial respiration, and defibrillation in the event of
cardiac arrest. In addition, the coronary
care nurse must also handle the emotional responses of patients to their
"heart attack" which may be manifested as hostility, depression, anxiety, and
fear of death.

INTERMEDIATE CORONARY CARE UNIT

The incidence of sudden arrhythmic
death, usually secondary to ventricular
fibrillation, after the first 48 hours
varies from less than 1 per cent to 4
per cent of all acute myocardial infarctions (Laurie et al., 1968; Dhurandhar et
al., 1971; Saunamaki, 1976). In an attempt to prevent such deaths, some
centers have instituted intermediate
or step-down coronary care units
equipped with the usual lifesaving
measures in the event of serious arrhythmias or other complications and

with nurses and personnel trained in
ECG techniques and resuscitation
(Grace and Yarvote, 1970). The use of
telemetric electrocardiographic monitoring of patients transferred from the
coronary care unit to a general care floor
has also been helpful in detecting
serious later-stage arrhythmias.

ANTIARRHYTHMIC THERAPY

The therapy of arrhythmias following
acute myocardial infarction may be
considered in two phases: 1) therapy
prior to the appearance of any arrhythmia and 2) therapy following their
onset in both pre-hospital and in-
hospital phases.

Recognition that a high percentage of
patients have a significant incidence of
serious arrhythmias in the early stage of
acute myocardial infarction (<1 hour)
led Sarnoff and others to propose the
prophylactic use of atropine and/or lidocaine at the onset of pain if a facility
for electrocardiographic monitoring
and treatment is not available. Support
for this concept is provided by Valentine et al., who, in a randomized study
of 269 patients with acute myocardial
infarction, found that 7 per cent of untreated patients compared with 1.9 per
cent of patients treated with intramuscular lidocaine developed ventricular
fibrillation prior to coming under active
care including resuscitative equipment.
However, increasingly rapid response
times and development of mobile coronary care units have, to some extent,
reduced the requirement for this form
of prophylactic treatment.

Once the patient comes under active
monitoring, either in the mobile unit or
in the coronary care unit, several attempts at prophylactic treatment using
quinidine, lidocaine, and procainamide to prevent lethal primary arrhythmias have been utilized. Careful
monitoring during the administration
of these drugs in therapeutic doses has
shown a significant decrease in the

number of premature ventricular contractions as compared to control groups (Kock-Weser, 1969; Mogensen, 1970). Lie et al., 1974, utilized lidocaine intravenously in a consecutive randomized series of 212 patients. Ventricular fibrillation did not occur in patients given lidocaine, while nine control patients did develop ventricular fibrillation. However, eight of nine patients were successfully defibrillated and only one patient, who eventually proved resistant to antiarrhythmic treatment, could not be resuscitated. All other deaths were related to pump failure or cardiac rupture. Lidocaine had significant side effects in 15 per cent of patients. The reason for the similarity in overall survival is clearly that careful monitoring and rapid institution of defibrillation or antiarrhythmic treatment, to a considerable extent, obviates the need for prophylactic therapy. Thus, although prophylactic antiarrhythmic treatment may be of value in the absence of, or prior to, monitoring and availability of definitive treatment, it is probably not necessary in a coronary care unit.

Factors predisposing to the production of arrhythmias should be controlled: chest pain, anxiety, hypotension, hypoxia, and acid-base disturbances must be aggressively treated. Ayres and Grace (1969) have reported hypoxemia and alkalemia in more than 40 per cent of their patients in the coronary care unit. Metabolic acidosis and the combination of hypoxia, alkalemia, and hypokalemia all predispose to arrhythmias that are difficult to terminate until the derangement is corrected. Left heart failure occurs in many patients with acute infarction and may both lead to and be aggravated by arrhythmias.

Supraventricular Arrhythmias

In general, no treatment is necessary for occasional premature contractions.

However, if the beats assume trigeminal or bigeminal form, or if short runs of atrial tachycardia are noted, evidence of left ventricular failure and treatment with digitalis and/or diuretics is the treatment of choice. If this approach proves unsuccessful, quinidine sulfate (200 to 400 mg every 4 to 6 hours, by mouth) or procainamide (500 to 750 mg every 3 to 4 hours, intramuscularly or by mouth) should be added (see Chapter 23).

In atrial fibrillation, digitalis should be administered in sufficient dosage to effectively slow the ventricular rate to 70 to 90 beats per minute. If atrial fibrillation with rapid ventricular response persists for several hours despite therapy, a small dose of propranolol, 0.5 to 1.0 mg intravenously or 10 mg orally, may occasionally be needed to slow the heart rate. Electric countershock should be employed if hemodynamics are clearly compromised secondary to the heart rate.

Digitalis is also indicated in the treatment of atrial flutter to slow the ventricular rate and, hopefully, convert flutter to fibrillation. Frequently, if the flutter persists, control with digitalis may be difficult and small doses of propranolol may prove efficacious in obtaining a controlled ventricular response. If the ventricular rate is unduly rapid, and hemodynamics is adversely affected, electrical conversion is the treatment of choice, followed by specific antiarrhythmic treatment.

Ventricular Arrhythmias

Premature ventricular contractions are the most common arrhythmia observed in patients with acute myocardial infarction (see Tables 15–1 and 15–2). Although it is clear that warning or premonitory arrhythmias frequently do not terminate in ventricular fibrillation (see above), the appearance of frequent ventricular premature contractions, groups or salvos, multifocal or "R on

T," merits promp treatment. Lidocaine administered intravenously (50–100 mg bolus), repeated one to two times if the arrhythmia persists, is the treatment of choice. It is then given in a constant intravenous drip at the rate of 1 to 4 mg per minute. Recurrence or persistence of frequent premature ventricular contractions warrants additional therapy. Intravenous procainamide is then utilized (50 mg per minute) to a total of 1.0 g, or rhythm control with a 1 to 5 mg per minute drip (see below). If this is unsuccessful, diphenylhydantoin, propranolol, and overdrive pacemaker suppression may be required (see Chapter 11). Ventricular ectopic activity usually diminishes or disappears after two to four days, so that oral antiarrhythmics are frequently not required (Kimball and Killip, 1968). If, however, the arrhythmia persists, therapy with an oral agent such as procainamide, quinidine sulfate, or disopyramide phosphate may be required.

Drug therapy for intermittent, nonsustained ventricular tachycardia is essentially the same as the treatment for premature ventricular contractions. On the other hand, sustained ventricular tachycardia is often associated with an immediate and severe compromise of systemic pressure and cardiac output, and prompt termination is necessary. If no response occurs after administering a 50 to 100 mg bolus and then a second 100 mg bolus of lidocaine, immediate electrical conversion is indicated. Ventricular tachycardia associated with circulatory collapse should be treated immediately with electric countershock. Time should not be wasted on manual cardiopulmonary resuscitation, drug administration, or even attempts at synchronizing the electrical discharge with the R wave. Immediately following a successful resuscitation from ventricular tachycardia or fibrillation, a dose of lidocaine should be given and maintenance therapy started with lidocaine in a continuous intravenous drip.

Bradyarrhythmias

Sinus bradycardia requires specific treatment if associated with hypotension or ventricular arrhythmias. If it is well tolerated, no treatment need be instituted. Atropine, the drug of choice, 0.6 mg administered intravenously in two to three doses within a two to three hour period, has beneficial effects in 90 per cent of patients.

If atropine is ineffective, the safest method for treating recurrent bradycardia is by pervenous pacing. Its major disadvantage is that ventricular pacing eliminates the atrial kick, which in the setting of an acute myocardial infarction provides an important supplement to cardiac output (Rahimtoola, 1975).

Atrioventricular Heart Block (see Chapter 12)

In first degree A-V heart block (P-R interval measuring greater than 0.20 second) treatment is not usually required. However, the patients should be carefully monitored for further progression of A-V heart block.

Wenckebach type II block in the patient with an inferior myocardial infarction often requires no specific treatment. Only if progression to third degree block with associated hypotension or arrhythmias occurs is treatment indicated. Small doses of atropine may suffice; however, if this fails, pacing is indicated.

Mobitz II A-V block or bilateral bundle branch block with anterior myocardial infarction is an absolute indication for transvenous pacing (see Chapter 12).

Patients who have a pre-existent bundle branch block may be monitored without need for a standby pacemaker. In general, appearance of new RBBB with or without LAHB or LBBB (i.e., bilateral BBB; see Chapter 24) in the setting of an anterior wall myocardial infarction is an absolute indication for standby ventricular pacer. However, left axis deviation per se, even in anterior myocardial infarction, is not considered an indication for pacemaker insertion.

REFERENCES

Abbott, S.A., and Scheinman, M.M.: Nondiagnostic electrocardiogram in patients with acute myocardial infarction. Clinical and anatomic correlations. Am. J. Med. 55:608, 1973.

Adgey, A.A.J., Geddes, J.S., Webb, S.W., Allen, J.D., James, R.G.G., Zaidi, S.A., and Pantridge, J.F.: Acute phase of myocardial infarction. Lancet 2:501, 1971.

Arbeit, S.R., Rubin, I.L., and Gross, H.: Dangers in interpreting the eletrocardiogram from the oscilloscope monitor. J.A.M.A. 211:453, 1970.

Atkins, J.M., Leskin, S.J., Blomquist, G., and Mullins, C.B.: Ventricular conduction blocks and sudden death in acute myocardial infarction. Potential indications for pacing. N. Engl. J. Med. 288:281, 1973.

Ayres, S.M., and Grace, W.J.: Inappropriate ventilation and hypoxemia as causes of cardiac arrhythmias. Amer. J. Med. 46:495, 1969.

Barber, J.M., et al.: Mobile coronary care. Lancet 2:133, 1970.

Battle, W.E., Naimi, S., Avitall, B., Brilla, A.H., Banas, J.S., Bete, J.M., and Levine, H.J.: Distinctive time course of ventricular vulnerability to fibrillation during and after release of coronary ligation. Am. J. Cardiol. 34:42, 1974.

Bellet, S., DeGuzman, N., Kostis, J., Roman, L., and Fleischmann, D.: Effect of cigarette smoke inhalation on ventricular fibrillation threshold in normal dogs and dogs with acute myocardial infarction. Amer. Heart J. 83:67, 1972.

Bigger, J.T., Dresdale, R.J., Heissenbuttel, R.H., Weld, F.M., and Wit, A.L.: Ventricular arrhythmias in ischemic heart disease: Mechanism, prevalence, significance and management. Prog. C-V Dis. 19:255, 1977.

Bloomfield, S.S., Romhilt, D.W., Chou, T.-C., and Fowler, N.O.: Quinidine for prophylaxis of arrhythmias in acute myocardial infarction. N. Engl. J. Med. 285:979, 1971.

Chadda, K.D., Banka, V.S., and Helfant, R.H.: Rate dependent ventricular ectopia following acute coronary occlusion. The concept of an optimal antiarrhythmic heart rate. Circulation 49:654, 1974.

Chadda, K.D., Lichstein, E., Gupta, P.K., Choy, R.: Bradycardia–Hypotension syndrome in acute myocardial infarction. Am. J. Med. 59:158, 1975.

Chapman, J.M., and Massey, F.J.: The interrelationship of serum cholesterol, hypertension, body weight, and risk of coronary disease. Results of the first ten years' follow-up in the Los Angeles heart study. J. Chronic Dis. 17:933, 1964.

Chiang, B.N., et al.: Predisposing factors in sudden cardiac death in Tecumseh, Michigan. A prospective study. Circulation 41:31, 1969a.

Chiang, B.N., Perlman, L.V., Ostrander, L.D., and Epstein, R.H.: Relationship of premature systoles to coronary heart disease and sudden death in the Tecumseh epidemiological study. Ann. Intern. Med. 70:1109, 1969b.

Cobb, L.A., and Werner, J.A.: Antiarrhythmic therapy, ventricular premature depolarizations and sudden cardiac death: The tip of the iceberg. Circulation 59:864, 1979.

Cobb, L.A., Baum, R.S., Alvarez, H., and Schaffer, W.A.: Resuscitation from out-of-hospital ventricular fibrillation: 4 years follow-up. Circulation 52(6 suppl 3):223, 1975.

Coronary Drug Project: Clofibrate and niacin in coronary heart disease. J.A.M.A. 231:360, 1975.

Crampton, R.S., Aldrich, R.F., Gascho, J.A., Miles, J.R., and Stillerman, R.: Reduction of prehospital, ambulance and community coronary death rates by the community-wide emergency cardiac care system. Am. J. Med. 58:151, 1975.

Cranefield, P.F.: The conduction of the cardiac impulse. Mount Kisco, N.Y. Futura 1975.

Cristal, N., Szwarcberg, J., and Gueron, M.: Supraventricular arrhythmias in acute myocardial infarction. Prognostic importance of clinical setting: Mechanism of production. Ann. Intern. Med. 82:35, 1975.

Day, H.W.: Effectiveness of an intensive coronary care area. Amer. J. Cardiol. 15:51, 1965.

Dhurandhar, R.W., Macmillan, R.L., and Brown, K.W.G.: Primary ventricular fibrillation complicating acute myocardial infarction. Am. J. Cardiol. 27:347, 1971.

Durrer, D., VanLier, A.A.W., and Buller, J.: Epicardial and intramural excitation in chronic myocardial infarction. Am. Heart J. 68:765, 1964.

Elharrar, V., and Zipes, D.P.: Cardiac electrophysiologic alterations during myocardial ischemia. Am. J. Physiol. 233:H329–H345, 1977.

El-Sherif, N., Lazzara, R., Hope, R.R., and Scherlag, B.J.: Reentrant ventricular arrhythmias in the late myocardial infarction period. I. The conduction characteristics in the infarction zone. Circulation 55:656, 1977.

Epstein, S.E., Goldstein, R.E., Redwood, D.R., Kent, K.M., and Smith, E.R.: The early phase of acute myocardial infarction: Pharmacologic aspects of therapy. Ann. Intern. Med. 78:918, 1973.

Frink, R.J., and James, T.N.: Normal blood supply to the human His bundle and proximal bundle branches. Circulation 47:8, 1973.

Gertler, M.M., White, P.D., Cady, L.D., and Whiter, H.H.: Coronary heart disease—a prospective study. Amer. J. Med. Sci. 248:377, 1964.

Godman, M.J., Lassers, B.W., and Julian, D.G.: Complete bundle branch block complicating acute myocardial infarction. N. Engl. J. Med. 282:237, 1970.

Grace, W.J., and Chadbourn, J.A.: The first hour in acute myocardial infarction. Observations in 50 patients. Circulation 41/42 III-160, 1970.

Grace, W.J., and Chadbourn, J.A.: The mobile coronary care unit. Dis. Chest. 65:452, 1969.

Gunnar, R.M., et al.: Myocardial infarction with shock. Hemodynamic studies and results of therapy. Circulation 33:753, 1966.

Han, J.: Mechanisms of ventricular arrhythmias associated with myocardial infarction. Amer. J. Cardiol. 24:800, 1969.

Han, J., Millet, D., Chizzonitti, B., and Moe, G.K.: Temporal dispersion of recovery of excitability in atrium and ventricle as a function of heart rate. Amer. Heart. J. 71:481, 1966.

Han, J., and Moe, G.K.: Nonuniform recovery of excitability in ventricular muscle. Circ. Res. 14:44–60, 1964.

Harris, A.S.: Potassium and experimental coronary occlusion. Am. Heart. J. 71:797, 1966.

Harris, A.S., and Rojas, A.G.: The initiation of ventricular fibrillation due to coronary occlusion. Expt. Med. Surg. 1:105, 1943.

Jewitt, D.E., Raftery, E.B., Balcon, R., and Ovam, S.: Incidence and management of supraventricular arrhythmias after acute myocardial infarction. Lancet 2:734, 1967.

Killip, T., and Kimball, J.T.: A survey of the coronary care unit: concept and results. Prog. Cardiovasc. Dis. 11:45, 1968.

Kimball, J.T., and Killip, T.: Aggressive treatment of arrhythmias in acute myocardial infarction: Procedures and results. Prog. Cardiovasc. Dis. 10:483, 1968.

Koch-Weser, J.: Antiarrhythmic prophylaxis in acute myocardial infarction. N. Engl. J. Med. 285:1024, 1971.

Koch-Weser, J., Klein, S.W., Foo-Canto, L.L., et al.: Antiarrhythmic prophylaxis with procainamide in acute myocardial infarction. N. Engl. J. Med. 281:1253, 1969.

Kurien, V.A., and Oliver, M.F.: A cause for arrhythmias during acute myocardial hypoxia. Lancet 1:813, 1970.

Lassers, B.W., et al.: Hemodynamic effects of artificial pacing in complete heart block complicating acute myocardial infarction. Circulation 38:308, 1968.

Lawrie, D.M., Higgins, M.R., Godman, M.J., Oliver, M.F., Julian, P.G., and Donald, K.W.: Ventricular fibrillation complicating acute myocardial infarction. Lancet 2:523, 1968.

Levine, J.H.: Pre-hospital management of acute myocardial infarction. Amer. J. Cardiol. 24:826, 1969.

Levites, R., Banka, V.S., and Helfant, R.H.: Electrophysiologic effects of coronary occlusion and reperfusion: Observations of dispersion of refractoriness and ventricular automaticity. Circulation 52:760–765, 1975.

Liberthson, R.R., Salisbury, K.W., Hutter, A.M., and DeSanctis, R.W.: Atrial tachyarrhythmias in acute myocardial infarction. Am. J. Med. 60:956, 1976.

Lichstein, E., Ribas-Meneclier, C., Gupta, P.K., and Chadda, K.D.: Incidence and description of accelerated ventricular rhythm complicating acute myocardial infarction. Am. J. Med. 58:192, 1975.

Lie, K.I., Wellens, H.J.J. Downar, E., Durrer, D.: Observations on patients with primary ventricular fibrillation complicating acute myocardial infarction. Circulation 52:755, 1975.

Lie, K.I., Wellens, H.J.J., VanCapelle, F.J., and Durrer, D.: Lidocaine in the prevention of primary ventricular fibrillation. N. Engl. J. Med. 291:1324, 1974.

Lown, B.: Approaches to sudden death from coronary heart disease. (Lewis A. Conner Memorial Lecture, Amer. Heart Assoc. 43rd Scientific Sessions, presented Nov. 12, 1970). Circulation 41–42:III-37, 1970.

Lown, B., Klein, M.D., and Hershberg, P.J.: Coronary and precoronary care. Am. J. Med. 46:705, 1969.

Lutnegger, F., Giger, G., Fuhr, P., Raeder, E.A., Burkart, F., Schmitt, H., Gradel, E., and Burkhart, D.: Evaluation of aortocoronary bypass grafting for prevention of cardiac arrhythmias. Am. Heart J. 98:15, 1979.

Massumi, R.A., Mason, D.T., Amsterdam, E.A., Demaria, A., Miller, R.R., Scheinman, M.M., and Zelis, R.: Ventricular fibrillation and tachycardia after intravenous atropine for treatment of bradycardias. N. Engl. J. Med. 287:336, 1972.

Mogensen, L.: Ventricular tachyarrhythmias and lignocaine prophylaxis in acute myocardial infarction: A clinical and therapeutic study. Acta Med. Scand. (Suppl) 513:1, 1970.

Moss, A.J., Davis, H.T., DeCammilla, and Bayer, L.W.: Ventricular ectopic beats and their relation to sudden and non-sudden cardiac death after myocardial infarction. Circulation 60:998, 1978.

Moss, A.J., Goldstein, S., Greene, W., DeCamilla, J.: Prehospital precursors of ventricular arrhythmias in acute myocardial infarction. Arch. Intern. Med. 129:756, 1972.

Myerburg, R.J., Conde, C., Sheps, D.S., Ceppel, R.A., Kiem, I., Sung, R.J., and Castellanos, A.: Antiarrhythmic drug therapy in survivors of pre-hospital cardiac arrest. Circulation 59:855, 1979.

Norris, R.M.: Heart block in posterior and anterior myocardial infarction. Ann. N.Y. Acad. Sci. 167:911, 1969.

Norris, R.M., and Mercer, C.J.: Significance of idioventricular rhythms in acute myocardial infarction. Prog. C-V Dis. 16:455, 1974.

Pantridge, J.F., and Adgey, A.A.J.: Pre-hospital coronary care: Mobile coronary care unit. Amer. J. Cardiol. 24:666, 1969.

Pantridge, J.F., Adgey, A.A.J., Geddes, J.S., and

Webb, S.W.: The Acute Coronary Attack. New York, Grune and Stratton, 1975.

Pantridge, J.F., and Geddes, J.S.: A mobile intensive care unit in the management of myocardial infarction. Lancet 2:271, 1967.

Rahimtoola, S.H., Ehsani, A., Sinno, M.Z., Loeb, H.S., Rosen, K.M., and Gunnar, R.M.: Left atrial transport function in myocardial infarction. Importance of its booster pump function. Am. J. Med. 59:686, 1975.

Rose, R.M., Lewis, A.J., Fenkes, J., Clifton, J.F., and Criley, J.M.: Circulation 49/50 III-121, 1974.

Rothfield, E.L., Zucker, R.I., Parsonnet, V., and Alinsonorin, C.A.: Idioventricular rhythm in acute myocardial infarction. Circulation 37:203, 1968.

Rutenberg, H.L., Pamintuan, J.C., and Soloff, L.A.: Serum free fatty acids and their relation to complications after acute myocardial infarction. Lancet 2:559, 1969.

Saunamaki, K.I., and Pedersen, A.: Significance of cardiac arrhythmias preceding first cardiac arrest in patients with acute myocardial infarction. Acta Med. Scand. 199:461, 1976.

Scheinman, M.M., and Abbott, J.A.: Clinical significance of transmural versus nontransmural electrocardiographic changes in patients with acute myocardial infarction. Am. J. Med. 55:602, 1973.

Scherlag, B.J., El-Sherif, N., Hope, R., and Lazzara, R.: Characterization and localization of ventricular arrhythmias resulting from myocardial ischemia and infarction. Circ. Res. 35:372, 1974.

Scherlag, B.J., Helfant, R.H., Haft, J.I., and Damato, A.N.: Electrophysiology underlying ventricular arrhythmias due to coronary ligation. Am. J. Physiol. 219:1665, 1970.

Schroeder, J.S., Lamb, I.H., and Hu, M.: The prehospital course of patients with chest pain. Analysis of the prodromal symptomatic, decision making, transportation and emergency room periods. Am. J. Med. 64:742, 1978.

Schulze, R.A., Rouleau, J., Rigo, P., Bowers, S., Strauss, H.W., and Pitt, B.: Ventricular arrhythmias with late hospital phase of acute myocardial infarction. Circulation 52:1006, 1975.

Stock, R.J., and Macken, D.L.: Observations on heart block during continuous electrocardiographic monitoring in myocardial infarction. Circulation 38:993, 1968.

Sutton, R., and Davies, M.: The conduction system in acute myocardial infarction complicated by heart block. Circulation 38:987, 1968.

Wallace, A.G., and Klein, R.F.: Role of catecholamines in acute myocardial infarction. Amer. J. Med. Sci. 258:139, 1969.

Waugh, R.A., Wagner, G.S., Haney, T.L., Rosati, R.A., and Morris, J.J.: Immediate and remote prognostic significance of fascicular block during acute myocardial infarction. Circulation 47:765, 1973.

Webb, S.W., Adgey, A.A.J., and Pantridge, J.F.: Autonomic disturbance at onset of acute myocardial infarction. Br. Med. J. 3:89, 1972.

Williams, D.O., Scherlag, B.J., Hope, R.R., El-Sherif, N., and Lazzara, R.: The pathophysiology of malignant ventricular arrhythmias during acute myocardial ischemia. Circulation 50:1163, 1974.

Sudden Death

Sudden death has been defined as death due to natural causes occurring within 24 hours of the beginning of the fatal event in an apparently previously well patient. Despite the latitude of the definition, it should be emphasized that most sudden fatalities due to coronary artery disease occur within minutes or hours of the onset of the terminal infarction or arrhythmia. The cause of sudden death in most instances is thought to be the abrupt onset of ventricular fibrillation or asystole. It is likely that many of these events could be reversed through the immediate application of appropriate therapeutic measures. However, it is difficult to identify susceptible patients, and easily applied preventive or therapeutic measures are not available.

ETIOLOGY

In a large necropsy study from Westchester County, New York, Spain et al. (1960) reported that of fatalities occurring within 1 hour of onset of symptoms, 91 per cent in men and 48 per cent in women were due to coronary heart disease. Other cardiovascular diseases (valvular, aortic aneurysm) accounted for 5.2 per cent, and cerebrovascular diseases accounted for 1.2 per cent. It is of interest that Moritz and Zamcheck (1946) found that approximately one half of sudden deaths in soldiers between 18 and 40 years of age were due to heart disease and that about 85 per cent of the victims had atherosclerosis. Reichenbach et al. (1977) compared pathologic findings in 87 patients who died suddenly to an age-matched group of 55 patients who died of traumatic causes and found a dramatically higher incidence of atherosclerotic heart disease in the group in which sudden death was due to natural causes. The same authors also found that only 5 per cent of patients who died suddenly had necropsy evidence of acute myocardial infarction. Others have reported frequencies of 0 to 33 per cent. These data are limited, however, by lack of conclusive pathologic evidence of acute myocardial infarction in the first 12 hours.

Recent studies in Seattle and Miami have shown that 16 to 31 per cent of patients resuscitated from ventricular fibrillation have evidence of acute transmural myocardial infarction associated with the acute event, and an additional third have ischemic ST and T changes (Cobb et al., 1975; Liberthson et al., 1974). Thus, a significant number of victims of sudden death do not manifest evidence of transmural myocardial infarction. The immediate cause of the ventricular fibrillation in such patients is unclear. Suggested mechanisms include transient ischemia due to platelet plugs or coronary spasm, with the resultant electrophysiologic changes predisposing to arrhythmia or neurogenic mechanisms (see Chapter 21). It is clear, however, that the vast majority of sudden deaths result from coronary heart disease, the terminal event being ventricular fibrillation. In an epidemiologic study in Tecumseh, Michigan, of those who died suddenly from coronary heart disease, 50 per cent had a history of clinical heart disease, 27.8 per cent had a history of hypertension, and 11.4 per cent had a history of diabetes (Chiang et al., 1969).

RISK FACTORS

As would be expected from the close relationship between coronary heart disease and sudden death, many of the risk factors that predispose to coronary heart disease also predispose to sudden death. These include age, sex, family history, elevated serum cholesterol, diabetes mellitus, hypertension, cigarette smoking, and abnormalities of the ECG, including ST segment depression and conduction abnormalities. Other factors that are suspected include lack of physical exercise and hyperactive or Type A personality. Despite these statistical relationships, however, only a small percentage of patients with one or more of these factors die suddenly. In the Tecumseh study, only 8 of 85 with diabetes mellitus and 6 of 67 with hypertensive cardiovascular disease died suddenly (Chiang, 1970). Moreover, 51 per cent of persons dying suddenly had two or more risk factors; however, 27 per cent of the population also had two or more. The Framingham study (Kannel et al., 1975) painted an even more dismal picture by pointing out that identification of even one third of potential sudden deaths would require identifying 10 per cent of the general population. Thus, accurate identification of the *individual* prone to sudden death presents major difficulties.

Recognition that most immediate causes of sudden death result from ventricular fibrillation has led to increasing emphasis on the significance of ventricular premature complexes and other ventricular arrhythmias as an index of underlying electrical instability in the patient with coronary heart disease. Approaches to detect the presence and severity of ventricular premature complexes have included stress testing and long-term monitoring (see Chapter 14). Such studies have focused on ventricular premature complexes in patients with known coronary heart disease or in older age groups where the likelihood of coronary heart disease is substantially increased. Thus, these data *cannot* be extrapolated to the patient *without* coronary heart disease.

Chiang et al. (1969) found that 10 of 45 persons who died suddenly had antecedent ventricular premature complexes on previous electrocardiograms. Conversely, of 165 with ventricular premature complexes, 10 died suddenly, a significantly higher per cent than in people without ventricular premature complexes. (It should be noted that of the 10 people who died suddenly, five had manifestations of coronary heart disease independent of ventricular premature complexes). Hinkle et al. similarly found an association between ventricular premature complexes and sudden death. This study also indicated, however, that such ventricular premature complexes are usually associated with other evidence of coronary heart disease, such as angina or old myocardial infarction. Thus, the significance of ventricular premature complexes without evidence of coronary heart disease remains questionable. Indeed, Kannel (1975), using prognostic data obtained in Framingham and Albany, concluded that ventricular premature complexes were not significant prognostic findings in persons without clinically manifested heart disease.

Considerable attention has been directed to the character and grade of ventricular premature complexes. As noted above, Lown proposed that more severe grades of arrhythmia were associated with a higher risk of ventricular fibrillation in acute myocardial infarction. A similar concept has been proposed for the patient with chronic coronary heart disease.

Data from the Coronary Drug Project (1973) showed that although frequent ventricular premature complexes are associated with sudden death, ventricular premature complexes in pairs, multiform, or bigeminy did not carry a higher risk and only suggested that prematurity of the ventricular premature complex might be of significance. Kotler et al. (1973) followed 160 patients for a period ranging from 30 to 54

months and found 14 sudden deaths. Holter recordings revealed no or infrequent ventricular premature complexes in two of the patients, frequent unifocal ventricular premature complexes in five, and multiform ventricular premature complexes in another five. Conversely, no sudden deaths occurred in 30 patient with paired or coupled ventricular ectopics or in 27 patients with parasystolic rhythm. Others, however, have found a relationship between more frequent and complex ventricular arrhythmias and cardiac mortality late after acute myocardial infarction (Moss et al., 1977). However, Moss et al. (1978) recently compared 66 patients with documented ventricular tachycardia prior to discharge after myocardial infarction to patients without ventricular tachycardia and found no significant difference in overall mortality or sudden death after 48 months follow-up. It is of interest that functional classification indicating left ventricular failure was much more predictive of mortality in chronic coronary heart disease.

The relationship between the extent of myocardial infarction, left ventricular dysfunction, and ventricular arrhythmia has also received increasing attention. Scheinman and Abbott (1973) found that the incidence of ventricular arrhythmias in the acute phase was similar in patients with transmural and nontransmural (no new Q waves) myocardial infarction.

In contrast, major differences in prognosis appear after discharge. Lopes et al. (1974) followed 169 patients with acute ST and T changes without enzyme elevations or Q waves for an average of 17.9 months. Twenty-three (13.6%) cardiac deaths, including 10 sudden deaths, occurred. Cannon et al. compared 148 patients with transmural myocardial infarction to 40 patients with nontransmural infarcts. In-hospital mortality was 16.8 per cent compared to 7.5 per cent. After discharge, however, 15.1 per cent of patients with transmural myocardial infarction died suddenly compared to 33.3 per cent who died suddenly after nontransmural myocardial infarction.

Clearly, patients with an increased number of obstructed coronary arteries and more severe left ventricular dysfunction have a worse prognosis. Calvert et al. (1977) examined the characteristics of ventricular premature complexes in 84 patients with coronary heart disease of varying severity. Overall, they found that 86 per cent of patients with coronary heart disease had ventricular premature complexes, while 67 per cent of normal patients had them. However, more complex arrhythmias were seen in 75 per cent of patients with coronary disease but in only 25 per cent of normals. In addition, 81 per cent of patients with obstructions of two or three coronary vessels had frequent or complex ventricular premature complexes but only 52 per cent of patients with single vessel coronary obstructive disease had them. In addition, more marked left ventricular dysfunction was also found to be closely related to more severe ventricular arrhythmias. Schulze et al. (1977) found that patients with more complex arrhythmias had more severe coronary heart disease, characterized by a greater number of obstructed vessels, a higher incidence of prior infarction, and more extensive left ventricular dysfunction. Thus, it seems apparent that ventricular premature complexes are associated with a higher incidence of sudden death in patients with coronary heart disease. It is equally apparent that the risk of sudden death is intimately tied to the presence and severity of coronary heart disease. This carries serious implications for treatment, since it implies that a secondary approach directed solely at the arrhythmia will lead to only limited success. To date no studies are available that have systematically evaluated the effect of antiarrhythmic treatment in patients with coronary artery disease and ventricular premature complexes.

Another concern in patients with coronary heart disease is the significance of fascicular block in relationship to sudden death. Waugh et al. (1973) followed 386 survivors of acute myocardial infarction for 1 year and found that a significant percentage of patients with fascicular block, particularly if associated with AV block, died suddenly. Atkins et al. (1973) reported similar data. These data suggest that prophylactic ventricular pacemaker therapy may be of value in these patients. However, although it has been presumed that heart block is the mechanism of death, it is also conceivable that ventricular fibrillation is responsible. Further delineation of the role of pacing will require a prospective randomized trial.

TREATMENT

Therapeutic approaches to sudden death are limited by several major problems. Although statistical delineation of a population at higher risk is now possible, as indicated above, identification of the specific patient who is prone to sudden death is limited. Moreover, even if accurate identification were possible, the appropriate medical or surgical approach is unclear.

In view of this, a major effort in dealing with sudden death has been directed toward more rapid out-patient management. This has involved a multifaceted approach, one facet of which is community-wide education concerning the problem, including teaching the techniques of cardiopulmonary resuscitation (CPR). As a result there has been marked improvement in the rapidity of initiation of cardiopulmonary resuscitation to potential victims of sudden death. This, in turn, has resulted in improved survival of these individuals. In addition to a community-wide education program, a critical supplemental element has been the deployment of rapid response vehicles such as ambulances or fire rescue or police vehicles, which include paramedical and/or medical personnel with resuscitative equipment and the capability of communicating directly with a remote facility such as a hospital emergency room for direction in the administration of specific cardiac drugs. Use of this approach, as developed in Belfast for more rapid treatment of acute myocardial infarction, is becoming increasingly more common. However, there are limitations involved in the use of these vehicles, such as difficulties in attaining response times of less than 5 minutes in heavily congested areas and appropriate deployment of units in more widespread and less heavily populated communities. It is clear, however, based on reported experiences in Miami and Seattle, that such an approach is workable and will result in successful resuscitation in a significant percentage of sudden death victims. Most important, in many cases these patients leave the hospital to live normal lives.

Difficulties with long term prophylactic therapy to prevent or reduce the risk of sudden death are highlighted by survivors of pre-hospital cardiopulmonary resuscitation. Such patients clearly manifest a high risk for sudden death in the months immediately following the initial resuscitation; indeed, patients who have undergone several successful resuscitations from sudden death have been reported (Schaffer and Cobb, 1975). Yet, various pharmacologic approaches attempted on an individual basis have met with limited success.

Appropriate treatment of frequent or complex ventricular arrhythmias in patients with coronary heart disease, who are thus considered at high risk for sudden death, is also unclear. The most common approach is to initiate antiarrhythmic therapy in these patients. To date, two studies have been reported which show a reduction in the incidence of sudden death with the use of new beta blockers, practolol and alprenolol. However, practolol has since been precluded from clinical use because of its significant side effects. The future role of alprenolol is unclear at this time. Use of procainamide, quin-idine, disopyramide, and other soon-to-be-released antiarrhythmics is limited by the lack of data indicating their role in preventing sudden death. Moreover, significant side effects may limit their usefulness. Other pharmacologic approaches, including aspirin and sulfinpyrazone, are currently under investigation.

The advent of coronary artery bypass grafting has raised the hope that this procedure might reduce the incidence of sudden death. Unfortunately, data to this time have not shown significant reduction in the incidence of ventricular premature complexes, severity of ventricular arrhythmias, or sudden death. Soyza et al. (1978) found a similar frequency and severity of ventricular premature complexes and sudden death in patients treated medically or surgically. In another report, Sami et al. (1978) found that aneurysmectomy for prevention of recurrent ventricular tachycardia or fibrillation failed to eliminate these arrhythmias; of 10 patients, two died suddenly within 1 1/2 and 7 months, while the 8 survivors continued to show runs of ventricular tachycardia or multifocal ventricular premature complexes. Thus, aortocoronary bypass surgery and/or aneurysmectomy appear at this time to have limited effectiveness as a preventive approach to sudden death.

Other approaches have included the use of an implantable defibrillator that would both automatically sense the onset of ventricular fibrillation and defibrillate the patient. Technical problems appear to limit its application. Another approach currently under investigation is transtelephonic resuscitation. This would depend on community-wide training in cardiopulmonary resuscitation and availability to the individual considered at risk of a briefcase containing a defibrillator and an acoustic coupler which would permit a physician remote from the scene to diagnose and treat (and defibrillate) the patient over the telephone.

REFERENCES

Atkins, J. M., Leshin, S. J., Blomquist, G., and Mullins, C. B.: Ventricular conduction blocks and sudden death in acute myocardial infarction. Potential indications for pacing. N. Engl. J. Med. 288:281, 1973.

Calvert, A., Lown, B., and Gorlin, R.: Ventricular premature beats and anatomically defined coronary heart disease. Am. J. Cardiol. 39:627, 1977.

Cannon, D. S., Levy, W., and Cohen, L. S.: The short- and long-term prognosis of patients with transmural and nontransmural myocardial infarction. Am. J. Med. 61:452, 1976.

Chiang, B. N., Perlman, L. V., and Fulton, et al.: Predisposing factors in sudden cardiac death in Tecumseh, Michigan. A prospective study. Circulation 41:31, 1970.

Chiang, B. N., Perlman, L. V., Ostrander, L. D., and Epstein, F. H.: Relationship of premature systoles to coronary heart disease and sudden death in the Tecumseh epidemiological study. Ann. Intern. Med. 70:1109, 1969.

Cobb, L. A., Baum, R. S., Alvarez, H., and Schaffer, W. A.: Resuscitation from out-of-hospital ventricular fibrillation: 4 year follow-up. Circulation 51/52:III-223, 1975.

Coronary Drug Project Research Group: Prognostic importance of premature beats following myocardial infarction. J.A.M.A. 223:1116, 1973.

Engel, G. L.: Psychologic stress, vasodepressor (vasovagal) syncope, and sudden death. Ann. Intern. Med. 89:403, 1978.

Hagstrom, R. M., Federspiel, C. F., and Ho, V. C.: Incidence of myocardial infarction and sudden death from coronary heart disease in Nashville, Tennessee. Circulation 44:884, 1971.

Kannel, W. B., Doyle, J. T., McNamara, P. M., Quickenton, P., and Gordon, T.: Precursors of sudden coronary death. Factors related to the incidence of sudden death. Circulation 51:606, 1975.

Kotler, M. N., Tabatznik, B., Mower, M. M., and Tominaga, S.: Prognostic significance of ventricular ectopic beats with respect to sudden death in the late post infarction period. Circulation 47:959, 1973.

Liberthson, R. R., Nagel, E. L., Hirschman, J. C., and Nussenfeld, S. R.: Prehospital ventricular fibrillation. N. Engl. J. Med. 291:317, 1974.

Lown, B., Graboys, T. B., Podrid, P. J., Cohen, B. J., Stockman, M. B., and Gaughan, C. E.: Effect of a digitalis drug on ventricular premature beats. N. Engl. J. Med. 296:301, 1977.

Lopes, M. G., Spivack, A. P., Harrison, D. C., and Schroeder, J. S.: Prognosis on coronary care unit noninfarction cases. J.A.M.A. 228:1558, 1974.

Mirowski, M., Mower, M. M., Staewen, W. S., Tabatznik, B., and Mendeloff, A. I.: Standby automatic defibrillation: An approach to prevention of sudden coronary death. Arch. Intern. Med. 126:158, 1970.

Moritz, A. R., and Zamcheck, N.: Sudden and unexpected deaths of young soldiers. Arch. Path. 42:459, 1946.

Moss, A. J., DeCamilla, J. J., Davis, H. P., and Bayer, L.: Clinical significance of ventricular ectopic beats in the early posthospital phase of acute myocardial infarction. Am. J. Cardiol. 29:635, 1977.

Multicentre International Study. Improvement in prognosis of myocardial infarction by long-term beta-adrenoceptor blockade using practolol. Brit. Med. J. 3:735–740, 1975.

Reichenbach, D. D., Moss, N. S., and Meyer, E.: Pathology of the heart in sudden death. Am. J. Cardiol. 39:865, 1977.

Ricks, W. B., Winkle, R. A., Shumway, N. E., and Harrison, D. C.: Surgical management of life-threatening ventricular arrhythmias in patients with coronary artery disease. Circulation 56:38, 1977.

Ruberman, W., Weinblatt, E., Goldberg, J. D., Frank, C. W., and Shapiro, S.: Ventricular premature beats and mortality after myocardial infarction. N. Engl. J. Med. 297:750, 1977.

Sami, M., Chaitman, B. R., Bourassa, M. G., Charpin, D., and Chabot, M.: Long term follow-up of aneurysmectomy for recurrent ventricular tachycardia or fibrillation. Am. Heart J. 96:303, 1978.

Schaffer, W. A., and Cobb, L. A.: Recurrent ventricular fibrillation and modes of death in survivors of out-of-hospital ventricular fibrillation. N. Engl. J. Med. 293:259, 1975.

Scheinman, M. M., and Abbott, J. A.: Clinical significance of transmural vs nontransmural electrocardiographic changes in patients with acute myocardial infarction. Am. J. Med. 55:602, 1973.

Schulze, R. A., Humphries, J. O., Griffith, L. S. C., Ducci, H., Achuff, S., and Baird, M. G.: Relationship to ventricular irritability in the late hospital phase of acute myocardial infarction. Circulation 55:839, 1977.

Sharma, S. D., Ballantyne, F., and Goldstein, S.: The relationship of ventricular asynergy in coronary artery disease to ventricular premature beats. Chest 66:358, 1974.

Soyza, N. de, Murphy, M. L., Bissett, J. K., Kane, J. J., and Doherty, J. E.: Ventricular arrhythmia in chronic stable angina pectoris with surgical or medical treatment. Ann. Intern. Med. 89:10, 1978.

Spain, D. M., Bradess, V. A., and Mohr, C.: Coronary atherosclerosis as a cause of unexpected and unexplained death. J.A.M.A. 174:384, 1960.

Waugh, R. A., Wagner, G. S., Haney, T. L., Rosati, R. A., and Morris, J. J.: Immediate and remote prognostic significance of fascicular block during acute myocardial infarction. Circulation 47:765, 1973.

Wilhelmsson, C., Vedin, J. A., Wilhemsen, L., Tibblin, G., and Werko, L.: Reduction of sudden deaths after myocardial infarction by treatment with alprenolol. Lancet 2:7890, 1974.

16

VALVULAR, MYOCARDIAL, AND PERICARDIAL DISEASE

MONTY M. BODENHEIMER, M.D.
RICHARD H. HELFANT, M.D.

Certain arrhythmias have been found to be commonly associated with valvular, myocardial, and pericardial disease. This chapter will deal with these arrhythmias and their significance in the setting of the specific disease state. Although specific antiarrhythmic therapy is often necessary, treatment should be directed primarily toward the underlying cardiac disorder.

RHEUMATIC MITRAL VALVE DISEASE

Mitral stenosis or combined mitral stenosis and insufficiency is usually caused by rheumatic carditis. These valvular lesions result in increased left atrial pressure and left atrial enlargement with fibrosis of the left atrial myocardium. The combination of left atrial dilatation and fibrosis is apparently responsible for the fact that there is a high incidence of atrial arrhythmias in these patients. By far the most common atrial arrhythmia is atrial fibrillation, although atrial flutter is not uncommon. The other supraventricular arrhythmias occur less frequently.

Wood (1954) found that 39 per cent of

patients manifested established *atrial fibrillation*, while paroxysmal atrial fibrillation was seen in 6 per cent. The incidence of atrial fibrillation in patients with pure mitral regurgitation was 30 per cent. In addition, there appeared to be an age relationship in that the average age of patients with atrial fibrillation was 41 compared with an average age of 33 in those with sinus rhythm. Rowe and co-workers (1960) followed 250 patients with mitral stenosis for 10 to 20 years. Initially, they found that 21 per cent had established atrial fibrillation, while 9 per cent had paroxysmal atrial fibrillation. These authors also found, as did Wood, that atrial fibrillation was more frequent in the older patients; 76 per cent were more than 40 years old. Over the first 10 years, 33 per cent of the patients had persistent atrial fibrillation and 12 per cent had paroxysmal fibrillation. Many authorities believe that the development of atrial fibrillation in these patients signals progressive disease; however, Wood did not find any relationship between atrial fibrillation and rheumatic activity or the degree of mitral stenosis and Rowe et al. noted that survival of patients with and without atrial fibrillation was similar when related to age and severity of disease.

The importance of atrial fibrillation in patients with mitral stenosis and mitral regurgitation relates to the hemodynamic effects of the tachycardia and the incidence of systemic and pulmonary emboli (see Chapter 8). Hemodynamically, the appearance of rapid atrial fibrillation results in a decrease in diastolic filling time, a loss of atrial contribution, and a further increase in left atrial pressure. This not infrequently results in a worsening of existing symptoms and may even precipitate pulmonary edema. Indeed, this may mark the first time that symptoms of heart failure occur. Control of atrial fibrillation alleviates or may at times even eliminate symptoms if the mitral valve lesion itself is still relatively mild.

A serious manifestation of mitral valve disease is the occurrence of systemic and pulmonary emboli. In the series of Rowe et al., all patients with pulmonary emboli and 15 of 17 with systemic emboli prior to the first visit had atrial fibrillation. During a follow-up period of 10 years, all 30 patients with arterial emboli and 14 of 16 with pulmonary emboli had atrial fibrillation. Thus, almost all embolic phenomena in this series were associated with atrial fibrillation.

Treatment of atrial fibrillation is directed toward control of the ventricular response with digitalis, often with the addition of quinidine and occasionally propranolol (see Chapter 8). In view of the high incidence of emboli, patients with atrial fibrillation and mitral valve disease are usually anticoagulated unless specific contraindications exist. Electrical cardioversion is generally not performed owing to both the high failure rate and the high incidence of recurrences (see Chapter 25). It should be emphasized that mitral valve surgery is predicated on the symptoms and clinical state of the patient and not on the presence or absence of atrial fibrillation per se.

MITRAL VALVE PROLAPSE

The mitral valve prolapse syndrome has attracted considerable interest in recent years. It is characterized clinically by symptoms of atypical chest pain, dizziness, palpitations, fatigue, and lightheadedness. Its diagnosis rests on the auscultatory findings of one or more mid or late systolic clicks followed by a systolic murmur. This may be confirmed by the presence of mitral valve prolapse either on echocardiography or cineventriculography. Mitral valve prolapse is considered to be due to an abnormality of the mitral valve apparatus which permits the valve leaflets (most commonly the posterior leaflet) to balloon into the left atrium during ventricular systole. Although no definitive information on the incidence of mitral valve prolapse in the general population is available, echocardiographic studies have shown an incidence of 6 to 10 per cent in asymptomatic young women (Procacci et al., 1975; Brown et al., 1975; Markiewicz et al., 1975) and of 1 to 7 per cent in males (Brown et al., 1975; Micolich et al., 1978).

Palpitation is a common manifestation of mitral valve prolapse. In an extensive review of the literature, comprising 423 patients, Swarz et al. (1977) found that 44.3 per cent had palpitations, 11.6 per cent had lightheadedness, and 4.0 per cent had syncope. In addition, *premature atrial* and/or *ventricular premature complexes* were seen in 54.8 per cent, including 44.9 per cent with ventricular premature complexes. DeMaria et al. (1976) compared the arrhythmias detected on a 10-hour tape recording of 40 normal patients and 31 patients with mitral valve prolapse. Patients with mitral valve prolapse averaged 45 years of age and included 17 women and 14 men. Of the patients with mitral valve prolapse, 18 of 31 (58 per cent) had ventricular arrhythmias, including 15 of higher grade (more than five per minute, multifocal, pairs; see Chapter 11). In contrast, only 10 of 40

TABLE 16–1 CLINICAL FEATURES ASSOCIATED WITH MITRAL VALVE PROLAPSE AND SUDDEN DEATH

1. Family history
2. QT interval prolongation
3. ST and T wave abnormalities
4. Low serum potassium
5. ? Quinidine toxicity
6. Left ventricular abnormalities

(25 per cent) normal patients had ventricular premature complexes on a 10 hour tape, and only 3 of 40 (8 per cent) were higher grade. Similarly, supraventricular arrhythmias were more common (35 per cent versus 10 per cent) and more severe. Others (Winkle et al., 1975; Criley et al., 1973) have found ventricular premature complexes in 75 per cent and 82 per cent, respectively, of patients with mitral valve prolapse. Winkle et al. (1975) found that of 24 such patients studied with 24 hour tapes, five had ventricular tachycardia. Leichtman et al. (1976) have reported a high incidence of sinus bradycardia, A-V block, and even asystole in a family with mitral valve prolapse.

Of major concern is the apparent relationship between mitral valve prolapse and life-threatening arrhythmias (ventricular tachycardia and ventricular fibrillation) and *sudden death*. Swarz et al. found that ventricular tachycardia was documented in 5.3 per cent and sudden death in 1.4 per cent (7) of the 589 reported patients.

The concern over the possibility of sudden death has, to some extent, clouded the general view that mitral valve prolapse is a benign entity. Closer examination of these reports of sudden death reveals that the patients frequently had other underlying features (Table 16–1; Fig. 16–1). In one of the earliest reports of this syndrome, Hancock and Cohn (1966) described a 29-year-old woman who died suddenly. Her baseline electrocardiogram revealed a prolonged QT interval and R on T phenomenon. In addition, at the time of death she was being treated with quinidine. Another patient with spells of unconsciousness also had a prolonged QT interval. Others have noted the relationship between sudden death and a prolonged QT interval in patients with mitral valve prolapse (Winkle et al., 1976; Wie et al., 1978; Jeresaty, 1976). Indeed, the incidence of QT prolongation in patients with mitral prolapse

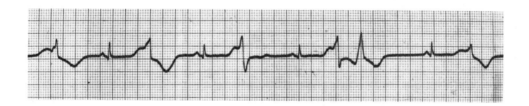

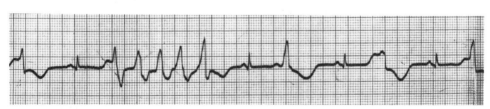

Figure 16–1 A patient with marked QT prolongation and frequent ventricular premature beats of varying coupling interval. Lower strip shows a VPC on the T wave (R on T) starting a short run of ventricular tachycardia.

has been reported to be from 26 per cent (DeMaria et al., 1976) to 60 per cent (Hancock and Cohn, 1966). Since QT prolongation is a recognized entity associated with sudden death, it should alert the physician. Indeed, Wie et al. (1978) reported on 60 consecutive patients referred for refractory ventricular tachycardia sufficiently severe to result in syncope, dizziness, or cardiac arrest. Of the 60 patients, 10 had mitral valve prolapse and of these 10 patients, four had ventricular fibrillation. It is of particular interest that two of the 10 also had coronary heart disease, five had a prolonged QT interval, and eight had prominent U waves.

Other findings associated with mitral valve prolapse and sudden death (Table 16–1) have been low serum potassium (Winkle et al., 1976; Jeresaty, 1976) and treatment of ventricular premature complexes with quinidine (Winkle et al., 1976). Jeresaty (1976), in a review of sudden death in mitral valve prolapse, noted a high incidence of mild to moderate cardiomegaly and ST and T wave changes, particularly in leads 2, 3, and aVF and less commonly the lateral precordial leads. Gulotta et al. (1974) have also noted a high incidence of left ventricular contraction abnormalities in patients with mitral valve prolapse. There are also several reports of patients with mitral valve prolapse, sudden death, and high familial incidence (Swarz et al., 1977; Leichtman et al., 1976).

Thus, sudden death in patients with mitral valve prolapse is predominantly seen in the *symptomatic* patient. Moreover, these patients frequently have a familial history of sudden death, have manifested associated abnormalities, including QT prolongation, hypokalemia, and abnormal left ventricular function and have been given quinidine therapy. The rare instance of sudden death in the absence of any of these known associated findings may be coincidental, in view of the high prevalence of mitral valve prolapse in the general population.

Treatment of arrhythmias is usually unnecessary in the vast majority of patients with this syndrome. In those who present with troublesome symptoms, the major goal should be to exclude other associated conditions, particularly coronary heart disease or cardiomyopathy, especially when the major manifestation is serious ventricular arrhythmia. When other features are present, including a family history, QT prolongation, decreased potassium, and marked ST and T wave abnormalities, a more aggressive approach is indicated. Propranolol has been found to be an effective antiarrhythmic agent for these patients (Winkle et al., 1976). At times, however, it may be of limited value by itself, and additional drugs may be required (Winkle et al., 1976). Treatment with conventional agents may at times be inadequate, and Wei et al. (1978) have reported success with a new antiarrhythmic, aprindine (see Chapter 23). Overdrive pacing has also been reported to be of value in rare cases (Ritchie et al., 1975).

AORTIC VALVULAR DISEASE

While the major symptoms of aortic stenosis and insufficiency are angina pectoris, syncope, and heart failure, overt arrhythmias occasionally are observed. Atrial arrhythmias are rare. In one consecutive series only one of 122 patients exhibited atrial fibrillation, and this patient had advanced congestive heart failure (Myler, 1968). Wood (1958) noted that 13 per cent of his patients with aortic stenosis had atrial fibrillation, and all had associated mitral valve disease.

Syncope has been described in approximately one third to one half of patients with aortic stenosis or combined aortic stenosis and insufficiency (Wood, 1958; Rotman, 1971; Finegan, 1969). Rotman et al. also found that 48 per cent of patients with aortic stenosis and insufficiency had syncope (however, only 8 per cent with pure aortic insufficiency manifested syncope). The incidence of *sudden death* has been described from as low as 3 per cent (Rotman) to 15 to 20 per cent (Ross and Braunwald). Patients are usually symptomatic (congestive heart failure and/or angina pectoris) prior to sudden death.

Syncope with or without sudden death may occur either at rest or during or immediately after physical effort (Flamm, 1967; Schwartz et al., 1969). Flamm studied six patients with aortic stenosis during treadmill exercise and found a decrease in systolic pressure of 20 mm Hg or more, with presyncope in two of six. Detailed study of one of these patients showed that during exercise cardiac output and blood pressure initially rose. However, with the appearance of near syncope, both parameters decreased and there was a reduced systemic vascular resistance commensurate with an increase in pulmonary wedge pressure. No arrhythmias were seen. This suggested that the symptoms were related to left ventricular failure and an inability to meet the required cardiac output.

Schwartz et al. (1969) performed continuous electrocardiogram monitoring on nine patients with aortic stenosis. During the initial stages of syncope, lasting 20 to 40 seconds, a regular rhythm (usually sinus) was noted, with loss of heart sounds or blood pressure (implying mechanical dissociation). If this state persisted, ventricular tachycardia, ventricular fibrillation, or electrical standstill appeared. These studies strongly suggest that both rest and effort syncope are primarily due to left ventricular failure. Arrhythmias thus appear to be a secondary phenomenon occurring if left ventricular failure with reduction in blood flow persists.

Conduction system abnormalities may also be seen in aortic valvular disease. Left bundle branch block has been described in 10 and 14 per cent (Finegan, 1969; Wood, 1957). Atrioven-

tricular block, usually first or second degree, has been described in as many as 18 per cent of patients in one series of older (more than 60 years of age) patients (Finegan, 1969). However, high grade block is rare.

PRIMARY MYOCARDIAL DISEASE (CARDIOMYOPATHY)

Congestive Cardiomyopathy

Congestive cardiomyopathy is characterized by a predominance of left ventricular dilatation with markedly increased left ventricular and later right ventricular volumes, a marked global diminution of contraction, and a small amount of muscular hypertrophy. The etiology in the majority of patients is unclear (accounting for its designation as a *primary* cardiomyopathy); however, excessive alcohol intake, viral illness, or a peripartum etiology has been implicated in a variable number of patients (Goodwin and Oakley, 1972). The major clinical features in patients with congestive cardiomyopathy regardless of etiology are left ventricular failure, systemic and pulmonary emboli, and arrhythmias.

Arrhythmias make up an important part of the clinical picture in patients with a congestive cardiomyopathy. Hamby (1970) found that in a series of 100 of these patients only 10 per cent presented with palpitations, while 39 per cent had congestive heart failure, 29 per cent had dyspnea, and 19 per cent had an increase in heart size. However, approximately 45 per cent complained of palpitations on initial examination. In his series, 63 per cent of the patients demonstrated arrhythmias, including chronic atrial fibrillation in 11 per cent, paroxysmal atrial fibrillation in 9 per cent, and atrial flutter in 3 per cent. Frequent ventricular premature complexes were present in 28 per cent and ventricular tachycardia in 5 per cent. Others have reported similar high incidences of arrhythmias, particularly *atrial fibrillation* (or flutter) and *ventricular arrhythmias.* Massumi et al. (1965) noted 22 instances of atrial fibrillation or flutter in 56 patients, while Sanders found nine of 27 prospectively studied patients had atrial fibrillation or flutter. Ventricular premature complexes and atrial premature complexes were seen in 84 per cent (Massumi, 1965), while McDonald et al. (1971) reported a 79 per cent incidence of ventricular premature complexes.

Treatment of arrhythmias in such patients is directed primarily at the underlying heart failure, with sodium restriction, digitalis, diuretics and vasodilators. The arrhythmias may require specific antiarrhythmic drug therapy, but the importance of optimal management of congestive heart failure in controlling arrhythmia cannot be overemphasized. Not infrequently, improvement in heart failure is followed by a marked reduction in both atrial and ventricular arrhythmias, thereby altogether obviating or reducing the need for specific antiarrhythmics. Careful attention to electrolyte balance, particularly potassium, is also required, since such patients frequently must take large amounts of diuretics. Conversely, rapid atrial fibrillation, which might initially result from worsening of congestive heart failure or emboli, may in turn further exacerbate the congestive heart failure. Control of the ventricular rate with digitalis is mandatory. (Electrical cardioversion is rarely required.)

Despite the high incidence of ventricular arrhythmias, most deaths in patients with congestive cardiomyopathy result from progressive congestive heart failure and low cardiac output states. Hamby (1970) found that only four of 35 deaths were sudden. Similarly, McDonald et al. (1971) found that three of 19 deaths were sudden, and Demakis et al. (1974) found only one unexplained and potential sudden death in 24 patients who died. Spain (1960), in a postmortem study of sudden death victims, found that only five of the 463 deaths were attributable to a cardiomyopathy (compared to 91 per cent that were attributable to coronary heart disease). Thus, sudden death is not a prominent feature in patients with a congestive cardiomyopathy.

Hypertrophic Cardiomyopathy

This entity includes idiopathic hypertrophic subaortic stenosis (IHSS), hypertrophic obstructive cardiomyopathy (HOCM), muscular subaortic stenosis (MSS), and asymmetric septal hypertrophy (ASH) and is associated with the following disorders: 1) left ventricular hypertrophy (primarily of the interventricular septum) and histologic findings of hypertrophied bizarrely shaped and disorganized myocardial cells (Epstein et al., 1974); 2) a resting or inducible systolic left ventricular outflow gradient in over 80 per cent of patients (Shah et al., 1974; Goodwin, 1974); 3) impaired diastolic filling; 4) a clear familial pattern in many patients (Clark et al., 1973); and 5) a highly variable clinical course characterized by dyspnea (76 per cent), angina pectoris (56 per cent), *palpitations* (45 per cent), and *syncope* (27 per cent).

Shah et al. (1974), in a cooperative study of 190 patients with IHSS and a systolic left ventricular outflow gradient, found arrhythmias in only 13 patients on the initial visit and in an additional 22 patients over an average follow-up period of 5.2 years. Of the 13 patients with arrhythmias on the initial visit, six had ventricular premature complexes, three had atrial premature complexes, and one had atrial tachycardia. Another 10 developed atrial tachycardia. Similarly, Frank and Braunwald (1968) found that 29 of 90 (32 per cent) patients with IHSS had rhythm disturbances, including 21 with ectopic beats. In contrast, Ingham et al. (1975) performed 24 hour tape recordings and found atrial premature complexes in 96 per cent, supraventricular tachycardia in 70 per cent, ventricular premature complexes in 96 per cent, and ventricular tachycardia in 15 per cent.

Atrial fibrillation is a relatively unusual arrhythmia, being seen initially in three of 190 patients by Shah et al. (1974) and in six of 123 patients by Frank and Braunwald (1969). During follow-up it appeared in an additional 6.8 per cent and 8 per cent of patients, respectively (Shah et al., 1975; Frank and Braunwald, 1968). Atrial fibrillation is of particular significance in these patients, however, since it generally leads to marked clinical deterioration with appearance of left ventricular failure. This is not surprising in view of the further impediment to diastolic inflow resulting from the increase in heart rate with reduction in diastolic filling time and loss of the atrial kick. This additional burden results in significant clinical deterioration independent of the initial clinical status (Frank and Braunwald, 1968). Treatment of such cases is directed toward management of the atrial fibrillation with digitalis and propranolol.

The major mode of death in patients with IHSS is *sudden death*. Frank and Braunwald (1968) had 10 deaths attributable to IHSS, of which six were sudden. Three of the sudden deaths were in boys aged 8 to 15 years with familial IHSS. The remaining three were adults. Of interest were the relatively low outflow gradients (23 mm Hg average) in these six patients compared to the other patients (56 mm Hg average). Similar data were reported by Shah et al. Of 132 patients treated either symptomatically or with beta blockers, 28 died, 23 of them suddenly. Only two had known ventricular tachycardia prior to death. With regard to possible warning factors, Shah et al. (1974) could find no relationship with initial or final clinical class, age, or length of follow-up. Syncope did not relate to sudden death. In addition, Maron et al. (1978) found that

the initial clinical symptom in 17 of 26 patients was sudden death, while the remaining 9 had only transient symptoms.

In young males a familial history of sudden death appears to portend high risk. Maron et al. (1978) found that one third of these patients who died suddenly had a history of sudden death of a first degree relative. In addition, Hardarson (1973) found that 19 of 39 patients with a positive family history died suddenly during an average follow-up period of 4½ years.

The mechanism or mechanisms of sudden death are unclear. It is conceivable that a sudden exacerbation of the outflow gradient with a sharp decrease in cardiac output is primarily responsible. Maron et al. (1978) found that 13 of 26 sudden deaths occurred during or just after moderate to severe exertion, while an additional seven were during mild exertion. However, treadmill exercise, while inducing arrhythmias (these have been relatively mild), did not result in syncope or other symptoms (Ingham et al., 1975). Conversely, the primary problem may be a decrease in diastolic inflow as a result of progression of the disease, with a consequent decrease in cardiac output. Alternatively, a sudden ventricular arrhythmia may be the primary mechanism. Maron found that five of 26 sudden deaths were in ventricular fibrillation immediately after collapse; however, it is not clear whether this was a primary or secondary arrhythmia.

Limitations in understanding the mechanism are reflected in uncertainty in approach to treatment. Medical treatment has centered on use of beta blockers. However, sudden death occurred in 18 per cent of those on propranolol and in 16 per cent of those receiving no treatment independent of clinical class. In addition, Ingham et al. (1975) found no reduction in arrhythmias with beta blockers. Others have reported success with high doses of beta blockers (Frank et al., 1978). Surgical treatment has been reported to reduce the incidence of sudden death to 5.2 per cent of patients; however, operative mortality was 26 per cent (Shah et al., 1974). In another series, Morrow et al. (1975) reported a much lower operative mortality of 7 per cent after left ventriculomyotomy and myectomy for relief of symptoms and reduction in left ventricular outflow gradient in patients with class III or IV symptoms. It is conceivable, therefore that *if* the mechanism of sudden death is an exacerbation of outflow obstruction, a surgical approach to prevent sudden death would be of value. However, this would have to be balanced against exposing many class I and II patients to a significant risk of operative mortality.

PERICARDIAL DISEASE

Acute pericarditis is characterized by an inflammatory process involving the pericardium, with variable involvement of the underlying epicardial surface of the myocardium. The proximity of the pericardium to the sinus node predisposes to sinus tachycardia, which is a common feature of this disease. James (1962), in a necropsy series, found that 26 of 38 patients (68 per cent) had arrhythmias. However, a large number of these patients had concomitant underlying cardiac disease. In a more recent prospective study, Spodick (1976) found that arrhythmias occur but are relatively uncommon. In a series of 100 patients referred with acute pericarditis of diverse etiology and evaluated using serial electrocardiograms, there were seven instances of arrhythmias, of which five were atrial fibrillation, one was junctional tachycardia, and one was atrial flutter. All seven occurred in 24 patients with known underlying heart disease. It is conceivable however, that with long-term monitoring more arrhythmias might have been detected (see Chapter 14).

In chronic constrictive pericarditis,

atrial arrhythmias are quite common. Dalton et al. (1956) found that 28 of 78 patients had chronic atrial fibrillation or flutter and another five had transient fibrillation or flutter. Similarly, Wood (1961) reported atrial fibrillation in 35 per cent and atrial flutter in another 10 per cent, with a relationship to the duration of the disease. It is of interest that postoperatively of 13 patients with atrial fibrillation prior to pericardiectomy, all persisted while 1 with preoperative atrial flutter converted to normal sinus rhythm (Dalton et al., 1956).

REFERENCES

Mitral Valve Disease and Aortic Valve Disease

Finegan, R. E., Gianelly, R. E., and Harrison, D. C.: Aortic stenosis in the elderly. N. Engl. J. Med. 281:1261, 1969.

Flamm, M. D., Braniff, B. A., Kimball, R., and Hancock, E. W.: Mechanisms of effort syncope in aortic stenosis. Circulation 35/36:II-109, 1967.

Mitchell, A. M., Sackett, C. H., Hunzecker, W. J., and Levine, S. A.: The clinical features of aortic stenosis. Am. Heart J. 48:684, 1954.

Myler, R. K., and Sanders, C. A.: Aortic valve disease and atrial fibrillation. Arch. Intern. Med. 121:530, 1968.

Noble, R. J., and Fisch, C.: Factors in the genesis of atrial fibrillation in rheumatic valvular disease. Cardiovasc. Clin. 5:(2) 97, 1973.

Rios, J. C., and Goo, W.: Electrocardiographic correlates of rheumatic valvular disease. Cardiovasc. Clin. 5:247, 1973.

Roberts, N. C.: The congenitally bicuspid aortic valve. A study of 85 autopsy cases. Am. J. Cardiol. 226:72, 1970.

Roberts, W. C., Perloff, J. K., and Costantino, T.: Severe valvular aortic stenosis in patients over 65 years of age. A clinicopathologic study. Am. J. Cardiol. 27:497, 1971.

Ross, J., and Braunwald, E.: Aortic stenosis. Circulation 37:V-61, 1968.

Rotman, M., Morris, J. J., Behar, V. S., Peter, R. H., and Kong, Y.: Aortic valvular disease: A comparison of types and their medical and surgical management. Am. J. Med. 51:241, 1971.

Rowe, J. C., Bland, E. F., Sprague, H. B., and White, P. D.: The course of mitral stenosis without surgery: Ten and twenty year perspectives. Ann. Intern. Med. 52:741, 1960.

Schwartz, L. S., Goldfischer, J., Sprague, G. J.,

and Schwartz, S. P.: Syncope and sudden death in aortic stenosis. Am. J. Cardiol. 23:647, 1969.

Spann, J. F., and Sand, M. J.: The incidence and significance of atrial dysrhythmias in rheumatic valvular disease. Cardiovasc. Clin. 5:(2) 115, 1973.

Takeda, J., Warren, R., and Holzman, D.: Prognosis of aortic stenosis. Arch. Surg. 87:931, 1963.

Wood, P.: An appreciation of mitral stenosis. Part I and II. Brit. Med. J. May 8, 1954, 1051–1113.

Wood, P.: Aortic stenosis. Am. J. Cardiol. 1:553, 1958.

Yater, W., and Cornell, H.: Heart block due to calcareous lesions of the bundle of His. Ann. Intern. Med. 8:777, 1935.

Mitral Valve Prolapse

Brown, O. R., Kloster, F. E., and DeMots, H.: Incidence of mitral valve prolapse in the asymptomatic normal. (abst) Circulation 57/58:II–229, 1978.

Criley, J. M., Zeilenga, D. W., and Morgan, M. T.: Mitral dysfunction: A possible cause of arrhythmias in the prolapsing mitral leaflet syndrome. Trans. Am. Clin. Climatol. Assoc. 85:44, 1973.

DeMaria, A. N., Amsterdam, E. A., Vismara, L. A., Nevmann, A., and Mason, D. T.: Arrhythmias in the mitral valve prolapse syndrome. Prevalence, nature and frequency. Ann. Intern. Med. 84:656, 1976.

Gulotta, S. J., Gulco, L., Padmanabhan, V., Miller, S.: The syndrome of systolic click, murmur and mitral valve prolapse — a cardiomyopathy? Circulation 29:717, 1974.

Hancock, E. W., and Cohn, K.: Syndrome associated with midsystolic click and late systolic murmur. Am. J. Med. 41:183, 1966.

Jeresaty, R. M.: Sudden death in the mitral valve prolapse — click syndrome. Am. J. Cardiol. 37:317, 1976.

Leichtman, D., Nelson, R., Gobel, F. L., Alexander, C. S., and Cohn, J. N.: Bradycardia with mitral valve prolapse. A potential mechanism of sudden death. Ann. Intern. Med. 85:453, 1976.

Markiewicz, W., Stoner, J., London, E., Hunt, S. A., and Popp, R. L.: Mitral valve prolapse in one hundred presumably healthy females. Circulation 52:II–77, 1925.

Mikolich, J. R., Darsee, J. R., Nicoloff, N. B., and Lesser, L.: Mitral valve prolapse in 101 presumably healthy young males. Circulation 57/58:II–229, 1978.

Procacci, P. M., Sauran, S. V., Schreiter, S. L., and Bryson, A. L.: Clinical frequency and implications of mitral valve prolapse in the female population.

Ritchie, J. L., Hammermeister, K. E., and Kennedy, J. W.: Refractory ventricular tachycardia and fibrillation in a patient with the prolapsing mitral leaflet syndrome: successful control with overdrive pacing. Am. J. Cardiol. 37:314, 1975.

Shappell, S. D., Marshall, C. E., Brown, R. E., and Bruce, T. A.: Sudden death and the familial occurrence of midsystolic click, late systolic murmur syndrome. Circulation 48:1128, 1973.

Swarz, M. H., Teichholz, L. E., and Donoso, E.: Mitral valve prolapse: a review of associated arrhythmias. Am. J. Med. 62:377, 1977.

Wei, J. Y., Bulkley, B. H., Schaeffer, A. H., Greene, H. L., and Reid, P. R.: Mitral valve prolapse syndrome and recurrent ventricular tachyarrhythmias. A malignant variant refractory to conventional drug therapy. Ann. Intern. Med. 89:6, 1978.

Winkel, R. A., Lopes, M. G., Fitzgerald, J. W., Goodman, D. J., Schroeder, J. S., and Harrison, D. C.: Arrhythmias in patients with mitral valve prolapse. 52:73, 1975.

Winkel, R. A., Lopes, M. G., Popp, R. L., and Hancock, E. W.: Life-threatening arrhythmias in the mitral valve prolapse syndrome. Am. J. Med. 60:961, 1976.

Cardiomyopathy

Dalton, J. C., Pearson, R. J., and White, P. D.: Constrictive pericarditis: A review of long-term follow up of 78 cases. Ann. Intern. Med. 45:445, 1956.

Demakis, J. G., Proskey, A., Rahimtoola, S. H., Jamil, M., Sutton, G. C., Rosen, D. M., Gunnar, R. M., and Tobin, J. R.: The natural course of alcoholic cardiomyopathy. Ann. Intern. Med. 80:293, 1974.

Goodwin, J. F.: Congestive and hypertrophic cardiomyopathies. Lancet 1:731, 1970.

Goodwin, J. F.: Prospects and predictions for the cardiomyopathies. Circulation 50:210, 1974.

Goodwin, J. F., and Oakley, C. M.: The cardiomyopathies. Br. Heart J. 34:545, 1972.

Hamby, R. I.: Primary myocardial disease. A prospective clinical and hemodynamic evaluation in 100 patients. Medicine 49:55, 1970.

James, T. N.: Pericarditis and the sinus node. Arch. Intern. Med. 110:305, 1962.

Massumi, R. A., Rios, J. C., Gooch, A. S., Nutter, D., DeVita, V. T., and Datlow, D. W.: Primary myocardial disease. Report of 50 cases and review of the subject. Circulation 31:19, 1965.

McDonald, C. S., Burch, G. E., and Walsh, J. J.: Alcoholic cardiomyopathy managed with prolonged bed rest. Ann. Intern. Med. 74:681, 1971.

McMartin, D. E., and Flowers, N. C.: Clinical-electrocardiographic correlations in diseases of the myocardium. Cardiovasc. Clin. 8B:191, 1977.

Sanders, V.: Idiopathic disease of myocardium. Arch. Intern. Med. 112:661, 1963.

Spodick, D. H.: Arrhythmias during acute pericarditis. A prospective study of 100 consecutive cases. J.A.M.A. 235:39, 1976.

Stapleton, J. F., Segal, J. P., and Harvey, W. P.: The electrogram of myocardiopathy. Prog. C/V Dis. 13:217, 1970.

Wood, P.: Chronic constrictive pericarditis. Am. J. Cardiol. 77:48, 1961.

Idiopathic Hypertrophic Subaortic Stenosis

Clark, C. E., Henry, W. L., and Epstein, S. E.: Familial prevalence and genetic transmission of idiopathic hypertrophic subaortic stenosis. N. Engl. J. Med. 289:709, 1973.

Epstein, S. E., Henry, W. L., Clark, C. E., Roberts, W. C., Maron, B. J., Ferrans, V. J., Redwood, D. R., and Morrow, A. G.: Asymmetric septal hypertrophy. Ann. Intern. Med. 81:650, 1974.

Frank, M. J., Abdulla, A. M., Canedo, M. E., and Saylors, R. E.: Longterm medical management of hypertrophic obstructive cardiomyopathy. Am. J. Cardiol. 42:993, 1978.

Frank, S., and Braunwald, E.: Idiopathic hypertrophic subaortic stenosis. Clinical analysis of 126 patients with emphasis on the natural history. Circulation 37:759, 1968.

Goodwin, J. F.: Congestive and hypertrophic cardiomyopathies. Lancet 1:731, 1970.

Goodwin, J. F.: Prospects and predictions for the cardiomyopathies. Circulation 50:210, 1974.

Hardarson, T., Curiel, R., Calzada, C. S. de la, and Goodwin, J. F.: Prognosis and mortality of hypertrophic obstructive cardiomyopathy. Lancet 2:1462, 1973.

Ingham, R. E., Rossen, R. M., Goodman, D. J., and Harrison, D. C.: Ambulatory electrocardiographic monitoring in idiopathic hypertrophic subaortic stenosis. (abst.) Circulation 51/52:II-93, 1975.

Ingham, R. E., Rossen, R. M., Goodman, D. J., and Harrison, D. C.: Treadmill arrhythmias on patients with idiopathic hypertrophic subaortic stenosis. Chest 68:759, 1975.

Maron, B. J., Roberts, W. C., Edwards, J. E., McAllister, H. R., Foley, D. D., and Epstein, S. E.: Sudden death in patients with hypertrophic cardiomyopathy: characterization of 26 patients without functional limitation. Am. J. Cardiol. 41:803, 1978.

Morrow, A. G., Reitz, V. A., Epstein, S. E., Henry, W. L., Conkle, D. M., Itscoitz, S. B., and Redwood, D. R.: Operative treatment in hypertrophic subaortic stenosis: Techniques and the results of pre- and postoperative assessments in 83 patients. Circulation 52:88, 1975.

Shah, P. M., Adelman, A. G., Wigle, E. D., Gobel, F. L., Burchell, H. B., Hardarson, T., Curiel, R., Calzada, C. de la, Oakley, C. B., and Goodwin, J. F.: The natural (and unnatural) history of hypertrophic obstructive cardiomyopathy. Circ. Res. 34/35: II-179, 1974.

Teare, D.: Asymmetrical hypertrophy of the heart in young adults. Br. Heart J. 20:148, 1958.

ARRHYTHMIAS IN INFANTS, CHILDREN, AND THE FETUS

MONTY M. BODENHEIMER M.D.
RICHARD H. HELFANT, M.D.

Abnormalities of rhythm are not uncommon in infancy and childhood; however, they differ in many respects from those observed in adults. The principal differences are related to etiology and to the fact that infants and children have a less stable autonomic system and a greater facility of conduction through the AV junction, with resultant high heart rates. In addition, the types of arrhythmias, their incidence, course, prognosis, and therapeutic regimen differ somewhat from those encountered in adults.

One may observe the following: sinus arrhythmia, SA heart block, premature beats, shifting pacemaker from the SA to the AV node (this occurs rather commonly with increased vagal activity), atrial tachycardia and atrial flutter (Fig. 17–1) and arrhythmias arising in the AV junction (Fig. 17–2) or the bundle of His, and various degrees of AV heart block, although the higher degrees of block are less frequently encountered (Keith et al., 1967).

Arrhythmias observed in association with congenital cardiac anomalies depend largely on the type of anomaly

present. They are due to one or a combination of factors: 1) congenital malformation with disturbance in the normal distribution of the automatic centers in conduction tissue; 2) strain

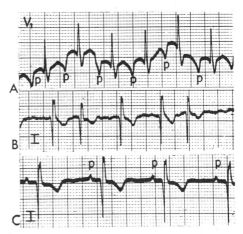

Figure 17–1 Atrial flutter occurring in a child, age 6, with tetralogy of Fallot. Conversion to normal sinus rhythm.

(A) (V_1). Note the presence of atrial flutter with a 2:1 A-V conduction. The ventricular rate is 130 per minute and the atrial rate is 260 per minute. (B) (Lead I). Shows conversion to atrial fibrillation by digitalis. (C) (Lead I). Shows restoration of normal sinus rhythm.

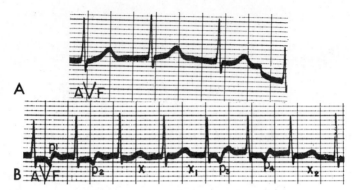

Figure 17-2   A-V junctional rhythm with retrograde conduction and Wenckebach phenomenon, taken from a child, 2½ years of age.

(*A*) The cardiac rate is 100 per minute. Note the absence of P waves, probably the result of an A-V junctional rhythm.

(*B*) Note the absence of P waves in cycles X, X_1, and X_2. Note the retrograde P waves (P_1, P_2, P_3, and P_4). These are due to retrograde conduction in the presence of an A-V junctional rhythm. The R-P interval is short in the cycle with P_3 and longer with P_4 (Wenckebach phenomenon, so-called retrograde Wenckebach).

on various chambers of the heart because of septal and valvular defects with resulting hypertrophy or dilation of the cardiac chambers; 3) inflammatory changes with fibrosis; 4) hypoxia, especially after effort or excitement; 5) surgical correction of congenital anomalies.

ETIOLOGY AND INCIDENCE

Etiologic factors to be considered are congenital defects, pre-excitation syndromes (see Chapter 13), rheumatic heart disease, viral infections, malnutrition, cardiomyopathies, endocrine disorders, acid-base disturbances, and neurogenic disturbances. Head trauma and cardiac surgery are occasional factors. A frequent association has been observed between neonatal arrhythmias and mothers who are elderly and primiparous (Lunberg, 1963). The incidence of digitalis toxicity is minor; and degenerative states, including hypertension and coronary artery disease, which are of such prime importance in the genesis of arrhythmias in adults, are virtually absent.

Familial occurrence of certain ar-

rhythmias has been observed in successive generations. The arrhythmias may appear in conjunction with congenital anomalies or independent of other clinical manifestations. This, however, does not rule out the possible presence of microscopic abnormalities in some of the conduction pathways.

Arrhythmias that have a familial occurrence include sinus tachycardia, atrial fibrillation, supraventricular tachycardia, and multifocal premature ventricular complexes (Harris, 1970). In addition, the familial occurrence of several other arrhythmias has been linked to either a gross or a microscopic cardiac lesion. These include bradycardia and Stokes-Adams seizures, impaired AV conduction, and bundle branch block. The pathologic lesions in these cases vary from such well-recognized anomalies as atrial septal defect to rare anomalies, such as complete absence of the AV node or hypoplasia of the bundle branches. There does not appear to be a pattern of inheritance common to all familial occurrences of arrhythmias. Each case seems to be individual, and the modes of inheritance vary from sex linked recessive to autosomal dominant.

ARRHYTHMIAS IN CONGENITAL HEART DISEASE

Congenital AV Heart Block

Atrioventricular conduction disturbances are not infrequent in infants and children (Ayers, 1966; Nakamura and Nadas, 1964). The normal upper limit for the PR interval varies from 0.14 seconds in infancy to 0.18 seconds in adolescence. Prolongation of the PR interval beyond this range constitutes first degree AV heart block.

First degree heart block is commonly associated with acute rheumatic fever with myocardial involvement, occasionally with diphtheria, and in viral diseases such as mumps and rubella. Some types of congenital heart disease are associated with 1 degree AV block, including patent ductus arteriosus, atrial septal defect, endocardial cushion defects, Ebstein's anomaly, and corrected transposition of the great vessels.

Second degree AV block in infants and children is usually of the Mobitz type I form (see Chapter 12). Etiologies are similar to those for first degree AV block. Mobitz type II is rare, having been reported after cardiac surgery and in the rare case of infantile coronary sclerosis. Clinical manifestations of first and second degree block are related to the underlying etiology, the severity of the block, and the associated cardiovascular state. Therapy is dependent upon the underlying etiology and clinical manifestations. Specific therapy, especially for first and second degree and Mobitz type I block, is usually not required. Mobitz type II, when it does occur, is usually related to severe underlying disease and requires a pacemaker.

Congenital Complete AV Heart Block

Congenital complete heart block occurs in approximately 1 of 20,000 live births compared with an incidence of approximately 1 per cent for all congenital anomalies. Congenital origin may be difficult to establish if the condition is first diagnosed during childhood because of the possibility that an infection is responsible. In a large cooperative study by Engle and Ehlers (1975), an associated congenital malformation was present in 33 per cent of the patients. Corrected transposition of the great vessels was the most common, followed by patent ductus arteriosus. Other less commonly associated anomalies include ostium primum defects, single ventricle, and ventricular septal defect (especially if the membranous septum was involved). However, except for corrected transposition, no definite relation exists between these conditions and congenital heart block. In addition, a familial incidence has been shown.

The diagnostic criteria for congenital complete heart block are: 1) bradycardia noted at an early age; 2) AV heart block proven by ECG; 3) absence of history suggesting other causes, for example, diphtheria. In cases in which the conduction system has been studied histologically, congenital absence or fibrotic disruption in continuity has been observed between the AV junction and the His bundle. In addition, absence of the His bundle has been observed.

Clinical manifestations vary considerably. The ventricular rate at rest in congenital heart block is generally 40 to 80 beats per minute and the QRS complex is supraventricular (i.e., narrow) in form in over 90 per cent of patients, regardless of whether associated anomalies are present or absent (Engle and Ehlers, 1975). This would indicate that a pacemaker is located above the bifurcation of the bundle of His. Such patients, although their heart rates are characteristically slow, have compensatory increased stroke volume and normal cardiac output at rest. Exercise tolerance is frequently normal. In one study of such patients between the ages of 7 and 23 years, heart rate increased by 18 to 82 beats per minute, with the average being 45 beats per minute. Thus, this form of heart block differs from that usually seen in adults with acquired complete AV block, in whom only a slight acceleration in heart rate may occur with exercise (Ikkos et al., 1974).

In a large cooperative study of 418 infants and children with congenital complete heart block and no associated congenital anomalies, two thirds had reached the second decade of life (Engle and Michaelson, 1972). Thirty-two died, including 15 in the first week of life, all apparently from cardiac failure. Sixteen died after one year of age. Of the 14 who died suddenly, 5 had prior episodes of dizziness or syncope while 9 died suddenly and unexpectedly. Age at death in these 16 was evenly distributed from 1 through 15 years. Overall, 92.4 per cent were alive at the last follow-up, in comparison to only 71.3 per cent of those with congenital complete heart block and associated cardiac anomalies.

Possible risk factors for death in patients with congenital heart block were examined. Aside from coexisting heart disease, an enlarging heart was found to be of predictive value. Also, in infants without associated heart disease, only one of 23 with a ventricular rate of 55 or more and an atrial rate of less than 140 beats per minute died. In contrast, 17 of 58 (29%) with a ventricular rate of less than 55 beats per minute died. It is of interest that in a large cooperative study of causes of sudden death in children with known cardiovascular disease, only one case of congenital complete heart block was present (Lambert et al., 1974). This again indicates the low incidence of sudden death in such patients.

Primary treatment of congenital complete AV block is pacemaker implantation (see Chapter 24). Pacemaker therapy is indicated in the presence of cardiac failure unresponsive to digitalis, syncope, or Stokes-Adams (Engle,

1972). Ideally, insertion of pacemakers in all patients with congenital complete heart block, regardless of the absence of symptoms, might prevent the few instances of unexpected sudden death. However, in the absence of an ideal long term pacemaker (see Chapter 24), one is reluctant to use this approach in a patient whose condition may not require it for many years. However, pacemaker insertion is associated with considerable problems, particularly in infants and to a lesser extent children. Furman examined their results in 19 patients, including nine with congenital heart block. Pacers were inserted in six for syncope, two for low cardiac output, one for a complication of cardiac catheterization and seven with postoperative heart block. They found that 16 of 19 did well and three died, one as a direct result of pacemaker insertion. These authors also noted that under the age of two, problems with pacer size and patient growth are major limiting factors. In addition, Hofschire (1977) reported that although no deaths were attributable to heart block in patients with permanent pacers, 15 of 19 had pacer related complications and averaged one hospitalization per year for pacemaker induced problems. Thus, at this time, pacemakers are inserted at the appearance of Stokes-Adams, low cardiac output, or slow ventricular heart rates. In addition, temporary pacemakers are indicated at the time of anesthesia and surgery.

Postoperative Heart Block

A significant incidence of heart block is seen following surgical repair of congenital cardiac anomalies. Hofschire (1977) reported on 64 children, all of whom developed heart block in the immediate postoperative period that persisted for a minimum of 24 hours. Underlying lesions were ventricular septal defects in 42, tetralogy of Fallot in 15, atrial septal defect and/or ventricular septal defect in five, endocardial cushion defect in one, and transposition in one. In 28 patients, the heart block lasted less than 30 days and normal sinus rhythm appeared in 23. Twenty-six persisted for more than one month and were permanently paced.

Considerable interest has focused on the patient undergoing total repair for tetralogy of Fallot. Some studies have indicated that patients who develop bifascicular block (right bundle branch block and left anterior hemiblock) or trifascicular block (bifascicular block and PR prolongation) are at risk of complete heart block and sudden death. Steeg et al. (1975) found that 18 of 207 patients (8.7%) developed bifascicular block following surgery at an age range of four to 27 years. None of the 18 patients experienced symptoms, and no deaths occurred during a follow-up for more than 5 years of 13 of the patients. In contrast, Quattlebaum and co-workers (1976) evaluated 243 patients 6½ to 16½ years after repair of tetralogy. Seven died suddenly between 3 months and 5½ years after surgery. Of the seven, four had a right bundle branch block while three had trifascicular block. They also noted that in 18 patients with right bundle branch block or bifascicular block, progression to trifascicular block over a period of one month to seven years postoperatively occurred. Of interest was the finding that ventricular premature contractions were frequently seen, and the suggestion was made by these authors that the mechanism of death in some patients might be ventricular tachyarrhythmias.

It has been suggested that determination of the site of block might be of value. Godman et al. (1974) reported that HV prolongation accompanied right bundle branch block and left axis deviation in patients who underwent surgery for ventricular septal defect or tetralogy. Similarly, Hougen et al. (1978) showed that of 14 patients with bifascicular or trifascicular block or

transient complete heart block postoperatively, all had prolongation of the HV interval. However, they did not find any cases of sudden death over follow-up periods ranging from 18 months to 16 years. Thus, the value of His bundle electrocardiography in delineating the need for a pacemaker is unclear. At present, careful follow-up is indicated and pacemaker insertion is warranted with appearance of block progression or syncopal symptoms.

Sinus Node Arrhythmias

The normal sinus rate varies from 110 to 150 beats per minute in the newborn and gradually decreases to 60 to 100 beats per minute by the age of 6. A common variation is sinus arrhythmia characterized by a phasic increase during inspiration and a decrease during expiration. Persistent sinus bradycardia is unusual and most commonly is related to increased vagal tone. Pathologic states that may be causal include increased intracranial pressure, hypothyroidism, hypothermia, obstructive jaundice, typhoid fever, and drugs such as quinidine. In contrast, sinus tachycardia is common and may be seen in any stress state whether cardiac or noncardiac in origin.

A wandering atrial pacer may be seen and is characterized by a slow heart rate and a shift in contour of the P wave. It is generally benign. Sinoatrial block (see Chapter 5) may be seen; the possible causes are myocarditis, rheumatic fever, drugs such as digitalis and quinidine, and hyperkalemia.

SA node dysfunction, or sick sinus syndrome, may on occasion be seen, manifesting as in the adult with various forms of sinus bradycardia and/or block and associated atrial arrhythmias. Such arrhythmias have been observed following such cardiac surgery as the Mustard procedure, balloon septostomy, and closure of an atrial septal defect (Nugent et al., 1973).

Supraventricular Tachycardia

Although paroxysmal supraventricular tachycardia is relatively infrequent, it is probably the most common type of rapid heart action encountered in the newborn or the young child. It is usually not associated with underlying cardiac disease. Pre-excitation has been reported in approximately 50 per cent of such patients (Lundberg et al., 1973; Anderson et al., 1973). As a result of physiologic differences in the AV junction of children as compared with adults, supraventricular tachycardia in infants and children with atrial rates of as high as 300 will usually be conducted through an efficient AV junction with resulting 1:1 ventricular response.

About 10 per cent of the cases manifest no symptoms, and the tachycardia is discovered only during routine physical examination. However, the majority — especially very young infants — appear quite ill. Their color is often ashen gray, their skin is cold and damp, and cyanosis is frequently present. The infant is usually restless and irritable, and the respirations are rapid and labored. At times a hacking cough may appear and the abdomen may be distended. Fever may be present but usually indicates the existence of an infection that may have actually initiated the arrhythmia, or it may result from congestive failure with complicating pneumonitis. The clinical picture may closely resemble that of a severe pneumonia or septicemia. The heart is usually enlarged, and transient functional murmurs may appear. Congestive failure is a relatively common complication of paroxysmal supraventricular tachycardia in children.

The paroxysms often end spontaneously. An initial attempt to bring the rate to normal may be made by carotid sinus pressure. Digitalis is the drug of choice in infants and children and is successful in terminating 80 per cent of episodes (Keith et al., 1967). The digitalizing dose in infants under one year of age is 0.04 mg per pound of body weight. One half the calculated dose is given initially followed by one fourth dose at two consecutive four to six hour intervals. It should be noted, however, that long term prevention may be difficult with any agent. In older children, specific etiologies of supraventricular tachycardia, such as myocarditis and hyperthyroidism, should be considered. Vagal maneuvers may succeed in converting the rhythm, and digitalis is the treatment of choice in both acute and chronic cases.

Long term prognosis in such patients is good. Lundberg et al. (1973) followed 47 patients with paroxysmal supraventricular tachycardia beginning at less than 1 year of age (75% were under two months) for a minimum of 10 years. Recurrences decreased from 55 per cent in infancy to 17 per cent from ages two to 10 and 23 per cent in those more than 10 years old. Similarly, Anderson et al. (1973) found that of 28 cases beginning under one year of age, 15 had no recurrences after infancy, including 17 of 23 followed for more than five years. In contrast, 20 of 23 patients whose paroxysmal supraventricular tachycardia began in childhood continued to have recurrences. Pre-excitation appears to play an important role in such patients. Lundberg et al. (1973) found an incidence of 49 per cent, and Anderson et al. (1973) found an incidence of 56 per cent. Moreover, both found that the recurrences appeared mostly in patients with Wolff-Parkinson-White syndrome. Thus, Lundberg reported that between the ages of two and 10 years, 46 per cent of patients with WPW had recurrences, compared with only 6 per cent of those patients without pre-excitation.

An unusual form of tachycardia is persistent ectopic atrial tachycardia characterized by a heart rate of less than 200 beats per minute, an abnormal P wave vector, and marked chronicity lasting weeks to months and occasionally years. Keane et al. (1972) reported on 16 such patients and found an overall good prognosis; 13 patients became asymptomatic and only one died. Drug response is poor. Although digitalis is the treatment of choice and frequently succeeds in slowing the heart rate, conversion to normal sinus rhythm is unusual (Keane). It is of interest that none of these patients manifested pre-excitation.

Atrial Flutter

Atrial flutter is rare in the pediatric age group. Its classification has been based on age at presentation: at or immediately after birth or beginning weeks to months later. Episodes of atrial flutter that have an early onset tend to be better tolerated and to subside in the first year of life. In contrast, an onset weeks to months after birth is associated with cardiac decompensation and a worse prognosis. Etiologic factors include upper respiratory and other infections, diphtheria, pertussis, pneumonia, and bronchitis associated with otitis media. The manifestations of atrial flutter vary greatly; however, they are generally similar to those of paroxysmal tachycardia. When this arrhythmia accompanies an underlying congenital heart disease they produce a serious complication. The diagnosis is suspected clinically if a tachycardia (rate of 250/minute) is present and is definitely established by the finding of characteristic F waves on the electrocardiogram (see Chapter 7).

Digitalization is the initial treatment of choice. If the rhythm converts to atrial fibrillation, quinidine may be added. If normal sinus rhythm does not occur, electric countershock may be used.

Atrial Fibrillation

Atrial fibrillation in infants and children is rare. When it is present, it is almost always associated with severe myocardial disease (atrial fibrillation occurs in 1 to 2% of cases) (Paul, 1966), hypokalemia, congenital heart disease (especially atrial septal defect), thyrotoxicosis (Keith et al., 1967), and tumors of the atria.

Treatment usually entails full digitalization followed by quinidine in an attempt to convert to normal sinus rhythm. In refractory cases, or where conversion is considered urgent, direct-current countershock should be employed followed by quinidine to maintain normal sinus rhythm after conversion. The onset of this arrhythmia in children frequently has ominous prognostic implications. In one group, the average survival after the onset of atrial fibrillation was eight months in children between nine and 12 years of age and 30 months in adolescents (Gibson, 1941).

Ventricular Arrhythmias

Occasional ventricular premature contractions are of no significance and require no therapy. If more complex ventricular arrhythmias occur (multifocal, bigeminy, etc.), cardiomyopathy, rheumatic carditis, and metabolic derangements should be considered.

Ventricular tachycardia occurs infrequently in infants and children. Engle and Ehlers (1975) reported on 45 patients clustered in infancy (11 patients) or preadolescence (34 patients). Most presented with chest pain, palpitations, or dizziness. Eighteen (40%) had associated diseases including 10 with congenital anomalies and eight with a cardiomyopathy. Six died during the follow-up period. Treatment is directed at control of the rhythm acutely, using cardioversion if hemodynamic deterioration is present or intravenous therapy with lidocaine and procainamide, as in adults (see Chapter 11).

Sudden Infant Death Syndrome

This entity is generally seen in infant boys usually younger than six months old and most frequently two to four months old (Valdes-Dapena, 1967). Congenital cardiac anomalies were present in only 3.1 per cent (Valdes-Dapena, 1967). Various cardiac etiologies have been proposed. James (1976) suggested that there may be electrical instability partly resulting from the normal development process of the conduction system. However, Lie et al. (1976) could find no histologic abnormality that was confined to infants with sudden infant deaths compared to a control series. To date, the cause or causes of this syndrome are not defined.

Cardiac Arrest

Cardiac arrest arises nearly three times more frequently in infants than in all other age groups (Rackow et al., 1961). Because infants and children possess a high degree of vagal tone, they are likely to develop episodes of cardiac slowing accompanied by sinus pauses. Thus, surgery and anesthesia in infants are not uncommonly complicated by cardiac arrest. Emergency therapy in infants consists of closed-chest cardiac compression with both thumbs pressing on the midsternum. Flexing the lower extremities upon the chest has frequently been successful in

cardiac resuscitation in infants and children. Older children may be treated with cardiac compression techniques similar to those used in adults. Mouth-to-mouth ventilation should be applied simultaneously until positive pressure respiration is instituted. When these techniques are employed in the early stages before the occurrence of prolonged hypoxia, recovery with little or no neurologic impairment should result.

ELECTROCARDIOGRAMS OF THE FETUS

Fetal electrocardiography represents an objective method of studying the developing heart in the fetus and furnishes the cardiologist and obstetrician with an invaluable tool in the diagnosis of cardiac arrhythmia in the fetus before and during labor. Furthermore, the fetal electrocardiogram can help to reveal the presence of congenital heart disease and to determine whether a fetal malformation has occurred during the course of a maternal illness or infection.

With present techniques, the earliest demonstration of the fetal electrocardiogram has been at 11 weeks. Many other successful recordings have been

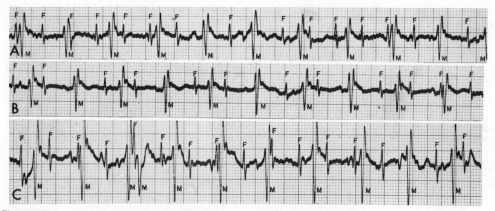

Figure 17–3   Fetal electrocardiogram. The maternal heart rate (M) is 92 per minute and the fetal heart rate (F) is 140 to 160 per minute. Note that the fetal beats are easily distinguishable from the maternal beats. (This tracing was taken by the technique of radioelectrocardiography.

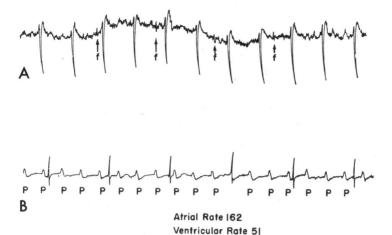

Figure 17-4 Antenatal diagnosis of complete heart block with the fetal electrocardiogram. (*A*) Fetal electrocardiogram showing fetal complexes occurring at a slow fixed rate, slower than the maternal rate. (*B*) The newborn electrocardiogram confirms the existence of heart block, showing complete A-V dissociation. (From Larks, S. D.: Fetal Electrocardiography: The Electrical Activity of the Fetal Heart, 1961. Courtesy of Charles C Thomas, Publisher, Springfield, Illinois.)

made at 12, 13, and 14 weeks, and increasing numbers at later periods of gestation (Fig. 17–3). The fetal electrocardiogram in the human is recorded through the intact maternal abdomen (Kendall et al., 1962).

ARRHYTHMIAS ENCOUNTERED IN THE FETUS

Transient bradycardias as low as 70 beats per minute or transient tachycardias up to 200 beats per minute are occasionally observed during the period of gestation and during labor. Atrioventricular junctional escape rhythm has been observed in the fetus during periods of sinus bradycardia. Paroxysmal tachycardia of supraventricular origin with heart rates ranging from 210 to 240 beats per minute has been observed (Urbach et al., 1966). Atrial fibrillation occurs only rarely in the fetus; however, it carries an extremely serious prognosis (Urbach et al., 1966). It is believed to be a primary factor in the death of the fetus.

Figure 17–4 demonstrates a case of complete AV heart block as diagnosed prenatally with the fetal electrocardiogram. Various degrees of AV block in the fetus occur most commonly during periods of vagal stimulation. There is evidence to suggest that AV block occurs normally in the fetus during vagal stimulation but may be indicative of congenital heart disease when it is sustained.

Bradycardia alone or in association with other fetal cardiac arrhythmias and tachycardia, in addition to alterations in the S-T segments and T waves of the fetal electrocardiogram, have been considered ominous signs.

Cardio-Auditory Syndrome

The cardio-auditory syndrome, also called the surdo-cardiac syndrome, presents a characteristic set of signs and symptoms with onset in infancy and childhood. These subjects suffer from congenital deafness and attacks of syncope (Stokes-Adams attacks) or milder episodes resembling angina pectoris. Two types have been described: 1) marked Q-T prolongation and deafness occurring in subjects with clinically normal hearts (most common); and 2) Q-T prolongation and deafness occurring in subjects with congenital heart disease. In addition, a third, very similar syndrome has been described in children and adults with no auditory impairment. These latter patients have a tendency to develop paroxysmal ventricular fibrillation.

Genetic Factors. The cardioauditory syndrome appears to be an autosomal recessive trait which occurs more commonly in situations of parental consanguinity. The syndrome without deafness is thought to be transmitted as a dominant trait (Barlow et al., 1964).

Clinical Findings. The syndrome is most commonly seen in females ranging in age from infancy to 12 years of age at the time of onset. Its initial appearance in adult life has also been described (James, 1967). The most common types associated with deafness characteristically developed their initial syncopal attacks in infancy and childhood. They suffered from repeated brief episodes and in many instances experienced a lessening of symptoms with increasing age (Jervell et al., 1966).

Various degrees of syncopal attacks have been observed: 1) episodes without loss of consciousness; 2) those with loss of consciousness and recovery; and 3) those terminating fatally. Mild attacks without loss of consciousness may cause the child to sit quietly, in evident pain, and hold his chest, mimicking an anginal episode.

In the series by Garza et al. (1969), four factors appeared capable of precipitating attacks that ended in death: 1) an increase in systemic blood pressure with pressure-induced extrasystoles; 2) an increase in serum potassium; 3) an early extrasystole (R on T syndrome); and 4) sinus tachycardia when the sinus impulse reaches the ventricles still in a depolarized state.

Electrocardiogram. The electrocardiogram shows characteristic findings. The Q-T interval is prolonged, often to a considerable degree; however, the prolongation may be transient. The Q-T interval is further prolonged by exercise, epinephrine, and quinidine and tends to decrease following digitalization. Sinus pauses have been noted in some cases (James, 1967). The T wave may be abnormal; it may be negative in leads I and aVL, diphasic in the precordial leads, and bizarre, often of considerable amplitude in leads II, III, aVF, V_1, V_2, and V_3. The T waves vary in appearance from one examination to another and usually become more abnormal with exercise.

Therapy. To date, therapy has generally proved to be unsatisfactory. Digitalis has been given to shorten the Q-T interval, but it is doubtful whether it has any actual effect on the other manifestations, and it may prove dangerous because it produces ventricular premature beats (James, 1969). Propranolol has been suggested to suppress the syncopal episodes and appears to be the most effective agent available (Vincent, 1974). Another therapeutic approach is based on the feeling that an abnormal adrenergic mechanism underlies this entity. Thus, canine studies have shown that the Q-T may be prolonged by right stellate gangliectomy or left stellate stimulation. An initial report by Moss et al. indicated that left stellate gangliectomy was beneficial. Sympathomimetic drugs aggravate the condition. A stress-free life is recommended because excitement or fright tends to precipitate the episodes. In addition, exercise has been shown to further prolong the Q-T interval. Because of this association, James has proposed the investigation of drugs known to suppress paroxysmal discharges from the central nervous system as well as to decrease cardiac automaticity, particularly phenobarbital and diphenylhydantoin (James, 1969). Children with repeated syncopal attacks have been treated by pacemaker implantation, but this procedure is relatively unsatisfactory because of the age of the patients and the danger (because of the long Q-T interval) of a pacemaker impulse falling in the vulnerable period.

Prognosis. The prognosis is poor, and sudden death is common. In cases with unimpaired hearing, the prognosis appears to be similar; however, some patients have survived to the fourth or fifth decade.

REFERENCES

Anderson, E. D., Jacobsen, J. R., Sandoe, E., Vibeback, J., and Wennevold, A.: Paroxysmal tachycardia in infancy and childhood. Acta Med. Scand. 62:341, 1973.

Ayers, C. R., Boineau, J. P., and Spach, M. D.: Congenital complete heart block in children. Amer. Heart J. 72:381, 1966.

Barlow, J. B., Bosman, C. K., and Cochrane, J. W. C.: Congenital cardiac arrhythmias. Lancet 2:531, 1964.

Campbell, M., and Emanuel, R.: Six cases of congenital complete heart block followed for 34–40 years. Brit. Heart J. 29:577, 1967.

Cohen, L. S., Samet, P., and Yeh, B. K.: Analysis of A-V conduction in children using His bundle electrograms. Circulation 41–42:III-80, 1970.

El-Said, G., Rosenberg, J. S., Mullins, C. E., et al.: Dysrhythmias after Mustard's operations for transposition of the great arteries. Am. J. Cardiol. 30:526, 1972.

Engle, M. A., and Ehlers, K. H.: Natural history of congenital complete heart block. In Morse, D. P., and Goldberg, H. (eds.): Important Topics in Congenital Valvular and Coronary Artery Disease. Mount Kisco, New York, Futura Publishing Co., 1975, p. 3.

Engle, M. A., and Ehlers, K. H.: Ventricular dysrhythmias. In Morse, D. P., and Goldberg, H. (eds.): Important Topics in Congenital, Valvular and Coronary Artery Disease. Mount Kisco, New York, Futura Publishing Co., 1975, p. 13.

Engle, M. A., and Michaelson, M.: Congenital complete heart block: An international study of the natural history. Cardiovasc. Clin. 4 (3):87, 1972.

Furman, S., and Young, D.: Cardiac pacing in children and adolescents. Am. J. Cardiol. 39:550, 1977.

Garza, L. A., et al.: Familial repolarization myocardiopathy. Amer. J. Cardiol. 23:112, 1969.

Gibson, S.: Auricular fibrillation in childhood and adolescence. J.A.M.A. 117:96, 1941.

Gleckler, W. J., and Lay, J. V. M.: Wolff-Parkinson-White syndrome and paroxysmal tachycardia in infancy. J.A.M.A. 150:683, 1952.

Godman, M. J., Roberts, N. K., and Izukawa, T.: Late postoperative conduction disturbances after repair of ventricular septal defect and tetralogy of Fallot. Analysis of His bundle recordings. Circulation 49:214, 1974.

Hofschire, P. J., Nicoloff, D. M., and Moller, J. H.: Postoperative complete heart block in 64 children treated with and without cardiac pacing. Am. J. Cardiol. 39:559, 1977.

Hougen, T. J., Dick, M. II, Freed, M. D., and Keane, J. F.: His bundle electrogram after intracardiac repair of tetralogy of Fallot: Analysis of data in 59 patients. Am. J. Cardiol. 41:552, 1978.

Ikkos, D., and Hanson, J. S.: Response to exercise in congenital complete atrioventricular block. Circulation 22:583, 1960.

James, T. N.: Congenital deafness and cardiac arrhythmias. Amer. J. Cardiol. 19:627, 1967.

James, T. N.: QT prolongation and sudden death. Mod Conc. Cardiovasc. Dis. 38:35, 1969.

James, T. N.: Sudden death of babies. Circulation 53:1, 1976.

Jervell, A., and Lange-Nielsen, F.: Congenital deaf-mutism, functional heart disease with prolongation of the Q-T interval and sudden death. Amer. Heart J. 54:59, 1957.

Jervell, A., Thingstad, R., and Endsjo, T.: The surdo-cardiac syndrome. Three new cases of congenital deafness with syncopal attacks and Q-T prolongation in the electrocardiogram. Amer. Heart J. 72:582, 1966.

Keane, J. F., Plauth, W. J., Jr., and Nadas, A. S.: Chronic ectopic tachycardia of infancy and childhood. Am. Heart J. 84:748, 1972.

Keith, J. D., Rowe, R. D., and Vlad, P.: Heart Disease in Infancy and Childhood. 2nd ed., New York, Macmillan, 1967, pp. 1049–1075.

Kelly, D. T., Brodsky, S. J., and Krovetz, L. J.: Mobitz-type II atrioventricular block in children. J. Pediatr. 79:972, 1971.

Kendall, B., Farrell, D. M., and Kane, H. A.: Fetal radioelectrocardiography: A new method of fetal electrocardiography. Amer. J. Obstet. Gynec. 83:1629, 1962.

Krongrad, E., Hefler, S. E., Bowman, F. O., Malm, J. R., and Hoffman, B. F.: Further observations on the etiology of right bundle branch block pattern following right ventriculotomy. Circulation 50:1105, 1974.

Lambert, E. C., Menon, V. A., Wagner, H. R., and Vlad, P.: Sudden unexpected death from cardiovascular disease in children. Am. J. Cardiol. 34:89, 1974.

Lie, J. T., Rosenberg, H. S., and Erickson, E. E.: Histopathology of the conduction system in the sudden infant death syndrome. Circulation 53:3, 1976.

Lundberg, A.: Neonatal asphyxia with atrial flutter. Acta Pediatr. 52:531, 1963.

Lundberg, A.: Paroxysmal tachycardia in infancy: followup study of 47 subjects ranging in age from 10–26 years. Pediatrics 51:26, 1973.

Moller, J. H., Davachi, F., and Anderson, R. C.: Atrial flutter in infancy. J. Pediatr. 75:643, 1969.

Morgan, B. D., and Guntheroth, W. B.: Cardiac arrhythmias in normal newborn infants. J. Pediatr. 67:1199, 1965.

Nakamura, F. F., and Nadas, A. S.: Complete heart block in infants and children. N. Engl. J. Med. 270:1261, 1964.

Nugent, E. W., Varghese, P. J., and Rowe, R. D.: Sluggish sinus node syndrome in children after open heart surgery for acyanotic congenital heart disease. Pediatr. Res. 7:298, 1973.

Paul, M. H.: Cardiac arrhythmias in infants and children. Prog. Cardiovasc. Dis. 9:136, 1966.

Quattlebaum, T. G., Varghese, J., Neill, C. A., and Donahoo, J. S.: Sudden death among postoperative patients with tetralogy of Fallot. Circulation 54:289, 1976.

Rackow, H., Salanitre, E., and Green, L. T.: Frequency of cardiac arrest associated with anesthesia in infants and children. Pediatrics 28:697, 1961.

Rodriguez-Coronel, A., Seublingvong, V., and Hastreiter, A. R.: Clinical forms of atrial flutter in infancy. J. Pediatr. 73:69, 1968.

Roy, P. R., Emanuel, R., Ismail, S. A., and El Tayib, M. H.: Hereditary prolongation of the Q-T interval. Am. J. Cardiol. 37:237, 1976.

Steeg, C. N., Krongrad, E., Davachi, F., Bowman, F. O., Malm, J. R., and Gersony, W. M.: Postoperative left anterior hemiblock and right bundle branch block following repair of tetralogy of Fallot. Circulation 51(6):1026, 1975.

Urbach, J. R., Zweizig, H. Z., Loveland, M. W., and Lambert, R. L.: Monitoring of fetal and neonatal arrhythmias. In Dreifus, L. S., Likoff, W., and Moyer, J. H. (eds.): Mechanisms and Therapy of Cardiac Arrhythmias. New York, Grune and Stratton, 1966.

Valdes-Dapena, M. A.: Sudden and unexpected death in infancy. A review of the world literature, 1954–1966. Pediatrics 39:123, 1967.

Vincent, G. M., Abidskov, J. A., and Burgess, M. J.: QT interval syndromes. Prog. Cardiovasc. Dis. 16:523, 1974.

White, R. I., Jr., and Humphries, J. O.: Direct current electroshock in the treatment of supraventricular arrhythmias. J. Pediatr. 70:119, 1967.

Wolff, G. S., Han, J., and Curran, J.: Wolff-Parkinson-White syndrome in the neonate. Am. J. Cardiol. 41:559, 1978. (Reports 8/16 with PSVT in neonate 8 had WPW type A).

18

DIGITALIS

VIDYA S. BANKA, M.D.
RICHARD H. HELFANT, M.D.

Since the original observations of William Withering two centuries ago, digitalis has been one of the most commonly used cardiotonic drugs. Digoxin was the fifth most common drug prescribed by physicians in the United States in 1971 (National Prescription Audit). In spite of a continuing uncertainty regarding the mechanism of action at the cellular level, digitalis is clearly an important therapeutic agent in the treatment of some arrhythmias as well as congestive heart failure. Since the margin of safety between therapeutic doses and toxic doses is relatively small, digitalis toxicity has been a frequent problem in therapy. In fact, several arrhythmias can be related specifically to digitalis toxicity.

PHARMACOKINETICS

Sources and Chemistry

The most commonly used cardiac glycosides are obtained from the leaves of the foxglove plants *Digitalis purpurea, Digitalis lanata* and *Strophanthus gratus* (Table 18–1). Cardiac glycosides are also present in the venom found in the skin glands of toads.

The basic chemical structure of cardiac glycosides (Figure 18–1) is characterized by the presence of 1) a steroid (cyclo-pentanoperhydrophenanthrene ring), 2) a lactone ring attached at position C_{17} of the steroid nucleus, and 3) a sugar moiety (digitoxose). The first two components of the chemical structure (i.e., the steroid nucleus and the lactone ring) form an aglycone or genin, which is mainly responsible for the pharmacologic activity of the cardiac glycoside. The sugars (digitoxose) have no intrinsic pharmacologic activity but they enhance the activity of the aglycone by increasing solubility or enhancing the ability of the drug to penetrate the cell membrane.

The most commonly used preparations are digoxin, digitoxin, lanatoside C (Cedilanid) and ouabain.

TABLE 18–1

Preparations
Digitalis purpurea
Digitoxin
Gitalin
Digitalis leaf
Digitalis lanata
Digoxin
Deslanoside
Lanatoside C
Strophanthus gratus
Strophanthin
Ouabain

255

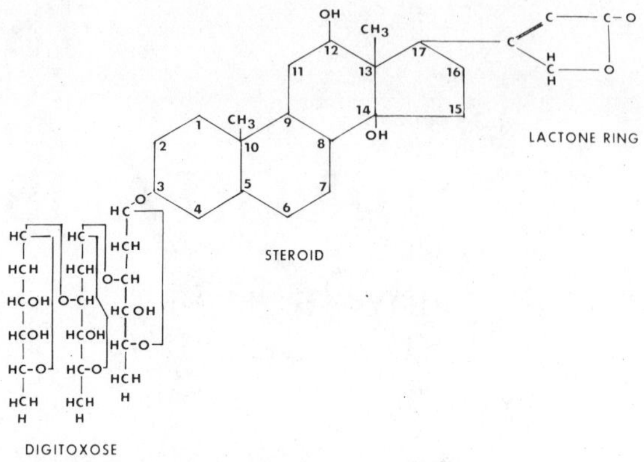

Figure 18–1 Structural formula for cardiac glycosides.

Absorption, Metabolism, and Excretion

The absorption, metabolism, and excretion of the digitalis glycosides have been extensively studied using radioactive tracer methods (Doherty, 1968, 1973). When administered orally, *digoxin* is 80 to 85 per cent absorbed from the gastrointestinal tract. The major site of absorption is the small intestine, although some gastric absorption is also reported (Hall and Doherty, 1971). The enterohepatic recycling of digoxin is only 6.8 per cent (Doherty et al., 1970). The dominant half life is approximately 33 hours. Regardless of the route of administration, the major excretory pathway for digoxin is renal, with much smaller amounts being recovered in the feces. Of the total body dose of digoxin, 33 per cent is excreted per day, 30 per cent as digoxin and 3 per cent as its metabolites (Doherty and Perkins, 1962).

Digitoxin is almost 100 per cent absorbed from the gastrointestinal tract. It is metabolized to cardio-inactive compounds before being excreted in the urine. Its enterohepatic recycling is fourfold higher than digoxin, approximately 26 per cent of digitoxin being recycled through the enterohepatic circulation. The dominant half life of digitoxin is considerably longer than that of digoxin. The radioactive serum turnover rates parallel the 4 to 6 day physiologic half times estimated by systolic time intervals (Weissler et al., 1966). Nearly 8 per cent of digitoxin is ultimately metabolized to digoxin. When drugs such as phenylbutazone or phenobarbital are administered along with digitoxin, there results an increased production of digoxin and thus the half life is considerably shortened (Solomon et al., 1971). Since digitoxin is principally excreted in the urine as cardio-inactive metabolites, it has been proposed as the preferred drug for patients with renal failure (Rasmussen et al., 1972). However, it has recently been demonstrated that in the presence of renal failure, increasing amounts of digitoxin are metabolized to digoxin, and thus the half life of digitoxin is somewhat shortened by augmentation of the metabolic pathway (Sorstein, 1973).

Factors That Alter Absorption, Metabolism, and Excretion

Several factors should be considered in the administration of digitalis glycosides.

Renal Failure. Several investigators (Doherty et al., 1964; Marcus et al., 1966; Bloom et al., 1966) have studied tritiated digoxin turnover in human subjects with renal failure and demonstrated reduced renal excretion, increased serum levels, and prolonged serum half life of digoxin without a compensatory increase in stool excretion. It has thus been proposed that the presence of renal failure is a major factor that leads to digitalis toxicity. It was observed that in patients with renal failure, the half life of the digoxin was approximately three times that in patients with congestive heart failure alone (Doherty et al., 1964). The ratio of digoxin clearance to creatinine clearance is approximately 1:1. Thus, with decreased creatinine clearance, digoxin clearance is proportionately decreased. Similarly, the higher the levels of blood urea nitrogen, the lower the digoxin clearance. The half life varies from 1.5 to 5.2 days, depending upon the degree of renal damage. (Neither hemodialysis nor peritoneal dialysis is capable of correcting digitalis toxicity in patients with renal failure, because neither can effectively alter the tissue digitalis concentrations.) The use of digitalis in a uremic patient is thus complex, and several calculations for administration of digoxin and digitoxin have been proposed (Jelliffe and Brooker, 1974). However, from a practical standpoint, approximately 41 per cent of the standard maintenance dose of digoxin can be administered to an anuric patient. When the creatinine clearance is diminished by 75 per cent, it is usually safe to administer 50 per cent of the regular maintenance dose of digoxin (Jelliffe and Blankenhorn, 1967).

Hepatic Failure. The excretion and half life of digoxin and digitoxin have been studied in patients with severely compromised liver function (Marcus and Kapadia, 1964; Okita, 1964). Since the excretion and half life of digoxin are not modified in the presence of severe liver dysfunction, no modification in dose is necessary. Because of significant extrahepatic metabolism, the same is true for digitoxin.

Thyroid Disease. Clinical observations have suggested that patients with hypothyroidism are sensitive to digitalis, while those with hyperthyroidism are resistant to the effects of digitalis. Experimental studies in the dog, however, do not show a significant difference in the digitalis uptake of the heart in hypothyroid, hyperthyroid, and euthyroid states (Doherty, 1968). Clinical observations indicate that patients with hyperthyroidism have lower serum levels of digitalis than those who are euthyroid (Doherty and Perkins, 1966). Smaller dosages are recommended if digitalization is indicated in patients with myxedema, while patients with hyperthyroidism require larger doses. This is particularly pertinent to patients who develop atrial fibrillation because of hyperthyroidism. It is difficult to control the ventricular response with digitalization alone, even though larger doses are administered, unless hyperthyroidism is corrected by antithyroid drugs. Propranolol is a useful adjunct in such patients.

Pulmonary Heart Disease (Chronic Cor Pulmonale). The tritiated digoxin turnover and excretion times in patients with pulmonary heart disease appear to be normal. However, clinically it has been observed that these patients are more sensitive to digitalis and develop digitalis toxicity more frequently. This may be attributed to 1) associated abnormalities of pH and/or electrolytes, 2) red cell mass, and 3) hypoxia and hypothermia that are frequently observed in patients with chronic cor pulmonale.

Malabsorption. Patients with malabsorption syndromes have impaired gastrointestinal absorption of digitoxin and digoxin. Heizer et al. (1971) reported faulty absorption of digoxin, necessitating large overdoses of the drug in patients with sprue. However, malabsorption related to pancreatic insufficiency does not affect digoxin absorption. The bioavailability of oral digoxin was not impaired in any of these patients who underwent jejunoileal bypass surgery (Marcus et al, 1977).

Electrolyte Disturbances. Electrolyte imbalance plays a major role in predisposing patients to digitalis toxicity (see Chapter 19). Hypokalemia, which often is produced by the concomitant use of diuretics, sensitizes the heart to digitalis intoxication (Steiness and Olesen, 1976). Increased sensitivity to digitalis consequent to potassium depletion frequently follows dialysis, steroid intake, diarrhea, and vomiting, and often occurs in renal disease. Conversely, *hyperkalemia* inhibits myocardial binding of digitalis and protects against digitalis toxicity.

Hypomagnesemia increases myocardial uptake of digoxin and sensitizes the heart to digitalis. Treatment with magnesium sulfate has been shown to suppress digitalis induced arrhythmias that are unresponsive to potassium therapy.

Calcium and digitalis have a synergistic effect on automaticity. At high serum calcium concentration (15 mEq/L) arrhythmias due to digitalis toxicity are produced with lower doses of digitalis (60–70% of control) than when serum calcium levels are within normal limits. Thus, the combination of these factors results in a summation effect: toxic effects may result from this combination (Nola et al., 1970).

Age. It is well recognized that older patients are more sensitive to digitalis than younger individuals. This is primarily due to renal function and the glomerular filtration rate. Since the glomerular filtration rate decreases with age, the serum levels of digitalis remain higher in older individuals, and thus these patients develop signs of digitalis toxicity more frequently.

Obesity. If the dosage of digoxin is calculated for body weight, it may be erroneously high in obese patients. Ewy et al. (1971) studied the serum concentration of digoxin after a single dose in five patients who had a mean loss of 102 pounds in weight. The serum digoxin concentrations were similar before and after weight reduction. It was thus concluded that fat free body weight is a more important determinant of blood digoxin concentration

than total body weight. Very low concentrations of tritiated digoxin have been found in the adipose tissue of man. Thus, the digitalis requirement of an obese patient is similar to that of a patient with relatively normal weight.

Drug Interaction. Concomitant use of other drugs may affect the pharmacokinetics of or sensitivity to digitalis. Pentobarbital, phenylbutazone, and phenytoin increase beta-hydroxylation of digitoxin, resulting in decreased plasma concentration and shortened plasma half life. One should also consider the concomitant use of diuretics, laxatives, insulin, salicylates, and steroids, which may cause hypokalemia and thus make a patient more digitalis sensitive. Recent studies indicate that concomitant use of quinidine and digoxin results in a decrease in total body and renal clearance of digoxin, with a resultant increase of serum digoxin concentrations (Hager et al., 1979). Quinidine probably causes displacement of digoxin from binding sites in the tissues. Use of neomycin may inhibit digoxin absorption to a modest degree, and thus higher dosages of digoxin may have to be administered. Caution should also be advised in withdrawing thyroid extract (see above).

Dosage and Administration

Administration of digitalis is carried out in two stages. Initial digitalization establishes body stores of the drug that are associated with its therapeutic effect. Subsequently, doses are given at regular intervals, the amount of each being adjusted to increase, maintain, or decrease the body glycoside stores as appropriate for each patient. The digitalizing dose varies considerably in different individuals (Table 18–2). The time course of onset and maximal effect also varies markedly for the different digitalis glycosides (Figure 18–2). Following initial digitalization, the patient is placed on a maintenance dose that will maintain relatively constant body

TABLE 18-2 DOSAGE SCHEDULES FOR DIGITALIS PREPARATIONS

Drug	Full Digitalization Dose Intravenously (Orally)	Daily Maintenance Dose
For Adults		
Digitalis Leaf	3 to 5 U.S.P. units (digalen)* (15 U.S.P. units; 1.3 gm.)	½ to 2 U.S.P. units (¾ to 3 gr.) (45 to 180 mg.)
Digitoxin	1.2 to 1.6 mg. (1.2 to 1.6 mg.)	0.05 to 0.2 mg.
Digoxin	0.75–1.5 mg. (1.5–3.0 mg.)	0.25 to 0.75 mg.
Desacetyl-lanatoside C (Cedilanid-D)	1.2–1.6 mg.	
Lanatoside C (Cedilanid)	1.2–1.6 mg. (5–10 mg.)	0.5 to 1.2 mg.
Gitalin	(5.5–6.0 mg.)	0.4 mg.
Ouabain	0.5 to 1.0 mg.	
For Children	**Dosage for Total Digitalization**	
Digitoxin	Digitoxin group—0.01 to 0.02 mg./lb. body weight, I.M., I.V. or orally.	
Digoxin	Orally: 0.02 to 0.03 mg./lb. I.M., or 0.01 to 0.02 mg./lb. I.V.	
Lanatoside A-B-C	0.01 to 0.02 mg./lb. I.M. or I.V.	
Strophanthin	.005 to .007 mg./lb. I.V.	
Ouabain	.003 to .006 mg./lb. I.V. (½ total dose) followed by $\frac{1}{10}$ of total dose every ½ hr. for five doses.	

*Not usually given by vein.

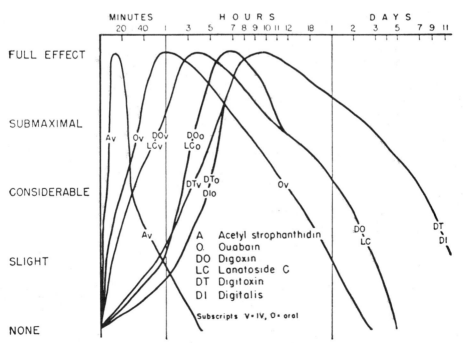

Figure 18-2 Approximate curves of accumulation and decline of the biological effects of single doses of cardioactive preparations in man. The curves of orally administered gitalin (amorphous) and of acetyl digitoxin, if plotted, would fall between those of oral digoxin and of oral digitoxin. (Kay, courtesy of Circulation.)

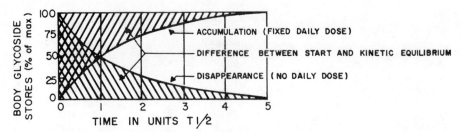

Figure 18-3 Cumulation of glycoside on a fixed daily dose, compared with disappearance of glycoside after therapy is stopped (1). Time is shown in units of drug half-life (T½). (From Jelliffe, R. W., et al., Ann. Intern. Med., 72:253, 1970.)

stores of digitalis (Figure 18–3). The duration of action of digitalis preparations is shown in Table 18–3.

There is no precise method of determining the proper digitalizing dose except in patients with atrial fibrillation. When a glycoside is administered to control the ventricular response in this arrhythmia, the maximal therapeutic effect is said to be obtained when the apical rate drops to about 70 per minute with elimination of the pulse deficit. Determining the optimal digitalizing and maintenance doses in patients with normal sinus rhythm is much more difficult.

Studies by Marcus and co-workers (1966) have indicated that a "loading" dose of digitalis is not really essential in patients in whom an immediate therapeutic effect is not required. They demonstrated that digoxin given as a daily dose without an initial loading dose would accumulate until a steady state

was reached in five to seven days. This pattern of glycoside accumulation is due to the pattern of drug elimination characterized by the excretion of a percentage of the daily amount of the body stores rather than excretion of a constant amount each day. Since approximately 33 per cent of the total body stores of digoxin are excreted per day, if 0.25 mg of digoxin is fully absorbed and one third of the accumulated dose is excreted daily, the amount remaining in the body at the end of the day is 0.17 mg. After the second dose of 0.25 mg, the total body load is 0.42 mg. One third of this amount is excreted during the next day, leaving a total body store of 0.28 mg. By these repetitive calculations, it is evident that a steady state is soon reached, characterized by an excretion equal to the drug absorption and reflected by a plateau of serum levels (Marcus, 1975). This concept of digitalization over a period of 5 to 7

TABLE 18-3   DURATION OF ACTION OF DIGITALIS PREPARATIONS

	Speed of Action			Duration of Action After Full Digitalization (days)
Drug	I.V.	Oral (hours)	Absorption (per cent)	
Whole leaf digitalis	–	12–24	20	14–21
Digitoxin	–	12–24	90–100	14–21
Digoxin	¼–1 hr.	2–6	70–85	3–5
Lanatoside C	10–30 min.	1–4	40	3–5
Ouabain	10–30 min.	–	–	1–2

In most arrhythmias, the rapidly acting forms, digoxin or lanatoside C, are used to bring the patient out of critical state. The longer-acting preparations may be used for maintenance therapy.

days without a loading dose has decreased the incidence of digitalis toxicity considerably.

Digitalis preparations can be administered orally, intramuscularly, or intravenously. The mode of administration is dependent upon the urgency of the situation. Doherty et al. (1968) studied serum levels of tritiated digoxin when administered orally, intramuscularly, and intravenously. By oral administration (in an alcoholic solution) the peak serum levels were obtained at 30 to 60 minutes and digoxin levels were demonstrable 6 minutes after administration. Intramuscular administration of the labeled glycoside produced peak serum concentrations later than did oral administration. However, tritiated digoxin was noted to produce a high early serum concentration and an earlier plateau when given intravenously than when given by either the oral or intramuscular route. With intravenous administration the tissue distribution and binding of the glycoside had a half time of 30 minutes compared to 50 minutes with oral administration.

Myocardial Effects

The salutary hemodynamic effects produced by digitalis glycosides in congestive heart failure result primarily from their direct effect on myocardial contractility. Studies of isolated muscle preparations have indicated that the glycoside can produce a positive inotropic effect before any evidence of failure is obtained. The positive inotropic effect is due to direct action of cardiac glycosides on the myocardial cells and can be demonstrated in the denervated heart, in the catecholamine depleted heart, and in the failing and non-failing heart. Braunwald and co-workers (1961) studied the effect of acute digitalization on the force of contractions of the non-failing human ventricle during cardiopulmonary bypass and showed increased

contractility in all patients. Evidence for a positive inotropic effect of digitalis in the non-failing human heart at cardiac catheterization has also been demonstrated (Sonnenblick et al., 1966). Experimentally, Banka et al. (1975) have shown that the inotropic effect increases progressively with increasing doses until toxic arrhythmias appear. Further suppression of arrhythmias with potassium, diphenylhydantoin, or sequential atrio-His bundle pacing allows still further increase in inotropy (Williams, et al., 1966; Helfant et al., 1967; Banka et al., 1975). The mechanism responsible for the positive inotropic effect of cardiac glycosides is not fully understood. Calcium apparently plays a major role. Many studies have demonstrated the effect of cardiac glycosides on calcium flux as well as on the uptake and release of calcium from subcellular structures (Smith and Haber, 1973; Schwartz et al., 1975; Fozzard, 1977). The relation between this effect and positive inotropism, however, has not been definitely established (Rhee et al., 1976). Data have also been presented suggesting that the positive inotropic effect and the inhibition of Na^+-K^+ ATPase may be an independent phenomenon. It is generally accepted that digitalis is a specific inhibitor of the sodium-potassium activated ATPase located primarily in the sarcolemmal membrane. Present evidence supports the concept that positive inotropic effects of digitalis are not seen unless inhibition of the enzyme and, therefore, of the sodium pump leads to a small increase of intracellular sodium. This leads to augmented activity of a sodium transport system that is coupled not to potassium but to calcium. Evidence for the existence of Na^+-Ca^{++} coupling at excitable membranes is accumulating. The possibility exists that digitalis induced inhibition of the Na^+-K^+ coupled system produces an increase in Na^+-Ca^{++} coupled transport and, thereby, an increase of influx of calcium to the myofilament, thereby increasing contractility (Langer, 1972).

Effect on Autonomic Nervous System

Studies in the denervated human heart have confirmed previous experimental observations in animals, indicating that the indirect action of digitalis on the sympathetic and parasympathetic nervous system influences its pharmacologic actions. Vagal activity is augmented both by central stimulation of the vagus nerve and by sensitization of the cardiac cells to the action of digitalis. Its effects on the sympathetic nervous system appear more complex. Digitalis in lower doses increases the sensitivity of the carotid sinus baroreceptors, thus, enhancing vagal tone and reducing sympathetic activity. Large doses of digitalis, however, increase central sympathetic outflow and may release endogenous catecholamines.

Electrophysiologic Effects

A knowledge of the electrophysiologic effects of therapeutic concentrations of digitalis is important to the understanding of its clinical role in various arrhythmias. The direct effects of digitalis in therapeutic concentrations on the sinoatrial node are minimal (Gillis et al., 1975). In the innervated heart, the slowing of sinus rate by digitalis is mediated mainly through its vagotonic effects as well as through the decrease in sympathetic tone. The latter effect is important subsequent to improvement in the failing heart. The effects on atrial tissue include a decrease in resting transmembrane potential, a decreased maximal rate of rise of phase zero of the sodium dependent action potential (V max), depressed conduction velocity, and a prolonged effective refractory period (ERP) (Rosen et al., 1975). These effects may be counterbalanced by the induced vagotonia and increased sensitivity of the atrial tissue to acetylcholine. Thus, as a net result, there may be no significant change or a shortening of the effective refractory period and increase of intra-atrial conduction. This effect is responsible for the clinically observed increase in atrial rate in patients with atrial flutter after digitalization. Vagal stimulation may enhance the temporal dispersion of atrial repolarization, thereby favoring the development of atrial fibrillation or conversion of atrial flutter to fibrillation (Abildskov, 1975).

The most important therapeutic effects of digitalis in patients with atrial flutter or atrial fibrillation result from its effects on the A-V node. Digitalis impedes conduction through the A-V node by decreasing conduction velocity and prolonging both effective and functional refractory periods. Since the impedance in conduction through the A-V node occurs at drug concentrations that have no effect on the A-V nodal action potential, it seems to result from a change in autonomic activity (i.e., vagotonia and withdrawal of sympathetic tone) (Toda and West, 1969). In the denervated transplanted heart, therapeutic digitalis concentrations cause only insignificant prolongation of the effective and functional recovery period (Goodman et al., 1975). Although digitalis increases the effective refractory period of the normal A-V node, the effective refractory period in the anomalous A-V pathways is decreased. Thus, it may preferentially facilitate conduction through the anomalous pathway in patients with Wolff-Parkinson-White syndrome, resulting in a potentially catastrophic ventricular response during atrial fibrillation (Wellens and Durrer, 1973).

The effects of digitalis on Purkinje fibers and ventricular muscle are variable. Low concentrations appear to cause a decrease in membrane potassium conductance and thus produce a small but variable prolongation of repolarization. Higher concentrations result in increased potassium conductance and acceleration of repolarization. The latter effect has, however, been considered toxic rather than therapeutic. Therapeutic concentrations of digitalis do not alter the refractoriness of the His-Purkinje system (Przybyla et al.,

1974). Isolated canine Purkinje fibers show an increase in the action potential duration that can be correlated with the electrocardiographic ST-T wave changes.

Although ouabain can enhance phase 4 depolarization in Purkinje fibers, thereby enhancing automaticity, it can also set the stage for triggered arrhythmias (Cranefield, 1977). It has been shown that the action potentials of Purkinje fibers exposed to ouabain develop delayed after-depolarization (Davis, 1973; Rosen et al., 1973; Ferrier and Moe, 1973). A premature impulse enhances the amplitude of after-depolarization and can bring the after-depolarization to threshold, causing a single premature beat or initiating a burst of non-driven premature impulses (Cranefield and Aronson, 1974; Ferrier et al., 1973). The amplitude of these delayed after-depolarizations increases with increasing calcium and decreasing potassium (Ferrier and Moe, 1973).

INDICATIONS FOR THE USE OF DIGITALIS IN TREATMENT OF ARRHYTHMIAS

Digitalis exerts the following major effects in the therapy of arrhythmias: 1) direct depression of A-V conduction, 2) reflex increase in vagal tone and decrease in sympathetic tone, and 3) inotropic effects. The combination of these effects is seen in the effect of digitalis on the S-A node, atrial muscle, and A-V junction. Since few or no vagal fibers are present in the human ventricle, the ventricular effects are usually considered solely the results of a direct action.

Digitalis is indicated in the treatment of supraventricular arrhythmias accompanied by rapid ventricular response, particularly in the presence of atrial fibrillation, atrial flutter, and supraventricular tachycardia (Figs. 18–4 and 18–5). Chronic atrial fibrillation or flutter is seldom reverted to sinus rhythm but the ventricular rate may be reduced by increased concealed conduction into the A-V node, decreased conduction velocity, and prolonged effective refractory period of the A-V node. Digitalis may also be of help in the treatment of ventricular premature beats accompanied by or resulting from congestive heart failure. Digitalis therapy is not, however, indicated in patients with ventricular tachycardia. The relative indications and contraindications to digitalis with respect to individual arrhythmia are discussed in greater detail in Chapter 23.

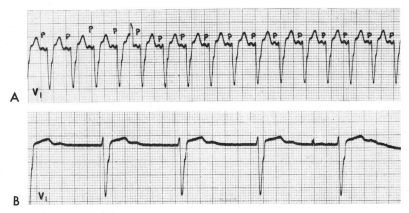

Figure 18–4 Effect of digitalis therapy in paroxysmal atrial tachycardia. (A) (V₁). Note the supraventricular tachycardia (rate 160 per minute). (B) *After digitalization,* note the presence of an A-V junctional rhythm with a rate of 47 per minute. The P waves are not observed; these may be buried in the QRS complexes(?). This probably denotes evidence of slight toxicity.

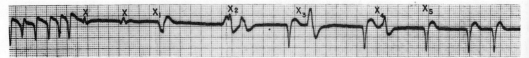

Figure 18–5 Atrial fibrillation with rapid ventricular rate (250 per minute): marked slowing after digitalis (lead III). Atrial fibrillation with a rapid ventricular rate is present in the initial part of the strip. Following the administration of Cedilanid (1.6 mg. in two divided doses given over a period of three hours), note the resumption of slow ventricular beating. Note the aberrant beats at X, X_1, and X_2 and the coupled beats at X_3 and X_4 as evidence of digitalis toxicity. Premature beats are absent at end of strip starting with X_5.

DIGITALIS TOXICITY

The diagnosis and treatment of digitalis toxicity continues to be one of the most frequent cardiac problems. The prevalence of digitalis toxicity in a hospital population has been reported variously from 7 per cent to 22 per cent (Sodeman, 1965; Rodensky, 1964). In a study reported by Beller et al. (1971), 15 per cent of all patients at Boston City Hospital admitted to the medical service were taking digitalis, and the prevalence of digitalis toxicity in these patients was 20 to 30 per cent. Many factors contribute to the development of digitalis toxicity, relating both to excessive digitalis accumulation (particularly in the heart) and to increased myocardial sensitization to digitalis (Table 18–4). Excessive digitalis accumulation may, on occasion, reflect an excessive dose, but more commonly it is due to diminished excretion.

Manifestations

The manifestations of digitalis toxicity are variable and can be conveniently divided into extra-cardiac and cardiac manifestations (Table 18–5). The classic extra-cardiac manifestations of digitalis toxicity include *anorexia*, nausea, vomiting, and diarrhea as well as *visual disturbances*. Lely and Van Enter (1970) have reported that loss of visual acuity (rather than yellow or green vision), *fatigue*, and weakness are major noncardiac symptoms of digitalis toxicity. In addition, psychic symptoms and headache have also been reported. These extra-cardiac effects are not life-threatening and, while frequently associated with more serious cardiotoxic effects of the drug, are by no means an

TABLE 18–4   FACTORS PREDISPOSING TO THE DEVELOPMENT OF DIGITALIS TOXICITY

Excessive accumulation
  High dosage
  Diminished excretion
    Renal disease
    Old age

Increased myocardial sensitivity
  Type of heart disease
    Myocardial ischemia
    Severe myocardial failure
    Acute or chronic cor pulmonale
    Cyanotic congenital heart disease

Electrolyte imbalance
  Hypokalemia
  Hypomagnesemia
  Hypocalcemia

Blood gas abnormalities
  Hypoxia
  Alkalosis

Metabolic disease
  Hypothyroidism

Autonomic nervous system abnormality
  Vagotonia
  Increased sympathetic tone

Drug interactions
  Catecholamines
  Reserpine
  Quinidine

High energy electrical current

Cardiopulmonary bypass

TABLE 18–5   MANIFESTATIONS OF DIGITALIS TOXICITY

	Common	Uncommon
Cardiac	Bradycardia, S-A block, sinus arrhythmias, all degrees of A-V block (sometimes with paroxysmal tachycardia), A-V junctional rhythm (including premature beats, coupled ventricular premature beats, and paroxysmal tachycardia)	Atrial fibrillation, atrial flutter, ventricular tachycardia and fibrillation, complete A-V heart block
Arrhythmias that have a high probability of being caused by digitalis toxicity	Multifocal ventricular premature beats, A-V junctional tachycardia, A-V dissociation, PAT with block	
Extracardiac		
Gastrointestinal	Anorexia, nausea, vomiting	Diarrhea
Visual	Alterations in color perception, scotomata, blurring, shimmering, micropsia, macropsia	Amblyopia
Neurologic	Headache, fatigue, insomnia, depression	Convulsions, delirium
Allergic	None	Urticaria, eosinophilia
Endocrine	None	Gynecomastia

invariable accompaniment. Although these effects frequently appear earlier than the cardiotoxicity, this does not pertain to all patients and cardiotoxicity may present as a sole manifestation.

Cardiac Toxicity

Cardiotoxic effects are potentially dangerous and can be fatal. However, serious toxicity can be avoided if digitalis therapy is carefully monitored. Cardiac toxicity can be divided into increasing *heart failure* and rhythm disturbances. Although clinical studies have suggested that aggravation of heart failure may occur even without the emergence of serious arrhythmias or the development of conduction defects, the mechanism of this observation is not fully understood. Experimentally, digitalis has a positive inotropic effect even in toxic doses (Banka et al., 1975). These studies, in fact, indicate that with continued digitalis infusion in toxic doses the positive inotropic effect of digitalis pre-exists until the onset of ventricular fibrillation (Williams et al., 1966; Helfant et al., 1967; Banka et al., 1975). Lown and Levine (1954) postulated subendocardial myocardial ischemia as a cause, but careful histologic studies in man have failed to substantiate this thesis.

The most serious consequence of digitalis intoxication is *cardiac arrhythmia*. The arrythmias induced by digitalis intoxication can be divided into 1) tachyarrhythmias due to either enhanced

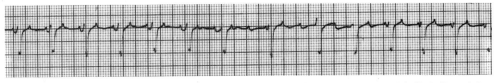

Figure 18–6   Rhythm strip showing atrial tachycardia with block in a patient with digitalis toxicity. The first seven beats show 2:1 A-V conduction. The last seven beats demonstrate high grade A-V block.

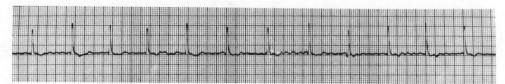

Figure 18–7   Rhythm strip showing atrial fibrillation with regularization of R-R intervals indicating non-paroxysmal junctional tachycardia as evidence of digitalis toxicity.

automaticity or re-entry, or both (atrial tachycardia with block, non-paroxysmal junctional tachycardia, ventricular premature complexes, ventricular tachycardia, ventricular flutter and fibrillation, bidirectional ventricular tachycardia, multiple ectopic rhythms; 2) depression of conductivity (type I first, second, or third degree A-V block); 3) depression of pacemakers (sinus bradycardia); 4) depression of conduction with ectopic pacemakers; 5) A-V dissociation due to either suppression of dominant pacemaker with escape of a subsidiary pacemaker or an inappropriate acceleration of a lower pacemaker (Fisch and Knoebel, 1970).

Although any type of arrhythmia can occur in patients with digitalis toxicity, some of the specific rhythm disturbances need special mention.

ATRIAL TACHYCARDIA WITH BLOCK

Atrial tachycardia with block is a classic digitalis toxic arrhythmia. This arrhythmia is caused by digitalis toxicity in 70 per cent of cases. However, it is less common than other forms of ectopic tachycardias induced by digitalis and, in particular, less common than non-paroxysmal junctional tachycardia (Dreifus et al., 1963; Soffer, 1962). In other patients it may be due to hypokalemia or the patient's own underlying heart disease and not to digitalis. These patients may benefit from administration of digitalis. The atrial rate varies from 150 to 230 per minute, with characteristic small P waves in the limb leads separated by an isoelectric line

(Fig. 18–6). The P-P interval is either constant or variable, and premature ventricular systoles are frequently seen.

NON-PAROXYSMAL JUNCTIONAL TACHYCARDIA

Non-paroxysmal junctional tachycardia also bears a definite relationship to digitalis toxicity (Pick and Dominguez, 1957; Pick et al., 1961; Dreifus et al., 1961). This arrhythmia, particularly seen in the presence of atrial fibrillation, is highly specific for digitalis toxicity (Fig. 18–7). Other conditions in which non-paroxysmal junctional tachycardia may occur are open heart surgery, inferior myocardial infarction, and, rarely, myocarditis and certain anesthetics (Fisch et al., 1969). Non-paroxysmal junctional tachycardia is a form of A-V dissociation due to acceleration of the lower (in this case junctional) pacemaker. It differs from paroxysmal junctional tachycardia in that it exhibits only a modest acceleration of the ventricular rate, usually between 70 and 130 beats per minute, and that it lacks a sudden onset or termination. It may co-exist with sinus rhythm, atrial tachycardia, atrial fibrillation, or flutter. In the absence of an exit block, the ventricular rate in non-paroxysmal junctional tachycardia is absolutely regular and the diagnosis is not difficult. If the degree of exit block is constant, the result may be a slow junctional rate, in which case an erroneous diagnosis of passive escape rhythm rather than an accelerated tachycardia will be made.

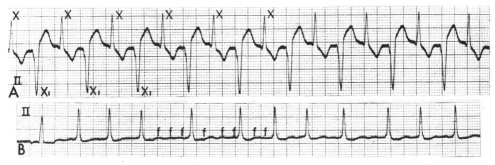

Figure 18–8 Junctional tachycardia (bidirectional type) resulting from toxic digitalis effects.

(*A*) Note that the upwardly directed deflection (X) has a relatively narrow QRS measuring 0.08 second. The downwardly directed complexes (X₁) have a slightly wider QRS width measuring 0.12 second. Note that the rhythm of the upwardly directed complexes is entirely regular at 75 per minute, and the same is true of the downwardly directed complexes, resulting in a regular ventricular rate, 150 per minute.

(*B*) After the omission of digitalis, note the presence of atrial fibrillation with the persistence of the upwardly directed complexes; the downwardly directed complexes have disappeared. These findings suggest that in *A* we are dealing with an A-V junctional rhythm with an ectopic focus occurring in some portion of the A-V node or bundle of His.

Occasionally, and usually in the presence of severe digitalis toxicity, the junctional tachycardia may be accompanied by alternation of intraventricular conduction, resulting in "bidirectional" ventricular tachycardia (Figs. 18–8 and 18–9). In most cases, bidirectional ventricular tachycardia is a result of alternation of intraventricular conduction. In other instances, this arrhythmia is a junctional tachycardia with ventricular bigeminy. Rarely, bidirectional ventricular tachycardia is the result of two alternating ventricular pacemakers or one ventricular focus activating the ventricle alternately in different directions. Rosenbaum, Elizari, and Lazarri (1969) strongly argue in favor of right bundle branch block with alternating block of the anterior and posterior division of the left bundle as the mechanism of many of the cases of bidirectional ventricular tachycardia. Regardless of mechanism, bidirectional ventricular tachycardia is a life threatening arrhythmia requiring urgent treatment.

ATRIOVENTRICULAR DISSOCIATION

Atrioventricular dissociation is frequently a manifestation of digitalis toxicity. The basic term implies that the atria and ventricles are driven by independent pacemakers. Atrioventricular dissociation can be due to presence of A-V block or, in the absence of block, can result from either slowing of the primary pacemaker (with an escape of a

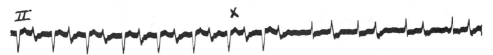

Figure 18–9 Bidirectional junctional tachycardia abolished by carotid sinus pressure (lead II).

The initial portion of the tracing shows a bidirectional junctional tachycardia that resulted from toxic digitalis effects. Following carotid sinus pressure at X, the rhythm is converted to atrial fibrillation, which was the original mechanism. It is of interest that the QRS complexes following the conversion possess a similar character and contour to those of the upright complexes of the paroxysm. The response to carotid sinus pressure suggests that the mechanism is junctional in origin.

lower pacemaker) or an inappropriate acceleration of a lower pacemaker (usually sinus and junctional).

VENTRICULAR PREMATURE COMPLEXES

Although ventricular premature complexes are the most common manifestations of digitalis toxicity, they are also the least specific. Ventricular premature complexes may arise from several foci and may be associated with fixed or variable coupling. It is difficult to differentiate between ventricular premature beats related or unrelated to digitalis toxicity; however, Pick (1957) describes the following criteria that suggest digitalis: 1) fixed coupling, 2) ventricular bigeminy, 3) runs of ventricular premature complexes on a rhythm strip showing other evidence of digitalis toxicity. Ventricular premature complexes with fixed coupling in the presence of atrial fibrillation strongly suggest the possibility of digitalis toxicity (Fig. 18–5), particularly in bigeminal patterns. The clinical setting in which such arrhythmias occur is decisive in the final analysis. Continued digitalis administration can result in bidirectional extrasystoles, ventricular tachycardia, and ultimately, ventricular fibrillation (Fig. 18–8).

VENTRICULAR TACHYCARDIA

Ventricular tachycardia is a common rhythm disturbance brought about by digitalis excess. It is generally caused by increased automaticity of a ventricular pacemaker as a result of increased slope of phase 4 diastolic depolarization of the His-Purkinje system. However, a re-entry mechanism can also be responsible. Digitalis toxicity is strongly suggested if the ventricular tachycardia manifests as a true *bidirectional ventricular tachycardia* (Figs. 18–8 and 18–9). Ventricular tachycardia in the presence of digitalis intoxication is a serious arrhythmia with a mortality rate of 65 to

90 per cent if the cause is not recognized (Dreifus et al., 1963; Dall, 1965). Ventricular fibrillation may frequently supervene.

VENTRICULAR FIBRILLATION

Ventricular fibrillation as a manifestation of digitalis toxicity (Fig. 18–10) is less commonly reported in man, since it is usually preceded by other relatively less serious arrhythmias (Von Capeller et al. 1959). The most frequent reports of ventricular fibrillation in this context have been instances in which cardioversion was attempted in patients with digitalis toxicity. There are very few documented reports of survival following digitalis induced ventricular fibrillation.

TYPE I ATRIO-VENTRICULAR BLOCK

Digitalis can cause varying degrees of A-V block by suppressing conduction through the A-V node both by its direct effect and by vagal action, causing prolongation of the refractory period of the A-V node. All degrees of A-V block may result. One of the most common electrocardiographic manifestations of digitalis toxicity is prolongation of the P-R interval, and if this is ignored, higher degrees of A-V block may occur (i.e., Wenckebach periodicity or complete A-V block). The ventricular rate in digitalis induced complete A-V block is usually 40 to 60 beats per minute, and Adam-Stokes seizures are rarely seen. Digitalis induced Mobitz type II block apparently does not occur (Kaufman et al., 1961).

Other Digitalis Arrhythmias

Sino-atrial block with or without the Wenckebach phenomenon, sinus arrhythmia, wandering pacemaker, sinus bradycardia, sinus tachycardia, atrial extrasystoles, reciprocal beating, and

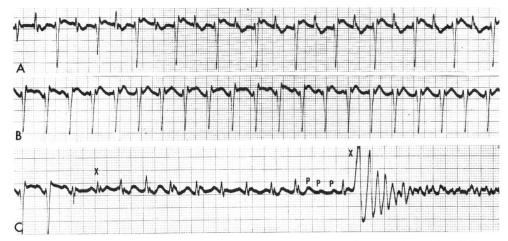

Figure 18–10   Male, age 60, with malignant hypertension, congestive failure, and renal insufficiency. BUN, 75 mgm. per cent.

(A) This patient had been receiving 0.1 mg. digitoxin for two months. In the week prior to this tracing, he had been receiving 0.5 mg. digoxin orally because of an irregular rhythm. After 0.4 mg. Cedilanid at 11:40 A.M., note the presence of a bidirectional junctional tachycardia.

(B) Probable ventricular tachycardia. The P waves occur at a slower rate and independently of the ventricular complexes.

(C) After 3 mg. of Pronestyl intravenously, note the occurrence of marked changes in the direction of the ventricular complexes, the appearance of atrial tachycardia in the cycle marked "X" with A-V block, probably due to toxic digitalis effects. Note the terminal ventricular flutter and ventricular fibrillation, illustrating that the initial beat of the terminal paroxysm occurs during the vulnerable period of the T wave.

concealed conduction are all additional rhythm disturbances that may be caused by digitalis.

Although digitalis is so beneficial in controlling the rapid ventricular response of atrial fibrillation or flutter, transient or permanent atrial fibrillations have on rare occasions been reported to be toxic manifestations. In our view, this rarely if ever occurs.

Arrhythmias Not Caused by Digitalis

While digitalis toxicity should be suspected in any patient who develops a rhythm change while on a glycoside, the following arrhythmias are generally believed *not* to be caused by digitalis administration: sinus (or other) exit block, type II heart block, bundle branch block, parasystolic rhythms, and probably atrial fibrillation and flutter.

Diagnosis of Digitalis Toxicity

The diagnosis of digitalis toxicity is primarily clinical, the problem being threefold: 1) suspicion of a specific arrhythmia, 2) differentiation of the arrhythmia from other rhythm disturbances, and 3) — and most important — a determination of whether digitalis is the cause. Digitalis toxicity should be strongly suspected in any patient receiving digitalis when congestive heart failure suddenly worsens or reappears without any obvious cause. A ventricular rate that becomes *faster* despite digitalis administration should also strongly suggest toxicity, as should a change in rhythmicity: either regular sinus rhythm becoming irregular or atrial fibrillation suddenly becoming rapid and/or regular. Once digitalis toxicity is suspected, careful monitoring of the patient is mandatory, for the abnormal response may initially be transitory and further digitalis could result in a serious rhythm disturbance within hours or days.

Serum Digitalis Levels

Since excessive accumulation of digoxin is a major factor in the development of toxicity and there is some constancy in myocardial serum digoxin ratio (Gullner et al., 1974; Hartel, 1976), several authorities have sought to determine whether serum digoxin levels would be useful in the diagnosis of digitalis toxicity (Smith, 1975; Ingelfinger and Goldman, 1976). In patients with clear-cut digoxin toxicity on clinical grounds, 87 per cent have been reported to have serum levels about 2.0 ng per ml. In those patients who are taking digitalis but have no clinical evidence of toxicity, 90 per cent had serum levels below 2.0 ng per ml (Smith and Haber, 1971). However, several studies indicate that there is a *significant overlap* of serum digitalis levels in patients with and without toxicity (Beller et al., 1971; Evered and Chapman, 1971; Fogelman et al., 1971; Doherty, 1973). This is probably due to differences in 1) myocardial sensitivity, 2) potassium imbalance, 3) acid-base status and oxygenation, 4) myocardial metabolism, and 5) underlying electrophysiologic status. Thus, based purely on digitalis levels, it is not possible to predict that an individual patient is digitalis toxic.

Digitalis levels thus are less important in determining the diagnosis of digitalis toxicity than are the clinical presentation and type of arrhythmia exhibited. In some patients with arrhythmias that suggest digitalis toxicity who are poor historians, the absence of digoxin in the serum rules out toxicity. Table 18–6 shows the commonly accepted levels of digoxin and digitoxin in patients with and without clinical toxicity (Doherty, 1973).

Treatment of Digitalis Toxicity

Most rhythm disturbances due to digitalis toxicity can be managed satisfactorily by simply stopping the drug. Correction of various factors that increase the sensitivity to digitalis, namely electrolyte disturbances (particularly hypokalemia), changes in pH, and hypoxia may be all that is required after drug cessation to effectively control the arrhythmia. However, more aggressive therapy is mandatory if the heart rate is either so rapid or so slow as to seriously compromise cardiac output and blood pressure or accelerate severe congestive heart failure and pulmonary edema. In addition, serious or premonitory arrhythmias should also be treated.

As a rule, low grade ventricular premature complexes, first and second degree A-V block (Wenckebach phenomenon), and A-V dissociation with an acceptable ventricular rate require no specific therapeutic measures other than discontinuing digitalis. More serious arrhythmias, particularly ventricular tachycardia, require administration of other drugs, such as potassium chloride (especially with hypokalemia), diphenylhydantoin (Dilantin), lidocaine, procainamide, propranolol, and bretylium, and overdrive suppression.

POTASSIUM

Potassium is a very effective agent for the suppression of digitalis induced

---

TABLE 18–6   SERUM LEVELS OF DIGOXIN AND DIGITOXIN

Glycoside	Therapeutic Levels	Toxicity Levels*
Digoxin	0.5–2.5 ng/ml	≥3.0 ng/ml
Digitoxin	20–30 ng/ml	≥45 ng/ml

*There is considerable overlap between therapeutic and toxic levels (see text).

arrhythmias and is frequently advocated as the first line of treatment, particularly in the presence of hypokalemia. There is considerable evidence that digitalis toxicity is aggravated by extracellular and probably intracellular depletion of potassium. This correlation between potassium depletion and increased sensitivity to digitalis is the rationale for the use of potassium in the treatment of digitalis induced tachyarrhythmias (Lown et al., 1952; Surawicz, 1966; Fisch and Knoebel, 1970). However, potassium slows conduction through myocardial as well as specialized conduction tissue via a direct effect, and this depression of conduction is potentiated by the presence of digitalis. Potassium should, therefore, be administered with caution (if at all) to patients with digitalis induced conduction disturbances (Fisch and Knoebel, 1970). In our view, potassium administration is contraindicated in digitalis induced high grade A-V block. The specific rhythm disturbances for which potassium administration has been considered useful are atrial tachycardia with block, frequent ventricular premature beats, and ventricular tachycardia. Since intracellular potassium concentration cannot be judged by serum potassium measurements, when such rhythm disturbances are present in the presence of digitalis toxicity, administration of potassium may be useful even though serum potassium levels are normal.

When the reversion of rhythm is not urgent and the patient is tolerating the rhythm disturbance well, oral administration of potassium may be undertaken. Potassium chloride may be administered in tomato juice or orange juice, 1 gram (13 mEq) every 4 hours. If oral medication is not feasible because of nausea, vomiting, or intolerance to the drug, one may give 40 mEq potassium chloride in 500 ml of 5 per cent glucose in water intravenously over a period of 3 to 4 hours. Before intravenous potassium therapy is undertaken, a urinary output of more than 20 ml per hour and a normal or low serum potassium level should be confirmed. Continuous electrocardiographic monitoring is mandatory during intravenous potassium administration. Under no circumstance should the rate of potassium administration exceed 0.5 mEq per kilogram per hour.

When the rhythm disturbance is atrial tachycardia with 2:1 or 3:1 A-V block, as a general rule, instant reversion is not required, since there is no hemodynamic instability.

OTHER ANTIARRHYTHMIC DRUGS

Ventricular tachycardia due to digitalis intoxication requires prompt treatment. In addition to potassium repletion, other antiarrhythmic drugs may have to be used to revert the arrhythmia to a normal sinus mechanism. This can be achieved by the administration of intravenous *lidocaine* or *diphenylhydantoin*. Occasionally, procainamide, propranolol, and bretylium are necessary. If reversion does not occur in a short period of time, overdrive suppression or, rarely, direct current cardioversion is indicated. Although all of the aforementioned drugs have been utilized to revert the ventricular ectopic rhythm to normal sinus mechanism, diphenylhydantoin has been particularly favored for the treatment of ventricular tachycardia due to digitalis intoxication. Diphenylhydantoin causes reversion of digitalis induced arrhythmias without causing significant depression of conduction (Helfant et al., 1967). The antiarrhythmic effect of the drug is probably due to a direct effect on the specialized myocardial tissue. Lidocaine is also very effective in the treatment of severe ventricular arrhythmias due to digitalis excess.

Propranolol is reportedly successful in the treatment of digitalis induced arrhythmias in 75 to 100 per cent of patients (Szekely et al., 1966; Turner, 1966; Stock, 1963). Of the various arrhythmias due to digitalis, atrial tachycardia with block and ventricular arrhythmias seem to respond best to propranolol. Its action depends chiefly on the beta blocking and quinidine-like effects. Although beneficial effects may be obtained, the use of propranolol entails certain risk due to 1) its negative inotropic effect, which may aggravate the patient's underlying heart failure, and 2) its tendency to slow A-V conduction, which may aggravate A-V block.

ATRIAL PACING

Recently, rapid right atrial pacing has been shown to be effective in terminating supraventricular tachycardia in patients receiving digitalis. No complications have been encountered with this technique, in contrast to the usually frequent occurrence to post countershock arrhythmias in digitalis toxicity.

VENTRICULAR PACING

In experimental animals, digitalis induced junctional or ventricular tachycardia can be completely abolished by ventricular pacing at appropriately rapid rates. The electrical stimulus is delivered at a more rapid rate than the frequency of the ectopic ventricular focus, thereby suppressing the ectopic pacemaker. In addition, the faster electrical pacemaker is capable of depressing the slope of diastolic depolarization of the ectopic focus. It is emphasized that ventricular pacing should only be employed when standard pharmacological measures have failed.

HEMOPERFUSION

Hemoperfusion using resin or activated charcoal appears to be effective in the management of massive digoxin overdose. As has been mentioned previously, both peritoneal dialysis and hemodialysis have no value in clearing excessive serum levels of digoxin from the blood. In patients who had accidentally ingested massive doses of digoxin,

Smiley and co-workers (1978) have been able to decrease serum digoxin levels considerably with the help of 5 hour hemoperfusion with resin or with activated charcoal. Such a measure is, of course, indicated only when massive doses of digoxin have been ingested and is of little value in the routine treatment of patients with digitalis toxicity.

DIGOXIN-SPECIFIC ANTIBODIES

Considerable interest has recently been focused on the use of digoxin-specific antibodies for the treatment of digitalis toxicity (Butler, 1970; Schmidt and Butler, 1971). However, the use of immune serum is accompanied by allergic reactions and serum sickness. A recent report has demonstrated promising results in patients with severe digitalis toxicity by using less allergic fragments of antibodies (Smith et al., 1976). Currently, the use of digoxin-specific antibodies can be considered only in life threatening situations where massive doses of digoxin have been ingested.

REFERENCES

Abildskov, J. A.: The nervous system and cardiac arrhythmias. Circulation 52(6 Suppl 3):116, 1975.

Banka, V. S., Scherlag, B. J., and Helfant, R. H.: Contractile and electrophysiological responses to progressive digitalis toxicity. Cardiovasc. Res. 9:65, 1975.

Beller, G. A., Smith, T. W., Abelmann, W. H., et al.: Digitalis intoxication. A prospective clinical study with serum level correlations. N. Engl. J. Med. 284:989, 1971.

Bloom, P. M., Nelp, W. B., and Tuell, S. H.: Relationship of the excretion of tritiated digoxin to renal function. Am. J. Med. Sci., 251:133, 1966.

Braunwald, E., Bloodwell, R. D., Goldberg, L. I., and Morrow, A. G.: Studies on digitalis: IV. Observations in man on the effects of digitalis preparation on the contractility of the non-failing heart and on total vascular resistance. J. Clin. Invest. 40:52, 1961.

Brest, A. N., Durge, N. G., and Goldberg, H.: Conversion of atrial fibrillation to atrial flutter as a manifestation of digitalis toxicity. Am. J. Cardiol. 6:682, 1960.

Butler, V. P., Jr.: Digoxin: Immunologic approaches to measurement and reversal of toxicity. N. Engl. J. Med. 283:1150, 1970.

Cranefield, P. F.: Action potential, after potentials and arrhythmias. Circ. Res. 41:415, 1977.

Cranefield, P. F., and Aronson, R. S.: Initiation of sustained rhythmic activity by single propagated action potentials in canine cardiac Purkinje fibers exposed to sodium-free solution or to ouabain. Circ. Res. 34:477, 1974.

Dall, J. L. C.: Digitalis intoxication in elderly patients. Lancet 1:194, 1965.

Davis, L. D.: Effect of changes in cycle length of diastolic depolarization produced by ouabain in canine Purkinje fibers. Circ. Res. 32:206, 1973.

Doherty, J. E.: Digitalis glycosides; pharmacokinetics and their clinical implications. Ann. Int. Med. 79:229, 1973.

Doherty, J. E.: The clinical pharmacology of digitalis glycosides: A review. Am. J. Med. Sci. 255:382, 1968.

Doherty, J. E., Flanigan, W. J., Murphy, M. L., et al.: Tritiated digoxin XIV. Enterohepatic circulation, absorption and excretion studies in human volunteers. Circulation 42:867, 1970.

Doherty, J. E., and Perkins, W. H.: Digoxin metabolism in hypo and hyperthyroidism. Studies with tritiated digoxin in thyroid disease. Ann. Int. Med. 64:489, 1966.

Doherty, J. E., and Perkins, W. H.: Studies with tritiated digoxin in human subjects after intravenous administration. Am. Heart J. 63:528, 1962.

Doherty, J. E., Perkins, W. H., and Wilson, M. C.: Studies with tritiated digoxin in renal failure. Am. J. Med. 37:536, 1964.

Dreifus, L. S., Likoff, W., and Bender, S. R.: Serious cardiac arrhythmias induced by digitalis. Prognosis and treatment. Circulation 24:922, 1961.

Dreifus, L. S., McGarry, T. F., and Kimbiris, D.: New concepts in the approach to digitalis therapy for atrial fibrillation. Dis. Chest 44:197, 1963.

Dreifus, L. S., McKnight, E. H., Katz, M., and Likoff, W.: Digitalis intolerance. Geriatrics 18:494, 1963.

Evered, D. C., and Chapman, C.: Plasma digoxin concentrations and digoxin toxicity in hospital patients. Brit. Heart. J. 33:540, 1971.

Ewy, G. A., Groves, B. M., Ball, M. F., Nimmo, L., Jackson, B., and Marcus, F.: Digoxin metabolism in obesity. Circulation 44:810, 1971.

Ferrier, G. R., and Moe, G. K.: Effects of calcium on acetylstrophanthidin induced transient depolarizations in canine Purkinje tissue. Circ. Res. 33:508, 1973.

Ferrier, G. R., Saunders, J. M., and Mendez, C.: A cellular mechanism for the generation of ventricular arrhythmias by acetylstrophanthidin. Circ. Res. 32:600, 1973.

Fisch, C., and Knoebel, S. B.: Recognition and therapy of digitalis toxicity. Prog. Cardiovasc. Dis. 13:71, 1970.

Fisch, C., Oehler, R. C., Miller, J. R., and Redish, C. H.: Cardiac arrhythmias during oral surgery with halothane-nitrous oxide-oxygen anesthesia. J.A.M.A. 208:1839, 1969.

Fogelman, A. M., LaMont, J. T., Finkelstein, S., Rado, E.: Fallibility of plasma digoxin in differentiating toxic from nontoxic patients. Lancet 2:727, 1971.

Fozzard, H. A.: Heart: Excitation-contraction coupling. Ann. Rev. Physiol. 39:201, 1977.

Friedberg, C. K., and Donoso, G.: Arrhythmias and conduction disturbances due to digitalis. Prog. Cardiovasc. Dis. 2:408, 1960.

Gillis, R. A., Pearle, D. L., and Levitt, B. (Editorial): Digitalis: A neuroexcitatory drug. Circulation 52:739, 1975.

Goodman, D. J. Rossen, R. M., Cannon, D. S., Dider, A. K., and Harrison, D. C.: Effect of digoxin on atrioventricular conduction: Studies in patients with and without cardiac autonomic innervation. Circulation 15:251, 1975.

Güllner, H. G., Stinson, E. B., Harrison, D. C., and Kalman, S. M.: Correlation of serum concentrations with heart concentrations of digoxin in human subjects. Circulation 50:653, 1974.

Hager, W. D., Fenster, P., Mayersohn, M., Perrier, D., Graves, P., Marcus, F. I., and Goldman, S.: Digoxin-quinidine interaction; pharmacokinetic evaluation. N. Engl. J. Med. 300:1238, 1979.

Hall, W. H., and Doherty, J. E.: Tritiated digoxin. XVI. Gastric absorption. Am. J. Dig. Dis. 16:903, 1971.

Härtel, G., Kyllönen, K., Merikallio, E., Ojala, K., Menninen, V., and Reissell, P.: Human serum and myocardial digoxin. Clin. Pharmacol. Ther. 19:153, 1976.

Heizer, W. D., Smith, T. W., and Goldfinger, S. E.: Absorption of digoxin in patients with malabsorption syndromes. N. Engl. J. Med. 285:257, 1971.

Helfant, R. H., Lev, S. H., Cohen, S. I., and Damato, A. N.: Effect of diphenylhydantoin on A-V conduction in man. Circulation 36:686, 1967.

Helfant, R. H., Scherlag, B. J., and Damato, A. N.: Protection from digitalis toxicity with the prophylactic use of diphenylhydantoin sodium: an arrhythmic-inotropic dissociation. Circulation 36:119, 1967.

Ingelfinger, J. A., and Goldman, O.: The serum digitalis concentration — does it diagnose digitalis toxicity? N. Engl. J. Med. 294:867, 1976.

Jelliffe, R. W., and Blankenhorn, D. A.: Improved method of digitalis therapy in patients with reduced renal function. Circulation 36:II-150, 1967.

Jelliffe, R. W., and Brooker, G.: A nomogram for digoxin therapy. Am. J. Med. 57:63, 1974.

Kaufman, J. G., Wachtel, F. W., Rothfield, E., and

Bernstein, A.: The association of complete heart block and Adams-Stokes syndrome in two cases of Mobitz type of block. Circulation 23:253, 1961.

Kleiger, R., and Lown, B.: Cardioversion and digitalis. II. Clinical studies. Circulation 33:878, 1966.

Langer, G. A.: Effects of digitalis on myocardial ionic exchange. Circulation 46:180, 1972.

Lely, A. H., and VanEnter, C. H. J.: Large-scale digitalis intoxication. Brit. Med. J. 3:737, 1970.

Lown, B., and Levine, S. A.: Current concept in digitalis therapy. N. Engl. J. Med. 250:771, 1954.

Lown, B., Kleiger, R., and Williams, J.: Cardioversion and digitalis drugs: Changed threshold to electric shock in digitalized animals. Circ. Res. 17:519, 1965.

Lown, B., Weller, I. M., Wyatt, N., Hoigne, R., and Merrill, J. P.: Effects of alterations of body potassium on digitalis toxicity. J. Clin. Invest. 31:648, 1952.

Lown, B., and Wittenberg, S.: Cardioversion and digitalis. III. Effect of change in serum potassium concentration. Am. J. Cardiol. 21:513, 1968.

Marcus, F. I.: Digitalis pharmacokinetics and metabolism. Am. J. Med. 58:452, 1975.

Marcus, F. I., Burkhalter, L., Cuccia, C., Pavlovich, J., and Kapadia, G. G.: Administration of tritiated digoxin with and without a loading dose. Circulation 34:865, 1966.

Marcus, F. I., and Kapadia, G. G.: The metabolism of tritiated digoxin in cirrhotic patients. Gastroenterology 47:517, 1964.

Marcus, F. I., Peterson, A. S., Sadel, A. F., et al.: The metabolism of tritiated digoxin in renal insufficiency in dogs and man. J. Pharmacol. Exp. Ther. 153:372, 1966.

Marcus, F. I., Quinn, E. J., Horton, H., Jacobs, S., Pippin, S., Stafford, M., and Zukoski, C.: The effect of jejunoileal bypass on the pharmacokinetics of digoxin in man. Circulation 55:537, 1977.

National Prescription Audit. 9th ed., Ambler, Pa., Gosselin and Co. 1972, p. 27.

Nola, G. T., Pole, S., and Harrison, D. C.: Assessment of synergistic relationship between serum calcium and digitalis. Am. Heart J. 79:499, 1970.

Okita, G. T.: Metabolism of radioactive cardiac glycosides (abstract). Pharmacologist 6:45, 1964.

Pick, A.: Digitalis and the electrocardiogram. Circulation 15:603, 1957.

Pick, A., and Dominguez, P.: Nonparoxysmal A-V nodal tachycardia. Circulation 16:1022, 1957.

Pick, A., Langerdorf, R., and Katz, L. N.: A-V nodal tachycardia with block. Circulation 24:12, 1961.

Przybyla, A. G., Paulay, K. L., Stein, E., and Damato, A. N.: Effects of digoxin on A-V conduction pathways in man. Am. J. Cardiol. 33:344, 1974.

Rasmussen, K., Jervell, J., Storstein, L., et al.: Digitoxin kinetics in patients with impaired renal function. Clin. Pharmacol. Ther. 13:6, 1972.

Rhee, H. M., Dutta, S., and Marks, B. H.: Cardiac Na, K-ATPase activity during inotropic and toxic actions of ouabain. Eur. J. Pharmacol. 37:141, 1976.

Rodensky, P. L., and Wasserman, F.: The possible role of sex in digitalis tolerance. Am. Heart J. 68:325, 1964.

Rosen, M. R., Gelband, H., and Hoffman, B. F.: Correlation between effects of ouabain on the canine electrocardiogram and transmembrane potentials of isolated Purkinje fibers. Circulation 47:65, 1973.

Rosen, M. R., Wit, A. L., and Hoffman, B. F.: Electrophysiology and pharmacology of cardiac arrhythmias. IV. Cardiac antiarrhythmic and toxic effects of digitalis. Am. Heart J. 89:391, 1975.

Rosenbaum, M. B., Elizari, M. V., and Lazarri, J. O.: The mechanism of bidirectional tachycardia. Am. Heart J. 78:4, 1969.

Schmidt, D. H., and Butler, V. P., Jr.: Reversal of digoxin toxicity with specific antibodies. J. Clin. Invest. 50:1738, 1971.

Schwartz, A., Lindenmayer, G. E., and Allen, J. C.: The sodium-potassium adenosine triphosphatase: Pharmacological, physiological and biochemical aspects. Pharmacol. Rev. 27:3, 1975.

Smith, T. W.: Digitalis toxicity: Epidemiology and clinical use of serum concentration measurements. Am. J. Med. 58:470, 1975.

Smith, T. W., and Haber, E.: Digitalis. N. Engl. J. Med. 289:945, 1010, 1063, 1125, 1973.

Smith, T. W., and Haber, E.: Digitalis intoxication: The relationship of clinical presentation to serum digoxin concentration. J. Clin. Invest. 49:2377, 1971.

Smith, T. W., Haber, E., Yeatman, L., and Butler, V. P., Jr.: Reversal of advanced digoxin intoxication with Fab fragments of digoxin-specific antibodies. N. Engl. J. Med. 294:797, 1976.

Smiley, J. W., March, N. M., and Guercio, E. T. D.: Hemoperfusion in the management of digoxin toxicity. J.A.M.A. 240:1736, 1978.

Sodeman, W. A.: Current concept — diagnosis and treatment of digitalis toxicity. N. Engl. J. Med. 273:35, 1965.

Soffer, A.: The changing clinical picture of digitalis intoxication. Arch. Int. Med. 107:681, 1961.

Soffer, A.: The changing clinical picture of digitalis intoxication. Arch. Int. Med. 104:422, 1962.

Solomon, H. M., Reich, S. D., Spirt, N., et al.: Interactions between digitoxin and other drugs in vitro and in vivo. Ann. N.Y. Acad. Sci. 179:362, 1971.

Sonnenblock, E. H., Williams, J. F., Jr., Glick, G.,

and Mason, D. T.: Studies on digitalis. XV. Effects of cardiac glycosides on myocardial force-velocity relations in the non-failing human heart. Circulation 34:532–539, 1966.

Sorstein, L.: The influence of renal function on the pharmacokinetics of digitoxin. In Proceedings of the International Symposium on Digitalis. Oslo, Gyldendal Forlag.

Steiness, E., and Olesen, K. H.: Cardiac arrhythmias induced by hypokalemia and potassium loss during maintenance digoxin therapy. Brit. Heart J. 38:167, 1976.

Stock, J. P. P., and Dale, N.: Beta-adrenergic receptor blockade in cardiac arrhythmias. Brit. Med. J. 2:1230, 1963.

Surawicz, B.: Role of electrolytes in etiology and management of cardiac arrhythmias. Prog. Cardiovasc. Dis. 8:364, 1966.

Szekely, P., Jackson, F., Wynne, N. A., Vohra, J. K., Batson, G. A., and Dow, W. I. M.: Clinical observations on use of propranolol in disorders of cardiac rhythm. Am. J. Cardiol. 18:426, 1966.

Toda, N., and West, T. C.: The action of ouabain on the function of the atrioventricular node in rabbits. J. Pharmacol. Exp. Ther. 169:287, 1969.

Turner, J. B. R.: Propranolol in the treatment of digitalis induced and digitalis resistant tachycardias. Am. J. Cardiol. 18:450, 1966.

Von Capeller, D., Copeland, G. D., and Stern. T. N.: Digitalis intoxication. Arch. Intern. Med. 104:422, 1962.

Wellens, H. J., and Durrer, D.: Effect of digitalis on AV conduction and circus movement tachycardia in patients with Wolff-Parkinson-White syndrome. Circulation 47:1229, 1973.

Weissler, A. M., Synder, J. R., Schoenfeld, C. D., et al.: Assay of digitalis glycosides in man. Am. J. Cardiol. 17:768, 1966.

William, J. F., Jr., Klocke, F. J., and Braunwald, E.: Studies on digitalis. XIII. A comparison of the effects of potassium on the inotropic and arrhythmia-producing actions of ouabain. J. Clin. Invest. 45:346, 1966.

SUPPLEMENTARY READING

Bigger, J. T.: The quinidine-digoxin interaction. What do we know about it? N. Engl. J. Med. 301:779, 1969.

Doherty, J. E.: How and when to use the digitalis serum levels. J.A.M.A. 239:2594, 1979.

Hager, W. D., Fenster, P., Mayersohn, M., Perrier, D., Graves, P., Marcus, F. I., and Goldman, S.: Digoxin-quinidine interaction. Pharmacokinetic evaluation. N. Engl. J. Med. 300:1238, 1979.

Okada, R. D., Hager, W. D., Graves, P. E., Mayersohn, M., Perrier, D. G., and Markus, F. I.: Relationship between plasma concentration and dose of digoxin in patients with and without renal impairment. Circulation 58:1196, 1978.

19

DISTURBANCES OF ELECTROLYTE BALANCE

MICHAEL S. FELDMAN, M.D,
RICHARD H. HELFANT, M.D.

INTRODUCTION

Electrolyte abnormalities have become an increasingly important cause of arrhythmias due to the widespread use of high potency diuretics, chronic dialysis, complex surgery (including open heart surgery), and potassium sparing diuretics. Clinically, it is particularly important that the role of electrolyte disturbances in the etiology of an arrhythmia be recognized since 1) the efficacy of standard antiarrhythmic agents is often attenuated in this circumstance (particularly with hypokalemia), 2) the toxic effects of cardiotonic agents (particularly digitalis) are often increased in the presence of electrolyte disturbances, 3) severe electrolyte abnormalities can result in fatal arrhythmias if uncorrected, and 4) conversely, the majority of these arrhythmias are readily reversible with correction of the electrolyte disturbance.

POTASSIUM

Hyperkalemia

Etiology. Excess serum potassium (i.e., concentrations above 5.5 mEq per liter) can be derived from either endogenous or exogenous sources. A shift of

276

potassium from the intracellular to the extracellular space may result from 1) increased tissue destruction, such as gangrene, crush-syndrome, and intravascular hemolytic reactions; 2) acidosis, which is associated with an increased tissue metabolism and shift of potassium ions from the intracellular to the extracellular space; 3) hypoxia, which leads to a similar shift in potassium; 4) hyperglycemia, particularly in patients with hypoaldosteronism; and 5) dehydration and shock.

Clinical Manifestations. Hyperkalemia causes generalized weakness and flaccid paralysis of the skeletal muscles. These manifestations are frequently accompanied by listlessness, mental confusion, numbness, tingling of the extremities, a sense of weakness and heaviness in the legs, pallor, and a sensation of coldness. Severe hyperkalemia may also cause peripheral vascular collapse and hypotension with poor heart sounds as a result of the direct depressant effect of potassium on cardiac muscle contraction and an accompanying peripheral vasodilatation.

Electrocardiographic Manifestations. The classic initial electrocardiographic manifestation of hyperkalemia is *peaking of the T wave*. This usually occurs before any measurable alterations in the

QRS are evident. The T wave contour is characteristically tall, sharp, narrow, and symmetrical with a diminished or absent ST segment (Fig. 19–1) (Weidman, 1955). However, the effect of hyperkalemia depends not only on the serum concentration but also on the rapidity of its development. Thus, large peaked T waves may not be present in patients with mild hyperkalemia (serum potassium concentrations between 5.5 and 6.5 mEq per liter). Conversely, alterations in T wave amplitude are often nonspecific and can be seen in bradycardia, aortic insufficiency, psychiatric disorders, or subendocardial ischemia (Braun, Surawicz, and Bellet, 1955).

Tall peaked T waves are almost invariable at serum concentrations above 7 mEq per liter. In addition, an *increase in the duration of the QRS complex* usually occurs together with an *increase in P wave duration and a decrease in P wave amplitude*. Atrial myocardium is more sensitive to potassium than are the specialized conduction fibers or ventricular myocardium. Consequently, at potassium levels above 8 mEq per liter, atrial activity may not be seen on the surface ECG even though conduction from the

Figure 19–1 Electrocardiographic effects of hyperpotassemia; reversal by molar sodium lactate.

10:35 A.M.: (Serum K, 9.9 mEq./L.) Note widened QRS to 0.16 second and absence of P waves. The absence of the P waves is probably due to sinoventricular conduction. This returns to normal A-V conduction as the K+ concentration decreases.

10:40 A.M.: (After 150 ml. of molar sodium lactate.) Note narrowing of QRS to 0.08 second, peaking of waves and return of P waves.

10:52 A.M.: (After 300 ml. of molar sodium lactate in 17 minutes.) Note still further narrowing of QRS with return of P waves.

11:07 A.M.: (Serum K, 8.9 mEq./L.) Note continuous improvement.

11:50 A.M.: (Serum K, 7.7 mEq./L.) Note narrowing of QRS with P waves present.

6:30 P.M.: (Serum K, 5.9 mEq./L.) Note still further narrowing in QRS, with less peaking of T waves and shorter P-R interval. (From Bellet, S., and Wasserman, F.: Arch. Intern. Med., *100*:565, 1957.)

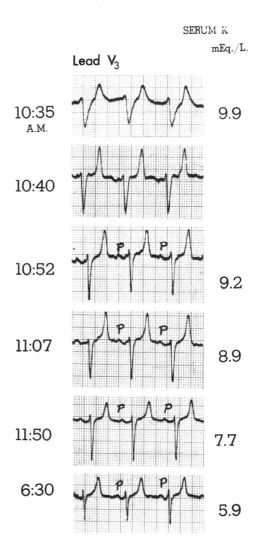

SERUM K
mEq./L.

Lead V$_3$

10:35 A.M.   9.9

10:40

10:52   9.2

11:07   8.9

11:50   7.7

6:30   5.9

S-A node to the ventricles is occurring through specialized conduction pathways. The term *sino-ventricular conduction* has been used to describe this phenomenon (Fig. 19–2) (DeMello and Hoffman, 1960; Bashour and Cheng, 1973). If hyperkalemia progresses, the QRS duration increases further, becoming progressively slurred, while the initially peaked and narrowed T waves become wider and of lesser amplitude (probably because of severe abnormalities of intraventricular conduction and depolarization, with repolarization beginning in some areas at the same time that other areas are still being depolarized). Under these circumstances, a *"sine wave"* electrocardiogram may be seen (Fig. 19–3) (Ettinger, 1974). Occasionally, in advanced hyperkalemia, ST segment alterations from the baseline simulating an acute pattern of injury may also be present. These ST segment deviations are most likely due to the increase in QRS duration. They revert to an isoelectric pattern with hemodialysis (Levine, Wanzer, and Merril, 1967; Arnsdorf, 1976; Shaw, 1978).

Electrophysiologic Abnormalities. Initially, an increase in extracellular potassium lowers the transmembrane resting potential (the transmembrane resting potential becomes less negative). Consequently, the velocity of phase 0 of the action potential is decreased and conduction is slowed (see Chapter 2). Elevations of extracellular potassium above 6 mEq per liter result in shortening of the action potential duration, predominantly because of the decrease in phase 2 and an increase in the velocity of repolarization. Phase 4 depolarization is also decreased. The effect on the action potential, and consequently on the surface electrocardiogram, is progressive and roughly parallels successive elevations in extracellular potassium.

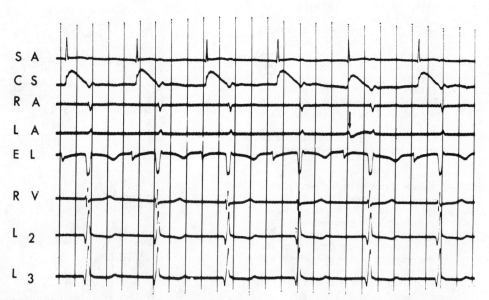

Figure 19–2 Sinoventricular conduction. Sinus impulses propagate regularly to the coronary sinus and the ventricles in absence of activity in the other atrial leads and with complete absence of the P wave. The arrow shows a single activation of the left appendage. SA trace retouched to show rapid deflections. Paper speed 100 mm./sec.; time lines at intervals of 100 msec. (SA: sinus node; CS: coronary sinus; RA: right atrial musculature; LA: left atrial musculature; EL: unipolar record obtained through the catheter lead in right atrium; RV: epicardial surface of right ventricle; L_2: standard Lead II; L_3: standard Lead III.) (From Vassalle, M., and Hoffman, B. F.: Circ. Res., *17*:285, 1965.)

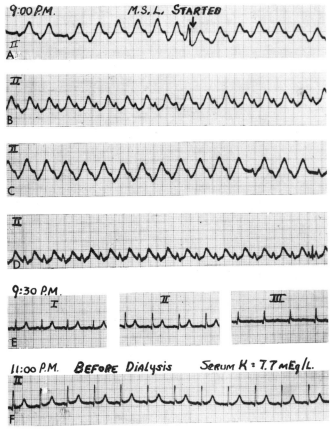

Figure 19-3   Electrocardiographic effect in hyperpotassemia showing reversal by molar sodium lactate.

(A) (Lead II) Taken at 9:00 P.M., when the patient was in coma and circulatory collapse. Bizarre ventricular beats resembling ventricular flutter are present. The serum potassium was 10.7 mEq./L. Molar sodium lactate was started slowly as indicated.

(B) (Lead II) Taken at 9:10 P.M. after 60 mEq. of molar sodium lactate was given intravenously in ten minutes. The rhythm still appears to be ventricular flutter but is somewhat less bizarre.

(C) (Lead II) Taken at 9:14 P.M. after 50 ml. of 50 per cent dextrose with 80 units of regular insulin had been given intravenously two minutes previously. No additional lactate was given. Note further deterioration of the complexes compared to strip B above.

(D) (Lead II) Taken at 9:25 P.M., five minutes after an additional 110 ml. of molar sodium lactate was given rapidly in two minutes. The QRS complexes have narrowed significantly; the ventricular rate is regular at 137 per minute. No P waves are discernible.

(E) (Leads I, II, and III) Taken at 9:30 P.M. Sinus rhythm has been restored. The rate has slowed to 100 per minute. The QRS complexes have narrowed to approximately 0.06 sec.

(F) (Lead II) Taken at 11:00 P.M., shows a relatively normal electrocardiogram. The Q-T interval (0.36 second) is slightly prolonged for the heart rate. (From Bellet, S., and Wasserman, F.: Arch. Intern. Med., 100:565, 1957.)

Arrhythmias Induced by Hyperkalemia. The profound abnormalities of conduction, depolarization, and repolarization occurring with advanced hyperkalemia (levels exceeding 9–10 mEq per liter) result in a variety of tachy- and bradyarrhythmias. *Supraventricular tachycardia* and atrial fibrillation may occur in addition to severe ventricular arrhythmias.

As the level of extracellular potassium rises, localized areas of intraventricular block may occur, with ventricular depolarization and repolarization becoming so fragmented that re-entrant arrhythmias develop that can progress to *ventricular tachycardia* and *ventricular fibrillation*. Conversely, hyperkalemia can also cause *ventricular arrest* resulting from both failure of conduction from S-A node and suppression of automaticity in the subsidiary cardiac pacemakers (Vasalle and Hoffman, 1965).

The N region of the A-V node is more resistant to elevated extracellular potassium levels than is atrial, His-Purkinje, or ventricular tissue (possibly because the predominant determinant of conduction in this region is the slow calcium channel). Therefore, spontaneous hyperkalemia rarely, if ever, produces advanced A-V block. However, at extreme ranges of hyperkalemia, the absence of discernible atrial activity may simulate A-V block and make correct diagnosis difficult (Fisch, 1970).

Treatment. Treatment should be both prophylactic and active. Prophylactic therapy includes early recognition and careful management of patients in whom renal insufficiency is suspected. In particular, potassium sparing diuretics should be avoided in these patients, and close observation is necessary during the immediate postoperative period. Avoidance of high potassium intake in the diet may also be useful.

The treatment of hyperkalemia includes one or more of the following: 1) the use of alkalinizing agents (such as sodium bicarbonate); 2) calcium infusion; 3) glucose and insulin infusion; 4) cation exchange resins; and 5) dialysis. In occasional patients with extremely slow heart rates, the temporary insertion of an artificial pacemaker may be necessary.

Hypokalemia

Etiology and Clinical Manifestations. There are a number of conditions associated with a depletion in potassium that can be manifested in the intracellular compartment or plasma concentration, or both. These include 1) the use of high potency diuretics; 2) potassium loss from the gastrointestinal tract during prolonged vomiting or diarrhea, ileostomy with intestinal drainage, or biliary fistulae; 3) urinary loss associated with salt losing nephritis or the diuretic phase of acute renal failure urinary loss may also be iatrogenically induced; 4) the use of insulin (as in the treatment of diabetic ketoacidosis), which shifts potassium from the serum to the cells, especially in skeletal muscle and liver; 5) excess use of alkalinizing agents, such as sodium bicarbonate and molar sodium lactate, resulting in alkalosis with a shift of potassium into the cells and an increase in its elimination through the kidneys; 6) hormone administration (particularly steroids); 7) initiation of B_{12} therapy (leading to a K^+ shift into cells); 8) poisoning with pesticides containing barium salt (leading to a K^+ shift into cells); and 9) lack of potassium intake (normal being 50–100 mEq or 2 to 4 grams/day).

The clinical manifestations of hypokalemia include weakness, tachycardia, hypotension, hypoperistalsis, and a polyuric "nephropathy" (with a frequent complication being pyelonephritis in addition to the arrhythmias).

Electrocardiographic Manifestations. The classic ECG manifestations of hypokalemia include exaggeration of the *U wave* with an accompanying depression of the ST segment and a decrease in the amplitude of the T wave. While the presence of a U wave per se does not necessarily indicate hypokalemia (left ventricular hypertrophy, digitalis and/or quinidine may cause similar changes) when the U wave amplitude exceeds that of the T wave, it is highly suggestive. With progressive hypokalemia, the U wave may become fused to the T wave and the QT interval can no longer be accurately measured. Under these circumstances, the surface electrocardiogram may mistakenly be interpreted as showing a *prolonged QT interval.* In some patients, the P and QRS amplitude and duration may increase and the PR interval may be prolonged. This increase in QRS duration is seen only in severe hypokalemia and rarely exceeds 0.2 second in most adults (Surawicz and Gettes, 1971). It presumably is due to generalized slowing of intraventricular conduction.

Attempts have been made to quantitatively evaluate the electrocardiographic changes with progressive hypokalemia (Surawicz, 1957). The criteria used include 1) depression of the ST segment by greater than 0.5 mm; 2) a U wave amplitude of greater than 1 mm; and 3) a U wave amplitude greater than that of the T wave in the same lead. Using these criteria, the electrocardiogram was found to be typical for hypokalemia in 78 per cent of patients with plasma potassium concentrations of 2.7 mEq per liter or less and was deemed compatible in an additional 11 per cent. However, an electrocardiogram for "typical" hypokalemia was present in only 10 per cent of the patients in whom the plasma potassium concentration was between 3 and 3.5 mEq per liter. Severe hypokalemia may increase the sensitivity to vagal tone, resulting in sinus bradycardia or A-V transmission defects (Chung, 1972; Chang, 1974).

Since alterations in extracellular potassium significantly affect the intracellular-extracellular potassium ratio (and therefore the potassium concentration gradient), it is generally accepted that the extracellular potassium concentration, rather than total body or intracellular potassium, accounts for the electrocardiographic changes. Patients with large decreases in total body potassium have been found to have normal electrocardiograms if the plasma concentration remains normal (Davidson and Surawicz, 1967). Other investigators have not been able to correlate the severity of hypokalemia and ECG abnormalities.

Electrophysiologic Abnormalities. With decreasing levels of serum extracellular potassium, phase 0 of the action potential of nonautomatic cells shows an increase in amplitude, duration, and upstroke velocity. These changes may be attributed to the hyperpolarization of the cell membrane; that is, an increase in resting membrane potential. This results in an increasing amount of voltage change needed to reach the threshold potential in a spontaneously generated action potential (i.e., a decrease in excitability). Phase 2 of the action potential is progressively shortened, and phase 3 is progressively prolonged as the serum potassium diminishes. The prolonged duration of repolarization facilitates re-entry (see Chapter 2). In automatic cells, a decrease in potassium concentration increases the slope of diastolic depolarization (phase 4) and decreases the threshold of maximum diastolic resting potential in automatic cells. These effects tend to increase automaticity (Gettes, Surawicz, and Shine, 1962).

Arrhythmias Induced by Hypokalemia. Hypokalemia may result in *premature beats* and tachyarrhythmias, presumably by enhancing automaticity and/or promoting re-entry. It can also cause arrhythmias by increasing the sensitivity to vagal tone, thereby decreasing the rate of depolarization of the dominant pacemakers. Hypokalemia commonly is associated with *supraventricular* and *ventricular arrhythmias,* with *ventricular fibrillation* occurring in more severe hypokalemic states (Kunin and Surawicz, 1962). In one study of 81 patients with serum potassium levels of less than 3.2 mEq per liter and no digitalis therapy, 22 per cent exhibited supraventricular beats and 28 per cent had ventricular premature beats. Arrhythmias characteristic of digitalis excess have also been reported, such as junctional or atrial tachycardia with block (Davidson and

Surawicz, 1967). Disturbances of intraventricular and atrioventricular conduction have also been reported, although they are usually mild (Fisch, 1966).

In patients receiving digitalis, mildly reduced serum potassium levels that do not per se usually precipitate arrhythmias have been found to potentiate the arrhythmogenic actions of the glycoside. The synergistic effect of digitalis and reduced serum potassium on automaticity and conduction probably accounts for the fact that patients receiving digitalis preparations appear to be particularly prone to arrhythmias in the presence of hypokalemia (Surawicz and Gettes, 1971).

Treatment.   When possible, oral replacement of potassium is the preferential means of correcting hypokalemia. Parenteral administration may be necessary for patients who are unable to handle oral intake. When parenteral potassium is used, care must be taken to carefully control the rate of administration, since the potassium depleted myocardium is often sensitive to sudden increases in cation concentration. The generally recommended maximum rate of infusion is 1 mEq per kg per hour. However, it is our suggestion that the rate of infusion not exceed 0.5 mEq per kg per hour except in an emergency situation. When oral preparations are used, those containing potassium chloride are preferable to other potassium salts. Care should be taken to correct other electrolyte and acid-base disturbances, particularly the alkalosis that frequently accompanies hypokalemia.

Factors Modifying Tolerance to Potassium

The tolerance of cardiac tissue to abnormal potassium concentrations varies considerably in different patients. Consequently, the electrocardiographic pattern is often a more important indicator of cardiac toxicity than is the serum potassium level per se. Sensitivity to potassium ion fluctuation depends on 1) the rapidity with which the changes occur; 2) the degree of underlying cardiac abnormality; 3) the age of the patient (those in the older age groups are more sensitive); and 4) the serum levels of other electrolytes, particularly calcium and sodium. These two electrolytes act as antagonists to potassium, so that when their levels are low there is a relatively increased effect of the potassium ion in potassium ion concentration (and vice versa).

CALCIUM

Hypercalcemia

Etiology and Clinical Manifestations.   Hypercalcemia is observed in primary hyperparathyroidism, hypervitaminosis D, multiple myeloma, sarcoidosis, and metastatic carcinoma. In man, spontaneous elevations of serum calcium are usually gradual and rarely imperil the heart. However, following the therapeutic administration of calcium salts by intravenous injections, sudden transient increases in concentration may occur resulting in very high levels: 15 to 20 mEq per liter.

Occasionally, death results from such rapid and substantial elevations in calcium concentration. This occurs most often in patients with previous heart disease. In a digitalized patient, the danger of ventricular fibrillation appears to increase with a rising calcium level either because of synergism or a combination of increased calcium levels associated with underlying heart disease in these patients.

Electrocardiographic Changes in Arrhythmias.   The classic change on the surface ECG caused by hypercalcemia is a *shortened Q-T interval* with a shortened ST segment. This, however, is seen only when the serum calcium level is elevated by more than 50 per cent of normal. During severe hypercalcemia, the QRS duration may be prolonged, and A-V block may develop (Surawicz, 1971). High serum calcium levels tend to oppose the effect of hyperkalemia, whereas they enhance the effect of hypokalemia. Although there is experimental evidence that hypercalcemia initiates ectopic beats which may eventuate in ventricular fibrillation, the incidence of premature beats in patients with hypercalcemia does not appear to be increased (Surawicz, 1971). Thus the role of calcium in clinical cardiac arrhythmias remains unclear. The effects of alterations in serum calcium concentration on calcium dependent slow channel conduction (apparently present in the S-A node, in the N region of the A-V node, and possibly in areas of diseased conduction in the Purkinje and ventricular myocardium) have not been well defined.

Depression of conduction and extrasystoles due to hyperkalemia can be reversed by the administration of calcium. (This effect is probably related to an increase in transmembrane resting potential.) Hypercalcemia has also been implicated in the induction of cardiac extrasystoles in conjunction with digitalis therapy at levels of digitalization that would not normally be associated with an increase in ectopic activity.

Electrophysiological Changes. Extreme elevations in calcium concentrations may result in a decrease in excitability and in the rate of spontaneous activity. However, hypercalcemia has also been found to increase the rate of diastolic depolarization seen in the sino-atrial and nodal fibers of rabbits (Tempte and Davis, 1967; Seifen, 1964). High calcium concentrations also tend to shorten phase 2 of the action potential, thus decreasing its duration as well as the effective refractory period. This decrease in refractory period theoretically predisposes to arrhythmias (see Chapter 2).

Hypocalcemia

Etiology and Clinical Manifestations. The clinical conditions in which hypocalcemia are most common include 1) chronic renal failure (uremia

associated with retention of phosphorus); 2) malabsorption syndromes; 3) the postoperative period following partial parathyroidectomy; 4) pseudohypoparathyroidism; 5) acute pancreatitis; 6) respiratory and metabolic alkalosis; 7) idiopathic hypoparathyroidism; 8) high urinary calcium loss (essential hypercalciuria and renal tubular acidosis); 9) high intestinal loss (vitamin D deficiency, diarrhea); and 10) low calcium intake. Occasionally, hypokalemia and hypocalcemia occur simultaneously during alkalosis; that is, in association with upper intestinal obstruction.

The symptoms of hypocalcemia include increased nervous irritability, tremor, and convulsions. More marked abnormalities are associated with hypotension.

Electrocardiographic Changes. The ECG patterns seen in hypocalcemia depend on the degree to which the disorder involves a pure hypocalcemic state or occurs simultaneously with other electrolyte abnormalities, particularly those involving potassium. The classic ECG manifestation of hypocalcemia is a *prolonged Q-T interval,* which closely parallels the lowering of serum calcium. This prolongation disappears with an increase in calcium concentration. Aside from hypothermia, hypocalcemia is the only metabolic abnormality capable of producing prolongation of the ST segment without changing the duration of the T wave. In extreme cases, the T wave may become flattened or inverted despite the normal serum potassium and magnesium concentration. A recent report suggests T wave alternans may also be elicited by severe hypocalcemia (Navarro-Lopez et al., 1978). The effects of calcium and potassium are antagonistic. If a decrease in potassium accompanies the decrease in calcium, the effects are minimized. Alterations of the calcium ion concentration in reverse of potassium will also enhance the effect of the latter.

Electrophysiologic Changes. Significant hypocalcemia prolongs phase 2 of the action potential in various cardiac fibers. This prolongation increases the duration of the action potential as well as the effective refractory period. It also most likely accounts for the increased duration of the ST segment and Q-T interval observed on the surface ECG (Hoffman, 1956; Surawicz, 1963). In dogs the increased duration of the Q-T interval corresponds roughly with the total increase in mechanical systole.

Arrhythmias. Clinically significant levels of hypocalcemia do not appear to produce an increase in ventricular premature beats or in fibrillation. In experimentally isolated rabbit hearts, less than 1/20 of the normal perfusing solution is necessary to produce an increase in ventricular premature beats (Weiss, 1966). Although it has been suggested that digitalis induced premature beats can be abolished by lowering the serum calcium concentrations (with EDTA), the relationship between digitalis and calcium remains somewhat unclear (Surawicz et al., 1971).

MAGNESIUM

Hypomagnesemia

Etiology and Clinical Manifestations. There are several clinical conditions in which low serum magnesium is found. These include 1) malignancy; 2) during recovery from diabetic acidosis; 3) hyperthyroidism; 4) eclampsia. Its occurrence has also been reported during the polyuric phase of recovery from acute renal failure as well as in the malabsorption syndrome, chronic alcoholism, dehydration states, hyperparathyroidism, primary aldosteronism, and hepatic cirrhosis (Seller and Moyer, 1969). Of clinical significance is the fact that many diuretics lower not only potassium levels but also magnesium levels (Seller, 1970). Clinically, hypomagnesemia is manifested by varying degrees of neuromuscular irritability

which can progress to frank tetany. In some cases grand mal seizures have been reported.

Electrocardiographic Changes. Isolated abnormalities of serum magnesium concentration usually cannot be detected on the surface electrocardiogram. Those that reportedly occur are nonspecific, and at times resemble hypokalemia.

Electrophysiological Effects. The effects of magnesium on the action potential are very closely related to an interplay between calcium and potassium ions. If the calcium concentration is normal, elevation or reduction of magnesium alone produces very little effect on Purkinje fibers. Increasing calcium concentration renders the fibers relatively insensitive to changes in magnesium concentration. Only the presence of a low calcium concentration allows variations in magnesium to alter the action potential. Under these circumstances, a decrease in the level of magnesium increases the duration of phase 2.

Arrhythmias. *Ventricular arrhythmias* have been reported to result from low serum magnesium concentrations (Loeb et al., 1968). Recent evidence also suggests that hypomagnesemia may also predispose to *digitalis toxicity*. Only 70 per cent of the dose of digitalis necessary to cause an arrhythmia experimentally in a dog with a normal serum magnesium concentration is needed for arrhythmia production if the dog is made hypomagnesemic (Seller, 1969). In addition, experimental digitalis induced arrhythmias can be corrected rapidly by magnesium infusion. A deficiency of magnesium combined with the action of digitalis may also promote excessive loss of intracellular potassium.

Hypermagnesemia

Hypermagnesemia is usually due to 1) renal retention, 2) excess ingestion of magnesium, or 3) dehydration. Serum levels of 6.0 mEq per liter are associated with progressive depression of cardiac conduction as well as of neuromuscular activity. As with hypomagnesemia, direct cardiovascular effects of hypermagnesemia have rarely been found clinically in man, although hypotension has been reported.

Occasionally, when large amounts of intravenous magnesium salts are given to man, an initial bradycardia may develop that is often followed by a tachycardia. The P-R interval may increase, and if administration is continued, intraventricular conduction is slowed and T wave changes may occur (Seller and Moyer, 1969). Significant elevations of extracellular magnesium ion concentration levels ranging from 3 to 5 mEq per liter have been reported to depress atrioventricular and intraventricular conduction. At significantly higher levels, cardiac arrest has reportedly occurred.

SODIUM

Alterations in serum sodium concentrations have little clinical effect on electrophysiology, arrhythmias, or surface ECG. This is because the levels necessary to alter the action potential experimentally are incompatible with life.

REFERENCES

Ammon, R. A.: Glucose induced hyperkalemia with normal aldosterone levels. Studies in a patient with diabetes mellitus. Ann. Int. Med. 89:349, 1978.

Arnsdorf, M. R.: Electrocardiogram in hyperkalemia: Electrocardiographic pattern of anteroseptal myocardial infarction mimicked by hyperkalemic induced disturbances of impulse conduction. Arch. Int. Med. 136:1161, 1976.

Bashour, T., and Cheng, T.: Evidence for specialized atrioventricular conduction in hyperkalemia. J. Electrocardiology 8:65, 1978.

Bellet, S.: The electrocardiogram or electrolyte imbalance. Arch. Int. Med. 96:618, 1955.

Braun, H. A., Surawicz, B., and Bellet, S.: T waves in hyperpotassemia. Am. J. Med. Sci. 230:147, 1955.

Chalmers, L. J., Burgess, M., and Abildskov, J. A.: Effects of acute hyperkalemia on cardiac excitability. Am. Heart. J. 94:955, 1977.

Chawla, K. K., Cruz, J., Kramer, N., and Towne, W.: Electrocardiographic changes simulating acute myocardial infarction caused by hyperkalemia. Am. Heart J. 95:637, 1978.

Chung, E. K.: Electrocardiographic findings in hypokalemia. Postgrad. Med. 51:285, 1972.

Cohen, H. C., Rosen, K. M., and Pick, A.: Disorders of impulse conduction and impulse formation caused by hypokalemia in man. Case Report. Am. Heart J. 89:591, 1975.

Davidson, S., and Surawicz, B.: Ectopic beats and atrioventricular conduction disturbances in patients with hypopotassemia. Arch. Intern. Med. 120:280, 1967.

DeMello, W. C., and Hoffman, B. R.: Potassium ions and electrical activity of specialized cardiac fibers. Am. J. Physiol. 199:1125, 1962.

Dinari, L., and Aygen, M. M.: Sinoventricular conduction. N. Engl. J. Med. 289:1238, 1973.

Ensellberg, R. D., Simmons, H. G., and Mintz, A. A.: The effects of potassium on the heart with special reference to the possibility of treatment of toxic arrhythmias due to digitalis. Am. Heart J. 39:713, 1950.

Ettinger, P. O., Regan, T. T., and Oldewurtel, H. A.: Hyperkalemia, cardiac conduction and the electrocardiogram. A Review. Am. Heart J. 88:360, 1974.

Fisch, C.: Effect of potassium on A-V conduction. Circulation 41:575, 1970.

Fisch, C., Knoebel, S. B., Feigenbaum, H., and Greenspan, K.: Potassium and the monphasic action potential, electrocardiogram, conduction and arrhythmia. Prog. Cardiovasc. Dis. 8:387, 1966.

Fisch, C., Martz, B. L., and Priebe, F. H.: Enhancement of potassium induced AV block by toxic doses of digitalis drugs. J. Clin. Invest. 35:1885, 1960.

Gettes, L. S., Surawicz, B., and Shine, J. C.: Effect of high K+, low K+ and quinidine on QRS duration and ventricular action potential. Am. J. Physiol. 203:1135, 1962.

Hoffman, B. F., and Cranefield, P. R.: Electrophysiology of the heart. New York: McGraw-Hill, 1960.

Hoffman, B. F., and Sackling, E. F.: Effects of several cations on transmembrane potentials of cardiac muscle. Am. J. Physiol. 186:317, 1956.

Kahil, M. E., Parrish, T. E., Simons, E. L., and Brown, H.: Magnesium deficiency and carbohydrate metabolism. Diabetes 15:734, 1966.

Kunin, A. S., Surawicz, B., and Sims, E. A. H.: Decrease in serum potassium concentrations and appearance of cardiac arrhythmias during infusion of potassium with glucose in potassium depleted patients. N. Engl. J. Med. 266:228, 1962.

Levine, H. D., Wanzer, S. H., and Merril, J. P.: Dialyzable currents of injury in potassium intoxication resembling acute myocardial infarction or pericarditis. Circulation 13:29, 1956.

Loeb, H. S., Pietras, R. J., Gunnar, R. M., and Tobin, R.: Paroxysmal ventricular fibrillation in two patients with hypomagnesemia. Circulation 47:210, 1968.

Lown, B., Weiler, J. M., Wyatt, N., et al.: Effects of alteration of body potassium on digitalis toxicity. J. Clin. Invest. 31:618, 1952.

Nardone, D. A., et al.: Mechanisms of hypokalemia: Clinical correlation. Medicine 57:435, 1978.

Navarro-Lopez, F., Cinca, J., et al.: Isolated T wave alternans elicited by hypocalcemia in dogs. J. Electrocardiography 11:102, 1978.

Paes de Carvallo, A., and Langan, W. B.: Inference of extracellular potassium levels on atrioventricular transmission. Am. J. Physiol. 205:375, 1963.

Seifen, E., Schaer, H., and Marshall, J. M.: Effect of calcium on the membrane potentials of single pacemaker fibers and atrial fibers in isolated rabbit atria. Nature 202:1223, 1964.

Seller, R. H., and Moyer, J. H.: Magnesium and digitalis toxicity. Heart Bull. 18:32, 1969.

Surawicz, B.: Effects of calcium on duration of Q-T interval and ventricular systoles in dogs. Am. J. Physiol. 205:785, 1963.

Surawicz, B.: Relationship between electrocardiogram and electrolyte. Am. Heart J. 73:814, 1967.

Surawicz, B., Braun, H. A., Crum, W. B., Kemp, R. L., Wagner, S., and Bellet, S.: Quantitative analysis of the electrocardiographic pattern of hyperpotassemia. Circulation 16:750, 1957.

Surawicz, B., and Gettes, L. S.: Effect of electrolyte abnormalities on the heart and circulation. In Conn, H. Z., and Horowitz, D. (eds.): Cardiac and Vascular Disease. Philadelphia, Lea and Febiger, 1971.

Tempte, J. N., and Davis, L. D.: Effect of calcium concentration on the transmembrane potentials of Purkinje fibers. Circ. Res. 20:32, 1967.

Trautwein, W.: Generation and conduction of impulses to the heart as affected by drugs. Pharm. Rev. 15(2), June, 1963.

Vassalle, M., and Hoffman, B. R.: The spread of sinus activation during potassium administration. Circ. Res. 17:285, 1965.

Walker, W. J., Elkins, J. T., and Wood, E. W.: Effect of potassium in restoring myocardial response to a subthreshold cardiac pacemaker. N. Engl. J. Med. 271:597, 1969.

Weaver, W. R., and Burchell, H. B.: Serum potassium and electrocardiogram in hypokalemia. Circulation 21:505, 1960.

Weidmann, S.: The effect of the cardiac membrane potential on the rapid availability of the sodium carrying system. J. Physiol. 127:213, 1955.

Weiss, D. L., Surawicz, B., and Rubenstein, I.: Myocardial lesions or calcium deficiency causing irreversible myocardial failure. Am. J. Path. 48:653, 1965.

SUPPLEMENTARY READING

Bridge, J., and Langer, G.: Calcium dependent sodium efflux in heart muscle. Circulation 60:II–223, 1979.

Dyckner, T., and Webster, P. O.: Ventricular extrasystoles and intracellular electrolytes before and after potassium and magnesium infusion in patients on diuretic treatment. Am. Heart J. 97:12, 1979.

Isner, J. M., Sours, H. E., Paris, A. L., Ferrous, V. J., and Roberts, W. C.: Sudden, unexpected death in avid dieters using the liquid protein modified fast diet. Circulation 60:1401, 1979.

Kronhaus, K. D., Spear, J. F., Kline, R. P., and Moore, E. N.: Relationship between sinoatrial node membrane potential and extracellular potassium accumulation after vagal stimulation. Circulation 60:II–109, 1979.

20

ANESTHESIA AND SURGERY

MICHAEL S. FELDMAN, M.D.
RICHARD H. HELFANT, M.D.

The increasing frequency and complexity of surgical procedures performed on elderly and chronically ill patients as well as the widespread use of cardiothoracic surgery re-emphasize the importance of arrhythmias in the anesthetized patient. Electrolyte and acid-base disturbances (especially hypokalemia) that occur during anesthesia and surgery, alterations in vagal and sympathetic tone, and in cardiac surgery the wide spread use of hypothermia, and cardioplegia all predispose to the development of cardiac arrhythmias. The anesthetic agents themselves, intubation, and visceral manipulations are also arrhythmogenic. Furthermore, pre-existing cardiac and respiratory diseases all affect the frequency of rhythm disturbances during surgical stress. When continuous electrocardiographic monitoring is used, the overall evidence of intraoperative arrhythmias can be as high as 80 per cent (Katz and Bigger, 1970). However, the great majority of these arrhythmias are clinically insignificant and rarely require antiarrhythmic therapy.

INTUBATION

Intraoperative arrhythmias most frequently occur at the time of tracheal intubation and extubation. These procedures cause sympathetic and parasympathetic stimulation, usually with resultant increases in cardiac rate and blood pressure. Although induced tachycardias are generally well tolerated in young, healthy individuals, in the elderly and chronically ill (particularly those on chronic diuretic or digitalis medication), significant supraventricular arrhythmias may bring about severe hemodynamic abnormalities. Paradoxically, patients who have impaired sympathetic responses may develop severe bradycardias during or following intubation, tracheal suction, or extubation as a result of hypoxia and a relatively unopposed increase in vagal stimulation (Mathias, 1976). Since the arrhythmogenic tendencies of intubation may be further complicated by premedication with cholinergic blocking agents, such as atropine or glycopyrronium, many authorities currently feel that routine atropine premedication is unnecessary (Mirakhur, 1978; Eikard, 1977).

INHALATIONAL ANESTHETICS

The commonly used inhalational anesthetic agents have both direct and indirect cardiac effects (Katz and Ep-

287

stein, 1968). They have a direct depressant effect on cardiac function and, in addition, cause dilatation of peripheral vessels by 1) central depression of vasomotor tone and 2) alterations in baroreceptor reflexes. However, cyclopropane, diethylether, and several other agents are capable of precipitating large increases in circulating catecholamines and sympathetic nerve activity, frequently resulting in a net increase in cardiac output. While the increased catecholamine concentrations often compensate for the cardiac depression and peripheral vasodilatatory effects, there is also a concomitant increase in the tendency toward arrhythmias. Halothane, in particular, sensitizes the myocardium to the actions of catecholamines (Khan et al., 1977) (an effect that appears to be diminished by premedication with barbiturates) (Andersen, 1978) or beta blocking agents (Pöntinen, 1978). Aminophylline administration adds to the propensity for ventricular tachycardias when used in patients receiving halothane anesthesia (Roizen and Stevens, 1978).

The inhalational agents may also alter cardiac rhythms by inducing changes in intracardiac conduction and/or automaticity (Atlee and Rosy, 1972). Halothane, in particular, causes disturbances in depolarization of the pacemaker cells as well as decreased conduction at the atrial, A-V nodal, His-Purkinje, and/or ventricular levels. Therefore, varying degrees of A-V and intraventricular conduction block as well as re-entrant tachycardias can result.

Ancillary medications commonly administered in conjunction with the inhalational agents may also be arrhythmogenic. Muscle relaxants, such as pancuronium and gallamine, now in common use may induce sinus tachycardia. Succinylcholine, on the other hand, may produce an increase in vagal tone with resultant bradycardia (Sagarminaga and Wynauds, 1963), an effect that is more pronounced in young, healthy individuals than in the elderly.

Occasional episodes of asystole have been reported with this agent (McLeskey et al., 1978). While bradycardia may be avoided with the prophylactic use of atropine, the price may be serious ventricular arrhythmias in as many as 15 to 30 per cent of patients (Mirakhur et al., 1978). In addition, severe hyperkalemia has also been reported following administration of succinylcholine, particularly in patients with demyelinating nerve disorders or massive burns.

HYPOXIA

Hypoxia is a major factor contributing to arrhythmias during anesthesia, since most of the agents used are potent respiratory depressants. A decrease in arterial oxygen tension takes place regardless of the anesthetic used or whether ventilation is controlled or spontaneous. This effect is largely due to atelectasis and can be minimized by ventilating the patient with periodic large tidal volumes. The vulnerability to hypoxia is increased during anesthesia because the anesthetic agents modify the patient's own homeostatic mechanisms and impair the body's ability to adequately respond with secondary compensatory mechanisms. The major additional causes of hypoxia include 1) intrapulmonary shunting, which is often severe and refractory to oxygen therapy; 2) decreased alveolar oxygen tensions (resulting in decreased oxygen gradients with decreased pulmonary capillary oxygen tension); and 3) decreased mixed venous oxygen content due to increased metabolic rate, decreased cardiac output, and/or arterial oxygen content.

ELECTROLYTE DISTURBANCES

Hypokalemia

Acute hypokalemia is often observed during anesthesia as a result of iatrogenic hyperventilation (Edwards et al.,

1977). Under these circumstances, there is usually no significant tendency toward cardiac arrhythmias so long as the serum potassium concentration remains above 2.5 mEq per liter. However, patients who are chronically hypokalemic and alkalotic as a result of long term diuretic therapy are especially sensitive to serum pH changes with resultant changes in serum potassium. The combination of alkalosis and hypokalemia can produce significant arrhythmias that are only transiently ablated with potassium alone unless there is a concomitant return to normocapnia (Edwards et al., 1977).

Some additional causes of chronic hypokalemia include 1) gastrointestinal disorders resulting in electrolyte loss, 2) chronic steroid therapy, and 3) systemic diseases, such as hyperaldosteronism and renal tubular dysfunction.

Hyperkalemia

The development of acute hyperkalemia during surgery often results in brady- as well as tachyarrhythmias (Fisch, 1973). Hyperkalemia may be caused by 1) hypoventilation with resultant respiratory acidosis (Katz and Epstein, 1968); 2) inappropriate administration of potassium chloride; 3) administration of old blood with an elevated serum potassium level; 4) the use of succinylcholine in severely burned or traumatized or cord injured patients; and 5) malignant hyperthermia — a condition in which there is a defect in calcium transfer leading to an elevated intracellular calcium level and resultant hypermetabolism in the muscle.

Acid-Base Disturbances

Alkalosis often occurs and may produce significant physiologic alterations. Cardiac output tends to be increased and catecholamine responses enhanced. Atrial, junctional, and ventricular arrhythmias can occur and are often refractory to drug treatment until the alkalosis is corrected (Winnie and Edwards, 1977). Serum potassium may be reduced, and increased sensitivity to digitalis may result.

Metabolic acidosis is occasionally seen, particularly in patients with diabetes mellitus, thyrotoxicosis, starvation, heart failure, hypovolemia, hyperpyrexia, convulsions, and violent muscle contractions. Metabolic acidosis may also be produced during moderate or profound hypothermia. When it does occur, there is an increase in the extracellular potassium ion concentration and a decrease in the cellular membrane resting potential leading to an increased sensitivity to cardiac arrhythmias and ventricular fibrillation.

ADDITIONAL FACTORS PREDISPOSING TO ARRHYTHMIAS

The risk of surgery in the *elderly* is proportionately increased because of the increased incidence of associated diseases and their decreased ability to tolerate complications. Supraventricular arrhythmias are particularly common in elderly patients with chronic lung disease. Because atrial fibrillation frequently occurs during surgery, prophylactic digitalization has been advocated for this group. However, in our view, digitalis prophylaxis is not to be recommended except in situations where frequent atrial premature complexes are seen prior to surgery. If atrial fibrillation does occur with a rapid ventricular response, carotid massage may be particularly dangerous in the elderly, since carotid sinus sensitivity may be present with resultant severe bradycardias and asystole. Elderly patients also frequently undergo cataract surgery, at which time stimulation of the oculocardiac reflex can also result in asystole. While intracardiac conduction disturbances and sinus node dysfunction are also more commonly seen in the elderly, temporary pacemaker insertion is no longer routinely recommended for patients with bifascicular block even in the presence of increased P-R intervals unless a second degree A-V block has been documented or symptoms suggesting episodic complete heart block are present (Pastore et al., 1978).

Cardiac patients, regardless of age, are also at higher risk to develop serious arrhythmias. Many of these patients come to surgery medicated with a combination of digitalis, diuretic, antianginal, antihypertensive, and antiarrhythmic preparations. The incidence of intraoperative arrhythmias may be as much as two to four times greater in patients with coronary heart disease than in the general population (Kimbrough et al., 1975). The surgical mortality in these patients is highest in the initial 6 week period following an acute myocardial infarction and decreases progressively with time until 6 months, at which time the patient's risk appears to be similar to that of the general population. Similarly, patients with unstable angina pectoris, uncontrolled heart failure, or pre-existent arrhythmias are all at higher risk for arrhythmias during surgery and should have these abnormalities corrected whenever possible prior to operation (Goldman et al., 1977).

SURGERY

Non-cardiac Surgery

Although there is a high incidence of isolated supraventricular and ventricular ectopic beats with general anesthesia (80–90%), serious arrhythmias are relatively uncommon. Clinically significant rhythm disturbances most often occur in elderly patients and those with previous cardiac disease or other predisposing factors such as chronic obstructive pulmonary disease. In addition, however, certain operative procedures are associated with increased frequency of significant arrhythmias. Neurosurgical, ophthalmo-

logic, dental, and non-cardiac thoracic procedures are particularly arrhythmogenic. Patients undergoing intracranial surgery frequently suffer from intracranial hypertension with resultant central nervous system stimulation and may develop a marked bradycardia, atrial and ventricular premature complexes, a marked widening of the Q-T interval and an increased risk of re-entrant tachyarrhythmias. When the patient is operated on in the sitting position, stimulation of cranial nerves and air embolization are particularly likely to occur, resulting in serious ventricular arrhythmias (Slbin et al., 1976). Halothane anesthesia used in conjunction with neurosurgical procedures results in a markedly increased tendency toward arrhythmias, which is potentiated by local infiltration with epinephrine (to decrease bleeding and maintain a clear visual field). Epinephrine induced arrhythmias can often be prevented by the simultaneous use of lidocaine (Horrigan et al., 1978).

Patients undergoing ophthalmologic surgery have an unusually high incidence of supraventricular arrhythmias (greater than 70%). The majority of these are bradyrhythms resulting from stimulation of the oculocardiac reflex and occur predominantly in younger, healthier individuals. They can be prevented with small doses of atropine. Isolated premature ventricular contractions are also common in all patients, although only 6 per cent of patients have serious ectopic cardiac rhythm disorders (Alexander, 1975). Supraventricular tachycardia as well as rhythms frequently occurs during dental procedures because of stimulation of the autonomic nervous system via the fifth cranial nerve. Supraventricular and ventricular ectopic beats are common (Ostroff et al., 1977; Alexander, 1975).

Supraventricular and ventricular arrhythmias are also common in patients undergoing non-cardiac thoracic surgery, particularly pneumonectomy and lobectomy. The most common arrhythmias are multiple multifocal atrial ectopic beats, supraventricular tachycardia, atrial flutter, and atrial fibrillation. A retrospective study of 574 patients who had undergone resectional lung surgery revealed atrial fibrillation or flutter in 3.1 per cent with lobectomies and 19.4 per cent with pneumonectomies. The incidence of sustained atrial fibrillation or atrial tachycardia can be significantly decreased by prophylactic digitalization (Järvinen et al., 1978). In addition, there is also a significant incidence of ventricular arrhythmias, with 20 to 30 per cent of patients displaying frequent premature ventricular complexes during the course of surgery.

Cardiac Surgery

Intra- and postoperative arrhythmias occur in virtually all patients during open heart surgery (Gürsel et al., 1976). Ventricular premature complexes are the most frequent type of arrhythmias encountered, occurring in approximately 80 per cent of patients (Thormann and Schwarz, 1976). In addition to the previously mentioned general predisposing factors, surgical trauma to the heart, hypothermia, cardioplegic solutions, anoxic arrest, psychological trauma, and severe underlying cardiac disease all play contributing roles that are unique to open heart surgery. The induction of hypothermia is associated with marked prolongation of the Q-T interval, pronounced sinus bradycardia, varying grades of block and an increased sensitivity to calcium infusion (Martinez-Lopez, 1976). However, the arrhythmias associated with hypothermia or cardioplegic solutions are usually transient and disappear following reperfusion and warming.

Although all cardiac patients have an increased likelihood of developing significant rhythm disorders, specific abnormalities in cardiac function are particularly sensitive to the hemodynamic consequences of the various arrhythmias. Patients with aortic stenosis have severely noncompliant left ventricles and, hence, loss of sinus rhythm and its "atrial kick" postoperatively can result in disastrous hemodynamic consequences. These patients may also develop A-V conduction abnormalities, such as Mobitz type II block due to trauma to the His-Purkinje network resulting from removal of calcium that has infiltrated into the conduction pathways (Fukuda et al., 1976). In these patients it is vital to have atrial as well as ventricular electrodes implanted so that in the presence of S-A arrest, A-V dissociation, or junctional rhythms, atrial or A-V synchronous pacing can be used to maintain the atrial contribution to cardiac output. Sinus tachycardia can be tolerated for short periods; however, because of the decreased compliance, severe bradycardias are not accompanied by resultant increases in stroke volume and low cardiac output, and decreased perfusion can occur.

Patients with volume overload lesions, such as aortic insufficiency and mitral regurgitation, tend to be sensitive to the hypotensive effects of anesthetic agents. The decrease in diastolic pressure seen with these agents may result in marked impairment of coronary perfusion pressure. In these patients, bradycardia should be avoided as it can result in undue ventricular distention with elevation of atrial pressure and pulmonary congestion. Patients with mitral stenosis, on the other hand, tolerate tachyarrhythmias poorly because of impaired diastolic filling (McIntosh et al., 1964). In these patients, digitalis therapy should probably be continued up to the time of surgery. The maintenance of atrial synchrony is not nearly as important in patients with mitral stenosis or mitral regurgitation as in those with aortic stenosis.

Patients with coronary heart disease have an increased tendency to severe arrhythmias, and the frequency and severity of ventricular arrhythmias are even greater when an intraoperative infarction occurs. Anoxic arrest is commonly used during coronary artery bypass surgery in order to facilitate anastomosis of the distal arteries and help minimize damage to the myocardium (Adappa et al., 1978).

In the immediate postoperative period, several arrhythmogenic factors persist: 1) hypothermia (which may be present for several hours postoperatively); 2) electrolyte imbalance (particularly hypokalemia due to cardiopulmonary bypass); 3) continued ventilatory support, with its attendant stimuli (intermittent suction, with subsequent vagal stimulation and hypoxemia); and 4) in some patients, catecholamine infusion (which is occasionally necessary during the initial postoperative period to support the blood pressure).

TREATMENT OF ARRHYTHMIAS

Arrhythmias that occur during anesthesia are best approached prophylactically. This means correcting the predisposing factors previously mentioned prior to anesthesia administration. In addition, appropriate intubation and induction techniques substantially reduce the incidence and severity of arrhythmias. During the surgical procedure, continuous monitoring of the electrocardiogram, blood pressure, respiration, oxygen and carbon dioxide tension, blood, and potassium are all necessary in order to prevent serious arrhythmias from developing. When an arrhythmia does occur during anesthesia it will often respond to lightening of the anesthesia, improving the oxygenation, and correcting the electrolyte and acid-base status. Antiarrhythmic agents play a secondary role. When the need for antiarrhythmic medications does occur, treatment should be based on the same principles and guidelines that govern their administration under other clinical circumstances.

REFERENCES

Abou-Madi, M. N., Keszler, H., and Yacoub, J. Y.: Cardiovascular reactions to laryngoscopy and tracheal intubation following small and large intravenous doses of lidocaine. Can. Anaesth. Soc. J. 24(1):12, 1977.

Adappa, M. G., Jacobson, L. B., Hetzer, R., Hill, J. D., Kamm, B., and Kerth, W. J.: Cold hyperkalemic cardiac arrest versus intermittent aortic crossclamping and topical hypothermia for coronary bypass surgery. J. Thoracic Cardiovasc. Surg. 75(2):171–178, 1978.

Alexander, J. P.: Reflex disturbances of cardiac rhythm during ophthalmic surgery. Br. J. Ophthalmol. 59(9):518–524, 1975.

Andersen, J. R., and Eikard, B.: Arrhythmias during halothane anesthesia. III. The influence of barbiturates. Acta Anaesthesiol. Scand. 22(4):430–436, 1978.

Angelini, P., Feldman, M. I., Lufschanowski, R., and Leachman, R. D.: Cardiac arrhythmias during and after heart surgery: Diagnosis and management. Prog. Cardiovasc. Dis. 16(5):469–495, 1974.

Apivor, D., Ravi, P. K., and Little, L.: Cardiac effects of intravenous atropine. Electrocardiographic studies during ketamine anesthesia. Anaesthesia 33(6):542–545, 1978.

Atlee, J. L., III, and Rosy, B. F.: Halothane depression of A-V conduction studied by electrograms of the bundle of His in dogs. Anesthesiology 36:112–118, 1972.

Bonfim, V., Kayser, L., and Olin, C.: Myocardial protection during aortic valve replacement. Physiological and metabolic effects of selective coronary perfusion on the fibrillating heart. Scand. J. Thorac. Cardiovasc. Surg. 12(3):207–212, 1978.

Bradshaw, E. G.: Dysrhythmias associated with oral surgery. Anaesthesia 31(1):13–17, 1976.

Brandt, M. R., and Viby-Gogeuseu, J.: Halothane anesthesia and suxamethonium III. Atropine 30 s before a second dose of suxamethonium during inhalation anaesthesia: Effects and side-effects. Acta Anaesthesiol. Scand. (Suppl.) 67:76–83, 1978.

Edwards, R., Winnie, A. P., and Ramamurthy, S.: Acute hypocapneic hypokalemia: An iatrogenic anesthetic complication. Anesth. Analg. 56(6):786–792, 1977.

Eikard, B., and Andersen, J. R.: Arrhythmias during halothane anaesthesia. II: The influence of atropine. Acta Anaesthesiol. Scand. 21(3):245–251, 1977.

Eikard, B., and Skovsted, P.: Effects of respiratory acidosis on the arrhythmia threshold during Fluroxene and halothane anesthesia. Acta Anaesthesiol. Scand. 19(2):120–126, 1975.

Eikard, B., and Sorenson, B.: Arrhythmias during halothane anesthesia. I: The influence of atropine during induction with intubation. Acta Anaesthesiol. Scand. 20(4):296–306, 1936.

Falkoff, M., Stowe, S., Ong, L. S., Heinle, R. A., and Barold, S. S.: Unusual complication of bifascicular block during surgery under general anesthesia. PACE 1(2):260–264, 1978.

Fisch, C.: Relation of electrolyte disturbances to cardiac arrhythmias. Circulation 47:408–419, 1973.

Föex, P.: Preoperative assessment of patients with cardiac disease. Br. J. Anaesth. 50(1):15–23, 1978.

Fukuda, T., Hawley, R. L., and Edwards, J. E.: Lesions of conduction tissue complicating aortic valvular replacement. Chest 69(5):605–614, 1976.

Futral, J. E.: Postoperative management and complications of coronary artery bypass. Heart Lung 6(3):477–486, 1977.

Geer, R. T.: Anesthetic management of patients with cardiac disease. Surg. Clin. North Amer. 55(4):903–912, 1975.

Goldman, L., Caldera, D. L., Nussbaum, S. R., Southwick, F. S., Krogstad, D., Murray, B., Burke, D. S., O'Malley, T. A., Goroll, A. H., Caplan, C. H., Nolan, J., Carabello, B., and Slater, E. E.: Multifactorial index of cardiac risk in noncardiac surgical procedures. N. Engl. J. Med. 297(16):845–850, 1977.

Goldman, L., Caldera, D. L., Southwick, F. S., Nussbaum, S. R., Murray, B., O'Malley, T. A., Goroll, A. H., Caplan, C. H., Nolan, J., Burke, D. S., Krogstad, D., Carabello, B., and Slater, E. E.: Cardiac risk factors and complications in non-cardiac surgery. Medicine (Baltimore) 57(4):357–370, 1978.

Gotta, A. W., Sullivan, C. A., Pelkofski, J., Kangwalklai, S. K., and Kozan, R.: Aberrant conduction as a precursor to cardiac arrhythmias during anesthesia for oral surgery. J. Oral Surg. 34(5):421–427, 1976.

Gürsel, G., Karamehmetoğlu, A., Bozer, A. Y., and Saylam, A.: Postoperative arrhythmias in open heart surgery — a study on fifty cases. Vasc. Surg. 10(1):30–37, 1976.

Horrigan, R. W., Eger, E. I., and Wilson, C.: Epinephrine induced arrhythmias during anflurane anesthesia in man: a nonlinear dose response relationship and dose dependent protection from lidocaine. Anesth. Analg. (Cleve.) 57(5):547–550, 1978.

Järvinen, A., Mattila, T., Appelgvist, P., Meurala, H., and Mattila, S.: Cardiac disturbances after pneumonectomy — The value of prophylactic digitalization. Ann. Chir. Gynaecol. 67(2):77–81, 1978.

Katz, R. L., and Bigger, J. T.: Cardiac arrhythmias during anesthesia and operation. Anesthesiology 33:193–213, 1970.

Katz, R. L., and Epstein, R. A.: The interaction of anesthetic agents and adrenergic drugs to produce cardiac arrhythmias. Anesthesiology 29:763–784, 1968.

Khan, A. A., Miletich, D. J., and Albrecht, R. F.: Direct "sensitization" of myocardial muscle cells to epinephrine by halothane. Abstracts of scientific papers, annual meeting of the American Society of Anesthesiologists, p. 93, 1977.

Kimbrough, H. M., Jr., Crampton, R. S., and

Gillenwater, J. Y.: Cardiac rhythm in men during cystoscopy. J. Urol. 113(6):846–849, 1975.

Kouchoukos, N. T., and Karp, R. B.: Management of the post-operative cardiovascular surgical patient. Am. Heart J. 92(4):513–531, 1976.

Lloyd, E. L., and Mitchell, B.: Factors affecting the onset of ventricular fibrillation in hypothermia. Lancet 2(7392):1294, 1974.

Martinez-Lopez, J. I.: Induced myothermia: electrocardiographic abnormalities. South. Med. J. 69(12):1548–1550, 1976.

Mathias, C. J.: Bradycardia and cardiac arrest during tracheal suction—mechanisms in tetraplegic patients. Europ. J. Intensive Care Med. 2(4):147–156, 1976.

McIntosh, H. D., Yihong, K., and Mossie, J., Jr.: Hemodynamic effects of supraventricular arrhythmias. Am. J. Med. 37:712, 1964.

McLesky, C. H., McLead, D. S., Hough, T. L., and Stallworth, J. M.: Prolonged asystole after succinylcholine administration. Anesthesiology 49(3)208–210, 1978.

Meyer, J., Reul, G. J., Jr., Sandiford, F. M., Wukasch, D. C., Norman, J. C., Hallyan, G. L., and Cooley, D. A.: The value of moderate hypothermia during anoxic cardiac arrest for coronary artery surgery. J. Cardiovasc. Surg. 16(5):465–469, 1975.

Mirakhur, R. K., Clarke, R. S., Elliot, J., and Dundee, J. W.: Atropine and glycopyrronium premedication. A comparison of the effects on cardiac rate and rhythm during induction of anesthesia. Anesthesia 33(10):906–912, 1978.

Moffitt, E. A.: Anesthesia for patients early after infarction. Anesth. Analg. (Cleve.) 55(5):640–642, 1976.

Mulder, D. G., Olinger, G. N., McConnell, D. H., Maloney, J. V., Jr., and Buckberg, G. D.: Myocardial protection during aortic valve replacement. Ann. Thoracic Surg. 21(2):123–130, 1976.

Ostroff, L. H., Goldstein, B. H., Pennock, R. S., and Weiss, W. W., Jr.: Cardiac dysrhythmias during outpatient general anesthesia — a comparison study. J. Oral Surg. 35(10):793–797, 1977.

Pastore, J. O., Yurchak, P. M., Janis, K. Y., Murphy, J. D., and Zir, L. M.: The risk of advanced heart block in surgical patients with right bundle branch block and left axis deviation. Circulation 57(4):677–680, 1978.

Pöntinen, P. J.: Cardiovascular effects of local adrenaline infiltration during halothane anesthesia and adrenergic beta receptor blockade in man. Acta Anaesthesiol. Scand. 22(2):130–144, 1978.

Pöntinen, P. J.: Cardiovascular effects of local adrenaline infiltration during neurolept analgesia and adrenergic beta-receptor blockade in man. Acta Anaesthesiol. Scand. 22(2):145–153, 1978.

Reisner, L. S., and Lippmann, M.: Ventricular arrhythmias after epinephrine injection in enflurane and in halothane anesthesia. Anesth. Analg. (Cleve.) 54(4):468–470, 1975.

Roizen, M. F., and Stevens, W. C.: Multiform ventricular tachycardia due to the interaction of aminophylline and halothane. Anesth. Analg. (Cleve.) 57(6):738–741, 1978.

Ryhanen, P., Saarela, E., Saukkonen, J., and Hollmen, A.: Circulatory responses to laryngoscopy and endotracheal intubation in patients with and without cardiovascular disease. Effect of prophylactic practolol. Ann. Chir. Gynaecol. 66(6):294–298, 1977.

Sagarminaga, J., and Wynauds, J. E.: Atropine and the electrical activity of the heart during induction of anesthesia in children. Can. Anaesth. Soc. J. 10:328–342, 1963.

Sapala, J. A., Ponka, J. L., Duvernay, W. F.: Operative and nonoperative risks in the cardiac patient. J. Am. Geriatric Soc. 23(12):529–534, 1975.

Schachner, A., Schimert, G., Lajos, T. Z., Lee, A. H., Montes, M., Chaudhry, A., Schafer, P., Vladutin, A., and Siegel, J. H.: Selective intracavitary and coronary hypothermic cardioplegia for myocardial preservation. Clinical, physiologic and ultrastructural evaluation. Arch. Surg. 111(11):1197–1209, 1976.

Siedleck, J.: Disturbances in the function of cardiovascular system in patients following endotracheal intubation and attempts of their prevention by pharmacological blockade of sympathetic system. Anesth. Resusc. Intensive Ther. 3(2):107–123, 1975.

Slbin, M. S., Babinski, M., Maroon, J. C., and Jannetta, P. J.: Anesthetic management of posterior fossa surgery in the sitting position. Acta Anaesthesiol. Scand. 20(2):117–128, 1976.

Sliwinsti, M., Rydlewska-Sadowska, W., Hoffman, M., Soczek-Michalska, J., Holdrowicz, M., Falencik, M., Kaminski, P., and Biederman, A.: Arrhythmia during mitral commissurotomy. Anesth. Resusc. Intensive Ther. 3(4):315–324, 1975.

Tarhan, S., White, R. D., and Moffitt, E. A.: Anesthesia and post-operative care for cardiac operations. Ann. Thoracic Surg. 23(2):173–193, 1977.

Thomas, V. J., Thomas, W. J., and Thurlow, A. C.: Cardiac arrhythmia during outpatient dental anesthesia: The advantages of a controlled ventilation technique. Br. J. Anaesth. 48(9):919–922, 1976.

Thormann, J., and Schwarz, F.: Long term observations of cardiac arrhythmias during and after cardiac surgery. I. Acquired heart disease. Scand. J. Thorac. Cardiovasc. Surg. 10(1):31–35, 1976.

Thormann, J., and Schwarz, F.: Long term observation of cardiac arrhythmias during and after cardiac surgery. II. Congenital heart disease. Scand. J. Thorac. Cardiovasc. Surg. 10(2):149–155, 1976.

Vourch, G., and Tannieres, M. L.: Cardiac arrhythmia induced by pneumoencephalography. Br. J. Anaesth. 50:833–839, 1978.

Winnie, A. P., and Edwards, R.: Anesthesia, alkalosis and arrhythmias. Surg. Ann. 9:75–82, 1977.

Wynands, J. E.: Arrhythmias in the operating room. Refresher courses in anesthesiology. American Society of Anesthesiologists. 6:199–214, 1978.

21

BRAIN AND HEART RELATIONSHIPS

MONTY M. BODENHEIMER, M.D.

It has been known for many years that the central nervous system plays a significant role in cardiovascular regulation. The older concepts about localization of regulatory centers in the medulla have given way to new ideas about the complex interrelationships existing among the higher centers of the brain and the peripheral effector cells. The result has been the establishment of a cause-and-effect relationship between functional and organic disturbances in the brain and the cardiac manifestations that often accompany them.

ELECTROCARDIOGRAPHIC EFFECTS AND ARRHYTHMIAS RESULTING FROM EXPERIMENTAL STIMULATION OF VARIOUS PARTS OF THE BRAIN

Profound electrocardiographic effects result from electrical and chemical stimulation of various parts of the brain. The hypothalamus can exert an influence over the medullary level of cardiovascular control, and it in turn is influenced by higher centers in the cerebral cortex and limbic systems (Bard,

1960). In cardiovascular regulation the role played by the hypothalamus is only one link in a complex, integrated neural chain of control. Stimulation of portions of the hypothalamus produces ischemia-like electrocardiographic changes and serious arrhythmias through sympathetic and parasympathetic effects. The alterations noted include T wave inversion, S-T interval changes, widening of the QRS complex, ectopic beats, A-V dissociation, and bouts of paroxysmal tachycardia (Attar et al., 1963). Depressor effects may be accompanied by no change in rate, by bradycardia, or by tachycardia (Smith et al., 1960). Some of the effects are due to an increase in catecholamine response, which tends to increase the cardiac output and atrial and ventricular contractility (Fig. 21–1). Intense, prolonged, and repeated lateral stimulation enhances the development and persistence of the electrocardiographic changes. Bilateral stimulation can produce the pathologic picture of acute myocardial infarction.

In dogs, electrical stimulation of the diencephalon and mesencephalon resulted in ventricular arrhythmias, including ventricular tachycardia and fibrillation (Hockman et al., 1966).

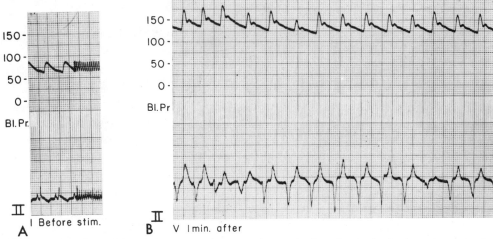

Figure 21-1   Effect of hypothalamic stimulation on the production of arrhythmias (experiment in the cat).

(A) Control before stimulation. Blood pressure is 85/60, and electrocardiogram shows normal sinus rhythm.

(B) 1 minute after stimulation. Note rise in blood pressure to 175/135. An idioventricular pacemaker now controls the heart rhythm. Note the widened QRS complexes and the irregularity in rhythm. Normal rhythm returned after cessation of the stimulation. (From Attar, H. J., Gutierrez, M. T., Bellet, S., and Ravens, J. R.: Circ. Res., 12:14, 1963.)

Sectioning of the vagi had no effect; however, propranolol prevented appearance of the arrhythmias.

RETICULAR FORMATION

Stimulation of the reticular formation, central gray substance of the midbrain, or the ventromedial region of the thalamus causes sinus tachycardia, followed by ventricular fusion beats, ventricular premature contractions (frequently multifocal and coupled to the preceding normal sinus complex, in bigeminal and trigeminal patterns), ventricular tachycardia, and sometimes ventricular fibrillation, always in that order, as the intensity of stimulation increases. Bilateral vagotomy does not affect the response but propranolol completely abolishes it. Thus, the action of norepinephrine at sympathetic neuroeffector sites in the myocardium may be responsible for these arrhythmias.

THE EFFECT OF ARRHYTHMIAS IN ALTERING CEREBRAL FUNCTION

We have discussed the effect of alterations in the brain on the production of arrhythmias; however, it is also known that certain arrhythmias may produce a decrease in cerebral blood flow, resulting in cerebral ischemia (Walter et al., 1970). This may occur in bradycardia accompanied by hypotension, with extremely rapid ventricular rates, or during Stokes-Adams attacks. Patients, particularly in the older age groups following the development of atrial fibrillation with rapid ventricular rate or ventricular tachycardia, may develop syncopal attacks or epileptic seizures. These episodes cease as the heart rate returns to normal. Moreover, routine clinical evaluation including an electrocardiogram is often unrevealing in detecting the caused arrhythmia. Walter et al. (1970), employing continuously recorded one hour electrocardiograms in 39 patients, observed periods of supraventricular tachycardia (7 patients) or high grades of A-V heart block (3 patients) that correlated with symptoms of cerebral ischemia. Goldberg et al. (1975) examined 130 patients with tape recordings; in 74 per cent of the group arrhythmias were considered the basis of the symptomatology. In addition, exercise testing was found to be relatively ineffective in detecting these arrhythmias. It should be remembered, however, that such patients frequently have associated obstructive lesions of the carotid or vertebral arteries (McHenry, 1976), which may underlie or actually be the basis of the episodes. It is, therefore, important to closely correlate the patient's symptoms with the presence of arrhythmias and not simply assume that occasional VPC's or APC's, which occur so frequently in the population in general, are causal.

THE EFFECT OF BRAIN DAMAGE OR DYSFUNCTION ON THE HEART AND CIRCULATION

The effect of certain types of brain damage or trauma has been correlated with various disturbances in circulatory function, including the production of arrhythmias. These include head trauma, subarachnoid and cerebral hemorrhage, cerebrovascular accidents, pneumoencephalography, and intracranial surgery.

It has been known for some time that severe head trauma may precipitate arrhythmias, particularly paroxysmal atrial fibrillation and premature beats. In experimental animals, moderate to severe concussion produces bradycardia, A-V junctional rhythms and a shortening of the Q-T_c (up to 38% reduction).

Following cerebrovascular accidents, a characteristic electrocardiographic pattern has been observed (Burch et al., 1954; Wasserman et al., 1956; Kreus et al., 1969). This consists of deep T wave inversion and lengthening of the Q-T segment. The most frequent changes occur in patients with subarachnoid hemorrhage (71.5%), followed by those with cerebral hemorrhage (57.1%) (Kreus et al., 1969). In contrast, only 41.1 per cent of patients with unclassified cerebrovascular accidents demonstrate electrocardiographic alterations consisting predominantly of prominent U waves. Estanol and Marin (1975) reported ventricular tachycardia in two patients with subarachnoid hemorrhage while being monitored and postulated that sudden death in such patients may be related to arrhythmias. Vander Ark (1975), in a series of 100 patients with acute subdural hematomas, found a high incidence of atrial arrhythmias (atrial flutter, fibrillation, and supraventricular tachycardia) and ventricular arrhythmias, including ventricular tachycardia and fibrillation. It was of interest that sinus tachycardia as well as bradycardia was seen in patients with evidence of a tentorial pressure cone.

The mechanism(s) whereby alterations in brain function can produce electrocardiographic changes and arrhythmias is unclear. Some pathology studies have not found any abnormalities in the myocardium at postmortem, while others have noted subendocardial hemorrhages. In addition, contraction bands or myofibrillar degeneration similar to that seen after catecholamine infusion have been described. It is possible that alteration in sympathetic tone, which can affect changes in ST-T waves and Q-T interval, may be responsible.

PSYCHOLOGICAL FACTORS

General Considerations

The effect of the mind and emotions on the heart has been recognized for many years. Psychological factors may precipitate ectopic rhythms in individuals with normal hearts as well as in those with structural disease. While similar factors are operative in both groups, patients with cardiac abnormalities are more vulnerable. Cardiac irregularities often accompany or follow an emotional episode. The patient may complain of heart consciousness, of his heart "jumping out of his throat," of dizziness or syncopal attacks. In the sensitive individual, awareness of premature beats or other arrhythmias may be quite disturbing.

Etiologic Factors

Arrhythmias associated with psychological disorders result from the interaction of many factors. Basic is the personality pattern and the life situation of those patients who tend to develop disturbances in cardiac rhythm. Studies in these subjects have shown that the most commonly observed emotional traits are chronic anxiety, excessive hostility, inadequate expression of hostility, compulsiveness, and a ready susceptibility to depression. While the chronic stress of the individual's life situation is considered the basic underlying factor, an acute exacerbation may precipitate an added degree of tension, with the resultant production of arrhythmias in susceptible subjects. The stress or tension may result from a variety of factors, such as sudden fear, anger, loss of sleep with excessive fatigue, or the excitement of watching a sporting event.

The relationship between psychological factors, arrhythmias, and *sudden death* is difficult to evaluate (Engel, 1971, 1976). Experimental studies in animals indicate that psychological stress can reduce the fibrillation threshold in dogs (Matta et al., 1976) and cause ventricular arrhythmias, sudden death, and pathologic abnormalities in pigs (Johanson et al., 1974). In man, it is clear that stressful situations can induce arrhythmias. Indeed, psychologic stress has been shown to induce serious ventricular arrhythmias in patients with previously known high grade ventricular arrhythmias (Lown et al., 1978). These patients generally had coronary heart disease. It is unclear, however, whether, except in a rare instance (Lown et al., 1976), psychologic factors can induce lethal arrhythmias in a patient without underlying heart disease.

The mechanism(s) of arrhythmia induction are also unclear. It is conceivable that stress exerts its effect via alterations in sympathetic and parasympathetic tone. On the other hand, neuropsychological factors may be mediated by inducing coronary spasm or causing platelet aggregation with resultant ischemia. Although the ischemia would be worse if an underlying coronary artery obstruction were present, a combination of ischemia and stress could possibly lead to arrhythmias even in the absence of anatomic obstruction. It should be emphasized that, to date, psychologic factors per se appear only rarely to result in ventricular fibrillation (Lown, 1976), since the overwhelming majority of patients who die suddenly are found to have significant coronary heart disease or other pathology (see Chapters 11 and 15). However, the role of psychologic factors in the context of coronary disease may be of greater significance. Thus, the exact role of neuropsychologic influences as a risk factor in sudden death, while provocative, awaits clarification.

REFERENCES

Abildskov, J. R.: Electrocardiographic wave form and the nervous system. Circulation 41:371, 1970.
Abildskov, J. R., Millar, K., Burgess, M. J., and Vincent, W.: The electrocardiogram and the central nervous system. Prog. Cardiovasc. Dis. 13:210, 1970.
Attar, H. J., Gutierrez, M. T., Bellet, S., and

Ravens, J. R.: The hypothalamus and the reticular activating system in the control of cardiac rhythm. Circ. Res. *12*:14, 1963.

Bard, P.: Anatomical organization of the central nervous system in relation to control of the heart and blood vessels. Physiol. Rev. *40*:3, 1960.

Benedict, R. B., and Evans, J. M.: Second degree heart block and Wenckebach phenomena associated with anxiety. Am. Heart J. *43*:626, 1952.

Burch, G. E., Colcolough, H., and Giles, T.: Intracranial lesions and the heart. Am. Heart J. *80*:574, 1970.

Burch, G. E., Meyers, R., and Abildskov, J. A.: A new electrocardiographic pattern observed in cerebrovascular accidents. Circulation *9*:719, 1954.

Combs, J. J., Jr., Bryant, G. N., Bodgonoff, M. D., and Warren, J. V.: The effect of induced anxiety and hostility on cardiovascular functions. J. Clin. Invest. *37*:885, 1958.

Connor, R. C. R.: Myocardial damage secondary to brain lesions. Am. Heart J. *78*:145, 1969.

Corday, E., and Irving, D. W.: Effect of cardiac arrhythmias on the cerebral circulation. Am. J. Cardiol. *6*:803, 1960.

Delgado, J. M.: Circulatory effects of cortical stimulation. Physiol. Rev. *40*(Suppl 4):146–171, 1960.

Engel, G. L.: Sudden and rapid death during psychological stress: Folklore or folk wisdom? Ann. Int. Med. *74*:771, 1971.

Engel, G. L.: Psychologic factors in instantaneous cardiac death. N. Engl. J. Med. *294*:664, 1976.

Estanol, B. V., and Marin, O. S. M.: Cardiac arrhythmias and sudden death in subarachnoid hemorrhage. Stroke *6*:382, 1975.

Goldberg, A. D., Raftery, E. B., and Cashman, P. M. M.: Ambulatory electrocardiographic records in patients with transient cerebral attacks or palpitations. Br. Med. J. *4*:569, 1975.

Hillis, L. D., and Braunwald, E.: Coronary artery spasm. N. Engl. J. Med. *299*:695, 1978.

Hockman, C. H., Mauck, H. P., and Hoff, E. C.: ECG changes resulting from cerebral stimulation. Am. Heart J. *71*:695, 1966.

Hoff, E. C., Kell, J. F., and Carroll, M. N.: Effects of cortical stimulation and lesions on cardiovascular function. Physiol. Rev. *43*:68–114, 1963.

James, T. N., Froggatt, P., and Marshall, T.: Sudden death in young athletes. Ann. Int. Med. *67*:1013, 1967.

Johansson, G., Jonsson, L., Lannek, N., et al.: Severe stress-cardiopathy in pigs. Am. Heart J. *87*:451, 1974.

Korteweg, B. C. J., Boeles, T. F., and Tencate, J.: Influence of stimulation of some subcortical areas on electrocardiogram. J. Neurophysiol. *20*:100–107, 1957.

Kreus, K. E., Kemila, S. J., and Takala, J. K.: Electrocardiographic changes in cerebrovascular accidents. Acta Med. Scand. *185*:327, 1969.

Lown, B. L., DeSilva, R. A., and Lenson, R.: Roles of psychologic stress and autonomic nervous system in provocation of ventricular premature complexes. Am. J. Cardiol. *41*:979, 1978.

Lown, B. L., Teinte, J. V., Reich, P., Gaughan, C., Regestein, Q., and Hai, H.: Basis for recurring ventricular fibrillation in the absence of coronary heart disease and its management. N. Engl. J. Med. *294*:623, 1976.

Lown, B. L., Verrier, R., and Corbalan, R.: Psychologic stress and threshold for repetitive ventricular response. Science *182*:834, 1973.

McHenry, L. C., Toole, J. F., and Miller, H. S.: Long term EKG monitoring in patients with cerebrovascular insufficiency. Stroke *7*:264, 1976.

Matta, R. J., Lawler, J. E., and Lown, B. L.: Ventricular electrical instability in the conscious dog. Effects of psychologic stress and beta adrenergic blockade. Am. J. Cardiol. *38*:594, 1976.

Selye, H.: The physiology and pathology of exposure to stress. Montreal, Acta Inc. 1950.

Smith, O. A., Jr., Suhayi, J., Rushmer, R. F., and Lasher, E. P.: Role of hypothalamic structures in cardiac control. Physiol. Rev. *136*:40, 1960.

Tzivoni, D., and Stern, S.: Pacemaker implantation based on ambulatory ECG monitoring in patients with cerebral symptoms. Chest *67*:274, 1975.

Vander Ark, G. D.: Cardiovascular changes with acute subdural hematoma. Surg. Neurol. *3*:305, 1975.

Walter, P. F., Reid, S. O., and Wenger, N. K.: Transient cerebral ischemia due to arrhythmia. Ann. Intern. Med. *72*:471, 1970.

Wasserman, F., Choquette, G., Cassinelli, R., and Bellet, S.: Electrocardiographic observations in patients with cerebrovascular accidents. Am. J. Med. Sci. *231*:502, 1956.

SUPPLEMENTARY READING

DeBusk, R. F., Taylor, C. M., and Agras, W. S.: Comparison of treadmill exercise testing and psychologic stress testing soon after myocardial infarction. Am. J. Cardiol. *43*:907, 1979.

Orr, W. C., Stahl, M. L., Whitsett, T., and Langevin, E.: Physiological sleep patterns. Cardiac arrhythmias. Am. Heart J. *97*:128, 1979.

22

INFECTIOUS DISEASES AND OTHER DISEASE STATES

MONTY M. BODENHEIMER, M.D.
RICHARD H. HELFANT, M.D.

INFECTIOUS DISEASES

The heart is involved in varying degrees by systemic infections. The degree and severity of involvement depend on the etiologic agent, its predilection for the heart, and the susceptibility of cardiac tissue to the organism. The involvement of the heart is usually diffuse and may include the atria, ventricles, and the specialized conduction system.

Certain bacterial and rickettsial infections show a marked affinity for the heart, affecting it by either direct involvement or toxic factors. *Diphtheria* results in a severe myopathy with a dilated myocardium. A prominent feature is development of heart block, which may progress to complete A-V block and which is associated with a poor prognosis. Tuberculous involvement of the myocardium may be a part of either the miliary form of the disease or an otherwise asymptomatic tuberculous nodule which may be associated with cardiac arrhythmias. *Typhoid fever* may be associated either with tachycardia or bradycardia.

Myocarditis results in varying degrees of cardiac dysfunction and may result in severe heart failure. Even upon subsidence of the infection, several months may pass before the cardiovascular state returns to normal. Occasionally the abnormalities produced are permanent. Serial electrocardiograms frequently reveal marked changes. Tachycardia, bradycardia, T wave inversion, and R-ST segment deviations may be recorded; Q-T interval prolongation and varied arrhythmias are not uncommon.

The arrhythmias most commonly associated with these diseases are premature beats; however, sinus tachycardia (or bradycardia, especially in diphtheria), paroxysmal atrial or ventricular tachycardia, and varying degrees of A-V conduction disturbance are also encountered. A-V junctional rhythm, atrial fibrillation, and ventricular fibrillation are less common. These arrhythmias usually respond poorly to therapy, particularly digitalis.

Bacterial endocarditis is primarily characterized by the severity of the valvular destruction and secondary complications of embolization and congestive heart failure. Serious arrhythmias, although usually not a prominent feature, may appear, particularly with in-

300

volvement of the myocardium by abscess formation or coronary emboli. Garvey and Neu (1978) found three cases of complete heart block in their series. Wang et al. (1972) reported six patients with complete heart block. All had aortic valve involvement, with extension of the infection to adjacent myocardium. In such cases, insertion of a transvenous pacemaker is indicated.

Syphilitic heart disease rarely if ever produces a diffuse myocarditis, and thus is usually associated with arrhythmias arising from myocardial dysfunction associated with aortic insufficiency, narrowing of the orifices of the coronary arteries, cardiomegaly, and congestive heart failure, or rarely gummatous involvement of the A-V conduction system.

Viral diseases are now recognized to be a significant cause of cardiovascular disease. Coxsackie B appears to have a particular predilection for the heart, resulting in both pericardial and myocardial involvement. Clinically, the patient may show congestive heart failure and/or pericarditis. The electrocardiogram is generally abnormal, and Smith (1970), in a series of 42 patients, reported arrhythmias in 31 per cent, including atrial fibrillation, ventricular premature contractions with one instance of ventricular fibrillation, and two patients with temporary complete heart block. Pathologic changes in the heart (notably myocarditis) have also been observed in viral hepatitis, infectious mononucleosis, poliomyelitis, roseola (measles), and influenza. This cardiac involvement produces various electrocardiographic changes (e.g., elevation or depression of the S-T segment, T wave flattening, and inversion), and is occasionally associated with arrhythmias. These include premature beats, sinus tachycardia, and, very commonly, A-V conduction disturbances.

Certain *parasitic diseases*, including trichinosis, schistosomiasis, echinococcus disease, and particularly Chagas' disease (trypanosomiasis), are associated with myocardial pathology which leads to arrhythmias. Direct cardiac involvement underlies the pathology of these diseases. Various electrocardiographic alterations and arrhythmias (commonly, premature beats) are observed. The most striking are the A-V conduction disturbances caused by Chagas' disease. This disease causes progressive A-V heart block, and all stages of bundle branch block leading to trifascicular heart block may be seen.

INFILTRATIVE DISEASES

Infiltrative diseases of the heart are relatively infrequent. However, they cause a secondary cardiomyopathy with serious cardiac dysfunction and arrhythmias. Chew et al. (1975) found that of all cardiomyopathies, amyloid made up 1.7 per cent, sarcoid 1 per cent, neuromuscular 1.5 per cent, collagen vascular disease 1.5 per cent and hemochromatosis 0.25 per cent. These diseases may be the cause of heart disease of obscure etiology, particularly in the older age group, and not infrequently have associated arrhythmias and atrioventricular conduction abnormalities.

Sarcoid

Sarcoidosis is a systemic disease characterized by the presence of granulomas and fibrosis. Cardiac involvement has been found in from 5.1 to 27 per cent of patients with sarcoid (Mayock et al., 1963; Silverman et al., 1978) and may involve the pericardium, myocardium, or endocardium, the most common being the left ventricular free wall (Roberts et al., 1977).

In a necropsy study of 89 patients with sarcoid heart disease, Roberts et al. (1977) found that the major clinical manifestations were *ventricular arrhythmias, conduction disturbances,* and *sud-*

den death. Overall, 19 (21%) patients had ventricular tachycardia and 25 (28%) had complete heart block. Pathologically, there was significant involvement of either the ventricular myocardium or the A-V conduction system, with granuloma and/or fibrous tissue. Sixty of the 89 patients (67%) died suddenly, with a minority (23%) dying in congestive heart failure. In 10 of the 60 sudden deaths, this was the first manifestation of disease. Of the remaining 50 patients, 20 had prior complete heart block while 12 had prior ventricular tachycardia.

Treatment of patients with sarcoid heart disease is difficult. Steroids are utilized with variable response (Brit. Med. J., 1972). Specific antiarrhythmic therapy for ventricular arrhythmias is clearly indicated; however, control of the arrhythmias is often difficult and may require multiple antiarrhythmics.

Amyloid

Amyloid involvement of the heart may be primary or secondary. It is characterized by varying degrees of amyloid deposition in the myocardium and specialized tissue. Brandt et al. (1968) found that of 42 patients with amyloidosis, cardiac involvement was evident in 28 (67%). They also noted that either primary amyloidosis or amyloid in association with myeloma had cardiac involvement in 90 per cent of patients, while secondary amyloid had cardiac involvement in 54 per cent.

The dominant clinical feature of cardiac amyloidosis is *congestive heart failure*. In addition, arrhythmias are a common occurrence. Ridolfi et al. (1977) found *atrial arrhythmias* in 39 per cent, including 17 per cent with atrial fibrillation, while Farrok et al. (1964) found atrial fibrillation in 28 per cent and *VPC's* in 85 per cent. Atrioventricular block, including complete heart block and fascicular block, is also common; however, Ridolfi et al. (1977) were not able to attribute this finding to amyloid infiltration of the conduction system in the majority of instances.

Cardiac deaths are generally attributable to progressive heart failure. Sudden death occurs uncommonly (Buja et al., 1970; Brandt et al., 1968) and is presumably related to ventricular arrhythmias.

Hemochromatosis

Hemochromatosis is most commonly seen in patients with chronic anemia of varying etiology who have received large numbers of transfusions. Buja and Roberts (1971), in a necropsy study, found that of 135 patients, 19 had iron deposits in the heart, and of these seven were extensive. The clinical picture is characterized by *congestive heart failure* and to a lesser extent arrhythmias. Engle et al. (1964), in a series of 41 patients, found *atrial arrhythmias* (supraventricular tachycardia, atrial fibrillation, and flutter) in 46 per cent and *ventricular arrhythmias* in 29 per cent, including three with repetitive ventricular tachycardia. In addition, atrioventricular heart block ranging from PR prolongation to complete A-V block (Engle et al., 1964; Schellhammer, 1967) and fascicular block are reported.

Neuromuscular Diseases

Involvement of cardiac muscle in progressive muscular dystrophy and Friedreich's ataxia is not uncommon. The degenerative myocardial lesions that are observed may be the cause of the atrial and ventricular premature beats and A-V conduction delays encountered.

Thyroid Disease

Hyperthyroidism is often accompanied by cardiac arrhythmias (Table 22–

TABLE 22–1 THYROID DISEASE

Hyperthyroidism
 — Sinus tachycardia
 — Atrial fibrillation
 — Atrioventricular
   conduction abnormalities

Hypothyroidism
 — Sinus bradycardia
 — Atrioventricular
   conduction abnormalities

1). Most commonly, *sinus tachycardia* is noted in such patients. Other common arrhythmias include *atrial fibrillation* in 23 per cent (Rosenblum and Delman, 1963). Hoffman and Lowrey (1960) found that atrial fibrillation was present in 12 per cent; however, only 2.2 per cent of patients under 40 had atrial fibrillation, while it was seen in 18 per cent of those over 40. Importantly, any patient who presents with atrial fibrillation should be evaluated for hyperthyroidism in view of the clear therapeutic implications. Paroxysmal atrial tachycardia and ventricular arrhythmias are rare. Occasionally, patients will exhibit first degree or higher atrioventricular block.

Hypothyroidism is associated with *bradycardia,* which at times may be marked. Ventricular tachyarrhythmias are generally seen only in myxedema coma. Atrioventricular conduction abnormalities are occasionally seen.

Neoplastic Disease

Tumors involving the heart may be primary or metastatic, the latter being more common. Primary tumors are usually *myxomata,* which commonly produce *atrial arrhythmias* and only rarely A-V conduction delays. Sarcomata, the less frequently seen primary tumors, most commonly cause A-V heart block.

Hanfling (1960) found that 18.3 per cent of a series of patients with *metastatic cancer* had involvement of the

heart, which rose to 36 per cent if only lymphoma, leukemia, and myeloma were considered. The manifestations of metastatic cancer of the heart depend largely upon the location of the tumors; however, they generally produce *ectopic rhythms.* Atrial fibrillation, flutter, and PAT are common in this situation. The sudden appearance of arrhythmias in a patient with a primary neoplasm outside the heart is highly suggestive of cardiac metastasis.

Cor Pulmonale

Cor pulmonale is characterized predominantly by right-sided heart enlargement resulting from disease of the pulmonary parenchyma and/or vascular bed. Arrhythmias that accompany acute cor pulmonale may be either atrial or ventricular (Table 22–2). In a study of routine electrocardiograms in 122 patients with chronic cor pulmonale, Corazza and Pastor (1958) found predominantly *atrial arrhythmias* in 31 per cent; these included frequent APC's, VPC's, supraventricular tachycardia, and atrial fibrillation.

Hudson et al. (1973) reviewed standard electrocardiograms in 70 patients with acute respiratory failure and chronic obstructive lung disease. Forty-seven per cent had major supraventricular or ventricular arrhythmia, including atrial tachycardia (16%), atrial flutter or fibrillation (19%), *multifocal atrial tachycardia* (17%), and ventricular tachycardia (6%). Significantly, Holford and Mithoefer (1973) obtained 72 hour tape recordings in 35 patients admitted

TABLE 22–2 COR PULMONALE

Atrial Arrhythmias
 — Atrial premature contractions
 — Supraventricular tachycardia
 — Atrial fibrillation
 — Multifocal atrial tachycardia
Ventricular Arrhythmias
 — Ventricular premature contractions
 — Ventricular tachycardia

with chronic obstructive lung disease including 16 with respiratory failure and found that the routine electrocardiograms seriously underestimated the frequency of arrhythmias. Fully 89 per cent had arrhythmias, including 57 per cent with either serious ventricular arrhythmias or atrial tachycardias. In comparison, only 31 per cent were detected by standard electrocardiogram.

The prognostic implications of these arrhythmias have been examined (Hudson et al., 1973). Of 37 patients with either sinus rhythm or rare arrhythmias, 22 per cent died during the follow-up period. In contrast, all the patients with serious ventricular arrhythmias died. These arrhythmias may simply reflect the severity of either the underlying lung disease or associated heart disease.

Recently, interest has focused on the relationship between the treatment of acute asthma with bronchodilators and the occurrence of arrhythmias. Grossman et al. (1976) obtained 24 hour electrocardiogram records on 20 patients with acute asthma being treated with aminophylline and isoproterenol inhalation. No supraventricular arrhythmias were seen. Five patients, all with underlying heart disease, had VPC's; of these, only two were frequent and none were of a serious grade. Of particular interest was the finding that the arrhythmias *decreased* with bronchodilator therapy. While it would thus appear that such therapy in appropriate doses is safe in such patients and may actually be beneficial, care should be utilized, particularly in patients with underlying heart disease.

ARRHYTHMIAS ASSOCIATED WITH VARIOUS RESPIRATORY MANEUVERS

Normal respiration and certain simple respiratory maneuvers affect the rhythm of the heart in various ways: 1) Vagal reflexes may be initiated by stimulation of stretch receptors in the visceral pleura or the lung parenchyma. From these receptors the impulse is transmitted via vagal afferent fibers and then vagal efferent (cardiac) fibers to complete the reflex arc. The normal variation of the cardiac rate between inspiration and expiration may represent the most common manifestation of this reflex. However, this phenomenon may be due to other factors, including 2) the effect of changing intrathoracic pressure and venous filling of the heart.

Breath-Holding

A deep breath held in maximal inspiration results in significant slowing of the heart rate as a result of the vagal reflex previously described. Other arrhythmias seen with breath-holding include transient cardiac arrest with ventricular escape, transitory A-V block without ventricular response, and changes in bundle branch conduction. It is of interest that this maneuver may at times convert W-P-W conduction to normal (Lamb et al., 1958). At the height of inspiration, certain subjects may develop premature ventricular systoles. These may occur regularly and without evidence of other cardiac arrhythmias. Following prolonged inspiration, releasing the breath may result in premature ventricular beats and occasionally in bigeminal rhythm (Lamb et al., 1958); occasionally, a rapid ectopic rhythm may be abolished.

Valsalva Maneuver

This respiratory maneuver consists of a forced expiration against a closed glottis. The hemodynamic changes in the Valsalva maneuver are due in part to the trapping of blood outside the thorax, thus impeding venous return to the right side of the heart.

One might expect cardio-inhibition during the Valsalva maneuver as a result of powerful vagal reflexes. Howev-

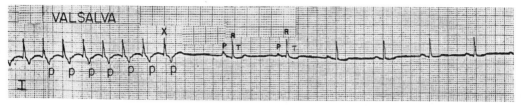

Figure 22–1 Shows the effect of the Valsalva maneuver in terminating supraventricular tachycardia (junctional). Note the tachycardia rate of 140 per minute with the QRS followed by an inverted P wave. Following the Valsalva maneuver at X, note the pre-automatic pause and the restoration of normal sinus rhythm (with a "warming-up" effect).

er, this is balanced by the "need" for a tachycardia (to compensate for the decreased venous return and decreased cardiac output) that outweighs the influence of pulmonary vagal reflexes. Upon release, the pressure overshoot is associated with a bradycardia. Bradycardia and frequent premature beats have been noted with the Valsalva maneuver; occasionally, the maneuver may abolish a supraventricular tachycardia (Fig. 22–1).

Hyperventilation

Hyperventilation is characterized by excessive breathing due to an increased rate or volume of respiration. In a normal subject, the biochemical result of hyperventilation is a decrease in the arterial pCO_2. If sufficiently prolonged, respiratory alkalosis may be observed: bigeminal or trigeminal rhythm following hyperventilation; transitory A-V dissociation with junctional tachycardia; irregular multifocal atrial complexes with rates up to 220 per minute, occasional transient episodes of atrial fibrillation, and ventricular fibrillation.

Cheyne-Stokes Respiration

Cheyne-Stokes respiration is a form of periodic breathing in which periods of hyperpnea alternate with periods of apnea. The apnea results from cerebral hypocapnia, which depresses the respiratory centers. Various arrhythmias are associated with this respiratory pat-

tern. Bradycardia may be due to sinus slowing, A-V junctional rhythm, or partial or complete A-V heart block. Other arrhythmias reported include premature beats, prolonged P-R interval, idioventricular rhythm, ventricular tachycardia, and electrical alternation of the heart (Scherf and Schott, 1953). Several instances have been reported in which A-V heart block appeared during apnea.

EFFECT OF CHANGES IN POSTURE ON HEART RATE, A-V CONDUCTION, AND THE PRODUCTION OF CERTAIN ECTOPIC RHYTHMS

Of 31 cases of partial A-V block, 26 revealed a shortening of the P-R interval when the patients changed from the recumbent to the upright position (Scherf and Dix, 1952). An increase in sympathetic tone and a reciprocal decrease in the vagal tone are assumed to be responsible for the shortening of the P-R interval in normal subjects and in patients with A-V block in standing positions.

ORTHOSTATIC PAROXYSMAL ACCELERATION OF THE HEART

Patients are occasionally encountered in whom the assumption of the upright position results in the production of a rapid ectopic rhythm: atrial tachycardia (Fig. 22–2), atrial flutter, or ventricular

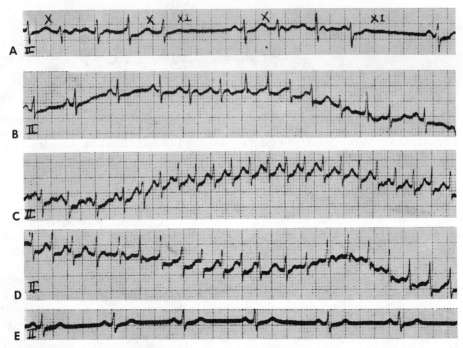

Figure 22–2 Postural atrial tachycardia.

(A) Control — supine. Note the presence of a normal sinus rhythm with occasional atrial premature beats at X and cycles of sinoatrial heart block at X_1.

(B) One minute after standing. Note frequent atrial premature beats and short paroxysms of supraventricular tachycardia.

(C) Three minutes after standing. Note the presence of supraventricular tachycardia.

(D) After 0.5 mg. neostigmine intramuscularly. It took seven minutes after standing for the tachycardia to appear.

(E) When maintained on neostigmine, no tachycardia resulted even on prolonged standing.

tachycardia. This may be the result of the following factors: 1) increased sympathetic tone in the upright position manifesting cardiac effects in those hearts that are vulnerable, and 2) fall in blood pressure and "inadequate venous return" to the right atrium due to pooling of abnormally large quantities of blood in the lower extremities with a decrease in coronary flow in addition to the compensatory increase in sympathetic tone.

REFERENCES

Barkve, R., and Stavem, P.: Cardiac arrhythmia associated with Cheyne-Stokes breathing. Acta Med. Scand. 180:395, 1966.

Benson, R., and Smith, J. F.: Cardiac amyloidosis. Brit. Heart J. 18:529, 1956.

Brandt, K., Cathcart, E. S., and Cohen, A. S.: A clinical analysis of the course and prognosis of forty-two patients with amyloidosis. Am. J. Med. 44:955, 1968.

Buja, L. M., Khoi, N. B., and Roberts, W. C.: Clinically significant cardiac amyloidosis. Clinicopathologic findings in 15 patients. Am. J. Cardiol. 26:394, 1970.

Buja, L. M., and Roberts, W. C.: Iron in the heart. Am. J. Med. 51:209, 1971.

Chew, C., Ziady, G. M., Raphael, M. J., and Oakley, C. M.: The functional defect in amyloid heart disease. The "stiffheart" syndrome. Am. J. Cardiol. 36:438, 1975.

Corazza, L. J., and Pastor, B. J.: Cardiac arrhythmias in chronic cor pulmonale. N. Engl. J. Med. 259:862, 1958.

Engle, M. A., Erlandson, M., and Smith, C. H.: Late cardiac complications of chronic severe refractory anemia with hemochromatosis. Circulation 30:698, 1964.

Farrok, L. A., Walsh, J. J., Massie, E.: Amyloid heart disease. Am. J. Cardiol. 13:750, 1964.

Fletcher, E., Brennan, C. F.: Cardiac complications of Coxsackie-virus infection. Lancet 1:913, 1957.

Garvey, G. J., and Neu, H. C.: Infective endocarditis — an evolving disease. A review of endocarditis of the Columbia-Presbyterian Medical Center. Medicine 57:105, 1978.

Grossman, J.: The occurrence of arrhythmias in hospitalized asthmatic patients. J. Allergy Clin. Immunol. 57:310, 1976.

Hanfling, S. M.: Metastatic cancer to the heart. Review of literature of 127 cases. Circulation 22:474, 1960.

Harvey, W. P.: Clinical aspects of cardiac tumors. Am. J. Cardiol. 21:329, 1968.

Hoffman, I., and Lowrey, R. D.: The electrocardiogram in thyrotoxicosis. Am. J. Cardiol. 6:893, 1960.

Holford, F. D., and Mithoefer, J. C.: Cardiac arrhythmias in hospitalized patients with chronic obstructive pulmonary disease. Am. Rev. Resp. Dis. 108:879, 1973.

Holmes, J. H., and Weill, D. R., Jr.: Incomplete heart block produced by changes in posture. Am. Heart J. 30:291, 1945.

Hudson, L. D., Kurt, T. L., Petty, T. L., and Genton, E.: Arrhythmias associated with acute respiratory failure in patients with chronic airway obstruction. Chest 63:661, 1973.

James, T. N., and Carrera, G. M.: Pathogenesis of arrhythmias associated with metastatic tumors of the heart. N. Engl. J. Med. 260:869, 1959.

Lamb, L. E., Dermksian, G., and Sarnoff, C. A.: Significant cardiac arrhythmias induced by common respiratory maneuvers. Am. J. Cardiol. 2:563, 1958.

McIntosh, H. D., Burnum, J. F., Hickam, J. B., and Warren, J. V.: Circulatory changes produced by the Valsalva maneuver in normal subjects, patients with mitral stenosis, and autonomic nervous system alterations. Circulation 9:511, 1957.

Massumi, R. A., and Nutter, D. O.: Arrhythmias with Cheyne-Stokes respiration. Bull. Johns Hopkins Hosp. 66:335, 1940.

Mayock, R. L., Bertrand, P., Morrison, C. E., and Scott, J. H.: Manifestations of sarcoidosis. Analysis of 145 patients with a review of 9 series selected from the literature. Am. J. Med. 35:67, 1963.

Reich, N. E.: The Uncommon Heart Disease. Springfield, Ill., Charles C Thomas, 1954.

Ridolfi, R. L., Bulkley, B. H., Hutchins, G. M.: The conduction system in cardiac amyloidosis. Clinical and pathologic features of 23 patients. Am. J. Med. 62:677, 1977.

Roberts, W. C., McAllister, H. A., and Ferrano, V. J.: Sarcoidosis of the heart. A clinicopathologic study of 35 necropsy patients (group I) and review of 78 previously described necropsy patients (group II). Am. J. Med. 63:86, 1977.

Rosenblum, R., and Delman, A. J.: First degree heart block associated with thyrotoxicosis. Arch. Int. Med. 112:488, 1963.

Sarcoid heart disease: Editorial. Brit. Med. J. 4:627, 1972.

Schellhammer, P. F., Engle, M. A., and Hagstrom, J. C.: Histochemical studies of the myocardium and conduction system in acquired iron-storage disease. Circulation 35:631, 1967.

Scherf, D., and Dix, J. H.: Effects of posture on A-V conduction. Am. Heart J. 43:494, 1952.

Scherf, D., and Schott, A.: Extrasystoles and Allied Arrhythmias. New York, Grune & Stratton, 1953.

Silverman, K. J., Hutchins, G. M., and Bulkley, B. H.: Cardiac sarcoid: A clinicopathologic study of 84 unselected patients with systemic sarcoidosis. Circulation 58:1209, 1978.

Smith, W. G.: Coxsackie B myopericarditis in adults. Am. Heart J. 80:34, 1970.

Surawicz, B., Mangiardi, M. L.: Electrocardiogram in endocrine and metabolic disorders. Cardiovasc. Clin. 8(3):243, 1977.

Wang, K., Gobel, F., Gleason, D. F., and Edwards, J. E.: Complete heart block complicating bacterial endocarditis. Circulation 46:939, 1972.

Wessler, S., and Freedberg, A. S.: Cardiac amyloidosis. Electrocardiographic and pathologic observations. Arch. Int. Med. 82:63, 1948.

Wildenthal, K., Fuller, D. S., and Shapiro, W.: Paroxysmal atrial arrhythmia induced by hyperventilation. Am. J. Cardiol. 21:436, 1968.

Woodward, T. E., McCrumb, F. R., Jr., Carey, T. N., and Togo, Y.: Viral and rickettsial causes of cardiac disease, including the Coxsackie virus etiology of pericarditis and myocarditis. Ann. Int. Med. 53:1130, 1960.

23

ANTIARRHYTHMIC AGENTS

MICHAEL S. FELDMAN, M.D.,
RICHARD H. HELFANT, M.D.

The great majority of cardiac arrhythmias are amenable to pharmacologic therapy. This is despite the fact that although several new drugs have been added to the pharmacopeia of antiarrhythmic agents none approaches the ideal. These drugs are all relatively short acting, display varying degrees of efficacy in individual patients, and often exhibit toxic cardiac and noncardiac side effects. The most satisfactory results are obtained when the goals of treatment are clearly defined, the arrhythmia is properly categorized, its clinical setting is identified, and attention is paid to correctable precipitating factors.

PHARMACOKINETICS

There is an important relationship between the plasma concentration of an antiarrhythmic agent and its pharmacologic effects. In general, bolus doses of an agent equilibrate relatively rapidly with the extravascular space, and plasma levels remain within therapeutic ranges for only a short period of time. On the other hand, a constant intravenous infusion results in a slow accumulation within the body and only gradual elevations in plasma concentration. Alterations in the rate of infusion

do not affect the time period over which the plateau levels are reached but result only in alterations in the absolute plateau level achieved (Harrison, 1977). Thus, a substantial amount of time is required to achieve therapeutic levels with infusions not preceded by a bolus. One can, however, rapidly achieve and maintain therapeutic concentrations by administering a bolus loading dose *and* simultaneously instituting a continuous infusion. This principle holds true for oral as well as intravenous administration. The optimal time interval between maintenance oral doses is determined by the half life of the agent. Since the objective is to achieve and maintain therapeutic plasma levels, the initial peak level is much less important than the concentration toward the end of each dose.

ELECTROPHYSIOLOGY

Attempts have been made to classify the major antiarrhythmic drugs into several groups according to their electrophysiologic effects. These categories, however, are only approximations and many drugs display electrophysiologic properties that cannot be accurately classified within one group (Vaughan, 1975). Group I agents include quinidine, procainamide, and disopyramide. In general, these drugs decrease automaticity, prolong action potential duration, prolong the refractory period, and decrease conduction velocity. Drugs in the group II category include lidocaine and diphenylhydantoin (phenytoin, DPH). Group II drugs also decrease automaticity but, in contrast to Group I agents, they shorten the action potential duration while prolonging its refractory period and decrease membrane responsiveness without having a significant effect on conduction velocity. Group III drugs include the beta blocking agents propranolol, tolamolol, and alprenolol. These drugs produce their antiarrhythmic effects by means of both beta-blocking activity and direct membrane effects. They slow sinus automaticity, decrease the slope of phase 0 depolarization, and prolong the effective refractory period of atrial and A-V nodal tissue. Propranolol in particular has direct membrane effects similar to both group I and group II agents at higher concentrations and may actually de-crease the action potential duration of Purkinje tissue.

Bretylium tosylate is the prototypical group IV agent. It has little direct membrane effect and exerts most of its effect through its antiadrenergic activity.

In addition, some of the newer drugs apparently have their primary action on the slow channel dependent portions of the action potential and have been classified as group V agents. Verapamil is the prototype antiarrhythmic drug in this category.

QUINIDINE

Electrophysiologic Effects

(Table 23–1)

Quinidine is the oldest and one of the most effective antiarrhythmic agents. Its electrophysiological properties may be explained by its effects on anion exchange across the cell membrane. It decreases phase 4 depolarization, decreases the rate of rise of phase 0 of the action potential, prolongs the action

TABLE 23–1   QUINIDINE: ELECTROPHYSIOLOGIC EFFECTS

Major Electrophysiologic Effects	Major Effects on Conduction	Major Effects on Electrocardiogram
Decreases rate of rise of phase 0	*S-A node* Decreases rate by a direct effect	Increases duration and induces notching of P wave at toxic doses
Decreases phase 4 depolarization	Indirectly increases rate by reflex sympathetic stimulation	Increases QRS duration
Increases action potential duration		Increases Q-T interval
Increases effective refractory period	May significantly slow rate in diseased tissue	May induce block in presence of diseased conduction system
	Atrial fibers Decreases conduction Decreases excitability	
	A-V node Minimal decrease at therapeutic levels	
	His-Purkinje fibers Decreases conduction	

potential duration, and increases the effective refractory period. These electrophysiological changes result in increased refractoriness thereby preventing arrhythmias that are dependent on re-entrant pathways.

The effects of quinidine are potentiated by an increase in extracellular potassium concentration and diminished by a decrease in this ion. At higher concentrations than are normally achieved clinically, threshold potential becomes more negative. Paradoxically, at these levels of quinidine concentration the rate of rise of phase 4 depolarization is increased, resulting in pacemaker acceleration. This may be one of the mechanisms underlying the development of ventricular arrhythmias associated with toxic doses of quinidine.

The effect of quinidine on sinus rate is unpredictable. It may accelerate the S-A node through reflex sympathetic stimulation in moderate doses (Cohen, 1977). However, higher doses usually produce a direct depressant effect, which is important in patients with abnormalities of sinus node function. Quinidine may also minimally decrease conduction through the A-V node, although therapeutic doses have been shown to have relatively little effect on A-V conduction. It can, however, accelerate the ventricular response during atrial fibrillation and flutter, most likely as a result of reduction in atrial impulses with a subsequent decrease in concealed conduction.

Direct Pharmacologic Effects on the Heart

Quinidine has a variable effect on myocardial contractility. The effect seen depends on the cardiac state and the dose of the drug. Some evidence suggests that quinidine has no depressant effect on contraction in therapeutic doses in individuals with normal cardiac function. It does, however, depress contraction when given in high doses or to patients with previously depressed function. This depressant effect may be related to altered calcium metabolism, that is, the exclusion of calcium from active regions of the actinomyocin molecule.

Effects on the Electrocardiogram

Quinidine induced changes on the electrocardiogram are a reflection of its electrophysiologic effects and are generally related to plasma concentration. Prolongation of the ventricular action potential is manifested by prolongation of the QT interval and the QRS duration. While the increase in the QRS duration usually is not significant at therapeutic drug concentrations, marked widening of the QRS complex is particularly dangerous since it may presage serious arrhythmias, such as ventricular tachycardia or fibrillation. Increases in the QRS interval to greater than 50 per cent of control in the absence of bundle branch block and 25 per cent in the presence of bundle branch block should be considered evidence of toxicity. In toxic doses, the P waves may also be affected, becoming somewhat widened and notched.

Pharmacology (Table 23–2)

The relationship between serum quinidine levels and the therapeutic effects of the drug is indirect, although a general correlation does exist. In most individuals a therapeutic effect is associated with plasma levels in the range of 2 to 6 mg per liter. At serum concentrations below 2 mg per liter, antiarrhythmic effects of the drug are rare. Conversely, toxic effects are generally noted at concentrations above 6 mg per liter, and at levels above 10 mg per liter are almost invariable. There is, however, significant variation between individuals, and plasma levels within the thera-

TABLE 23–2 QUINIDINE: PHARMACOLOGIC CONSIDERATIONS

Route of administration	Oral, IM IV (not recommended)
Dose	200–400 mg q4-6 hours (1.2–3.2 gm/day) Loading dose 2 times main- tenance dose
Therapeutic blood levels	2–6 μg/ml
Half life	3–10 hours (6 hours mean)
Protein binding	70–80%
Metabolism	10–40% excreted unchanged in the urine; remainder metabolized by liver

Major Toxic Manifestations

Hypotension	Allergic reactions
Cinchonism	Agranulocytosis
Nausea	QRS widening
Loose stools	Q-T prolongation

peutic range do not guarantee that toxic effects will not occur. Since a significant portion of quinidine is bound to serum protein, with 70 to 80 per cent being bound to albumin, hypoalbuminemia may decrease drug binding, and therapeutic effects may be seen at lower serum levels. Tissue binding of quinidine is greater than serum binding, and peak concentration in skeletal muscle, liver, kidney, and heart may be as much as 20 times that bound in the plasma.

In general, the plasma level of quinidine depends on the dose administered, the time elapsed since the last dose, and the rapidity with which the drug is metabolized and excreted. The peak plasma level following a single oral dose occurs in 1 to 2 hours. Quinidine usually has a half life of approximately 6 hours. There is, however, significant individual variability. There are some individuals in whom usual therapeutic doses may produce toxic serum levels and, conversely, others in whom large oral doses produce subtherapeutic blood levels.

The major portion of quinidine is hydroxylated in the liver and excreted by the kidney. Approximately 10 to 30 per cent of quinidine is excreted unchanged in the urine. High plasma levels of quinidine may occur when standard doses are given to patients with conditions that predispose to quinidine retention. However, significant changes in metabolism or excretion rates cannot be demonstrated in patients with severe heart failure and renal insufficiency. An occasional patient with heart failure will exhibit high serum levels after administration of normal doses of the drug. Similarly, while it has been suggested that the metabolism of quinidine may be significantly altered with liver disease, at least one study has found that this is not the case.

More recently, a relationship has been found between digitalis administration and quinidine, with a high incidence of drug toxicity possibly due to competitive myocardial binding and/or decreased renal clearance. Higher than expected serum digoxin concentrations have been observed during quinidine therapy. Thus, in the presence of digitalis, a given dose of quinidine is associated with a higher incidence of toxic side effects, and it has been suggested that the dose of digitalis be reduced by 30 to 50 per cent during quinidine administration (Doering, 1979).

Dosage and Administration

Although quinidine may be administered orally, intramuscularly, or intravenously, the oral route is the method of choice. The peak plasma concentration is reached sooner when quinidine is administered intramuscularly; however, injection is painful and produces tissue necrosis with elevated CPK levels. The intravenous infusion results in peak plasma levels almost immediately, but it is rarely used and is not recommended because of the unpredictable risk of severe hypotension.

Quinidine is available in various salts including quinidine sulfate, gluconate, and lactate. Quinidine sulfate is the preparation most commonly used. The gluconate and lactate salts differ from the sulfate in their gastrointestinal absorption. Since the absorption rate of a sulfate is twice that of the gluconate (Ochs, 1978), quinidine gluconate can be used as a longer acting agent and is frequently given before sleep to maintain adequate blood levels without the necessity of awakening patients. The average loading dose of quinidine sulfate is 600 mg and the maintenance dosage is 1.2 to 2.4 grams daily in divided doses.

Several methods can be utilized to rapidly achieve and maintain plasma concentrations with oral quinidine. A new method of acute drug testing has recently been proposed that may be a useful guide for determining the doses necessary for quinidine as well as other antiarrhythmic agents: administration of a large (600 mg) single oral dose with continuous electrocardiographic monitoring of the drug's antiarrhythmic effect and measurement of drug levels at times when the rhythm is altered or toxic effects are in evidence. The mean concentration achieved at the time of peak drug action with quinidine was reportedly 3.2 μg per ml, which is well within the accepted therapeutic range. With continued monitoring, trends of ectopic activity are followed, and blood sampling is performed at the precise stages of antiarrhythmic action. This method of quinidine administration is based on the concept that the key factor in antiarrhythmic therapy is the clinically therapeutic serum concentration, which is distinctive for each patient (Gaughen, 1976).

Toxic Manifestations

The most common non-cardiac adverse reactions are related to the gastrointestinal tract and central nervous system symptoms called cinchonism. Nausea, vomiting, and diarrhea may occur with even relatively small doses. Under the term cinchonism are grouped syncope—which reportedly occurs in 1.5% of patients and frequently is due to ventricular tachycardia or transient ventricular fibrillation (Luchi, 1978), impairment of hearing, ringing in the ears, vertigo, blurred vision, lightheadedness, and tremor (Cohen, 1977). Other less comon non-cardiac side effects include allergic reactions, skin rash, immune thrombocytopenia, agranulocytosis, fever, and hepatic toxicity.

The electrocardiographic signs of quinidine toxicity have been mentioned previously. Quinidine can cause ventricular arrhythmias that at times are life threatening, including ventricular tachycardia and fibrillation. These arrhythmias may be relatively independent of dose. Most episodes of ventricular tachycardia are self limited, although electrical conversion to sinus rhythm may be necessary. Most reported cases of ventricular tachycardia or ventricular flutter that occur with normal therapeutic dose ranges are associated with prolonged QT intervals and/or widening of the QRS complex. In addition, the majority of patients who develop ventricular tachycardia are concomitantly taking digitalis preparations.

Indications and Contraindications

Quinidine is indicated for the treatment of premature complexes of atrial, junctional, and ventricular origin and in the pharmacologic conversion of atrial flutter and fibrillation to normal sinus rhythm. It is also used to prevent recurrence of these arrhythmias.

Quinidine is contraindicated in the presence of partial or complete heart block, intraventricular conduction disturbances, or bundle branch block. It should be administered with caution in the presence of severe congestive heart failure, digitalis intoxication, or hyperkalemia.

Treatment of Quinidine Toxicity

To treat severe quinidine overdose, sodium bicarbonate or molar sodium lactate have been used to reduce the electrocardiographic toxicity by lowering the serum potassium concentration. Lidocaine may also be useful in the control of quinidine induced ventricular arrhythmias (Luchi, 1978). The increased pH level also increases the binding of free quinidine to albumin. Sympathomimetics or angiotensin (Luchi, 1978) are used to treat quinidine induced hypotension.

PROCAINAMIDE

Procainamide has been in clinical use since 1951 and remains a highly effective antiarrhythmic drug; it is administered both orally and parenterally in the treatment of ventricular and supraventricular tachyarrhythmias.

Electrophysiologic Effects (Table 23–3)

The electrophysiologic effects of procainamide are similar to those of quin-

TABLE 23–3 PROCAINAMIDE: ELECTROPHYSIOLOGIC EFFECTS

Major Electrophysiologic Effects	Major Effects on Conduction	Major Effects on Electrocardiogram
Decreases rate of rise of phase 0	*S-A node* Minimal effect on normal tissue	Occasionally prolongs PR interval
Decreases phase 4 depolarization	May slow the rate in diseased tissue or in toxic doses	Increases QRS duration
		Increases Q-T interval
Increases action potential duration	*Atrial fibers* Decreases conduction	Can induce block in presence of diseased conduction system
Increases effective refractory period	Decreases excitability	
	A-V node Minimal decrease at therapeutic levels	
	His-Purkinje fibers Decreases conduction	

idine. Procainamide causes a reduction in the excitability of atrial tissue and raises the threshold of electrical stimulation. High doses of the drug slow atrial conduction. In most instances it has no significant effect on the sinus rate. In therapeutic doses, the effect of procainamide on the A-V junction is also minimal, although higher doses do prolong A-V conduction time. Procainamide also depresses automaticity, prolongs the action potential duration and effective refractory period, decreases excitability, and decreases conductivity within the His-Purkinje system (Rosen, 1972).

Effect on Electrocardiograms

The effects of procainamide on the electrocardiogram are also similar to those of quinidine. The PR interval is occasionally slightly prolonged, as are the QRS and QT intervals. Widening of the QRS complex is a characteristic dose related effect, and when more than 25 per cent widening or a QRS of more than 0.14 second occurs, caution should be used in further administration. The drug should probably not be given if the QRS width exceeds 0.16 second or if its total prolongation is over 50 per cent.

Direct Cardiac Pharmacologic Effects

The hemodynamic effects of procainamide depend on the cardiovascular status of the patient and the route, rate, and dosage of administration. Rapid intravenous administration of procainamide may result in marked hemodynamic impairment with depressed function, peripheral vasodilatation, decreased cardiac output, and hypotension. Procainamide has anticholinergic actions and is capable of depressing the myocardium. However, the depressant effect of therapeutic plasma concentra-

tions of procainamide on myocardial tissue has been questioned. In our experience it rarely causes clinical manifestations when given orally and only occasional symptoms of cardiac depression when given by appropriately slow intravenous administration.

Pharmacology (Table 23–4)

Procainamide is rapidly and almost completely (75-95%) absorbed by the gastrointestinal tract following oral administration. Plasma levels peak at 60 to 90 minutes and then decrease by 10 to 20 per cent per hour, the average half life being 3 to 4 hours (Koch-Weser, 1971). Administration of identical oral and intravenous doses of procainamide will result in almost identical peak levels 1 hour after administration, followed by a similar rate of decline. Peak levels are also achieved within 30 to 60 minutes following intramuscular administration. In most individuals the therapeutic blood levels range from 4 to 8 μg per ml (Gey, 1974). Procainamide elimination occurs via both hepatic metabolism and renal excretion. Seventy-five to 90 per cent is eliminated in the urine, 30 to 60 per cent appearing as procainamide and the remainder as an active metabolite. Only 15 per cent of procainamide is bound to plasma (Koch-Weser, 1971). A metabolite of procainamide, NAPA, has been shown to have antiarrhythmic activity and a longer half life than procainamide.

Dosage and Administration

Procainamide may be administered intravenously by giving 100 mg slowly every 5 minutes until adverse reactions occur. Most arrhythmias are abolished before 1000 mg is given (occasionally 1500 mg or more may be given if toxicity does not occur). The rate of administration should never exceed 50 mg per minute (Koch-Weser, 1971) and blood

TABLE 23–4   PROCAINAMIDE: PHARMACOLOGIC CONSIDERATIONS

Route of administration	Oral IV
Dose	Oral—1 gm loading dose 250–750 mg q4 hours IV—500 mg–1 gm loading dose (administered slowly) 4–5 mg/min continuous infusion
Therapeutic blood levels	4–8 μg/ml
Half life	3–6 hours (4 hours mean)
Protein binding	15%
Metabolism	30–50% excreted unchanged in urine; remainder metabolized in liver

Major Toxic Manifestations

Hypotension	Allergic reactions
Anorexia	Lupus-like syndrome
Nausea	QRS widening
Loose stools	Q-T prolongation

pressure and electrocardiogram must be monitored continuously, since hypotension and QRS widening are indications to stop treatment. Maintenance intravenous doses are 4 to 5 mg per minute. This does may be tapered as long as rhythm control is maintained.

The recommended initial oral dose schedule is a 1 gram loading dose followed by a maintenance dose of 3 grams daily, administered either as 375 mg every 3 hours or 500 mg every 4 hours. If the drug is ineffective at this dosage it can slowly be increased to as high as 6 to 8 grams daily in divided doses if side effects do not occur.

Toxic Manifestations

The most commonly encountered cardiotoxic effects of intravenous procainamide include hypotension and QRS widening (McClendon, 1951). The most commonly reported side effects of oral procainamide are gastrointestinal (i.e.,

anorexia and vomiting). Procainamide also causes allergic side effects, such as skin rash, fever, and agranulocytosis.

A reversible clinical syndrome resembling systemic lupus erythematosus occurs in a fairly high percentage of patients receiving maintenance doses of procainamide (Blomgren, 1972). This appears to be related to the duration of therapy rather than to dose levels. The reported incidence has been between 20 and 70 per cent of patients on long term therapy. The most frequent clinical manifestations are arthralgias, pleural and pneumonic complaints, fever, pericarditis, hepatomegaly, and myalgia. The kidney is not involved. The most characteristic laboratory findings are the presence of antinuclear antibodies (100% of patients) and LE cells (94% of patients). In the majority of patients the symptoms abate within a week to a month after discontinuation of the drug. Procainamide induced lupus is reportedly distinguishable from systemic lupus by the lack of renal involvement and the absence of antibodies to DNA (Blomgren, 1972).

Indications and Contraindications

Procainamide is a highly effective antiarrhythmic agent that is useful in the treatment of atrial, junctional, and ventricular premature beats and tachyarrhythmias.

The contraindications to procainamide use are similar to those for quinidine. It depresses pacemaker automaticity and therefore is contraindicated in A-V block. It should be administered with caution in the presence of bundle branch block or hypotension (Scheinman, 1974). It should also be avoided if possible in patients with susceptibility to allergic responses as well as those with a history of bronchial asthma and myasthenia gravis, since serious side effects may be likely to occur.

DISOPYRAMIDE

Disopyramide phosphate is a new antiarrhythmic agent that has rapidly become an important addition to the antiarrhythmic armamentarium. The drug has been effective in the treatment of supraventricular and ventricular arrhythmias and tachycardias (Zipes, 1978). It has also been useful in the prevention of recurrent atrial fibrillation following cardioversion. The electrophysiologic effects of disopyramide (Table 23–5) are similar in many respects to those of quinidine and procainamide and it is considered a type I antiarrhythmic agent. These effects include 1) an increase in action potential duration, 2) an increase in the effective refractory period, 3) a decrease in phase zero depolarization, and 4) a decrease in phase 4 depolarization. As with other antiarrhythmic preparations, a decrease in serum potassium concentration tends to diminish the effects of the drug. Disopyramide also has potent anticholinergic properties as well. There is currently controversy as to whether it also has an effect upon the slow channel calcium dependent response because of its effect on phase 2 calcium influx into the cell (Zipes, 1978). If disopyramide does indeed have an effect on slow channel responses, this may in part at least explain its efficacy in treatment of ventricular arrhythmias refractory to quinidine. Disopyramide might also have other electrophysiologic effects primarily suggested by its local anes-

TABLE 23–5   DISOPYRAMIDE PHOSPHATE: ELECTROPHYSIOLOGIC EFFECTS

Major Electrophysiologic Effects	Major Effects on Conduction	Major Effects on Electrocardiogram
Decreases rate of rise of phase 0	*S-A node* Minimal effect on normal tissue	Prolongs P-R interval
Decreases phase 4 depolarization	May slow rate in diseased tissue or in toxic doses	Increases QRS duration
		Increases Q-T interval
Increases action potential duration	*Atrial fibers* Decreases conduction	Can induce block in presence of diseased conduction system
Increases effective refractory period	Decreases excitability	
	A-V node May decrease conduction	
	His-Purkinje fibers Decreases conduction	

TABLE 23-6   DISOPYRAMIDE: PHARMACOLOGIC CONSIDERATIONS

Route of administration	Oral IV—Clinical trial
Dose	Oral—200 mg loading dose 100–150 mg every 6 hours
Therapeutic blood levels	3–8 μg/ml
Half life	5–6 hours (at therapeutic blood levels) Degradation is nonlinear and concentration dependent
Protein binding	21–50%—increases with increased serum concentration

Metabolism	40–60% is excreted unchanged by
	  the kidney; remainder metabolized
	  by liver

Major Toxic Manifestations

Decreased myocardial contraction	
Nausea	Blurred vision
Urinary retention	QRS widening
Dry mouth	Q-T prolongation

thetic activity, the potency of which approaches that of lidocaine (Vismara, 1977). It prolongs the QT interval and QRS complex as well as occasionally increasing the P-R interval of the electrocardiogram. These effects are concentration dependent.

The drug is administered orally in a dosage ranging from 100 to 200 mg every 6 hours (Table 23–6). Occasionally higher doses are necessary. A loading dose of 200 to 400 mg is recommended. It is currently being investigated as an intravenous preparation. The therapeutic plasma concentration range is between 3 and 7 μg per ml, the half life being 5 to 6 hours (Hinderline, 1976).

Disopyramide appears to be almost completely absorbed from the GI tract (85%), with peak plasma levels occurring 2 to 3 hours after administration, and is primarily excreted by the kidneys, with 40 to 60 per cent being excreted unchanged. Albumin binding is reportedly 21 to 50 per cent at therapeutic blood levels but is concentration

dependent and varies between 5 and 65 per cent at concentrations of 1 to 10 μg per ml (Harrison, 1977).

Disopyramide can depress myocardial contractility. While at times this is a significant clinical problem, prior heart failure is not an absolute contraindication to its use. Other major side effects are primarily related to its anticholinergic effects. These include nausea, vomiting, constipation, urinary retention, blurred vision, and dryness of the mouth and eyes (Zipes, 1978). Comparative studies with quinidine, however, suggest that the side effects may be less severe and less frequent. Occasional widening of the QRS or prolongation of the QT interval can occur.

LIDOCAINE

Lidocaine is the most widely used intravenous agent for the treatment and prevention of ventricular arrhythmias after acute myocardial infarction. Although it is a remarkably effective and safe agent for ventricular arrhythmias, it is relatively ineffective in suppressing atrial arrhythmias.

Electrophysiology and Effects on Electrocardiogram (Table 23–7)

In contrast to quinidine, lidocaine decreases automaticity and increases the effective refractory period without prolonging the action potential or having a significant effect on conduction velocity.

In general, the electrophysiologic effects of lidocaine are more evident on the ventricle than the atria. There is a notable lack of effect on the sinus node rate in both normal subjects and patients with sinus node dysfunction, although isolated reports of S-A arrest have occurred. Lidocaine is generally considered to have little effect on A-V nodal or intraventricular conduction. However, there is evidence to suggest that lidocaine even at therapeutic blood levels increases conduction time in damaged infrahisian conduction fibers, and rare cases of complete heart block have been reported. Lidocaine decreases the capacity of ventricular fibers to follow rapid stimulation and causes a suppression of repetitive responses elicited by a premature beat.

There are no cardiac depressant effects in therapeutic doses and no significant effect on blood pressure, heart rate, cardiac output, or ventricular filling pressures. The effects on the electrocardiogram are generally negligible.

Pharmacology (Table 23–8)

Approximately 70 per cent of lidocaine is metabolized by the liver during its first passage. Following an initial bolus, the half life of the distributional phase is 8 minutes. With continuous infusion for up to 12 hours the half life has been found to be 90 minutes. After more than 24 hours the half life is as long as 3.2 hours. Lidocaine's metabolites have significant convulsive and emetic properties as well as antiarrhythmic effects. The therapeutic plasma level is between 1.4 and 6 μg per ml (Jewitt, 1968).

Indications and Methods of Administration

Lidocaine is the drug of choice for the intravenous treatment of premature ventricular complexes and ventricular tachycardia. Although most frequently used for arrhythmias that occur in acute myocardial infarction, it is also effective in other clinical contexts. Its use is

TABLE 23–7   LIDOCAINE: ELECTROPHYSIOLOGIC EFFECTS

Major Electrophysiologic Effects	Major Effects on Conduction	Major Effects on Electrocardiogram
Decreases phase 4 depolarization	S-A node Minimal	Minimal effect on QRS duration
Decreases or does not change action potential duration	Atrial fibers Minimal	Minimal effect on Q-T interval
Increases diastolic threshold	A-V node Minimal	May rarely induce block in presence of diseased tissue
Decreases ability of ventricular fibers to respond to repetitive stimuli	His-Purkinje fibers Minimal effect on normal tissue	
	May decrease conduction in diseased tissue	

TABLE 23–8   LIDOCAINE: PHARMACOLOGIC CONSIDERATIONS

Route of administration	IV
Dose	75–150 mg loading dose (1–2 mg/kg) 4 mg/min (15–45 μg/kg/min)
Therapeutic blood levels	1.4–6 μg/ml
Half life	10–20 minutes initial distribution 1½–3 hours after continuous infusion
Protein binding	40–60%
Metabolism	95% metabolism by liver
Major Toxic Manifestations	
CNS depression	Emesis
Convulsions Focal and grand mal seizures	Respiratory arrest
Dizziness	

restricted to the intravenous route and its rapid degradation by the liver necessitates a constant infusion, which must be carefully controlled.

The drug is administered in a bolus, which is followed by continuous intravenous infusion. The effective antiarrhythmic loading dose is 1 to 2 mg per kg (usually 50-100 mg). If no initial response is seen, a second dose may be given in 5-10 minutes. However, the total dose given over a short period should not exceed 5 mg per kg or 300 mg. If the arrhythmia in question is not controlled with 200 or 300 mg then it is presumed that lidocaine is ineffective and further administration is not indicated. If the arrhythmia is controlled, then constant infusion is given at a rate of 15 to 45 μg per kg per minute (usually 2-4 mg/min). If the arrhythmias recur, a small additional bolus of 25 to 50 mg may be given with a subsequent increase in infusion rate. In patients with severe hepatic disease the dose of lidocaine must be reduced by as much as 50 per cent (Stenson, 1971; Thomson, 1973). Serum lidocaine levels may occasionally be of value in the management of such patients.

Lidocaine has occasionally been given intramuscularly. Plasma levels within the range of 1 to 5 mg per liter are attained within 15 minutes and maintained for 60 to 120 minutes following the intramuscular injection of 300 mg of the drug.

Toxicity

The noncardiac effects of lidocaine are most common and are usually transient. These include emesis, central nervous system depression, dizziness, and focal and grand mal seizures. Respiratory arrest has rarely occurred.

DIPHENYLHYDANTOIN (PHENYTOIN, DPH)

Diphenylhydantoin is an antiarrhythmic agent that has been used in the treatment of supraventricular and ventricular arrhythmias. It is particularly efficacious in the treatment of tachyarrhythmias caused by digitalis toxicity (Helfant, 1967). It 1) lowers the threshold of stimulation, 2) increases conduction velocity, 3) decreases automaticity, 4) increases the effective refractory period, and 5) shortens A-V conduction. It does not affect the QRS complex and actually shortens the QT interval (Helfant, 1967). Its hemodynamic effects are minimal (Table 23–9).

When given orally, DPH is usually well absorbed from the GI tract, although this may be variable in some cases. A rapid decline in plasma level occurs within the first hour, the subsequent plasma half life being approximately 15 to 22 hours. Because of this, large initial doses are often required to maintain effective plasma concentrations. Metabolism, however, is nonlinear, being longer at higher blood levels and shorter at lower blood levels. Because DPH is metabolized by liver enzymes that can be affected by a number of drugs, including barbiturates, concomitant use of these agents requires larger doses of DPH. In the presence of hepatic dysfunction, toxic blood levels may occur because of the altered ability to metabolize the agent. It is 93 per cent plasma bound in normal patients.

Pharmacology and Administration
(Table 23–10)

Therapeutic antiarrhythmic blood levels of DPH occur between 10 and 18 μg per ml. The usual intravenous dose is 5-10 mg per kg, although as much as 1000 mg may be given if necessary and administered with appropriate precautionary measures. Intravenous therapy must be employed with caution and *never* administered at a rate faster than 50 mg per minute. The intravenous preparation is highly alkaline and may cause pain and thrombosis at the site of injection. This may be avoided by the use of an intravenous catheter into one of the large veins and with careful flushing of the catheter after the injection. Oral administration consists of a loading dose of 1000 mg on the first day, 500 to 600 mg on the second and third day, and a maintenance dosage of 400 mg daily thereafter.

Toxic Effects

The major side effects of DPH involve the cardiovascular and central nervous system. With intravenous use, the cardiovascular side effects relate more to the speed of administration than to the total dose given. Respiratory depression and arrest have been reported, as have severe hypotension, cardiac arrest, ventricular fibrillation, and death. Central nervous system effects include nystagmus, ataxia, tremors, cerebellar degeneration, diplopia, blurring of vision, ptosis, slurring of speech, fatigue and drowsiness, insomnia, and irritability. The hematologic effects that

TABLE 23–9   PHENYTOIN: ELECTROPHYSIOLOGIC EFFECTS

Major Electrophysiologic Effects	Major Effects on Conduction	Major Effects on Electrocardiogram
Increases rate of rise of phase 0	*S-A node* Minimal	Minimal effect on QRS
		Shortens Q-T interval
Decreases phase 4 depolarization	*Atrial fibers* Minimal	
Increases effective refractory period	*A-V node* Slight increase in conduction	
Decreases or does not change action potential duration	*His-Purkinje fibers* Minimal	
Decreases stimulation threshold		

TABLE 23–10 PHENYTOIN: PHARMACOLOGIC CONSIDERATIONS

Route of administration	Oral IV
Dose	IV—5–10 mg/kg (1 gm) loading Oral—500 mg–1 gm loading dose 400 mg daily
Therapeutic blood levels	10–18 μg/ml
Half life	15–22 hours—non linear and concentration dependent
Protein binding	93%
Metabolism	Metabolized by liver

Major Toxic Manifestations

Hypotension with IV administration	
Respiratory depression	Diplopia
Pancytopenia	Slurred speech
Megaloblastic anemia	Hepatitis
Nystagmus	Hyperplasia
Ataxia	Low PBI
Tremors	Depressed adrenocortical function

occur with longer term oral use include anemia, pancytopenia, megaloblastic anemia, and reticular endothelial disorders. Other toxic manifestations include gastrointestinal upset, hyperplasia of the gums, low total protein bound iodine, jaundice and hepatitis, and depressed adrenal cortical function.

Many of the side effects are related to the DPH blood level: nystagmus usually occurs at levels of approximately 20 μg per ml, ataxia at 30 μg per ml, and lethargy at 40 μg per ml. Because it is usually the first manifestation of toxicity, careful attempts should be made to detect the onset of nystagmus during intravenous administration, and the drug should be stopped when this occurs.

Clinical Use

Diphenylhydantoin is most effective in the treatment of arrhythmias pro-duced by digitalis excess. It has also been shown to be effective in the prophylaxis of post counter shock arrhythmias. The drug is not effective in conversion of atrial fibrillation or flutter to normal sinus rhythm and is of little efficacy in treating supraventricular arrhythmias that are not related to digitalis excess. Although DPH is not considered a first line antiarrhythmic drug, it is often very useful as a secondary agent or in a combined drug regimen in the treatment of refractory ventricular arrhythmias.

Contraindications

Diphenylhydantoin is contraindicated in the presence of hypotension, severe bradycardia, and A-V block. Because it is detoxified in the liver there are several drugs that will interact and therefore affect the serum half life of DPH. Dicumarol and certain sulfa drugs are detoxified by the same microenzyme system, and therefore increase the serum level of DPH. Phenobarbital, on the other hand, induces the same enzyme system and therefore increases DPH metabolism.

PROPRANOLOL

Electrophysiologic Effects
(Table 23–11)

At present, propranolol is the only beta blocking agent approved for antiarrhythmic use in the United States. Its antiarrhythmic action is based upon both specific beta blockade and direct "quinidine-like" effects. At lower dose levels, beta blockade appears to predominate, while at higher dose levels the direct effects are more important. In the S-A node, atria, A-V junction, and His-Purkinje system there is decreased automaticity and conduction velocity, with prolongation of the refractory period. Its effect on the automaticity of the A-V node appears to be independent of adrenergic influences. At present there is little evidence that propranolol has a direct membrane effect on the automaticity or conduction velocity of the His-Purkinje system.

Propranolol exerts a significant negative inotropic effect, the magnitude of which depends on the dose employed, the mode of administration, and the degree to which sympathetic tone is supporting cardiac function. Even in normal subjects, therapeutic doses of propranolol result in prolonged systolic ejection time, decreased velocity of shortening of myocardial fibers, slowed heart rate, and a diminution of cardiac output and left ventricular work. This may be important either in causing or worsening congestive heart failure in predisposed patients. On the surface electrocardiogram, the QT interval is usually shortened, with the PR interval being somewhat prolonged.

Pharmacology (Table 23–12)

Propranolol is metabolized by the liver and excreted by the kidney. After a single dose plasma concentrations in patients with severe renal dysfunction have been observed to be two to three times higher than in normal subjects. These findings suggest that less than usual doses be employed in patients with severe renal insufficiency. Patients with severe hepatic dysfunction should also receive less than the usual doses.

Indications

Propranolol is a useful agent when used in conjunction with digitalis and

TABLE 23–11   PROPRANOLOL: ELECTROPHYSIOLOGIC EFFECTS

Major Electrophysiologic Effects	Major Effects on Conduction	Major Effects on Electrocardiogram
Decreases rate of rise of phase 0	S-A node Decreases conduction velocity	Decreases sinus rate
		Prolongs P-R interval
Decreases phase 4 depolarization	Atrial fibers Decreases conduction velocity	Minimal effects on QRS duration
Increases effective refractory period	A-V node Decreases conduction velocity	Prolongs P-R interval
May decrease action potential duration of His-Purkinje tissue (at higher doses)	His-Purkinje fibers Decreases conduction velocity (minimal)	May occasionally induce heart block in presence of diseased conduction system

TABLE 23–12 PROPRANOLOL: PHARMACOLOGIC CONSIDERATIONS

Route of administration	IV Oral
Dose	1–5 mg IV 20–40 mg q6h oral
Therapeutic blood levels	50–200 nanogram/ml (approx)
Half life	3–6 hours
Protein binding	> 90%
Metabolism	99% metabolized by liver

Major Toxic Manifestations

Decreased myocardial contractility	
Bronchospasm	Nausea
Hypoglycemia	Fatigue

may be utilized to slow and maintain a physiologic rate in atrial flutter and fibrillation. The use of a combined drug regimen allows for a lesser dose of digitalis and a decreased likelihood of toxic effects. Propranolol is not a primary drug for this purpose, however, owing to its negative inotropic effects. It is also efficacious in the prophylaxis of supraventricular arrhythmias associated with Wolff-Parkinson-White syndrome, and it may be helpful in cases of repetitive tachycardias. Propranolol may also be a useful adjunctive drug for the control of ventricular premature complexes in situations where other antiarrhythmic agents such as quinidine, procainamide, or dysopyramide alone have been ineffective. However, propranolol is generally not considered a primary drug for the treatment of these arrhythmias except when the arrhythmia is associated with increased sympathetic activity. Although propranolol has also been recommended for the therapy of digitalis toxicity, it is not currently viewed as the drug of choice because of its negative inotropic effects as well as its effects on A-V conduction.

Doses and Methods of Administration

Propranolol is usually given orally, and experience has shown this to be relatively safe and reliable. Intravenously, propranolol has a much greater risk of serious cardiac depression and should be reserved for emergency situations. Effective oral doses range from 10 to 60 mg three to four times daily. In the rare instances in which intravenous propranolol is necessary, 1 to 3 mg may be administered initially with electrocardiographic and blood pressure monitoring. The rate of administration should not exceed 0.5 mg per minute. The total dose usually should not exceed 0.1 mg per kg.

Side Effects

The major electrocardiographic evidence of propranolol toxicity includes excessive bradycardia or less commonly heart block. In addition, it may precipitate or aggravate congestive heart failure because of its negative inotropic effects. Uncommonly, hypotension or even shock may occur. Through its beta blocking effects it may produce bronchial constriction and cause a sudden decrease in ventilatory function. This is of particular concern in patients with bronchial asthma. In addition, propranolol interferes with the normal physiologic response to hypoglycemia. This is important in patients prone to hypoglycemia, particularly unstable diabetics.

Contraindications

Propranolol is contraindicated in sinus bradycardia and A-V block, hypotension and shock, significant congestive heart failure, and bronchial asthma. In addition, it should be used with extreme caution in insulin dependent diabetics or those taking oral hypoglycemic agents.

BRETYLIUM

Bretylium tosylate is a drug that has been shown to inhibit release of norepinephrine from adrenergic nerve endings. It was initially used as an antihypertensive agent; however, because of poor absorption after oral dosing and rapid tolerance to its antihypertensive effect, it was deemed ineffective. Bretylium has been extensively studied as an antiarrhythmic agent, particularly for the treatment of life threatening ventricular arrhythmia, and has now been marketed in the United States for this indication.

Bretylium increases the action potential duration and prolongs the effective refractory period of isolated Purkinje fibers without altering the ratio of these parameters. In canine hearts the drug decreases the disparity of the action potential duration between normal and infarcted regions (Koch-Weser, 1979). It also increases the ventricular fibrillation threshold in dog hearts and has been shown to be antifibrillatory in

several experimental settings. In addition, the drug has an effect on adrenergic function that may also play a role in its antiarrhythmic actions.

Although bretylium has been found effective in the treatment of life threatening ventricular arrhythmias, it has been less impressive in suppressing more benign ectopic beats. The drug is also relatively ineffective in treating atrial arrhythmias. The presently approved indication for bretylium is treatment of life threatening ventricular arrhythmias that have failed to respond to adequate doses of first line antiarrhythmics, such as lidocaine or procainamide. At the present time, bretylium is not indicated for ventricular arrhythmias produced by digitalis excess (Koch-Weser, 1979).

Dose and Administration

Bretylium is available only as a parenteral agent in the United States. It may be given intravenously or intramuscularly, although a 20 minute to 1 hour delay in its onset of action can be expected after intramuscular injection. The usual dose is 5 to 10 mg per kg. Antiarrhythmic effects may last 6 to 12 hours after a single dose; however, a second dose may be given within 1 to 2 hours if the arrhythmia persists. Maintenance therapy is 5 to 10 mg per kg every 6 to 8 hours or 1 to 2 mg per minute by continuous drip. In patients with impaired renal function, the current recommendation is to decrease the dosage but no exact guide lines are available (Koch-Weser, 1979). Seventy to 80 per cent of the drug is excreted without change in the urine within 24 hours.

Toxic Effects

Bretylium is generally well tolerated. The non-antiarrhythmic actions of the drug are mostly related to its modification of adrenergic function. Occasional patients will have a moderate increase in blood pressure shortly after administration, owing to the adrenergic release of norepinephrine. A sinus tachycardia may also be observed in approximately 20 per cent of patients as a result of the same mechanism. The drug has also been found to exert a positive inotropic effect. However, because of its adrenergic blockade, 50 to 75 per cent of patients may develop a fall in mean arterial blood pressure; this is seldom more than 20 mm Hg in the recumbent position. Occasionally, more severe decreases in blood pressure have been observed. If vasopressor medication is necessary in patients receiving bretylium, a hypersensitivity to the catecholamine infusion may occur.

There has been concern regarding the interaction of bretylium with other antiarrhythmic medications, and several investigators have reported that it is more effective when used alone than in combination with other agents.

ANTAZOLINE

Antazoline is an antihistamine derivative that has electrophysiologic effects similar to quinidine. It has occasionally been efficacious in the therapy of certain supraventricular as well as ventricular arrhythmias. Although it has been successfully employed in occasional cases of atrial tachycardia, except for unusual instances it has relatively little efficacy in the conversion of atrial flutter or fibrillation to normal sinus rhythm. Although it has not attained an important role in the therapy of arrhythmias, it may have a role in those instances in which the patient manifests an intolerance or refractoriness to other antiarrhythmic drugs. The best results with this drug have been obtained in the treatment of premature ventricular beats and ventricular tachycardia.

The drug is administered orally and is generally well tolerated in doses of 100 to 200 mg three or four times daily. It is an antihistamine derivative and, as with other antihistamines, drowsiness may occur. The major toxic side effects include headache, nausea, vomiting, and diarrhea. Other side effects include a diffuse sensation of heat, facial flush, and occasional hypotension.

ATROPINE

Atropine is a naturally occurring belladonna alkaloid that blocks the parasympathetic effects on various organs, including the heart. It acts to competitively block acetylcholine, although its cardiac action is exerted directly on the receptor sites located on the effector cells of the conduction system and atrial muscle. Atropine exerts its effect on the sinus rate by blockade of acetylcholine and by affecting the interaction between acetylcholine and norepinephrine within the node.

The effect of atropine is dependent on the dose and the route and rapidity of administration as well as the age and physiologic state of the patient (particularly whether or not he is anesthetized). The parasympathomimetic blocking activity of the drug results in an increased sinus rate. However, when administered slowly in a small dose, direct parasympathomimetic effects may occur, decreasing the heart rate. This effect may last from 15 seconds to 15 minutes and can generally be avoided by administering an adequate dose (0.5 to 1 mg in a bolus form). Arrhythmias due to vagal hyperactivity can usually be partially or entirely abolished by atropine. Thus, it effectively increases ventricular rate (when due to vagotonia) in 1) sinus bradycardia, 2) sinus arrhythmia, 3) sinoatrial block, 4) atrial flutter and fibrillation associated with very slow ventricular responses, 5) partial A-V block (due to increased vagal tone), and 6) occasionally in digitalis intoxication with decreased ventricular responses through the A-V junction. Its effects are often transient, and systemic side effects may occur with the doses necessary to achieve these cardiovascular responses. Atropine may produce an undue increase in heart rate with deleterious effects when used during an acute myocardial infarction. Other side effects that are most commonly seen with atropine include flushing sensation, urinary retention, difficulty in swallowing, disturbed speech, headache, marked pupillary dilatation, and hallucinations. Questions have been raised as to the arrhythmogenic action of atropine during experimental coronary occlusion, although this has not been the clinical experience. The standard intravenous dose of atropine is 0.5 to 1 mg given intravenously in a bolus with additional 0.4 to 0.5 mg boluses to a maximum of 2 mg if the desired increase in heart rate has not occurred.

PARASYMPATHOMIMETIC AGENTS

The important parasympathomimetic agents that manifest antiarrhythmic action include acetylcholine, methycholine, neostigmine and edrophonium. Neostigmine and edrophonium are the most frequently used because they produce the least side effects. The major indication for these agents is in the occasional treatment of supraventricular tachycardias.

Neostigmine is usually injected in doses of 0.5 to 2.0 mg. Its therapeutic effect is often temporary. The onset of action occurs in about 20 minutes, reaching a peak in 1 hour and subsiding in 3 to 5 hours. Toxic effects with neostigmine include nausea, excess salivation, perspiration, dizziness, loose bowel movements, muscle aches and pains, abdominal cramps, and vomiting.

Edrophonium has a mechanism of action similar to that of neostigmine. However, its duration of action is shorter and it has limited use in the therapy of supraventricular arrhyth-

mias. It is administered in intravenous doses of 5 to 10 mg and has toxic effects similar to those of the other parasympathomimetic drugs. Rapid administration may cause excess slowing of the heart, transient hypotension, and increased bronchial secretions (all of which can be abolished by atropine).

NEWER ANTIARRHYTHMIC AGENTS

Tocainide

Tocainide is a promising oral lidocaine analog with similar electrophysiologic properties (Winkle, 1978). Sixty per cent of the drug dose is metabolized by the liver and 40 per cent is excreted unchanged from the kidneys (Harrison, 1977). Doses of 400 to 800 mg every 8 hours result in blood levels from 5 to 15 μg per ml. Tocainide in this concentration has been found very effective in the treatment of ventricular premature complexes and ventricular tachycardia (Winkle, 1976). Thus, ventricular arrhythmias have been reported to be successfully treated in as many as 80 per cent of patients. The drug is more than 50 per cent protein bound (Zipes, 1978). Its major side effects are GI and central nervous system symptoms as well as occasional skin rashes (Winkle, 1978).

Aprindine

Aprindine is another agent with local anesthetic effects. It is reportedly effective in the treatment of atrial and ventricular arrhythmias of several etiologies including digitalis toxicity and recurrent ventricular tachycardia. It also seems to affect "slow channel" induced arrhythmias (Zipes, 1978). Aprindine is 85 to 90 per cent protein bound (Danilo, 1979). Peak blood levels are achieved approximately 2 hours after an oral dose and the drug is predominantly metabolized by the liver. Aprindine has a significant effect on the A-V node, markedly increasing its refractory period. Studies in man have shown an increased A-H and H-V interval and an increase in QRS duration. It also increases the effective refractory period of the A-V node and ventricular conduction system. Its major side effects include tremors and heart block as well as widening of the QRS complex (Fasola, 1977). Cholestatic jaundice and agranulocytosis have also been reported (Danilo, 1979). The ratio between the therapeutic blood level and toxic dose appears to be small, and this may affect its clinical usefulness (Zipes, 1978).

MEXILETINE

Mexiletine is another primary analog of lidocaine with similar local anesthetic effects and antiarrhythmic properties. In man it has been shown to increase the effective refractory period of the A-V node and His-Purkinje system and to prolong the H-V interval (Roos, 1976). However, a similar study failed to show this effect (McComish, 1977). It has been used both intravenously and orally. Following oral administration, peak blood levels occur 2 to 4 hours after administration. The drug is metabolized by the liver, and less than 10 per cent is excreted in the urine. The major side effects reported include nausea, tremor, hypotension, convulsions, diplopia, and tremor (Zipes, 1978). It is administered in doses of 200 to 400 mg every 6 to 8 hours. The drug has been particularly effective in arrhythmias associated with acute myocardial infarction (Achuff, 1977).

AMIODARONE

Amiodarone has been reported to be effective in both atrial and ventricular arrhythmias in a variety of clinical situations and in the treatment of recurrent refractory ventricular tachycardia (Zipes, 1978; Olsson, 1973). It has also been found useful in patients with arrhythmias associated with the Wolff-Parkinson-White syndrome. Some reports suggest that amiodarone may be superior to standard antiarrhythmic therapy in the abolition of premature complexes. Its major side effects include skin discoloration, thyroid dysfunction, and corneal micro-deposits. It is slowly absorbed from the gastrointestinal tract and therefore may require days to weeks for its full antiarrhythmic effect.

VERAPAMIL

Verapamil is one of the first agents used clinically whose primary effect is to block "slow channel" arrhythmias. Clinically, this drug has been particularly useful in the treatment of supraventricular tachycardia and atrial fibrillation (Zipes, 1978). It has also been reported useful in tachycardias associated with the pre-excitation syndromes.

Verapamil given orally is rapidly and almost completely (90%) absorbed. It is rapidly metabolized by the liver and therefore its oral dose is five to eight times the intravenous dose. Electrophysiologic studies in man have shown that 10 mg given intravenously prolongs conduction time of the A-V node without increasing the H-V interval or increasing the QRS duration. In addition, it suppresses electrical activity in diseased atrial and ventricular muscle fibers that have diminished resting potentials. The sinus node slowing associated with this drug is only partially correctable by atropine. The intravenous dose is 5 to 10 mg, and oral dose is 40 to 120 mg every 8 hours. The major side effects of verapamil include decreased cardiac contractility, hypotension, and A-V block.

ETHMOZIN

Ethmozin is a phenothiazine derivative that has been used in clinical trials in the Soviet Union. It has been found effective in treating ventricular arrhyth-

mias, being less effective in atrial flutter, atrial fibrillation, and sinus tachycardia (Zipes, 1978). Relatively little has
been published concerning its pharmacology or electrophysiology. It is apparently effective orally in doses between 25 and 75 mg given three times
daily, with maximum effects being
achieved in doses of 5.5 mg per kg per
day, with a mean plasma concentration
of 0.8 μg per ml.

REFERENCES

Achuff, S. C., Pottage, A., Prescott, L. et al.:
Mexiletine in the prevention of ventricular arrhythmias in acute myocardial infarction. Postgrad. Med. J. 53:(Suppl. 1) 163–164, 1977.

Aronow, W. S., Turbow, M., Lurie, M., Whit-
taker, K., and Van Camp, S.: Treatment of
premature ventricular complexes with acebu-
tol. Am. J. Cardiol. 43:106–108, 1979.

Bigger, J. T., Dresdale, R. J., Heissenbuttel, R. H.,
Weld, F. M., and Wit, A. L.: Ventricular arrhythmias in ischemic heart disease: Mechanism, prevalence, significance, and management. Prog. Cardiovasc. Dis. 19(4):255–300,
1977.

Bigger, J. T., Schmidt, D. H., and Kutt, H.:
Relationship between the plasma level of diphenylhydantoin sodium and its cardiac antiarrhythmic effects. Circulation 38:363–374,
1968.

Blomgren, S. E., Condemi, J. J., and Vaughan, J.
H.: Procainamide induced lupus erythemato-
sus. Clinical and laboratory observations. Am.
J. Med. 52:338–348, 1972.

Bussmann, W. D., Müller, E., Hänel, H-J., and
Kaltenbach, M.: Orally administered prajmal-
ium bitartrate in acute and chronic ventricular
arrhythmias. Am. J. Cardiol. 41:577–583, 1978.

Chadda, K. D., Banka, V. S., and Helfant, R. H.:
Rate dependent ventricular ectopia following
acute coronary occlusion. The concept of an
optimal antiarrhythmic heart rate. Circulation
49:654–658, 1974.

Chiale, P. A., Przybylski, J., Halpern, M. S.,
Lazzari, J. O., Elizari, M. V., and Rosenbaum,
M. B.: Comparative effects of ajmaline on inter-
mittent bundle branch block and the Wolff-
Parkinson-White syndrome. Am. J. Cardiol.
39:651–657, 1977.

Cohen, I. S., Jick, H., and Cohen, S. I.: Adverse
reactions to quinidine in hospitalized patients:
Findings based on data from the Boston Col-
laborative Drug Surveillance Program. Prog.
Cardiovasc. Dis. 20(2):151–163, 1977.

Collinsworth, K. A., Kalman, S. M., and Harrison, D. C.: The clinical pharmacology of lidocaine as an antiarrhythmic drug. Circulation
50:1217–1230, 1974.

Coltart, D. J., Gibson, D. G., and Shaud, D. G.:
Plasma propranolol levels associated with sup-
pression of ventricular ectopic beats. Br. Med.
J. 1:490–491, 1971.

Conrad, K. A., Molk, B. L., and Chidsey, C. A.:
Pharmacokinetic studies of quinidine in patients with arrhythmias. Circulation 55:1–7,
1977.

Danilo, P., Jr.: Appraisal and reappraisal of cardiac therapy. Am. Heart J. 97:119–124, 1979.

Danilo, P., Jr., and Rosen, M. R.: Cardiac effects
of disopyramide. Am. Heart J. 92:532–536,
1976.

Dhingra, R. C., Amat-Y-Leon, F., Wyndham, C.,
Denes, P., Wu, D., Miller, R. H., and Rosen, K.
M.: Electrophysiologic effects of atropine on
sinus node and atrium in patients with sinus
nodal dysfunction. Am. J. Cardiol. 38:848–854,
1976.

Doering, W.: Quinidine-digoxin interaction:
pharmacokinetics, underlying mechanism and
clinical implications. N. Engl. J. Med. 301:400–
404, 1979.

Dreifus, L. S., and Ogawa, S.: Quality of the ideal
antiarrhythmic drug. Am. J. Cardiol. 39:466–
468, 1977.

Epstein, S. E., and Braunwald, E.: Beta-
adrenergic receptor blocking drugs. Mechanisms of action and clinical applications. N.
Engl. J. Med. 275:1106–1112, 1175–1183, 1966.

Fasola, A. F., Noble, R. J., and Zipes, D. P.:
Treatment of recurrent ventricular tachycardia
and fibrillation with aprindine. Am. J. Cardiol.
39:903–909, 1977.

Gaughan, C. E., Lown, B., Lanigan, J., Voukydis,
P., and Bresser, H. W.: Acute oral testing for
determining antiarrhythmic drug efficacy. I.
Quinidine. Am. J. Cardiol. 38:677, 1976.

Gey, G. O., Levy, R. H., Fisher, L., et al.: Plasma
concentration of procainamide and prevalence
of exertional arrhythmias. Ann. Int. Med.
80:718–722, 1974.

Gianelly, R., Vander Graeben, J. D., Spivack, A.
P., and Harrison, D. C.: Effect of lidocaine on
ventricular arrhythmias in patients with coronary heart disease. N. Engl. J. Med. 227:1215,
1967.

Gillis, R. A., Thibodeaux, H., and Barr, L.: Antiarrhythmic properties of chlordiazepoxide.
Circulation 49:272–282, 1974.

Hagemeijer, F.: Verapamil in the management of
supraventricular tachyarrhythmias occurring
after a recent myocardial infarction. Circulation
57(4):751–755, 1978.

Harrison, D. C., Meffin, P. J., and Winkle, R. A.:
Clinical pharmacokinetics of antiarrhythmic
drugs. Prog. Cardiovasc. Dis. 20(3):217–242,
1977.

Harrison, D. C., Sprouse, J. C., and Morrow, A.
G.: The antiarrhythmic properties of lidocaine
and procainamide. Circulation 28:486, 1963.

Helfant, R. H., Lau, S. H., Cohen, S. L., et al.:
Effects of diphenylhydantoin on atrioventricular conduction in man. Circulation 36:686–691,
1967.

Helfant, R. H., Seuffert, G., Patton, R., Stein, E., and Damato, A. N.: The clinical use of diphenylhydantoin (dilantin) in the treatment and prevention of arrhythmias. Am. Heart J. 77:315, 1969.

Hinderline, P. H., and Garrett, E. F.: Pharmacokinetics of the antiarrhythmic disopyramide in healthy humans. J. Pharm. Biopharm. 4:199–229, 1976.

Hoffman, B. F., Rosen, M. R., and Wit, A. L.: Electrophysiology and pharmacology of cardiac arrhythmias. VII. Cardiac effects of quinidine and procaine amide. Am. Heart J. 89:804–808, 1975.

Holder, D. A., Sniderman, A. D., Fraser, G., and Fallen, E. L.: Experience with bretylium tosylate by a hospital cardiac arrest team. Circulation 55(3):541–544, 1977.

Jewitt, D. E., Kishon, Y., and Thomas, M.: Lidocaine in the management of arrhythmias after acute myocardial infarction. Lancet 1:266–270, 1968.

Koch-Weser, J.: Drug therapy. Bretylium. Medical Intelligence 300(9):473–477, 1979.

Koch-Weser, J., and Klein, S. E.: Procainamide dosage schedules, plasma concentrations, and clinical effects. J.A.M.A. 215:1454–1460, 1971.

Luchi, R. J.: Intoxication with quinidine (editorial). Chest 73:129–131, 1978.

McComish, M., Robinson, C., Kitson, D., et al.: Clinical electrophysiological effects of mexiletine. Postgrad. Med. J. 53(1):85–91, 1977.

McClendon, R. L., Hansen, W. R., and Kinsman, J. M.: Hemodynamic changes following procaine amide administered intravenously. Am. J. Med. Sci. 222:375–381, 1951.

Nappi, J. M., Katz, M. H., and Thomsen, J. H.: Efficacy of disopyramide in treating arrhythmias. Drug Therapy May 1979, pp. 145–151.

Obayashi, K., Nagasawa, K., Mandel, W. J., Vyden, J. K., and Parmley, W. W.: Cardiovascular effects of ajmaline. Am. Heart J. 92(4):487–496, 1976.

Ochs, H. R., Greenblatt, D. J., Woo, E., et al.: Single and multiple dose pharmacokinetics of oral quinidine sulfate and gluconate. Am. J. Cardiol. 41:770–776, 1978.

Olsson, S. B., Brorson, L., and Varnauskas, E.: Antiarrhythmic action in man. Observations from monophasic action potential recordings and amiodarone treatment. Br. Heart J. 35:1255–1259, 1973.

Ranny, R. E., Dean, R. R., Karim, A., et al.: Disopyramide phosphate. Pharmacokinetic and pharmacologic relationship of a new antiarrhythmic agent. Arch. Int. Pharm. 191:162–170, 1971.

Roos, J. C., and Dunning, A. J.: Effects of lidocaine on impulse formation and conduction defects in man. Am. Heart J. 89:686–699, 1975.

Roos, J. C., Paalmau, A. C. A., and Dunning, A. J.: Electrophysiological effects of mexiletine in man. Br. Heart J. 38:62–72, 1976.

Rosen, M. R., Wit, A. L., and Hoffman, B. F.: Electrophysiology and pharmacology of cardiac arrhythmias. VI. Cardiac effects of verapamil. Am. Heart J. 89:665–673, 1975.

Rosenbaum, M. B., Chiale, P. A., Halpern, M. S., Nau, G. J., Przybylski, J., Levi, R. J., Lazzari, J. O., and Elizari, M. V.: Clinical efficacy of amiodarone as an antiarrhythmic agent. Am. J. Cardiol. 38:934, 1976.

Scheinman, M. M., Weiss, A. N., Shafton, E., Benowitz, N., and Rowland, M.: Electrophysiologic effects of procaine amide in patients with intraventricular conduction delay. Circulation 49:522–529, 1974.

Selzer, A., and Wray, H. W.: Quinidine syncope: Paroxysmal ventricular fibrillation occurring during treatment of chronic atrial arrhythmias. Circulation 30:17–26, 1964.

Shub, C., Gau, G. T., Sidell, P. M., and Brennan, L. A., Jr.: The management of acute quinidine intoxication. Chest 73:173–178, 1978.

Stenson, R. E., Constantino, R. T., and Harrison, D. C.: Inter-relationships of hepatic blood flow, cardiac output, and blood levels of lidocaine in man. Circulation 43:205–211, 1971.

Talbot, R. G., Julian, D. G., and Prescott, L. F.: Long-term treatment of ventricular arrhythmias with oral mexiletine. Am. Heart J. 91(1):58–65, 1976.

Thomson, P. D., Melmon, K. L., Richardson, J. A., et al.: Lidocaine pharmacokinetics in advanced heart failure, liver disease and renal failure in humans. Ann. Int. Med. 78:499–508, 1973.

Vaughan, W. M.: Classification of antidysrhythmic drugs. Pharm. Ther. 1:115–138, 1975.

Vismara, L. A., Mason, D. T., and Amsterdam, E. A.: Disopyramide phosphate: Clinical efficacy of a new oral antiarrhythmic drug. Clin. Pharmacol. Ther. 16:330–335, 1974.

Vismara, L. A., Vera, Z., Miller, R. R., and Mason, D. T.: Efficacy of disopyramide phosphate in the treatment of refractory ventricular tachycardia. Am. J. Cardiol. 39:1027–1034, 1977.

Watanabe, Y., and Dreifus, L. S.: Factors controlling impulse transmission with special reference to A-V conduction. Am. Heart J. 89(6):790–803, 1975.

Weiss, T., Lattin, G. M., and Engelman, K.: Vagally mediated suppression of premature ventricular contractions in man. Am. Heart J. 89(6):700–707, 1975.

Winkle, R. A., Alderman, E. L., Fitzgerald, J. W., and Harrison, D. C.: Treatment of recurrent symptomatic ventricular tachycardia. Ann. Int. Med. 85:1–7, 1976.

Winkle, R. A., Meffin, P. J., and Harrison, D. C.: Longterm tocainide therapy for ventricular arrhythmias. Circulation 57(5):1008–1016, 1978.

Zipes, D. P., and Troup, P. J.: New antiarrhythmic agents. Amiodarone, aprindine, disopyramide, ethmozin, mexiletine, tocainide, verapamil. Am. J. Cardiol. 41:1005–1024, 1978.

24

CARDIAC PACING

MICHAEL S. FELDMAN, M.D.
RICHARD H. HELFANT, M.D.

In the two decades since its inception, artificial pacing has become accepted as one of the most efficacious and reliable means of managing cardiac arrhythmias, particularly bradyarrhythmias. Currently there are over 250,000 patients with pacemakers in the United States alone, and as many as 40,000 to 50,000 new implantations yearly are predicted. It seems inevitable that the increasing sophistication of generator circuitry, as well as the increasing reliability of power sources and electrodes, will lead to a continued broadening of its application in the therapy of cardiac arrhythmias.

TEMPORARY PACING

Temporary artificial pacing is performed for a variety of diagnostic and therapeutic purposes. The site of entry chosen and the type of electrode utilized and generator employed vary with the indication and whether the implantation is being performed under emergency, urgent, or elective conditions.

Indications

While many indications for temporary pacing are clearly defined (Table 24–1), several areas, particularly in

acute myocardial infarction, are less uniformly agreed upon. In the latter circumstances, the need for temporary pacing is based on the patient's symptoms, the ventricular rate and rhythm, and the underlying etiologic and clinical circumstances. Generally accepted indications for temporary pacing include 1) symptomatic third degree or high grade A-V block, particularly in patients with syncope or near syncopal episodes (see Chapter 12); 2) symptomatic severe bradycardias; 3) life threatening ventricular arrhythmias resulting from a bradyarrhythmia; 4) overdrive suppression of refractory ventricular or supraventricular tachyarrhythmias; 5) hypotension and/or heart failure resulting from bradyarrhythmia; 6) symptomatic digitalis induced bradyarrhythmias.

TABLE 24–1 INDICATIONS FOR TEMPORARY PACING

Symptomatic bradycardias due to:
High grade A–V block
Second degree A–V block
Sick sinus syndrome
Carotid sinus syncope
Acute bundle branch block due to acute myocardial infarction
Determination of need for implantation of permanent pacemaker
Prophylaxis during open heart surgery
Drug resistant tachycardias

The indications for temporary pacing in acute myocardial infarction are determined by the location of the infarct, the hemodynamic consequences of the arrhythmia, associated life-threatening arrhythmias, patient symptomatology, the ventricular rate, and the site and degree of block present. In the presence of an inferior wall infarction, A-V block is generally of the type I variety, that is, within the A-V node. This is manifested by either first degree block, second degree block of the Wenckebach type, or third degree block (see Chapter 12). It is almost invariably transient and even in the presence of complete A-V block is generally associated with a relatively rapid junctional escape rate. Temporary pacing is usually not necessary under these conditions unless 1) the ventricular rate is less than 40 to 45 beats per minute, 2) ventricular premature complexes are present, 3) the patient is hypotensive, or 4) heart failure or signs of decreased cardiac output are present. Occasionally, a "brady-tachy" syndrome is associated with a diaphragmatic infarction, and it may be necessary to pace temporarily in order to properly treat the tachyarrhythmias.

Anterior wall myocardial infarctions are associated with second degree or complete A-V block less than one third as frequently as are inferior wall infarctions (DePasquale and Bruno, 1976). The block, when present, is almost always of the type II variety (i.e., in the His-Purkinje network) and usually involves the bundle branches. Second degree A-V block of the Mobitz II variety is usually associated with a wide QRS complex, and there is a high risk of complete A-V block, which is associated with a ventricular escape rhythm that is slower and less stable than that seen in inferior wall infarctions. Therefore, immediate insertion of a temporary pacemaker is indicated. Even with successful pacing, the mortality rate is high, approaching 75 to 90 per cent, since this type of block is usually associated with a massive infarction. Although less clearly defined, the acute onset of bilateral bundle branch block in the presence of an acute anterior wall infarction (even in the absence of second degree or complete A-V block) is considered an indication for temporary pacing by most authorities. Prophylactic pacemaker implantation with the onset of acute isolated left or right bundle branch block or with new right bundle branch block and left axis deviation (bifascicular block) is more controversial but is indicated in our view. There is no demonstrable value, however, in inserting pacemakers in patients with *pre-existing* right bundle branch block, left bundle branch block, or bifascicular block even in the presence of an acute infarction.

Technique

The technique of choice is endocardial pacing via an intravenous route to the right ventricular apex. Whenever possible, the temporary transvenous electrode should be positioned under direct x-ray visualization either in a cardiac catheterization laboratory or with the use of a portable image intensifier. Under certain circumstances, however, this is not practical, and a "blind technique" must be utilized, identifying the position of the electrode tip by means of electrocardiographic evidence alone. The preferred site of intravenous entry varies among physicians, and the brachial, subclavian, supraclavicular, internal jugular, and femoral approaches all have been advocated. Under absolute emergency conditions in which the immediate establishment of electrical activity is mandatory, a transthoracic approach through the subxiphoid area to the right ventricle has been used. This technique requires considerable experience.

There is a large variety of endocardial transvenous electrocatheters currently available, in sizes ranging from 5 to 7 French, having both unipolar and bipolar configurations, and varying in degrees of stiffness. In some instances, catheters with preformed curves for insertion are utilized from the femoral position. In general, bipolar electrodes are used in temporary pacing, although unipolar sensing is often superior. A new hexipolar catheter has been recently introduced for use in temporary A-V sequential pacing. This particular catheter has distal ventricular electrodes plus four electrodes which (under ideal circumstances) contact the atrial free wall and allow atrial as well as ventricular pacing.

The proper position of the electrode tip for ventricular pacing is at the apex of the right ventricle. This position is optimal for obtaining and maintaining maximal stability as well as satisfactory sensing and capture. In general current thresholds below 1 milliampere are indicative of good electrode position. Thresholds above this level are unacceptable, as there is an inordinate amount of subsequent electrode displacement.

Several external pulse generators are available, all of which have slightly different characteristics. Although the sensitivity of the units can be adjusted so that they function in a fixed rate or demand mode, the demand mode should be used. The external generator should be set at a milliamperage output that is a minimum of five times the threshold level obtained at implantation. When very low pacing thresholds are obtained, a minimum setting of 3 to 5 milliamperes is appropriate. Sensing difficulties are not uncommon with external generators, and for this reason high milliamperage output should be avoided when feasible, since the incidence of fibrillatory events increases at higher outputs, particularly with bipolar pacing (Chardock et al., 1969; Merx et al., 1975). All pacing should be cathodal with the distal electrode attached to the negative pole of the generator.

Complications of Temporary Pacing

The most common complication of temporary pacing is induced ventricular arrhythmias at the time of implantation. These can be minimized by proper lead placement and avoidance of undue pressure against the ventricular endocardial wall. Occasionally, even with proper positioning, the arrhythmias may persist and necessitate the use of antiarrhythmic agents. These agents are often ineffective in this setting, and if the ventricular irritability cannot be controlled, electrode repositioning must be considered.

Another common problem is electrode displacement. This can be minimized by positioning the catheter in the distal right ventricular apex under direct visualization, obtaining a stimulation threshold below 1.0 milliamps, and immobilizing the electrode with suture and tape.

Wound infection at the site of entry can be minimized by the use of sterile techniques at the time of implantation and the use of a topical antibiotic. Fortunately, phlebitis and/or endocarditis secondary to direct extension along the electrode from the wound site is uncommon. When phlebitis is present, the catheter should be removed and, if necessary, another intravenous site chosen.

Right ventricular perforation occurs occasionally, but is uncommon and is usually of minor consequence. Tamponade is extremely unusual when perforation does occur; however, hemopericardium and signs of tamponade should be watched for, particularly when anticoagulants have been used. Diaphragmatic and intercostal pacing are often associated with perforation, but they often occur in the absence of perforation.

PERMANENT PACING

Indications for Pacing
Bradyarrhythmias and Conduction
Abnormalities

Sick Sinus Syndrome. The most common current indication for permanent artificial pacing is not high grade heart block but the sick sinus syndrome (Furman, 1977) (see Chapter 5). The major indication for pacing in this syndrome is the presence of significant symptomatology, namely symptoms of syncope or near syncope, lightheadedness or dizziness, angina, low output state, or sensations of palpitations due to either brady- or tachyarrhythmias (Fig. 24–1).

Concomitant conduction abnormalities of the A-V junctional and His-Purkinje system are present in as many as 60 per cent of patients (Scarpa, 1976). In the majority of cases, therefore, pacing from a ventricular site is necessary. Ventricular synchronous pacing is adequate for most patients despite the fact that atrial or A-V sequential pacing has theoretical advantages in that: 1) atrial tachycardias may be more easily suppressed when atrial synchrony is maintained; 2) the atrial contribution to

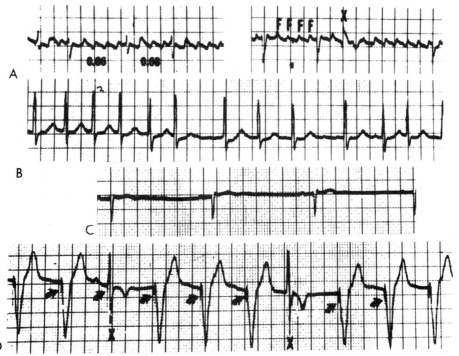

Figure 24–1 Use of pacemaker in treating brady-tachyarrhythmias. Tracing taken from a patient 71 years of age with episodes of coronary insufficiency that occurred at rapid ventricular rates and dizziness that occurred with slow heart rates.

(*A*) The first strip shows atrial flutter with varying degrees of A-V heart block (note cycle lengths). The second strip shows an aberrant beat (X).

(*B*) Atrial flutter-fibrillation. The initial five cycles show a rapid rate averaging 150 per minute. Thereafter, it becomes somewhat slower.

(*C*) Sinus bradycardia with normal sinus rhythm and a heart rate of 37 per minute.

(*D*) After insertion of a pacemaker (rate = 86 beats/minute) the dizzy spells disappeared; the patient was able to take digitalis, which improved the heart failure. At (X) is a normally conducted beat. Remaining widened QRS complexes are the result of the pacemaker; note the stimulus artifact (arrows).

cardiac output is preserved, providing enhanced cardiac function. Preservation of atrial synchrony is important, however, in patients with poor left ventricular function and borderline cardiac output. On occasion, pacing alone may not relieve the patient's symptoms and antiarrhythmic agents and digitalis may be necessary. Even with adequate pacing, patients with symptomatic sick sinus syndrome have a reported yearly mortality of one to two times that of patients paced for A-V block alone (15–30%) (Wohl et al., 1976).

Complete A-V Block. Although the Stokes-Adams syndrome with complete A-V heart block is the classic indication for permanent cardiac pacing (Fig. 24–2), currently it accounts for less than 20 per cent of permanent artificial pacemaker implantations (Furman, 1977). In our view, the presence of chronic complete A-V block is an indication for permanent pacing (a partial exception is congenital A-V block) regardless of the presence or absence of symptoms. Although ventricular demand pacing is adequate in most cases, when there is concomitant left ventricular dysfunction, A-V sequential, bifocal demand pacing is the preferred method to enhance cardiac performance.

Patients with congenital A-V block (most frequently adolescents) usually have ventricular complexes with a normal QRS duration and a rate that ranges between 50 to 60 beats per minute. In these patients, the ventricular pacing focus is located above the His bundle.

They frequently are asymptomatic and have an adequate increase in ventricular rate as a response to exercise. In the asymptomatic individual with congenital block, the need for ventricular pacing is unclear. Most physicians prefer to follow the patient and to treat only in the case of symptomatic disease. Many of these patients eventually become symptomatic and require permanent pacing. Occasionally, His bundle studies performed in patients with escape rates of 40 to 50 beats per minute and normal QRS complexes reveal block below or within the His bundle. These patients generally require permanent pacing.

Second Degree A-V Block — Mobitz Type II. The presence of type II second degree A-V block is generally accepted as an indication for permanent pacing. The area of conduction disease in Mobitz II block is below the His bundle and is usually progressive. These patients have an increased incidence of intermittent high grade A-V block, asystole, ventricular tachycardia, ventricular fibrillation, syncope, and sudden death. As with complete A-V block, demand ventricular synchronous pacing is usually appropriate.

Bifascicular Block. Many patients initially present with bifascicular block, that is, right bundle branch block with left anterior or left posterior division delay with or without first degree A-V block and no evidence of second or high grade block. In these individuals, the indication for permanent pacing is

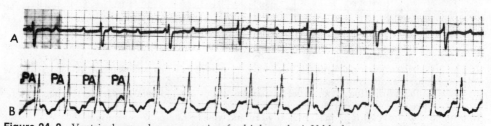

Figure 24–2   Ventricular synchronous pacing for high grade A-V block.
(A) High grade A-V block (atrial rate 94/min, ventricular rate 36/min). (B) Ventricular synchronous pacing at 79 per minute. Note the ventricular depolarization following each pacemaker discharge (PA).

controversial. Many authorities recommend permanent pacing for patients displaying bifascicular block with marked first degree A-V block, particularly if the major A-V conduction delay is below the His bundle, as demonstrated by a prolongation of the H-V interval on His bundle study. It is our opinion, however, that in the absence of documented second degree A-V block or symptoms suggestive of intermittent high grade block, pacing is not indicated, since the incidence of subsequent high grade block is low (McAnulty, 1978). Conversely, in the presence of recurrent symptoms suggestive of intermittent A-V block — lightheadedness or syncope — there is an increased incidence of progression to higher grades of A-V block and sudden death, particularly when the H-V interval is prolonged beyond 60 milliseconds on His bundle ECG. Permanent pacing is recommended in these individuals despite the inability to document second degree or higher grades of block (Altschuler et al., 1979). Similarly, the presence of alternating bundle branch block (i.e., intermittent right bundle and left bundle branch block) is indicative of bilateral bundle branch block and warrants permanent pacing regardless of symptomatology. However, patients with isolated left or right bundle branch block who are asymptomatic do not require permanent pacing.

Carotid Sinus Syncope. In patients with carotid sinus syncope that is not drug induced, permanent pacing is usually indicated. Demand ventricular pacing would appear to be adequate for these purposes except in the presence of severe left ventricular dysfunction.

Indications for Pacing Recurrent Ventricular and Supraventricular Tachyarrhythmias

Occasionally, patients with refractory paroxysmal ventricular or supraventricular tachycardia fail to respond to ag-gressive antiarrhythmic medication alone. The adjunctive use of temporary artificial overdrive suppression with pacing at a rate 10 to 25 per cent above the baseline ventricular rate has occasionally proven beneficial in suppressing these arrhythmias (Haft, 1974). If overdrive suppression is successful with temporary pacing and the arrhythmia is recurrent when the overdrive pacing is discontinued, permanent pacing is indicated.

The experience with overdrive pacing has indicated that 1) the rate of the overdrive does not have to exceed the tachycardia to prevent it; 2) a rate somewhat faster than the sinus rate can be effective; and 3) with paced rates greater than 100 beats per minute, complications are more likely to occur. As a rule, patients with recurrent ventricular tachycardia have significant disease of the myocardium as well as of the conduction tissue, and atrial, coronary sinus, or A-V sequential bifocal pacing may be necessary to preserve the atrial contribution to cardiac output. Although there is some controversy as to whether atrial or ventricular pacing is more effective in overdrive suppression when left ventricular function is relatively well preserved, standard demand endocardial right ventricular pacing is usually appropriate, since it has the advantage of more stable catheter positioning. Overdrive suppression is often inadequate without the use of concomitant antiarrhythmic medication. In the absence of bradycardia, there is question as to the efficacy of overdrive suppression of ventricular arrhythmias if the minimal effective rate is more than 20 per cent faster than the underlying cardiac rhythm. The frequency of premature ventricular contractions is diminished but the incidence of ventricular tachycardia may remain the same or even increase.

More recently, generators have been developed that are externally activated by radio-frequency controls. They have been specifically designed for use in the termination of recurrent episodic ventricular and supraventricular tachycardia (Fisher et al., 1978). The radiofrequency pacemaker appears to be a promising new mode of therapy, particularly in the control of supraventricular tachycardias in a select group of patients with accessory atrioventricular conduction in whom recurrent bouts of supraventricular tachycardia are disabling despite large doses of antiarrhythmic medication (Kahn et al., 1976).

Indications for Permanent Pacing After Myocardial Infarction

Permanent artificial pacing is rarely if ever required in the presence of an inferior wall infarction except in the occasional case of persistent sick sinus syndrome. In acute anterior wall infarctions, although there is some controversy (Ritter et al., 1976), we currently recommend permanent pacing for patients who display bilateral bundle branch block and associated second degree or higher grade block, however transient at the time of infarction. Patients who manifest isolated right bundle or left bundle branch block are not recommended for permanent pacemaker implantation, since there is no incontrovertible evidence to suggest an increase in survival (Hindman et al., 1978). Occasionally, refractory ventricular arrhythmias associated with either inferior or anterior wall infarction may temporarily or permanently necessitate overdrive pacing in conjunction with antiarrhythmic medication.

MODES OF ARTIFICIAL PACING

The rapid advances in electronic technology since the inception of artificial pacing, combined with an increasing awareness of the variable physiologic requirements of various clinical situations, has led to the development of a wide variety of pacemaker modalities. These include 1) asynchronous (fixed rate) stimulation; 2) noncompetitive (demand) stimulation, which may be of either R wave inhibited, R wave triggered, or R tracking varieties; 3) A-V synchronous stimulation; 4) A-V sequential stimulation; and 5) a variety of rapid stimulation pacemakers designed specifically for the overdrive conversion of recurrent supraventricular or ventricular tachyarrhythmias (other than atrial fibrillation).

Asynchronous (Fixed Rate) Pacing

The asynchronous (fixed rate) pacemaker is the simplest form of permanent generator. It stimulates the heart at a predetermined fixed cycle length regardless of the patient's underlying intrinsic rhythm (Fig. 24–3). The most serious drawback to fixed rate pacing is that competition can occur between the pacemaker stimulus and the patient's rhythm and, on occasion, can precipitate ventricular tachycardia or fibrillation. Currently, with the advent of cathodal stimulation and newer generators that utilize shorter pulse durations and lower milliamperage output, ventricular tachycardia may be more a theoretical than a practical problem in most patients. However, pacemaker induced ventricular tachycardia has been documented in the past in patients with ischemic heart disease or congestive heart failure. In view of the minimal practical advantages and the significant theoretical and practical disadvantages to this mode of pacing, most authorities feel that there is no indication for long term asynchronous pacing.

Ventricular Synchronous (Demand) Pacing

Ventricular demand pacing currently accounts for more than 90 per cent of all permanent pacemaker implants (Par-

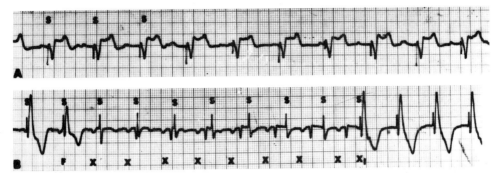

Figure 24–3 A normally functioning asynchronous pulse generator.

(A) Sinus rhythm is seen at a rate of 64 per minute. However, high grade block is present. The ventricle is being paced (S) at a rate of 71 per minute.

(B) The spikes marked S represent discharge from an asynchronous ventricular pulse generator. Those beats marked X are preceded by sinus P waves at a rate of 94 per minute. Note, however, the uninterrupted discharge of the pulse generator eventuating in a premature depolarization (X_1). The second beat represents a fusion beat (F).

sonnet, 1977). This type of generator stimulates the myocardium only when a normal ventricular depolarization does not occur within a predetermined interval. Generators are available with either R wave inhibited or R wave triggered circuitry (Fig. 24–4). The R wave inhibited variety has circuits that sense the patient's innate ventricular depolarization and produce a stimulus only

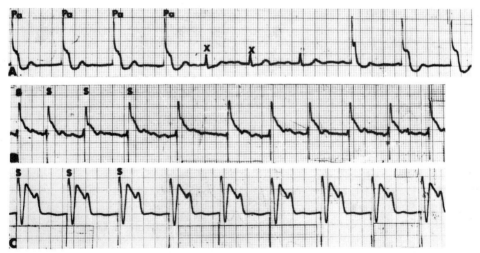

Figure 24–4 Normally functioning R wave inhibited and R triggered ventricular synchronous pacemakers.

(A) The complexes marked Pa represent ventricular activation stimulated by discharge of the pacemaker at a rate of 68 per minute. The beats marked (X) are preceded by sinus P waves and occur at a rate of 70 per minute. The pacemaker is sensing properly and hence has not discharged.

(B) The underlying rhythm is atrial fibrillation with a ventricular response varying between 70 and 130 per minute. The pacemaker is of the R triggered variety and hence discharges into the QRS complex (S).

(C) The same patient as in strip B. However, the ventricular response rate has now decreased and the ventricle is being activated by the pacemaker at regular intervals (68/min). Note also the difference in QRS and T wave contour between strips B and C.

when the patient's ventricle fails to depolarize within a predetermined period of time.

The R wave triggered variety, when sensing the patient's own intrinsic ventricular depolarization, produces a pulse stimulus that falls into the R wave of the QRS while the ventricle is refractory. Although the R wave triggered pacemaker produces a pulse artifact with each ventricular depolarization, it only stimulates the ventricle if the cardiac rate falls below that of the pacemaker's predetermined cycle length. All demand generators are preset to deliver a pulse stimulus at a given cycle length. Following discharge, all pacemakers are insensitive to incoming signals for a period of time during which a ventricular depolarization may not reset the generator. The refractory period varies with individual models and ranges from 200 to 400 milliseconds in duration. All demand generators also have a magnetic reed switch for external conversion to a temporary fixed rate mode and additional circuitry to detect electrical "interference," which allows them to convert to fixed rate pacing. A limited number of pacemaker generators have a built-in rate hysteresis allowing for a slightly greater cycle length between the last sensed depolarization (the patient's own intrinsic depolarization) and the first paced beat.

A variant of the R triggered pacemaker is the R tracking generator, which differs in that when ventricular depolarization is sensed, a low amperage non-depolarizing current is produced, thus allowing for an assessment of pacemaker function with low current drain.

The standard demand (R triggered or R inhibited) generators are used primarily for ventricular pacing. They are less frequently employed for atrial pacing because of the relatively low signal amplitude of atrial depolarization. Although high sensitivity generators are available, these units have also proved less than ideal in sensing atrial depolarization.

A-V Synchronous Pacing

Atrioventricular synchronous pacing was initially developed in order to maintain the atrial contribution to cardiac output as well as to allow for the physiologic sinus rate responses to exercise and other stimuli. In order to achieve synchronization, a sensing electrode is placed at the level of the atrium while a second pacing electrode is placed in the ventricle. Atrial depolarization is sensed and after a predetermined delay (120–250 milliseconds) ventricular depolarization is initiated by the pulse generator through the ventricular electrode (Fig. 24–5). In this generator design, the atrial electrode is incapable of driving the atrium, while the ventricular electrode has no sensing capability. These are serious limitations, although newer circuitry designs allowing for ventricular sensing as well as pacing are being developed. If after a predetermined interval no atrial depolarization is sensed, the pacemaker generates a pacing stimulus. As an additional safety feature, the circuits are designed so that in the presence of atrial rates greater than 150 beats per minute the generator is refractory and will revert to a fixed rate mode.

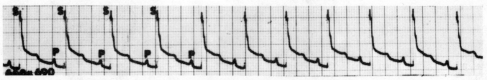

Figure 24–5 An atrial synchronous pulse generator. The sinus P waves (P) occur at intervals varying between 660 and 690 msec. The pacemaker senses the atrial depolarization and discharges (S) after a predetermined interval (180 msec), initiating ventricular activation.

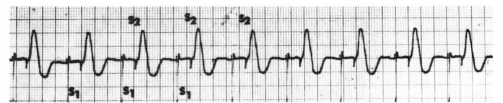

Figure 24–6 A normally functioning A-V sequential pacemaker. The pacemaker stimulated atrial depolarization (S₁) is followed after a predetermined interval (200 msec) by discharge of the ventricular electrode (S₂), resulting in ventricular depolarization.

A-V Sequential Pacing

Atrioventricular sequential pacing is a modification of A-V synchronous pacing designed for situations in which the atrial contribution is important and atrial activity is undependable. A double lead system in the atria and ventricle is again utilized, with electrode positioning similar to A-V synchronous pacing. The system designs differ, however, in that the atrial electrode is a pacing electrode with no sensing capabilities. The ventricular electrode has both pacing and sensing functions. The generator is preset at a predetermined rate with atrial stimulation timed to occur at a fixed interval after ventricular depolarization (Fig. 24–6). Following a delay of 120 to 250 milliseconds (predetermined for each generator), the ventricular electrode will initiate a stimulus, provided that ventricular depolarization does not occur in the interim.

Although some form of atrial synchronous pacing is potentially feasible in the majority of patients (75% of patients in complete heart block are in sinus rhythm), the use of A-V synchronous or A-V sequential pacing has been limited by 1) the relative bulk and unreliability of generator circuitry; 2) the relatively inefficient energy utilization with concomitant rapid depletion of previous power sources; 3) unreliability of atrial sensing; 4) the high incidence of atrial lead displacement (which has been reported to be as high as 50%) (Furman and Whitman, 1978); and 5) the questionable necessity for long term A-V sequential pacing in the majority

of patients requiring permanent pacemaker implantation.

Despite the fact that A-V synchronous contraction may increase the cardiac output by as much as 30 per cent in an acute setting, evidence suggests that with chronic pacing, patients with normal ventricular function are capable of compensating for the lack of A-V synchrony with virtually identical cardiac outputs using ventricular synchronous pacing alone (Benchimol et al., 1965). The addition of A-V synchrony does have significant physiologic effects in some individuals with left ventricular dysfunction, congestive heart failure, and low output states. It enhances their functional capability and may play a significant role in altering their survival. The advent of newer, longer-lived power sources and of more reliable and more compact pacemaker generators and circuitry has expanded the indications for permanent pacing in patients with left ventricular dysfunction. Important improvements in atrial electrode design will necessitate reevaluation and expansion of the indications and utilization of A-V sequential and synchronous pacing in the future.

Coronary Sinus and Right Atrial Pacing

Coronary sinus and right atrial pacing represent specialized forms of A-V synchronous pacing in which a single electrode system is utilized, the electrode being placed in the coronary sinus or right atrial appendage rather than the right ventricular apex (Fig.

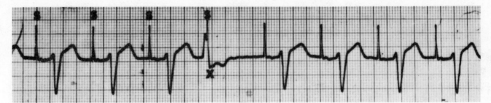

Figure 24-7 Pulse generator with the electrode implanted in the right atrium. Note the pacemaker initiated atrial depolarization (S) at a rate of 72 per minute. Ventricular depolarization occurs as a result of conduction from the atrium through the A-V junction. Note also the PVC (X), which is not sensed by the atrial electrode.

24–7). Less complicated generators can be utilized. Its usefulness in the past has been limited, however, by 1) the relative infrequency of isolated atrial abnormalities with no associated A-V junctional or subjunctional conduction impairment; 2) the questionable necessity for this mode of pacing in most patients; 3) the significant difficulties in sensing that are caused by the relatively small amplitude of atrial electrical depolarization; and 4) the high frequency of electrode displacement (20–30%). The system design difficulties have been partially corrected by the development of newer electrodes, which at least preliminarily have a lesser incidence of displacement, and pulse generators that have a higher sensing capability (Greenberg et al., 1978).

Radio Frequency Triggered Pacemakers

Various specially designed pacemakers have been introduced recently to control recurrent supraventricular and ventricular tachycardias (Peters, 1978). These pacemakers are designed to drive the ventricle at rates 125 per cent faster than the tachyarrhythmias, thus capturing the ventricles. With subsequent discontinuation of the pacing stimulus, there is a recurrence of the patient's normal rhythm. The pacemaker stimulus is initiated by the patient or physician through an external radio frequency transmitter. At the present time, use

of these generators should be considered more investigative than clinically established. Currently under evaluation are more sophisticated types that are capable of sensing the patient's ventricular complexes and firing either individual or paired stimuli at predetermined cycle lengths following the QRS. The clinical efficacy of these generators remains to be determined and, to date, only a small number have been implanted.

Programmable Pacemakers

Recent substantial advances in circuitry design now make it possible to independently and noninvasively reprogram the parameters of pacemaker rate, pulse duration, sensing capability, refractory period, current output, fixed or demand mode, and, in the case of A-V synchronous or A-V sequential pacing, P-R interval. This can be performed subsequent to implantation to meet the specific needs of each individual patient. The flexibility inherent in these pacemakers represents a significant advancement in pacemaker design, and more complex and physiologic programming capabilities may be expected in the future.

Endocardial Pacing

Transvenous endocardial pacing is relatively safe, can be performed under local anesthesia, and does not require a thoracotomy. For these reasons it is the preferred approach.

Electrode catheters are available for atrial, coronary sinus, or ventricular endocardial pacing. The catheters themselves vary in configuration and stiffness, whereas the electrodes employed differ in composition (platinum-iridium or cobalt-nickel alloy), surface area, contour, and unipolar versus bipolar configurations. The smaller-tipped electrodes, with a surface area of 8 to 10 square millimeters, are usually preferred for endocardial ventricular pacing because of their greater efficiency, while larger surface area electrodes are preferred in coronary sinus and atrial pacing because of their better sensing capabilities (Smyth et al., 1976). In the past, endocardial catheters were designed to passively adhere to the right ventricular endocardium; however, because of the problem of electrode displacement (particularly with coronary sinus and atrial pacing), catheters are now available that actively grasp the endocardial surface (Kleinert et al., 1977).

Regardless of the catheter chosen, proper positioning of the electrode at the time of implantation is imperative for adequate long term function. In order to ensure proper positioning, both anatomic location and electrical performance should be measured at the time of implantation. The electrical parameters that should be evaluated include current threshold (ideally less than 0.7 milliamperes; greater than 1.5 amperes is unacceptable), peak threshold (less than 1 volt), lead resistance (300–700 ohms), R wave sensing (greater than 4 millivolts), and generator performance (pulse width, rate, milliampere output and sensing capability). In order to ensure stability, the cephalic vein is the preferred site of entry, although the external or internal jugular vein can be used as alternative routes if necessary.

The complication most frequently seen with endocardial pacing is ventric-ular irritability. This occurs almost invariably at the time of implantation and can be minimized by proper visualization techniques and avoidance of undue catheter pressure on the endocardial wall. Occasionally, following implantation, ventricular irritability persists for 1 to 2 days and requires short term antiarrhythmic medication. However, long term antiarrhythmic therapy is not required in the vast majority of cases. When ventricular arrhythmias persist after several days, consideration must be given to repositioning of the electrode.

At present, the major drawback to endocardial pacing is the relatively high incidence of electrode displacement. This usually occurs during the first few days following implantation, before the electrical tip becomes firmly attached to the endocardial surface. Infection is also an important potential complication, reportedly occurring in 1 to 3 per cent of cases. When wound infection does occur, both systemic and topical antibiotics are usually ineffective and the pacing system has to be removed.

Other less common problems include venous thrombosis, pulmonary embolism, damage to the tricuspid valve, endocarditis, and air embolism.

Transthoracic Epicardial Pacing

Epicardial pacing has fallen into general disuse except under specialized circumstances because in the past it has required a thoracotomy with all its attending complications. More recently, however, sutureless electrodes have become commercially available which do not require a full thoracotomy. The leads can be implanted in the myocardium under local anesthesia if necessary, although general anesthesia is still preferred by most surgeons when using these electrodes, which have the disadvantage of requiring implantation into the left ventricle. In addition, epicardial atrial and A-V sequential pacing still necessitates a full thoracotomy. Standard sutureless electrodes are 6 millimeters in length and therefore inappropriate for right ventricular pacing. However, 4 millimeter electrodes are now available and have been used successfully on the right ventricle (although left ventricular implantation is still preferred).

Lead breakage does occasionally occur, but it is a less significant problem with epicardial electrodes than is displacement with endocardial leads.

STIMULATION THRESHOLD

Artificial pacing is dependent upon the ability of an electrical pacemaker to depolarize an area around its electrode tip that is sufficient to initiate a cardiac depolarization. The minimum stimulus required for this purpose is defined as the stimulation threshold and is characterized in terms of voltage, current, or energy. Threshold is an active rather than a static phenomenon, depending on numerous factors (Furman, 1977). These are enumerated below.

1. **Pulse Width.** Progressively shorter pulse widths require higher current amplitudes to achieve threshold. However, pulse durations of less than 0.2 to 0.4 milliseconds will not achieve threshold regardless of current strength. Conversely, there is a finite current level below which excitation will not occur regardless of pulse duration. The greatest variations in threshold occur at pulse durations between 0.5 and 2 milliseconds, and all pacemakers currently in clinical use produce pulses of 0.6 to 2.7 milliseconds duration.

2. **Electrode Surface Area and Configuration.** Electrodes with small surface area have lower current and charge thresholds than do larger electrodes. In addition, spherical electrodes have the highest chronic threshold factors and cylindrical electrodes have the smallest.

3. **Electrode to Myocardial Contact.** The initial position of the electrode in relation to excitable myocardium is critical, since thresholds increase rapidly as a function of distance between the electrode tip and excitable tissue. Several processes act to effectively increase this separation: Inflammatory processes that occur at the time of implantation produce elevations in the stimulation threshold to as much as 10 times the implantation threshold, reaching a maximum 5 to 10 days after implantation. This initial elevation is followed by a gradual diminution, with final stabilization occurring 3 to 4 weeks after implantation at two to five times the original threshold level. This level usually remains relatively stable subsequently. However, the increase in chronic threshold is larger relative to the acute threshold when electrodes of small surface area are used. Similarly, longer pulse durations also decrease the ratio between chronic and acute thresholds, although short pulse durations are more effective in terms of energy utilization.

4. **Unipolar versus Bipolar Pacing.** Although several reports have claimed that the threshold characteristics of bipolar electrodes are superior to those of unipolar electrodes (displaying more rapid stabilization and lower chronic pacing thresholds), the consensus of opinion at present is that there is probably no significant difference in the values achieved between the two.

5. **Cathodal versus Anodal Stimulation.** Cathodal stimulation is now used routinely, since as much as 16 times more energy is required to initiate ventricular contraction with an anodal pulse. In addition, pacemaker induced ventricular fibrillation has been observed in all cases but one with bipolar stimulation. This appears to be related to the anode of the bipolar electrode.

6. **Monophasic versus Biphasic Stimulating Pulses.** Monophasic pulses tend to produce marked tissue damage resulting in significant amounts of fibrosis, which is not seen in the presence

of biphasic pulses. All generators that are currently produced use biphasic stimulating pulses.

7. Physiologic Variables. Sleep may increase the stimulation threshold by as much as 30 to 40 per cent. Physical activity may decrease threshold by as much as 10 to 25 per cent from resting levels. Meals may increase thresholds by as much as 30 per cent. Acidosis and alkalosis both result in marked elevations of threshold. Hypoxia and hypercarbia have also been shown to increase stimulatory threshold.

8. Electrolyte Abnormalities. Both hyper- and hypokalemia have been reported to result in transient pacemaker malfunction. The absolute level of serum potassium is not as critical as the intracellular to extracellular ratio. On occasion a transient lowering of threshold can be produced with a slow continuous infusion of potassium even in the absence of hypokalemia. Rapid elevations in extracellular sodium concentrations can result in an increase in threshold; however, calcium has not been shown to have any significant effect on stimulation threshold.

9. Drug Effects. The sympathomimetic agents increase myocardial excitability and reduce the stimulation threshold (with the exception of isoproterenol, which at times may produce a paradoxical increase). Glucocorticoids lower threshold whereas mineralocorticoids raise it. Antiarrhythmic agents such as quinidine, procainamide, dysopyramide, propranolol, and verapamil in therapeutic doses increase stimulatory threshold by approximately 10 to 15 per cent. At toxic levels, this effect may be enhanced. Conversely, lidocaine and diphenylhydantoin have relatively little effect.

THE POWER SOURCES

Several power sources are now commercially available. These include zinc-mercury cells, rechargeable nickel-cadmium batteries, lithium (currently the most widely used power source), and radioisotopic cells.

Zinc-Mercury Cells

The early permanent implantable pacemakers were powered by zinc-mercury cells and the major experience in pacemaker longevity is derived from generators using this power source. The original zinc-mercury cells had an average longevity of approximately 18 to 22 months, with later improved versions showing mean survivals of 3 years (Furman, 1978).

Nickel-Cadmium Rechargeable Cells

Primarily because of the short survival time of pacemakers powered by zinc-mercury cells, a rechargeable cell powered by nickel-cadmium with an external recharger has been clinically available for several years. This power source has held up relatively well with more than 90 per cent survival 5 years after implantation. However, although available for a long period of time, it has not been popular, possibly because it requires frequent recharging. Recharging for 1 hour every 1 to 2 weeks is recommended, although 6 to 8 week lapses can occur before power drainage becomes excessive. Although a modified zinc-mercury cell that requires recharging at less frequent intervals has been tested in vivo and in vitro (Tyers et al., 1967), this has also been held in abeyance because of the availability of the newer lithium power sources.

Lithium Cells

Lithium power sources have virtually replaced the zinc-mercury batteries in permanently implanted pacing generators. The lithium power source has a higher energy density, forms a strongly reactive cation, which yields high cell voltages, has a variety of readily available cathodal materials, and is easily worked into a variety of shapes in its metallic state. At present, there are several lithium systems available, each having slight differences in function. Some are liquid and some are used in solid electrolyte systems. They all display a significant improvement in longevity over the zinc-mercury cells. Clinical experience to date has indicated more than a 90 per cent survival at 5 years after implantation (Parsonnet, 1977).

Nuclear Pacemakers

Radioisotopic power sources have been available for several years. They are designed to last from 10 to 70 years. Ten year survivals are expected to exceed 95 per cent confidence limits (Parsonnet, 1975). Although nuclear power sources appear to be reliable, they have not been popular because of difficulty with licensure in the United States and high cost. Furthermore, the fact that most pacemaker patients are 65 years of age or more makes the implantation of an extremely long-lived power source seem excessive. Although the availability of lithium generators with reliable 5 to 10 year life expectancies has further diminished the need for radioisotopic power generators in most patients, a selected group of relatively young, otherwise healthy patients may benefit from the longer life expectancy of the radioisotopic cells.

Generator Design

The improved performance of the newer model pacemakers is due not only to an improved power source but also to associated advances in circuitry design and the hermetic sealing of the electronic components within the generator.

The majority of pacemakers produced today have multicell batteries that may be interconnected in series, in parallel, or even in combination configurations to provide a backup power system should one of the cells fail. The lithium sources are generally two celled and are often designed to operate one cell at a time (a shift to the second cell is reflected by a change in pacemaker rate).

ABNORMALITIES IN PACEMAKER FUNCTION

Abnormalities in pacemaker function manifest themselves as alterations in 1) the pacing rate (acceleration, deceleration, or intermittent abrupt changes); 2) inappropriate sensing or failure to sense (intermittent or total); 3) failure to capture (intermittent or total); or 4) inappropriate pacing of the diaphragm, pectoral, or intercostal muscles.

Alterations in Pacemaker Rate

Decreases in Rate. Diminution in pacing rate due to depletion of the power source is the most common cause of generator replacement. At the present time, virtually all pacemakers are designed to display a decrease in rate as the end of generator life approaches and the power source energy supply diminishes. Occasionally, however, the pacemaker may show a decline prior to power source depletion. The most common non-power source rate decline is rate drift, a progressive constant rate decline that occurs over a period of time. The majority of pacemakers showing drift will restabilize at a slightly slower rate (within two to three beats of the original baseline). On occasion, however, the rate will continue to decline or function will abruptly cease, necessitating pacemaker replacement.

Changes in Rate. During the first several months following implantation, all pacemakers may develop minor accelerations or decelerations, which, however, rarely exceed one to two beats per minute, and the vast majority of pacemakers will then stabilize until the end of the generator's life. On rare occasions, however, a pacemaker may display significant further increases in rate (Lee, 1979) (Fig. 24–8). Although uncontrolled rate acceleration is still observed on rare occasions, it was much more frequent with the older models. This phenomenon is a true medical emergency, since ventricular tachycardia, fibrillation, and sudden death can occur. When early signs of pacemaker acceleration are seen, the pacemaker should be replaced with a new pulse generator.

The newer programmable pacemakers occasionally display abrupt changes in rate due to inadvertent reprogramming. The possibility of a "runaway" pacemaker has to be taken into consideration with these models. If inadvertent reprogramming has occurred, the pacemaker may be reset to a more appropriate stimulus interval by means of an external programmer.

Erratic Rates. Sudden fluctuations (acceleration and deceleration) with variations in rate of two to eight beats per minute have been reported in the generators of several manufacturers. Erratic rate changes, particularly those in which wide fluctuations are seen, may be a prodrome of more severe malfunction. Occasionally pacemakers displaying these phenomena will restabilize, but most of them require replacement.

Temperature Related Variations in Rate. Currently, several lithium power sources are available, some of which display temperature sensitive variations in rate. In these generators, small fluctuations may be part of the design. The changes in rate, however, rarely exceed one to two beats per minute. Wider variations should be observed closely, as more significant circuitry malfunction may be present.

Inappropriate Sensing

Inappropriate inhibition of demand pacemakers when there is no obvious ventricular depolarization has been reported due to inappropriate P or T wave sensing, intermittent separation of fractured epicardial leads, electromagnetic

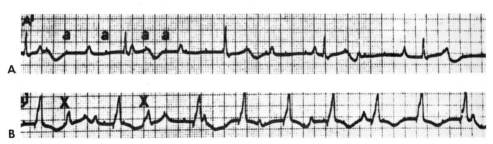

Figure 24–8 Runaway pacemaker in a 75 year old male patient with complete A-V heart block and arteriosclerotic heart disease. A permanent demand pacemaker was implanted 4 years earlier and the pacing rate set at 72 per minute. Owing to exhaustion of the battery, the pacemaker did not deliver adequate energy to stimulate the ventricle. In addition, the rate of the pacemaker was increased to 160 beats per minute (runaway pacemaker) and the demand system was not functioning. In (A), note pacemaker artifacts (a) (rate 160/min, which fails to activate the ventricle).

(B) A transvenous demand pacemaker was inserted in the same patient. It paced at the rate of 75 beats per minute. Note the difference in the ventricular complexes delivered by the new pacemaker, which captures the ventricles at 75 per minute. Note also that in this tracing, stimuli delivered by the old implanted pacemaker at X now produce ventricular complexes when they occur 500 to 580 msec after the stimulus of the newly inserted transvenous pacemaker. This may be due to supernormality resulting from the Wedensky effect.

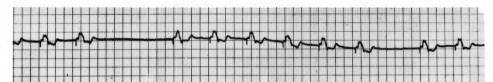

Figure 24–9 Inappropriate suppression of a ventricular synchronous R inhibited pacemaker. Note the normal pacing interval (70/min), which is interrupted by a long pause during which no atrial or ventricular activity is seen. The pause is too long to be accounted for by myopotential interference and represents an abnormality in the generator circuitry.

interference, or inhibition by non-cardiac muscle potentials. Inappropriate P wave sensing has been associated with lead displacement. Electromagnetic interference has become a much less significant problem with newer, better shielded pacemakers. At present, the most common sources of interference are microwave ovens, diathermy or, on occasion, radio or television transmitter antennas or commercial radar. Inhibition by non-cardiac muscle potentials is a frequent occurrence with unipolar pacemakers, the incidence being reported to be as high as 65 per cent (Ohm et al., 1974). This is rarely of clinical significance, however, and can be avoided by more frequent use of bipolar pacing. A less frequent, albeit more significant, problem is inhibition of demand pacemakers resulting in a prolonged stimulus interval that is not due to any of the above situations (Fig. 24–9). This strongly suggests malfunction in the sensing circuitry. Because patients who are paced frequently manifest suppression of their escape intrinsic foci, this can be a serious problem. Syncopal symptoms can recur in pacemaker dependent patients. When this occurs, replacement of the generator is required. Emergency therapy consists of induced fixed rate pacing by means of a magnetic reed switch.

Failure to Sense and Capture

Combined failure to sense and capture is almost invariably caused by displacement of the endocardial pacing electrode, lead fracture, improper contact between generator and lead, or, on occasion, marked fibrosis around the area of the electrode tip. Immediately after implantation, inflammatory responses may cause transient difficulties. Catheter displacement may be observed at any time; however, it is most commonly seen during the first several days to 1 month following implantation. Lead fracture and fibrosis are late phenomena. With the newer leads, fracture is relatively uncommon. Although sensing and capture abnormalities are occasionally complete (Fig. 24–10), more commonly they are intermittent.

When failure to sense occurs as an isolated event, it is usually intermittent as well and related to a poor electrical signal being delivered to the generator.

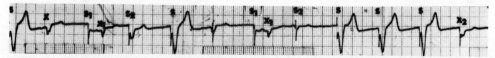

Figure 24–10 Intermittent lack of sensing and capture in an R wave inhibited ventricular synchronous pacemaker. Note the beats marked S, representing pacemaker discharge and ventricular depolarization. The beat marked X is sensed and results in a resetting of the pacemaker. The spikes marked S_1 are not followed by a ventricular response. Note also that the subsequent pacemaker spike (S_2) occurs early after an interposed QRS representing intermittent lack of sensing. The beat marked X_2 is a fusion beat.

Sensing abnormalities occur most frequently with the new, smaller tipped electrodes and in patients with myocardial fibrosis (Hughes et al., 1976). Sensing abnormalities are more common with bipolar systems, since generally the unipolar systems deliver a larger signal to the generator (DeCaprio et al., 1977).

Failure to sense is frequently associated with premature ventricular beats with shorter coupling intervals (Fig. 24–11). The abnormal wave of depolarization and the low frequency content associated with these beats occasionally result in an inability of the generator to sense the complex. When this occurs, competition may occur.

Failure to capture is also usually intermittent and associated with cathode displacement or fracture. However, isolated failure to capture has been reported with perforation of the endocardial electrode, fibrosis around the electrode tip (with elevations in threshold), fibrosis, hyperkalemia or hypokalemia, drug toxicity, and exit block from the ventricular site of electrode placement. Recurrence of the patient's original symptomatology frequently occurs, especially if the patient's intrinsic escape mechanism has been suppressed.

Other Problems

Pacing of the Intercostal, Diaphragmatic or Pectoralis Muscles. Pectoral muscle pacing is generally due to leakage at the generator-lead interface or turning over of unipolar generators so that they stimulate the muscle. Diaphragmatic and/or intercostal pacing may be due to perforation of the endocardial electrode through the right ventricular wall (although it has been reported without perforation). When perforation is present, the muscular pacing is often associated with failure to capture or an associated right bundle branch pattern. The sensing function of the pacemaker is frequently preserved. As an isolated finding, a right bundle branch block pattern associated with endocardial pacing is not necessarily an indication of perforation. Other findings that are associated with perforation include friction rub and, although uncommon, associated tamponade or pericardial effusion. However, friction rubs have occasionally been observed in patients without perforations (Glassman et al., 1977).

Displacement of the Pulse Generator. Migration of the artificial generator occasionally occurs, particularly in elderly individuals with inelastic skin. Endocardial electrode displacement or fracture may occur with a downward migration of the generator. On occasion the generator may rotate, resulting in current leakage at the interface between the generator and the electrode.

Pacemaker Related Cardiac Sounds. Pacemaker related cardiac murmurs are most commonly caused by a rupture of the ventricular septum or damage of the tricuspid valve due to laceration by the electrode. The most frequent auscultatory finding associated with permanent

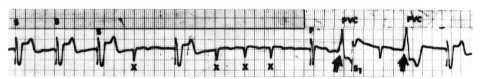

Figure 24–11 Intermittent lack of sensing in an R wave inhibited ventricular synchronous pulse generator. The beats marked S represent paced beats. The beats marked X are sensed appropriately in that the pacemaker is reset and does not discharge. However, the pacemaker fails to sense a premature beat (PVC) and the subsequent pacemaker spike (S₁) occurs while the ventricle is refractory. The second PVC is sensed by the pacemaker. Note also the fusion beat (F).

pacing is a high frequency presystolic click, which is currently thought to be produced by intercostal and diaphragmatic stimulation.

PACEMAKER FOLLOW-UP

The concept of pacemaker follow-up has evolved in an attempt to predict pacemaker failure, prolong the longevity of the generators by avoiding arbitrary replacement at preset intervals, and conversely prevent unpredicted emergency generator malfunctions. Proper care begins at the time of the implantation with the recording of essential data, such as the patient's name, manufacturer, model and serial number, electrode type, and electrical parameters and settings. However, the most significant advances have been in the area of long-term outpatient follow-up. Surveillance techniques vary from intermittent random electrocardiograms during routine office visits to sophisticated, computerized pacemaker clinics. To be considered adequate, any system must be capable of determining the pacemaker rate, cardiac response to the pacemaker impulse, and integrity of the sensing circuitry. At times it is beneficial to additionally evaluate the amplitude of the pacemaker artifact and the generator pulse duration. Proper evaluation of the data is imperative and can only be performed if a thorough knowledge of the mode of power source depletion and circuit design of each model being followed is understood, since design specifications vary from manufacturer to manufacturer and from model to model. Inadequate knowledge can result in failure to identify an improperly functioning unit or in false identification of malfunction.

Arbitrary replacement of the pacemaker at a preselected date is inappropriate because battery depletion is scattered over time. In addition, only about half of generator replacements are related to power source depletion and the remaining causes for removal are not taken into consideration. The more acceptable modes of long-term care include 1) evaluation of the pacemaker by electrocardiogram during a routine office examination; 2) evaluation of pacemaker function in a specialized pacemaker clinic; and 3) transtelephonic monitoring of pacemaker function.

Office Examination

Office evaluation alone is suboptimal. Electrocardiographic analysis of pacemaker function allows for the evaluation of sensing and capture; however, it is an inadequate means for determining early changes in rate which signify impending power source depletion. In addition, most physician's offices are not set up for a more detailed analysis of pacemaker problems. A further difficulty in office follow-up is the relative infrequency of examination and its inability to adequately monitor the pacing system at the time of incipient battery depletion when an accurate assessment of function is critical.

Pacemaker Clinics

Pacemaker clinics offer several advantages over the routine office examination while continuing to allow for the maintenance of adequate physician-patient relationship and direct patient observation. The electronic monitoring performed provides accurate and reliable information as to pacemaker function and includes determination of rate, wave form, refractory period, and the sensing and capture functions of the pacemaker. In addition, it provides a training ground for better patient understanding of pacemaker function. The disadvantages are that the patient is required to travel to the site of the clinic; data cannot be readily obtained at a time when the patient feels that there is a transient abnormality in pacemaker function; and there is a limitation in the number of follow-up visits that can be performed toward the end of the life of the generator. The clinic approach is also relatively expensive when compared with other follow-up systems.

Transtelephonic Monitoring

Telephone techniques can monitor rate accurately and identify capture and sensing function by both plethysmographic and electrographic techniques. The plethysmographic technique is adequate for many patients with ventricular synchronous pacing systems who do not have significant ventricular or supraventricular arrhythmias (Fig. 24–12). However, it has several shortcomings which do not allow for accurate interpretation of coronary sinus, atrial, or A-V sequential pacing systems. In addition, patients who have irregular rhythms, such as atrial fibrillation, flutter with varying block, and frequent premature atrial and ventricular contractions, require electrocardiographic analysis. Since all patient generators have magnetic reed switches that can be used to temporarily convert to fixed rate pacing, both demand and fixed rate pacing functions can be identified and interpreted by transtelephonic techniques.

Transtelephonic monitoring provides the advantage of allowing the patient to call into a central source if he suspects pacemaker malfunction regardless of when it occurs. In addition, it is convenient to patients, since it eliminates unnecessary travel time to and from the physician's office or clinic and allows more frequent re-examinations as the end of the pacemaker life approaches. The calling schedules vary in frequency, depending on the time lapse since implantation, suspected abnormalities in pacemaker function, the power source being utilized, and the pacemaker type.

REFERENCES

Altschuler, H., Fisher, J. D., and Furman, S.: Significance of isolated H-V interval prolongation in symptomatic patients without documented heart block. Am. Heart J. 97(1):19–26, 1979.

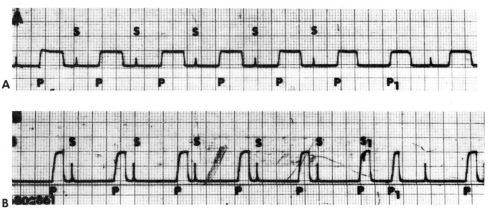

Figure 24–12 Plethysmographic recordings of normally functioning R wave inhibit and R triggered ventricular synchronous pacemakers. (A) Note the pacemaker spike (S) followed after a pause by a peripheral pulse (P). The relationship between the spike and pulse are evidence for capture of the ventricle by the pacemaker. The delay is caused by the transmission of the pulse to the periphery following ventricular depolarization. Note also the pulse marked P_1, which is not preceded by a pacemaker spike. The inhibition of the pacemaker is evidence for sensing.

(B) An R triggered ventricular pacemaker sensing and capturing appropriately. Note the relationship between the pacemaker spike (S) and peripheral pulse (P). Note also the early discharge (S_1) followed by the premature pulse (P_1), representing a sensed premature complex.

Benchimol, A., Ellis, J. G., and Dimond, E. G.: Hemodynamic consequences of atrial and ventricular pacing in patients with normal and abnormal hearts. Am. J. Med. 39:911–922, 1965.

Blaser, R., and Schaldach, M.: Susceptibility to interference of implantable cardiac pacemakers. In Thalen, H. J. (Ed.): Cardiac Pacing. Assen, The Netherlands, Van Gorcum, Publisher, 1973.

Chardock, W. M., Ishikowa, H., Fochler, F. J., Souther, S., and Gage, A. A.: Pacing and ventricular fibrillation. Ann. N.Y. Acad. Sci. 167:919, 1969.

DePasquale, N. P., and Bruno, M. S.: Incidence and implications of abnormal intraventricular conduction in the coronary care unit. Cardiology 61:215, 1976.

DeCaprio, V., Hurzeler, P., and Furman, S.: A comparison of unipolar and bipolar electrograms for cardiac pacemaker and sensing. Circulation 56(5):750, 1977.

Fisher, J. D., Mehra, R., and Furman, S.: Termination of ventricular tachycardia with bursts of rapid ventricular pacing. Am. J. Cardiol. 41:94–102, 1978.

Fontaine, G., Kevorkain, M., Welti, J. J., Ribot, A., and Petitot, J. C.: Comparison between endocardial versus myocardial and unipolar versus bipolar thresholds after long term pacing. In Thalen, H. J. (Ed.): Cardiac Pacing. Assen, The Netherlands, Van Gorcum, Publisher, 1973.

Furman, S., Garvey, J., and Hurzeler, P.: Pulse duration variation and electrode size as factors in pacemaker longevity. J. Thorac. Cardiovasc. Surg. 69:382, 1975.

Furman, S.: Cardiac pacing and pacemakers. I. Indications for pacing bradyarrhythmias. Am. Heart J. 93(4):523–530, 1977.

Furman, S., and Fisher, J. D.: Cardiac pacing and pacemakers. V. Technical aspects of implantation and equipment. Am. Heart J. 94(2):250–259, 1977.

Furman, S., Hurzeler, P., and Mehra, R.: Cardiac pacing and pacemakers. IV. Threshold of cardiac stimulation. Am. Heart J. 94(1):115–124, 1977.

Furman, S.: Cardiac pacing and pacemakers. VI. Analysis of pacemaker malfunction. Am. Heart J. 94(3):379, 1977.

Furman, S.: Cardiac pacing and pacemakers. VIII. The pacemaker follow-up clinic. Am. Heart J. 94(6):795–804, 1977.

Furman, S., and Whitman, R.: Cardiac pacing and pacemakers. IX. Statistical analysis of pacemaker data. Am. Heart J. 95(1):115–125, 1978.

Glassman, R. D., Noble, R. J., Tavel, M. E., Storer, W. R., and Schmidt, P. E.: Pacemaker induced endocardial friction rub. Am. J. Cardiol. 40:811, 1977.

Gould, L., Reddy, C. V., and Becker, W. H.: The sick sinus syndrome. A study of 50 cases. J. Electrocardiol. 11(1):11–14, 1978.

Greatbatch, W., Piersma, B., Shannon, F. D., and Calhoon, S. W., Jr.: Polarization phenomena relating to physiological electrodes. Ann. N.Y. Acad. Sci. 167:722, 1969.

Greenberg, P., Castellanet, M., Messenger, J., and Ellestad, M. H.: Coronary sinus pacing. Clinical follow-up. Circulation 57(1):98, 1978.

Haft, J. I.: Treatment of arrhythmias by intracardiac electrical stimulation. Prog. Cardiovasc. Dis. 16(6):539–568, 1974.

Hindman, M. C., Wagner, G. S., JaRo, M., et al.: The clinical significance of bundle branch block complicating acute myocardial infarction. Circulation 58:689, 1978.

Hughes, H. C., Brownlee, R. R., and Tyers, F. O.: Failure of demand pacing with small surface area electrodes. Circulation 54(1):128, 1976.

Hunter, S. W., Boldue, L., Long, V., et al.: A new myocardial pacemaker lead (sutureless). Chest 63:430, 1973.

Hurzeler, P., Furman, S., and Escher, D. J. W.: Cardiac pacemaker current thresholds versus pulse duration. In Silverman, H. T., Miller, I. F., and Salkind, A. J. (Eds.): Electrochemical Bioscience and Bioengineering. New Jersey, The Electrochemical Society, 1973.

Kahn, A., Morris, J. J., and Citron, P.: Patient initiated rapid atrial pacing to manage supraventricular tachycardia. Am. J. Cardiol. 38:200–204, 1976.

Kleinert, M., Bock, M., and Wilhemi, F.: Clinical use of new transvenous atrial lead. Am. J. Cardiol. 40:237, 1977.

Kosowsky, B. D., Scherlag, B. J., and Damato, A. N.: Re-evaluation of the atrial contribution to ventricular function. Am. J. Cardiol. 21:518–524, 1968.

Lee, H. J., Berman, G. M., and Ozolins, A. E.: Runaway demand pacemakers in two asymptomatic patients. Cardiovasc. Med. January 85–86, 1979.

Leinbach, R. C., Chamberlain, D. A., Kastor, J. A., and Hawthorne, W. J.: A comparison of the hemodynamic effects of ventricular and sequential A-V pacing in patients with heart block. Am. Heart J. 78(4):502, 1969.

Lichstein, E., Ribas-Menecker, C., Naik, D., Chadda, K. D., Gupta, P. K., and Smith, H., Jr.: The natural history of trifascicular disease following permanent pacemaker implantation. Significance of continuing changes in atrioventricular conduction. Circulation 54(5):780, 1976.

Lucieri, R. M., Furman, S., Hurzeler, P., and Escher, D. J. W.: Threshold behavior of electrodes in long-term ventricular pacing. Am. J. Cardiol. 40:184, 1977.

Merx, W., Han, J., and Yoon, M. S.: Effects of unipolar cathodal and bipolar stimulation on vulnerability of ischemic ventricles to fibrillation. Am. J. Cardiol. 35:37–42, 1975.

Moss, A. J.: Therapeutic uses of permanent pervenous atrial pacemakers: A review. J. Electrocardiol. 8(4):373, 1975.

McAnulty, J. H., Rahimtoola, M. B., Murphy, E. S., Kauffman, S., Ritzmann, L. W., Kanarek, P., and DeMots, H.: A prospective study of sudden death in "high risk" bundle branch block. N. Engl. J. Med. *299*(5):209, 1978.

Ohm, O. J., Bruland, H., Pedersen, O. M., and Waerness, E.: Interference effect of myopotentials on function of unipolar demand pacemakers. Br. Heart J. *36*:77, 1974.

Ohm, O. J., and Breivik, K.: Patients with high grade atrioventricular block treated and not treated with a pacemaker. Acta Med. Scand. *203*:521, 1978.

Parsonnet, V., Myers, G. H., Gilbert, L., Zucker, I. R., and Shilling, E.: Follow-up of implanted pacemakers. Am. Heart J. *87*(5):642, 1974.

Parsonnet, V., Myers, G. H., Gilbert, L., and Zucker, I. R.: Clinical experience with nuclear pacemakers. Surgery *78*:776, 1975.

Parsonnet, V.: Follow up of implanted pacemakers: an evaluation of methods. Cardiol. Dig. July 18–26, 1976.

Parsonnet, V.: Permanent pacing of the heart: 1952–1976. Am. J. Cardiol. *39*:250, 1977.

Parsonnet, V., Parsonnet, M., and Manhardt, M.: Cardiac pacing and pacemakers. VII. Power sources for implantable pacemakers. Part 1. Am. Heart J. *94*(4):517, 1977.

Pastose, J. O., Yurchak, P. M., Janis, K. M., Murphy, J. D., and Zir, L. M.: The risk of advanced heart block in surgical patients with right bundle branch block and left axis deviation. Circulation *57*(4):677, 1978.

Peleska, B., Vrana, M., and Netusil, M.: Optimal parameters for design of endocardial electrode. Proc. 8th Inter. Conf. Med. Biol. Eng. *29*:7, 1969.

Peters, R. W., Shafton, E., Frank, S., Thomas, A. N., and Scheinman, M. M.: Radiofrequency triggered pacemakers: Uses and limitations. A long term study. Ann. Int. Med. *88*:17, 1978.

Preston, T. A., Fletcher, R. D., Lucchesi, B. R., and Judge, R. D.: Changes in myocardial threshold: Physiologic and pharmacologic factors in patients with implanted pacemakers. Am. Heart J. *74*:235, 1967.

Preston, T. A.: Anodal stimulation as a cause of pacemaker induced ventricular fibrillation. Am. Heart J. *36*:366, 1973.

Ritter, W. S., Atkins, J. M., Blomqvist, C. G., and Mullins, C. B.: Permanent pacing in patients with transient trifascicular block during acute myocardial infarction. Am. J. Cardiol. *38*:205, 1976.

Roy, O. Z.: The current status of cardiac pacing. CRC Critical Reviews in Bioengineering *2*(3):259, 1975.

Rytand, D. A., Stinson, E., Kelly, J. J., Jr.: Remission and recovery from chronic established complete heart block. Am. Heart J. *91*(5):645, 1976.

Scarpa, W. J.: The sick sinus syndrome. Am. Heart J. *92*:648, 1976.

Siddons, H., and Sowton, E.: *In* Kugelman, I. N. (Ed.): Cardiac Pacemakers. Springfield, Ill., Charles C Thomas, 1967.

Smyth, N. P. D., Taryan, P. P., Chernoff, E., and Baker, N.: The significance of electrode surface area and stimulating thresholds in permanent cardiac pacing. J. Thorac. Cardiovasc. Surg. *71*(4):559, 1976.

Somerndike, J. M., and Ostermiller, W. E.: Sleeping threshold change causing failure of artificial cardiac pacing. J.A.M.A. *217*(6):980, 1971.

Spurrell, R. A. J., and Sowton, E.: Pacing techniques in the management of arrhythmias with emphasis on the tachycardias. J. Electrocardiol. *9*(1):89, 1976.

Stertzer, S. H., DePasquale, N. P., Bruno, M. S., and Cohn, L. J.: Early evaluation of a rechargeable pacemaker system. J. Electrocardiol. *9*(4):391, 1976.

Tyers, G. F. O., Hughes, H. C., Jr., Brownlee, R. R., Manley, N. F., and Gorman, I. N.: Rechargeable silver modified mercuric oxide zinc cell for cardiac pacemakers. Am. J. Cardiol. *38*:607, 1976.

Vera, Z., Mason, D. T., Awan, N. A., Hilliard, G., and Massumi, R. A.: Lack of sensing by demand pacemakers due to intraventricular conduction defects. Circulation *51*:815, 1975.

Vera, Z., Klein, R. C., and Mason, D. T.: Recent advantages in programmable pacemakers. Consideration of advantages, longevity and future expectations. Am. J. Med. *66*:473, 1979.

Wellens, H. J. J., Bar, F. W., Gorgel, A. P., and Muncharaz, J. F.: Electrical management of arrhythmias with emphasis on the tachycardias. Am. J. Cardiol. *41*:1025, 1978.

Wiggers, C. J., Wagria, R., and Pinero, B.: The effects of myocardial ischemia on the fibrillation threshold: the mechanism of spontaneous ventricular fibrillation following coronary occlusion. Am. J. Physiol. *131*:309, 1940.

Wohl, A. J., Laborde, J., Atkins, J. M., Blomqvist, C. G., and Mullins, C. B.: Prognosis of patients permanently paced for sick sinus syndrome. Arch. Int. Med. *136*:406, 1976.

Wyndham, C. R., Wu, D., Denes, P., Sugarman, D., Levitsky, S., and Rosen, K. M.: Self initiated conversion of paroxysmal atrial flutter utilizing a radiofrequency pacemaker. Am. J. Cardiol. *41*:1119, 1978.

Young, M. W., Meia, H., Furman, S., et al.: Effects of lidocaine and ouabain on myocardial threshold to pacer stimuli. Circulation *43*(Suppl. III):209, 1970.

25

DEFIBRILLATION AND ELECTRIC COUNTERSHOCK

VIDYA S. BANKA, M.D.

A defibrillator is an instrument that delivers an electric shock to the heart for the purpose of converting ventricular fibrillation to normal sinus rhythm. The current, which is applied directly to the heart or through the intact chest wall, may be AC or DC and may have a variety of wave forms. Countershock or cardioversion devices generally employ direct current, usually applied to the heart through the closed chest to convert various tachyarrhythmias to normal sinus rhythm. Although electrical cardioversion has been used most frequently to convert atrial fibrillation, the disappointingly low percentage of patients remaining in sinus rhythm has drastically reduced its application for this arrhythmia.

Reports to the medical society of Copenhagen suggest that precordial countershock was discovered as early as 1775 by Abildgaard, an astute veterinarian. He was successful in reviving hens that had been rendered lifeless by a shock to the head followed by shock to the chest from electrostatic glass jars (Driscol et al., 1975). Although Prevost and Batelli described the defibrillating effects of weak and strong currents on the heart in 1899, the first clinical application of defibrillation was provided by Zoll in 1956, who terminated ventricular fibrillation in man by externally applied countershock. Subsequent publications by Zoll and Linenthal and by Lown and co-workers in the early 1960's led to the widespread use of precordial shock not only for defibrillation but also for the conversion of supraventricular and ventricular arrhythmias to sinus rhythm (Zoll and Linenthal, 1962; Lown et al., 1962).

Defibrillation has assumed increasing importance in recent years because of the following: 1) recognition of the many factors that induce ventricular fibrillation; 2) the frequent onset of ventricular fibrillation in settings where immediate recognition and treatment are possible; 3) the use of defibrillators in many areas of the hospital and especially in coronary care facilities, where medical and nursing personnel are thoroughly trained in their use; 4) the advent of the mobile coronary care unit, which brings the defibrillator to the patient's home for use in emergency resuscitation; and 5) increasing experience which has shown that in many instances ventricular fibrillation is completely reversible.

SHOCKS INITIATING VENTRICULAR FIBRILLATION

Many investigators have shown that if stimuli exceeding a threshold value are delivered during the ventricular vulnerable period, which is present late in the relative refractory period of the cardiac cycle (Fig. 25–1), multiple extrasystoles or ventricular fibrillation results (Ferris et al., 1936; Lown et al., 1963). Although the exact mechanism of this phenomenon is not known, it is generally accepted that stimuli delivered during the vulnerable period encounter persisting areas of refractory myocardium and wander slowly through the tissue around these areas, forming multiple re-entrant paths, which result in self-perpetuating fibrillation.

SHOCKS TERMINATING VENTRICULAR FIBRILLATION

The immediate recognition of ventricular fibrillation and application of a defibrillating countershock can be lifesaving. Monitoring equipment for the recognition of this arrhythmia and vari-ous types of defibrillators are usually available in the hospital, especially in the coronary care facility, and often can be brought to the patient's home by a mobile coronary care unit or specially equipped ambulance. Even though closed-chest compression can circulate sufficient blood to sustain the brain and heart, the quicker the heart is defibrillated, the better is the chance for successful resuscitation.

OPTIMAL CONDITIONS FOR CLOSED CHEST DEFIBRILLATION

It is of utmost importance that all possible cardiopulmonary resuscitative measures (e.g., artificial respiration, closed chest cardiac compression) be instituted as quickly as possible, both before and during defibrillation. While both AC and DC countershocks of sufficient strength can effectively defibrillate most hearts, DC defibrillations are generally currently used (Fig. 25–2). Since fibrillating hearts in poor condition respond better to higher energy levels and since small currents are usually ineffective, discharges of 400

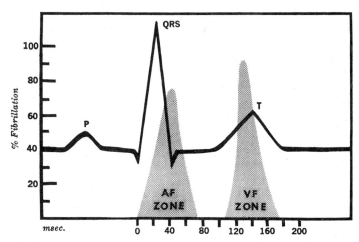

Figure 25–1 Fibrillation danger zones charted on the electrocardiogram. Shaded triangles represent zones where electroshock is most likely to produce atrial fibrillation (AF) or ventricular fibrillation (VF). (From Lown, B., Amarasingham, B., Neuman, J., and Berkovits, B. V.: J. Clin. Invest., 41:1381, 1962; courtesy of American Optical Corp.)

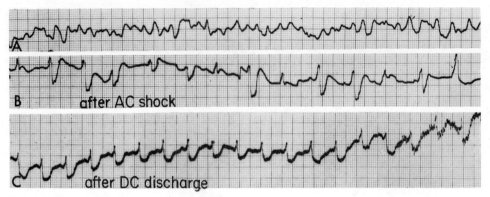

Figure 25–2 (*A*) Ventricular fibrillation.

(*B*) After AC shock, note the occurrence of occasional sinus beats; however, the rhythm is markedly abnormal due to varying types of aberration.

(*C*) After DC discharge, note the return to normal rhythm.

watt-seconds have been routinely employed in closed chest defibrillation. While some have recently argued that the defibrillation threshold depends on the body weight, this is controversial (Adgey, 1978). The highest energy setting should be utilized because valuable time may be lost in delivering ineffective shocks at low energy settings. If the first shock fails, repeated shocks should be delivered because the first shock may lower the skin resistance and therefore allow subsequent shocks to deliver a higher energy discharge to the myocardium. If the ventricular fibrillation remains refractory, correction of acidosis by administration of intravneous sodium bicarbonate, intracardiac injection of epinephrine (1 ml, 1:1000 dilution) or intravenous bolus of lidocaine (50–100 mg) or bretylium (5 mg/kg) followed by countershock may be helpful in restoring sinus rhythm (see chapter 26). For terminating ventricular fibrillation, the use of unsynchronized DC precordial shock is the procedure usually employed.

To define the factors that influence the success of emergency ventricular defibrillation, Kerber and Sarnot (1979) found no difference between groups that could or could not be successfully defibrillated regarding the following parameters; body weight, heart weight,

energy per kg of body weight or energy per gram of body weight. Factors that militated against successful defibrillation included a prolonged delay before the first defibrillatory shock, acidosis, and hypoxia. These three conditions tended to occur together in individual patients. In another study, it was observed that patient age, weight, delivered energy, duration of pulse wave, and duration of ventricular fibrillation had little, if any, effect on the defibrillation success rate (Gascho et al., 1979). Patients with acute myocardial infarction and primary ventricular fibrillation or with coronary disease and no myocardial infarction defibrillated more easily than patients with acute myocardial infarction and secondary ventricular fibrillation or with no coronary disease. Ventricular fibrillation in a terminal patient defibrillated less often than ventricular fibrillation in other clinical situations (Gascho et al., 1979).

ELECTIVE CARDIOVERSION

Mechanism

Conversion of certain tachyarrhythmias to sinus rhythm can be achieved by applying a synchronized direct current shock to the heart either directly or through the chest wall. The pulse discharge is synchronized with the R wave of the electrocardiogram (i.e., the absolute refractory period), thereby avoiding the ventricular vulnerable period at the peak of the T wave. The shock depolarizes all fibers that are excitable at the instant of stimulation, resulting in fusion of all wavelets and abolition of all available re-entry pathways. Simultaneous depolarization of the entire heart is necessary to terminate arrhythmias.

In addition to the direct effects of electric countershock in depolarizing all myocardial cells simultaneously, it also produces stimulation of the cardiac autonomic nervous system. Excitation of the intracardiac sympathetic nerves by countershock and by other forces of electrical stimulation has been shown to cause local release of norepinephrine. In addition, countershock is frequently followed by bradycardia, suggesting a parasympathetic release effect as well.

The immediate restoration of normal sinus rhythm after countershock depends not only upon the ability of the sinoatrial node to initiate impulses normally but also upon the integrity of the atrial muscle or intra-atrial conduction pathways to conduct these impulses. Post-countershock arrhythmias are usually related to the degree of sympathetic activation and, hence, to the strength of the shock or energy level setting on the cardioverter. Therefore, to avoid post-countershock arrhythmias, one should employ the lowest possible energy that will terminate the arrhythmia.

Factors Favoring Simultaneous Depolarization

Simultaneous depolarization of the entire heart is necessary to terminate arrhythmias. Therefore, before cardioversion is attempted, the levels of serum potassium and arterial pO_2 and pH (if disturbed) should be restored to normal. This restitution in some cases may be sufficient to terminate the arrhythmia.

Clinical Regimen for Cardioversion

The regimen must provide appropriate analgesia, antiarrhythmic medication if indicated, and a plan for choosing the intensity and duration of shocks to be delivered. The following is a suggested routine for the conversion of atrial fibrillation and other arrhythmias.

Maintenance antiarrhythmic therapy is begun prior to the procedure. The purpose is to establish an adequate plasma level in order to prevent prompt recurrence of the arrhythmia, to lower the incidence of conversion-induced arrhythmias, to facilitate conversion of arrhythmias at a lower energy level, and to determine whether the agent used is well tolerated. In fact, 10 to 20 per cent of patients with atrial fibrillation revert to normal sinus rhythm on "pretreatment" with quinidine alone.

Digitalis intoxication may prevent successful conversion and can precipitate severe post-countershock (PCS) arrhythmias including ventricular fibrillation (Fig. 25–3). Therefore, digitalis

AFTER 200 WATT SECS COUNTERSHOCK

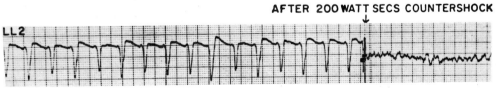

Figure 25–3 Ventricular fibrillation following countershock in the presence of digitalis toxicity. (Lead II) Control shows paroxysmal junctional tachycardia (rate, 150 per minute), probably the result of digitalis toxicity. Note occurrence of ventricular fibrillation following countershock at arrow.

therapy is discontinued prior to countershock, and whenever the preconversion electrocardiogram shows abnormalities suggestive of digitalis overdose, elective cardioversion should be postponed. In emergencies in which immediate conversion is mandatory and the patient has received large doses of digitalis, cardioversion should be attempted at an initially low energy level or by intra-atrial stimulation by a catheter electrode. (Lister et al., 1968; Pittman et al., 1973).

In patients with a previous history of *embolic phenomena* and/or rheumatic mitral valve disease, or with other indications that there is significant risk of an embolic episode, prophylactic anticoagulation is indicated. This measure significantly reduces the occurrence of post-countershock embolization.

Mild anesthesia may be achieved by using one of the following agents: diazepam, sodium pentobarbital, sodium thiopental, sodium methohexital, or methoxyflurane. Diazepam is the most common drug in current use for providing analgesia. It is administered in doses of 2 to 5 mg intravenously every 5 minutes until the patient is somnolent but can easily be aroused. Careful observation of the respiratory rate and pattern avoids undue respiratory depression. In an occasional patient, intubation may be necessary if respiratory depression occurs. The dose of diazepam may have to be decreased in older patients with congestive heart failure, while alcoholics may require a high total dose (Forsell et al., 1975). Although the patient may convulse or cry during application of countershock, he generally develops an amnesia for the event. Immediately after the procedure, the patient may sleep for a short duration and should be carefully monitored for post-countershock arrhythmias or the development of hypotension or left ventricular failure.

One should be prepared for complications and have ready a defibrillator, a pacemaker, lidocaine, and other antiarrhythmic drugs. Before the procedure, the accuracy of the synchronized circuit should be checked several times. The electrode paddles should be liberally covered with conductive paste. The electrodes are placed, one in the second or third interspace over the right of the sternum and the other in the mid back between the scapulae. An alternate placement is one paddle placed in the right parasternal area and the other placed in the left interspaces in the mid-axillary line.

The procedure should be *initiated* at low energy levels of 25 to 50 watt-seconds, with further shocks administered in increasing strength until sinus rhythm is restored. Countershock at levels above 400 watt-seconds are generally not used, and seldom are more than four shocks given in a series. Starting at a low level and increasing the energy of discharge in increments enables one to employ the minimal level necessary to restore normal sinus rhythm.

For atrial fibrillation and other arrhythmias, quinidine maintenance (Södermark et al., 1975) is continued in the doses employed prior to countershock; the first dose is administered 4 hours after conversion, and further doses are given every 6 hours thereafter. Long-acting preparations work very well for this purpose (Normand et al., 1976). Blood levels of quinidine may be determined, particularly in patients with congestive heart failure or renal insufficiency.

The *arrhythmias* that occur immediately following cardioversion may be divided into the following categories: 1) The majority are atrial in origin and are usually of minor significance — they consist of single or multiple premature atrial beats, which are usually transient. 2) Partial A-V block occurs frequently, usually indicating disease of the A-V junction or the effects of digitalis. 3) Delayed function or disease of the S-A node (i.e., sick sinus syndrome) may be manifested by a slow A-V junctional rhythm, sinus bradycardia, or A-V junctional escape. This is

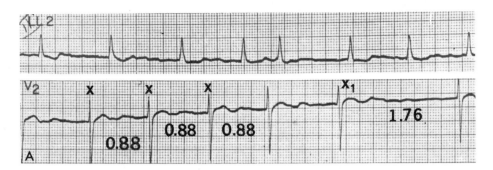

AFTER 200 WATT SECS COUNTERSHOCK

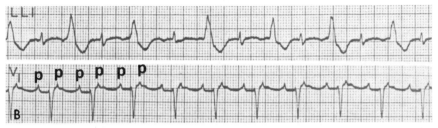

Figure 25–4   Countershock in atrial fibrillation; production of toxic digitalis effects in post-conversion period.

(*A*) Atrial fibrillation. Note that complexes at X have the same cycle length (0.88 sec.) (nodal rhythm). Cycle 4 is twice the regular cycle X. Exit block(?).

(*B*) After 200 watt-secs. countershock. Note upper strip (LI) with the occurrence of coupled ventricular premature beats. Lower strip (VI) shows an atrial tachycardia with a rate of 200 per minute with 2:1 block. These arrhythmias are probably due to toxic digitalis effects.

noted in 5 per cent of patients in whom atrial fibrillation was present for less than a year and in 45 per cent of patients in whom atrial fibrillation was present over 10 years. 4) Ventricular arrhythmias are less frequent but more serious (Figs. 25–4 and 25–5).

Drugs Employed to Prevent Post-Countershock (PCS) Arrhythmias

Electric countershock is an effective therapy for terminating many cardiac arrhythmias. The technique is simple

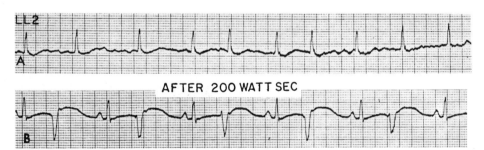

Figure 25–5   Conversion of atrial fibrillation to normal sinus rhythm. Note coupled premature ventricular beats.

(*A*) Atrial fibrillation with a ventricular rate averaging 75 per minute.

(*B*) Following cardioversion, note the presence of coupled premature ventricular beats.

and direct and usually does not result in significant complications. The primary problem usually is maintenance of normal sinus rhythm once conversion has been effected.

Various drugs help maintain the patient in sinus rhythm after conversion. Quinidine, procainamide, and lidocaine are the drugs usually employed; diphenylhydantoin is occasionally effective for this purpose (Helfant, 1968). These agents must be used with caution in patients prone to PCS sinus bradycardia because the drugs may prevent resumption of sinus rhythm by causing further depression of the sinus pacemaker.

Immediate Results. Normal sinus rhythm is initially restored in approximately 90 per cent of all patients receiving countershock. In a series of 1039 patients, 87 per cent (717 cases) of 820 episodes of atrial fibrillation were successfully converted to sinus rhythm (Figs. 25–6 and 25–7), whereas 96 per cent (107) of 111 cases of atrial flutter were converted (Bellet, 1971). In 42 cases of supraventricular tachycardias, 83 per cent (35) were converted, and in 66 cases of ventricular tachycardia 97 per cent (64) were converted (Bellet, 1971) (Fig. 25–8).

Long-Term Results. From 20 to 50 per cent of patients with atrial fibrillation treated by electric countershock remain in sinus rhythm for follow-up periods of 12 to 18 months. This varia-

tion is due to many factors: 1) the clinical status of the patient, 2) the type and extent of cardiac involvement, and 3) the method of administering quinidine. Quinidine is most effective when the doses are taken regularly by the patient and when long-acting preparations are used in appropriate cases.

In a typical series of 100 patients in whom atrial fibrillation was restored to normal sinus rhythm by countershock, 16 reverted to atrial fibrillation in the first 24 hours, and by the end of the 12 month follow-up period, 60 were again in atrial fibrillation (Szekely et al., 1969). An inverse relationship exists between the duration of atrial fibrillation prior to cardioversion and the length of time the sinus rhythm was maintained afterward. Those patients who have been in atrial fibrillation for less than a year have a much lower incidence (33%) of return to the arrhythmias after 12 months than those who had been in atrial fibrillation for more than a year (89%) (Szekely et al., 1969).

Normal sinus rhythm can be maintained for long periods of time, chiefly in patients with only slight cardiac enlargement who have hemodynamically minor heart disease and in those patients who have undergone ameliorative surgery. Marked atrial dilatation associated with severe underlying pathology is associated with frequent recurrence of the arrhythmias. Recur-

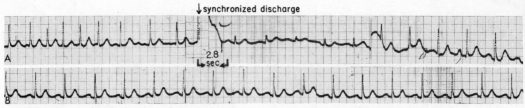

Figure 25–6 Reversion of atrial fibrillation to normal sinus rhythm. Male, 65 years old, with arteriosclerotic heart disease and atrial fibrillation of seven years' duration with borderline congestive heart failure.

(A) (Lead II) Shows atrial fibrillation. Synchronized discharge was applied at arrow and the resulting normal sinus rhythm is shown. The electrocardiogram was unreadable for 2.8 seconds, after which time normal sinus rhythm could be seen.

(B) Shows the tracing 10 minutes later with regular sinus rhythm.

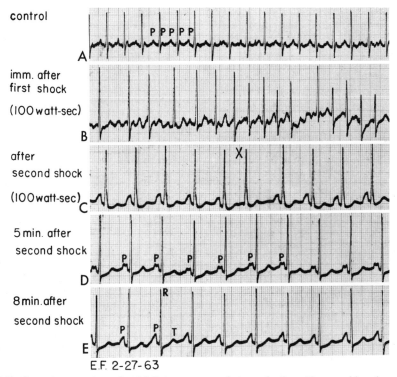

Figure 25-7 Steps in reversion of atrial flutter to normal sinus rhythm, 53-year-old male.

(A) Control. Shows 2:1 atrial flutter.

(B) After first synchronized discharge, atrial fibrillation with rapid ventricular response appears.

(C) After second synchronized discharge normal sinus rhythm is restored. Note the tall and broad P waves. A premature junctional beat is noted at X.

(D) Five minutes later the P waves become transiently notched.

(E) Eight minutes after the second shock the configuration of the P waves tends to become more normal.

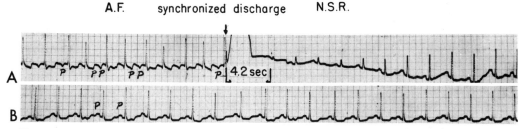

Figure 25-8 Reversion of atrial flutter to normal sinus rhythm. Male, 57 years old, with arteriosclerotic heart disease and mild congestive heart failure.

(A) (Lead II) Shows the reversion from atrial flutter to normal sinus rhythm. The electrocardiogram was unreadable for 4.2 seconds.

(B) Shows the tracing 10 minutes after reversion.

rence is also more common in subjects over the age of 55. The value of electrical conversion appears to be limited in patients with chronic atrial fibrillation associated with stable or progressive heart failure.

Hemodynamics Following Conversion of Atrial Fibrillation

Conversion to normal sinus rhythm improves the hemodynamics in most patients with atrial fibrillation. Numerous studies show that there is a progressive return of cardiac output and ventricular rate to normal levels for several days to several weeks after successful cardioversion. With atrial fibrillation, ventricular filling may be 30 per cent below normal because of the loss of the atrial contribution, and, consequently, ventricular contraction is less effective. The irregular cycle lengths also cause variable ventricular function, stroke volume, blood pressure, and cardiac output.

As a result of conversion, the ventricular rate decreases and does not rise excessively in response to exercise with the restoration of the atrial contribution, the stroke volume rises and remains at a fairly constant level, and the cardiac output is significantly greater both at rest and during exercise.

Hemodynamics Following Conversion of Other Rapid Arrhythmias

In tachyarrhythmias other than atrial fibrillation, the immediate post-conversion benefits are derived both from the ability of countershock to decrease the heart rate and from restoration of the atrial contribution. In patients with atrial flutter, atrial tachycardia, junctional tachycardia, and ventricular tachycardia of varying duration, a significant improvement in cardiac output averaging 11 per cent and an increase in stroke output of al-

most 100 per cent has been observed by Wright et al. (1970). The magnitude of increase in cardiac output is proportional to the heart rate prior to conversion, so that the advantageous effects of countershock will be relatively greater in the patients with more rapid tachyarrhythmia.

Echocardiographic studies have also indicated that reversion to sinus rhythm enhances the atrial transport mechanism, but this change does not always produce increases in systemic blood flow (DeMaria at al., 1975). Patients with depressed cardiac output are more likely to show improvement, while those with normal output may show no change.

Indications for Countershock

Countershock is generally indicated in the more severe arrhythmias associated with a deteriorating clinical state. Under these circumstances, countershock is generally indicated for the following arrhythmias: 1) acute onset of atrial fibrillation (Figs. 25–6, 25–7, 25–8); 2) atrial flutter; 3) paroxysmal atrial and junctional tachycardias; 4) other supraventricular tachycardias, particularly those associated with the W-P-W syndrome; and 5) ventricular tachycardia (Fig. 25–9). Although other methods of therapy may be tried initially, countershock remains the method of choice when drug therapy has been unsuccessful and when the patient is severely ill.

Contraindications to Countershock

Although the technique is simple and direct, there are several definite contraindications to countershock: 1) In supraventricualr arrhythmias with complete heart block — the existing hemodynamic changes cannot be reverted to sinus rhythm and little benefit can be achieved by countershock. 2) In digital-

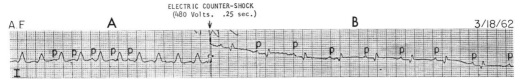

Figure 25-9 Effect of electric countershock in a patient with ventricular tachycardia refractory to drug therapy. (Lead I)

(*A*) Taken from a patient, age 75, with a ventricular tachycardia refractory to the usual methods of therapy. Note the ventricular rate of 145 per minute with markedly widened QRS complexes and P waves occurring at a slower rate independent of the ventricular complexes complete A-V dissociation.

(*B*) After the electric countershock (480 volts, 0.25 second). Note the restoration of a normal sinus rhythm with a P-R interval of 0.24 second. (From Medow and Dreifus: Amer. J. Cardiol.)

is toxicity — countershock is not indicated for arrhythmias due to digitalis toxicity inasmuch as countershock for digitalis-induced supraventricular arrhythmia is associated with a significant incidence of complications (Helfant, 1968). Preferred therapy consists of withdrawal of digitalis and use of lidocaine or diphenylhydantoin. 3) Inability to tolerate quinidine in patients who have a predisposition for the recurrence of the atrial fibrillation. These circumstances make the return of the arrhythmia a virtual certainty, despite using other drugs for maintenance therapy. 4) When atrial fibrillation or other arrhythmias recur immediately after repeated countershock despite adequate quinidine therapy, subsequent countershock is contraindicated.

RELATIVE CONTRAINDICATIONS

In some instances cardioversion is unlikely to be beneficial; the advisability of using this modality should be carefully considered for each patient in the following instances:

1. The recent onset of supraventricular arrhythmia if the patient is clinically stable is not an indication for immediate countershock, since other simpler measures for therapy are available. Electrical conversion should be deferred until drug therapy has been proven ineffective.
2. Electric countershock is usually of little efficacy in patients with repetitive tachycardias.

3. When atrial fibrillation is present, cardioversion should be used cautiously under the following conditions:
   a. Candidates for cardiac surgery should undergo the appropriate surgical procedures before conversion is considered.
   b. In postoperative cardiac patients, there is a high rate of recurrence of atrial fibrillation when countershock is employed either at the time of surgery or immediately thereafter. Electrical conversion should be deferred for 8 to 12 weeks until postoperative convalescence is nearly complete.
   c. A majority of patients with atrial fibrillation associated with hyperthyroidism will revert to sinus rhythm spontaneously when the euthyroid state is achieved. There is also a low success rate in maintaining normal rhythm in hypermetabolic patients. Electrical conversion should not be considered until after the hyperthyroid patient has been returned to the euthyroid state.
   d. A patient who has suffered a recent systemic embolism should not be considered for countershock unless it is an emergency procedure.
4. Cardioversion is not indicated for sinus tachycardia or normal sinus

rhythm with atrial, junctional, or ventricular premature beats.

5. In general, countershock should not be employed when a critical evaluation of the factors argues against the probability of maintenance of sinus rhythm after conversion.

Complications of Countershock

The major complications of countershock encountered include: 1) ventricular tachycardia and fibrillation, which occur in 1 to 2 per cent of patients treated; 2) pulmonary or systemic emboli, which occur in 1 to 2 per cent of patients who are not properly anticoagulated, but in less than 1 per cent of those who are; 3) pulmonary venous congestion with episodes of pulmonary edema (1 to 2 per cent); 4) elevation of serum glutamic-oxaloacetic transaminase, lactic dehydrogenase, and creatine phosphokinase may occur in 20 per cent or more of patients, as a result of the skeletal muscle damage associated with countershock, while MB-CPK is elevated in only 6 per cent of patients (Ehsani et al., 1973); and 5) various electrocardiographic changes may occur, especially transient S-T segment elevation in the precordial leads. These electrocardiographic changes, however, do not appear to affect morbidity or mortality (Resnekov and McDonald, 1967). Other less significant or very infrequent complications include: 1) hypoventilation, myocardial depression, and cardiac irritability associated with anesthesia; 2) drug reactions (potentiation of digitalis and quinidine toxicity); 3) A-V junctional rhythm; 4) severe bradycardia; 5) multiple premature ventricular beats immediately following cardioversion; 6) rarely, cardiac arrest.

Place of Countershock in Therapy

Electric countershock occupies an important place in the treatment of life-threatening and/or refractory tachyar-rhythmias. It has the following advantages: rapidity of conversion, relative safety, and avoidance of delay, uncertainty, and possible toxic effects of drugs.

Countershock is the method of choice in the conversion of ventricular tachycardia, atrial flutter, and atrial fibrillation when these arrhythmias are causally related to a deteriorating clinical state. However, the original enthusiasm for its use in patients with chronic atrial arrhythmias, particularly atrial fibrillation, has largely disappeared.

References

Aberg, H., and Cullhed, I.: Direct-current countershock complications. Acta Med. Scand. 183:415, 1968.

Adgey, A. A., Patton, J. N., Campbell, N. P., and Webb, S. W.: Ventricular defibrillation: Appropriate energy levels. Circulation 60:219, 1979.

Bell, H., Pugh, D., and Dunn, M.: Failure of cardioversion in mitral valve disease. Arch. Intern. Med. 119:257, 1967.

Bellet, S.: Clinical Disorders of the Heart Beat. 3rd ed., Philadelphia, Lea & Febiger, 1971.

Bjerkelund, C., and Orning, O. M.: An evaluation of DC shock treatment of atrial arrhythmias. Acta Med. Scand. 194:481, 1968.

Cobb, F. R., Wallace, A. G., and Wagner, G. S.: Cardiac inotropic and coronary vascular responses to countershock. Circ. Res. 23:731, 1968.

DeMaria, A. N., Lies, J. F., King, F. J., Miller, R. R., Amsterdam, E. A., and Mason, D. T.: Echocardiographic assessment of atrial transport, mitral movement and ventricular performance following electroversion of supraventricular arrhythmias. Circulation 51:273, 1975.

Driscol, T. E., Ratnoff, O. D., and Nygaard, D. F.: The remarkable Dr. Abilgaard and countershock. The bicentennial of his electrical experiments on animals. Ann. Int. Med. 83:878, 1975.

Ehsani, A. A., Ewy, G. A., and Sobel, B. E.: CPK isoenzyme elevations after electrical countershock (Abst). Circulation 48(IV):129, 1973.

Ferris, L. P., Spence, P. W., King, B. G., and Williams, H. B.: Effect of electric shock on the heart. Electrical Engineering 55:498, 1936.

Forsell, G., Hardlander, R., Nyquist, O., and Orinius, E.: Diazepam in cardioversion. Acta Med. Scand. 197:255, 1975.

Gascho, J. A., Crampton, R. S., Cherwek, M. L., Sipes, J. N., Hunter, F. P., and O'Brien, W. M.: Determinants of ventricular defibrillation in adults. Circulation 60:231, 1979.

Gilbert, R., and Cuddy, R.: Digitalis intoxication following conversion to sinus rhythm. Circulation *32*:58, 1965.

Härtel, G., Louhija, A., and Konttinen, A.: Disopyramide in the prevention of recurrence of atrial fibrillation after electroconversion. Clin. Pharmacol. Ther. *15*:551, 1974.

Helfant, R. H., Scherlag, B. J., and Damato, A. N.: Diphenylhydantoin prevention of arrhythmias after direct current cardioversion. Circulation *37*:424, 1968.

Helfant, R. H., Scherlag, B. J., and Damato, A. N.: Electrophysiological effects of direct current countershock before and after ouabain sensitization and after diphenylhydantoin desensitization. Circulation *22*:615, 1968.

Kerber, R. E., and Sarnat, W.: Factors influencing the success of ventricular defibrillation in man. Circulation *60*:226, 1979.

Kleiger, R., and Lown, B.: Cardioversion and digitalis. Part II. Clinical studies. Circulation *33*:878, 1966.

Kouwenhoven, W. B., Milnor, W. R., Jude, J. R., Knickerbocker, G. G., and Chestnut, W. R.: Closed chest defibrillation of the heart. Surgery *42*:550, 1957.

Lister, J. W., Cohen, L. S., Bernstein, W. H., and Samet, P.: Treatment of supraventricular tachycardias by rapid atrial stimulation. Circulation, *38*:1044, 1968.

Lown, B., Amarasingham, R., and Newman, J.: New method for terminating cardiac arrhythmias: Use of synchronized capacitor discharge. J.A.M.A. *182*:548, 1962.

Lown, B., Bey, S. L, Perlroth, M., and Abe, T.: Comparative studies of ventricular vulnerability to fibrillation. J. Clin. Invest. *42*:953, 1963.

Lown, B., Kleiger, R., and Williams, J.: Cardioversion and digitalis drugs: Changed threshold to electric shock in digitalized animals. Circ. Res. *17*:519, 1965.

Lown, B., Newman, J., Amarasingham, R., and Berkovits, B. V.: Comparison of alternating current with direct current electroshock across closed chest. Am. J. Cardiol. *10*:223, 1962.

Normand, J. P., Legendre, M., Kahn, J. C., Bourdarias, J. P., and Mathivat, A.: Comparative efficacy of short-acting and long-acting quinidine for maintenance of sinus rhythm after electrical conversion of atrial fibrillation. Brit. Heart J. *38*:381–387, 1976.

Peleska, B.: Srdecni Defibrillator. Sbornik vynalezu a zlepsovacich navrhu ve azrarotnictvi *3*:33, 1955.

Pittman, D. E., Makar, J. S., Kooros, K. S., and Joyner, C. R.: Rapid atrial stimulation: Successful method of conversion of atrial flutter and atrial tachycardia. Am. J. Cardiol. *32*:700, 1973.

Prevost, J. L., and Batelli, F.: Sur quelques effects des decharges electriques sur le coeur des mammifers. C.R. Acad. Sci. (D)(Paris) *129*:267, 1899.

Radford, M. D., and Evans, D. W.: Long-term results of DC reversion of atrial fibrillation. Brit. Heart J. *30*:91, 1968.

Resnekov, L., and McDonald, L.: Complications of 220 patients with cardiac dysrhythmias treated by phased direct current shock and indications for electroconversion. Brit. Heart J. *29*:926, 1967.

Södermark, T., Edhag, O., Sjögren, A., Jonsson, B., Olsson, A., Orö, L., Danielsson, M., Rosenhammer, G., and Wallin, H.: Effects of quinidine on maintaining sinus rhythm after conversion of atrial fibrillation or flutter: A multicenter study from Stockholm. Brit. Heart J. *37*:486–492, 1975.

Szekely, P., et al.: Direct current shock and digitalis. Brit. Heart J. *31*:91, 1969.

Wright, J. S., Fabian, J., Epstein, E. J.: Immediate effect on cardiac output of reversion to sinus rhythm from rapid arrhythmias. Brit. Med. J. *3*:315, 1970.

Zoll, P. M., and Linenthal, A. J.: Termination of refractory tachycardia by external countershock. Circulation *25*:596, 1962.

Zoll, P. M., Paul, M. H., Linenthal, A. J., Nomad, L. R., and Gibson, W.: Effects of external electric currents on heart: control of cardiac rhythm and induction and termination of cardiac arrhythmia. Circulation *14*:745, 1956.

Zoll, P. M., Linenthal, A. J., and Phelps, M. D., Jr.: Termination of refractory tachycardia by external electric countershock. Circulation *24*:1078, 1961.

Zoll, P. M., Linenthal, A. J., and Zarsky, L. R. N.: Termination of ventricular fibrillation in man by externally applied countershock. N. Engl. J. Med. *254*:427, 1956.

Zoll, P. M., Linenthal, A. J., and Zarsky, L. R. N.: Ventricular fibrillation: Treatment and prevention by external electric currents. N. Engl. J. Med. *262*:105, 1960.

26

CARDIAC ARREST

MONTY M. BODENHEIMER, M.D.,

GENERAL CONSIDERATIONS

The term "cardiac arrest" is usually used to designate the clinical cessation of cardiac activity, causing sudden and often unexpected failure of effective circulation. Since respiratory failure is an important causative factor of cardiac arrest and since it follows circulatory arrest within a matter of 20 to 30 seconds in any case, the more inclusive term "cardiopulmonary arrest" is preferable and is often employed (Jude, 1969).

The term "cardiac arrest" may be used in the literal sense, meaning cessation of electrical activity of the heart as determined by the electrocardiogram. Clinically, the term is applied to the syndrome characterized by the cessation of purposeful cardiac activity with no peripheral blood pressure. This may be the result of ventricular fibrillation or cardiac arrest in various combinations and sequences. In this section the term is used in one or the other connotation, but cardiac arrest (absence of electrical activity) occupies a prominent role.

Cardiac arrest has become a topic of prime importance because of the development of effective resuscitation methods and the experience that the prompt institution of therapy may avert a fatal outcome. Cardiac arrest is frequently the terminal mechanism in desperately ill patients. However, in this discussion we are primarily concerned with its sudden appearance, either associated with certain clinical conditions (e.g., myocardial infarction) or other unexpected circumstances in apparently healthy subjects or in the presence of minimal overt cardiac abnormalities.

TYPES OF CARDIAC ARREST

Cardiac arrest in man may be divided into the following categories: 1) primary cardiac arrest, 2) cardiac arrest as part of general circulatory failure, 3) cardiac arrest secondary to or coincident with respiratory failure, and 4) induced cardiac arrest during surgery.

INCIDENCE AND ETIOLOGY

Cardiac arrest is most commonly encountered during surgery and as a result of serious heart disease, either acute or chronic. It may also occur under totally unpredictable circumstances.

The factors that predispose to cardiac arrest include 1) pathologic states of the heart, particularly acute and chronic coronary heart disease such as acute myocardial infarction; 2) hypoxia and/or hypercapnia; 3) electrolyte disturbances, particularly hyperpotassemia and hypocalcemia; 4) acute conditions, such as severe chest trauma or overwhelming systemic infections; 5) drugs and anesthetic agents; 6) electric shock; 7) combinations of factors. In addition, cardiac arrest occurs without an apparent etiology.

In one study, the following etiologic factors were observed in 100 consecutive patients who developed cardiac arrest following admission to a medical intensive care unit: 1) myocardial infarction, 63 cases; 2) atherosclerotic, hypertensive, and valvular heart disease, 19 cases; 3) cerebrovascular disease, 4 cases; 4) pulmonary embolism, 4 cases; and 5) miscellaneous group, 10 cases (Linko et al., 1967).

Some of the important precipitating factors of unexpected cardiac arrest include the development of ectopic rhythms (e.g., ventricular tachycardia, ventricular fibrillation, sinus arrest); parasympathetic activity, from whatever cause (e.g., carotid sinus pressure), especially in the presence of hypoxia, hypercapnia, or hyperpotassemia, resulting in sudden depression of pacemaker activity with cardiac standstill or ventricular fibrillation; excitement or anxiety and severe mental stress in susceptible patients; Valsalva maneuver during defecation; early ambulation after prolonged periods of bedrest accompanied by a vasodepressor or postural type of hypotension; the effect of drugs (e.g., digitalis, quinidine, procainamide, potassium, and respiratory depressants); hypoglycemia, leading to ectopic rhythms; and convulsive seizures accompanying tetanus or epileptic forms of attack.

In addition, cardiac arrest may be precipitated unexpectedly during many therapeutic procedures. Cardiac arrest has been observed under the following circumstances: during angiography; during delivery and other gynecologic procedures; following rectal examination in elderly patients; during the rapid infusion of certain antiarrhythmic drugs; and during urologic examination (i.e., urethral catheterization) (Stephenson, 1969). Cardiac arrest also occurs in victims of drowning and other catastrophic accidents.

PATHOPHYSIOLOGY

The greatest danger of cardiac arrest lies in the extremely limited time within which the circulation may be safely restored, owing to the poor tolerance of certain cells to hypoxia. Cardiac arrest and its resultant hypoxia must be corrected in 3 to 4 minutes if residual neurologic changes are to be avoided. Profound hypothermia, as occurs during drowning in cold water, may prolong this period considerably and this should be considered in the decision to initiate resuscitation.

DIAGNOSIS

Cardiac arrest should be diagnosed if no peripheral pulses are palpable (particularly the carotid or femoral pulse), sounds are absent, and respirations have ceased. These episodes of unexpected cardiac arrest may be preceded by a convulsive seizure and appearance of cyanosis.

When a patient has no palpable pulses, heart sounds, or respiration, the diagnosis of cardiac arrest is usually made. However, electrocardiographic recordings show that the cardiac mechanism underlying cardiac arrest may be ventricular fibrillation, asystole or electromechanical dissociation, or a slow idioventricular rhythm without a palpable pulse or detectable blood pressure.

Studies in 132 critically ill patients who were continually monitored before and at the time of mechanical cardiac arrest showed ventricular fibrillation in 56 instances (43%) and ventricular standstill in 76 instances (57%) (Camarata et al., 1970). In such situations it is often suggested that the patient be defibrillated if no electrocardiographic records are available because time is of

TABLE 26–1   PROCEDURE FOR CLOSED CHEST CARDIOPULMONARY RESUSCITATION

1. Diagnosis
   Made on physical findings
   Do not delay initiation of resuscitation to obtain ECG

2. Call for assistance—note exact time

3. Deliver a direct and vigorous thump to precordium

4. Ventilation
   a. Check for and maintain an open airway
   b. Give artificial mouth to mouth ventilation. *Do not use endotracheal tube at this point due to time consumed in the procedure*
   c. If alone, ventilate five or six times and then begin cardiac compression; after each 15 compressions, ventilate twice
   d. When the anesthesiologist arrives, he continues artificial ventilation or assisted respiration by the technique indicated

5. External cardiac compression
   a. Place patient on a firm surface
   b. Compress lower one third of sternum 2 inches at a rate of 60 compressions per minute
   c. Carotid pulse should be used to monitor the efficacy of the compression

6. Drug therapy (When effective cardiorespiratory assistance has been established, drugs may be used to treat circulatory collapse):
   a. Open and maintain intravenous route(s) for rapid administration of drugs
   b. Agents to increase myocardial contractility
      1. Epinephrine
      2. Isoproterenol
      3. Norepinephrine
   c. Agents to reverse acidosis and increase ventricular beating
      1. Sodium bicarbonate
      2. Calcium gluconate

7. Definitive treatment
   a. Administer a cardioactive drug (see 6b)
   b. Establish electrocardiographic diagnosis (by ECG or Semler technique, Chapter 4)
      1. Beware of artifacts of precordial compression
      2. Asystole requires pacing (external or transvenous) (see Chapter 24)
      3. Fibrillation requires defibrillation (see Chapter 25)

8. Maintain post-resuscitative care
   a. Prevention of recurrence of cardiac arrest
   b. Maintenance of circulation
   c. Prevention of CNS damage

the essence. Many defibrillator paddles now serve as recording electrodes that display an electrocardiogram on an oscilloscope so that "instantaneous" knowledge of cardiac rhythm is available. Differentiation of ventricular fibrillation from asystole can thus be made instantly. This would obviate the application of the defibrillator to patients with asystole or slow idioventricular rhythm.

Since one has relatively little time in which to resuscitate the heart, therapy should be started immediately.

The outline of therapy for closed-chest cardiopulmonary resuscitation is discussed in Table 26–1. (See also Fig. 26–1).

The diagnosis of cardiac arrest during cardiac or thoracic operations is easy because the heart is either exposed or available to palpation. It should be diagnosed during any operative procedure when there occur cessation of the pulse, inaudible heart sounds, an absent blood pressure, and the development of apnea. It may occur completely without warning, but in most instances there may be some premonitory signs, such as bradycardia, tachycardia, or premature beats (Fig. 26–2). Early detection of changes in cardiac rhythm is possible by use of cathode ray oscilloscope or by continuous monitoring on tape.

TREATMENT OF CARDIAC ARREST

Cardiac arrest is a medical emergency for which effective treatment must be instituted within 3 to 4 minutes of onset in order to prevent permanent cerebral damage. Several developments, particularly the effective techniques for closed chest cardiac compression, the capacitor discharge defibrillator, and efficient pacing devices, have advanced treatment to the point that many patients may recover completely.

Because cardiac arrest can occur at

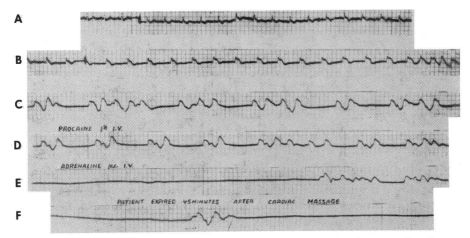

Figure 26–1. Evolution of electrocardiographic changes during the development of cardiac arrest at operation (continous Lead II).

(A) Taken prior to the beginning of cardiac arrest. Soon after the beginning of this strip, note the inversion of T waves followed by slight elevation of the S-T segment at the end of the strip.

(B) Shows increasing elevation of the S-T segment associated with atrial standstill. The ventricular rate increases toward the end of the strip.

(C) Note the increasing aberration of the ventricular complexes and irregularity of the ventricular rate.

(D) Further aberration of ventricular beats following administration of procainamide.

(E) Long periods of standstill with beginning ventricular fibrillation (after epinephrine).

(F) Long pause, two ventricular beats, and cardiac standstill.

any time, it is imperative that nurses, physicians, and other hospital personnel be taught the technique of treating cardiac arrest early in their training. Increasingly, training of the population at large has been instituted and shown to be a successful approach to reduce sudden cardiac arrest due to coronary heart disease. In Seattle, rapid bystander initiation of cardiopulmonary

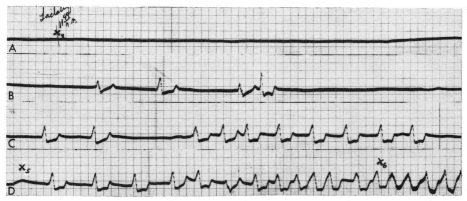

Figure 26–2. Patient, 73 years, manifesting terminal episodes of cardiac arrest. Following the infusion of molar sodium lactate, note resumption of idioventricular beats in B, which become more frequent in C and D. The rate increases in D although the complexes are bizarre. Although the electrocardiogram shows evidence of ventricular oscillations, the heart was in standstill at this time and showed only minute fibrillary twitchings. It should be emphasized that the presence of electrocardiogram deflections even of a relatively normal contour does not necessarily coincide with an effective ventricular contraction.

resuscitation has significantly reduced the incidence of sudden death in the community.

When the diagnosis of cardiac arrest has been made, the two primary responsibilities of a witness are to 1) maintain adequate ventilation and 2) effect adequate circulation. Opening and maintaining an adequate airway are critical to success. With the patient lying on his back, the head should be tilted backward and the mouth checked for foreign objects, including dentures. Artificial respiration, using the mouth to mouth approach, should be begun and adequacy of ventilation checked by observing chest movement. If this is not done, the airway must be reexamined and any foreign objects removed. Four quick full breaths should be administered and a quick check for appearance of a pulse either at the carotid or femoral locations should be made. If the pulse is still absent, then artificial circulation will have to be begun. This should be performed by compressing the lower portion of the sternum briskly at a rate of 60 per minute. If only one person is available to perform cardiopulmonary resuscitation, then the same person will have to carry out both ventilation and artificial circulation at a ratio of 15 compressions to two quick breaths. Cardiac compression alone will not result in adequate ventilation; therefore, both ventilation and cardiac compression should be continued in an uninterrupted manner until help arrives. If another person is present, the efficacy of cardiac compressions should be checked by palpating the carotid or femoral pulses. When help arrives, as in the form of an emergency health team, more definitive therapy, including diagnosis of the underlying rhythmn and appropriate treatment, either with cardioversion, intracardiac epinephrine, or other antiarrhythmic therapy, may be begun prior to transport to the hospital. It is of critical importance at this stage, particularly if resuscitation has been proceeding for more than 3 or 4 minutes, that

intravenous sodium bicarbonate be administered immediately in order to help reverse the marked metabolic and respiratory acidosis that occurs during cardiac arrest. This is of particular importance if initial cardioversion for ventricular fibrillation fails.

CARDIAC COMPLICATIONS

Closed-Chest. As many as half of the patients in whom closed-chest resuscitation is performed suffer some form of injury during or associated with this procedure. Rib fractures are most common, and sternal fractures occur with a roughly equal frequency. Fat emboli from bone marrow have been observed to occur in about 10 per cent of resuscitated patients (Baringer et al., 1961). More serious complications include trauma to the liver (which occurs in roughly 2 per cent of patients) and, less commonly, trauma to the spleen, inferior vena cava, and aorta (Nelson and Ashley, 1965; Paaske et al., 1968). Although complications are common, they generally do not have great significance. Approximately only 1 per cent of patients resuscitated in this manner showed serious complications that could have, in themselves, resulted in death (Paaske et al., 1968). While this consideration should be kept in mind, it should in no way restrict therapy.

Open-Chest. The complications of open-chest cardiac resuscitation are 1) direct trauma to the heart and 2) the operative risk involved in thoracotomy. Rupture or lacerations of the myocardium, pericardial tamponade, herniation of the heart, and epicardial hemorrhage have been reported (Stephenson, 1969).

CEREBRAL COMPLICATIONS OF CARDIAC ARREST

Brain damage due to thrombosis of cerebral vessels and brain damage due to hypoxia and subsequent disturbances in cerebral metabolism may occur after either method of resuscitation. The residual deficit may consist of loss of recent memory, inability to learn, emotional lability, and intellectual impairment with loss of integrative ability. In one series of 552 patients resuscitated by the closed-chest method, 11 subjects demonstrated irreversible cerebral damage. In most of these patients, the damage could be explained as caused by either delayed treatment or advanced age (Johnson et al., 1967).

Cardiac arrest is followed by various alterations in the mental and emotional state. Many patients demonstrate a mild to severe organic brain syndrome following resuscitation, which usually clears with the passage of time (Druss and Kornfeld, 1967). Serious cerebral complications have been estimated to occur in roughly 2 per cent of patients who are resuscitated successfully.

CRITERIA OF DEATH

Recent advances, particularly in the field of transplantation, including cardiac, have raised the question of what signs constitute definitive evidence of death. Several criteria have been proposed, particularly the combination of certain signs referable to the absence of central nervous system function — complete unresponsiveness to external stimuli, total absence of spontaneous movements, and total absence of reflexes for 24 hours. A persistent isoelectric electroencephalogram for 24 hours has been used as a criterion. However, since it cannot be interpreted with certainty, it is not a good criterion of death if the patient has ingested drugs such as barbiturates or is being treated by hypothermia. The aforementioned criteria are obviously far more rigorous than those commonly employed in the presence of cardiac arrest, since the signs of hypoxic cerebral damage discussed previously indicate a grave prognosis even in the presence of activity in the electroencephalogram. However, when ce-

rebral activity has been specifically depressed, as by an overdose of barbiturates, a flat electroencephalogram should not be considered evidence of cerebral death, since full mental recovery may occur.

PROGNOSIS FOLLOWING CARDIAC ARREST

The clinical diagnosis of cardiac arrest includes patients in whom the electrocardiogram demonstrates ventricular fibrillation as well as true arrest or asystole. In fact, most instances of acute arrest probably begin as ventricular fibrillation and progress to asystole with the passage of time. When asystole has supervened before resuscitation begins, the chance of successful resuscitation is much diminished (Adgey et al., 1969). Hollingsworth (1969) found that the probability of success was much greater with ventricular fibrillation, most failures being associated with asystole. Hollingsworth found that of 360 patients in whom resuscitation was attempted, 8.2 per cent survived to leave the hospital. Lemire and Johnson (1972) found that 230 (19.1%) of 1204 patients were resuscitated to be discharged with a 1 year survival rate of 74 per cent. Moreover, in a sample of these patients, they found that the majority showed no change in functional class. Only four were discharged with severe cerebral damage.

THE TERMINAL ELECTROCARDIOGRAM

The common pathophysiologic feature of terminal arrhythmias is the reduction of hemodynamic performance below that which is essential to provide adequate blood flow to the essential organs, especially the brain and the heart itself. In addition to ventricular fibrillation and asystole, disturbances of rhythm that cause inadequate blood flow consist of 1) severe tachyarrhyth-

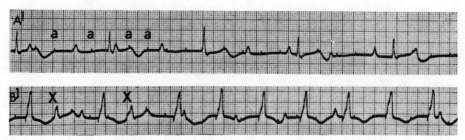

Figure 26–3. Runaway pacemaker in 75-year-old male patient with complete A-V heart block and arteriosclerotic heart disease. Because of battery exhaustion the current is inadequate to produce an effective contraction. A permanent demand pacemaker was implanted four years earlier and the pacing rate set at 72 per minute. Due to exhaustion of the battery, the pacemaker does not deliver adequate energy to stimulate the ventricle. In addition, the rate of the pacemaker was increased to 160 beats per minute (runaway pacemaker) and the demand system was not functioning. In (A¹), note pacemaker artifacts (a) (rate 160 per minute, which fails to activate the ventricle).

(B¹) A transvenous demand pacemaker was inserted in the same patient. It paced at the rate of 75 beats per minute. Note the difference in the ventricular complexes delivered by the new pacemaker which captures the ventricles at 75 per minute. Note that in this tracing stimuli delivered by the old implanted pacemaker at X now produce ventricular complexes when they occur 500 to 580 msec. after the stimulus of the newly inserted transvenous pacemaker. This may be due to supernormality resulting from the Wedensky effect.

mias, especially ventricular tachycardia, and 2) severe bradyarrhythmias, especially those with transient brief periods of ventricular asystole. Although death or at least neurologic dysfunction becomes inevitable after, at most, four minutes of total circulatory collapse, the period of circulatory arrest that can be tolerated is markedly reduced in individuals having severe pre-existing cardiac derangement.

The terminal mechanism is not easily determined unless one fortuitously has an electrocardiographic recorder connected to the patient at that time. Its elucidation has been facilitated by the use of continuous electrocardiographic monitoring.

The terminal cardiac mechanism depends principally upon whether 1) the arrhythmia occurs suddenly in an individual whose cardiac function has been at least minimally adequate or occurs at the termination of a progressively worsening cardiac derangement; 2) the subject had pre-existing conduction defects predisposing to ventricular asystole; 3) cardiovascular collapse is to some degree secondary to respiratory or peripheral vascular failure; and 4) the electrocardiogram is obtained promptly or is recorded after a period of delay.

Ventricular fibrillation or ventricular asystole is the usual terminal mechanism in most instances of sudden circulatory arrest. However, when death occurs slowly over a period of minutes or hours, the following sequence of events is frequently observed; 1) sinus slowing, leading to atrial standstill; 2) slow A-V junctional rhythm; 3) idioventricular rhythm with ventricular premature beats and occasionally ventricular tachycardia terminating in ventricular fibrillation, and finally ventricular standstill; or 4) with a slow idioventricular rhythm, the ventricular complex becomes more aberrant and widened, and the terminal mechanism is that of ventricular standstill (Fig. 26–3).

REFERENCES

Adelson, L.: A clinicopathologic study of the anatomic changes in the heart resulting from cardiac massage. Surg. Gynecol. Obstet. 104:513, 1957.
Adgey, A. A. J., et al.: Management of ventricular

fibrillation outside hospital. Lancet *1*:1169, 1969.

Ad Hoc Committee on Cardiopulmonary Resuscitation of the Division of Medical Sciences, National Academy of Sciences, National Research Council: Cardiopulmonary resuscitation. J.A.M.A. *198*:372, 1966.

American College of Cardiology, Conference Report: Training techniques for the coronary care unit. Am. J. Cardiol. *17*:736, 1966.

American College of Cardiology, Sixth Bethesda Conference: Early care for the acute coronary suspect. Am. J. Cardiol. *23*:603, 1969.

Baringer, J. R., Salzman, E. W., Jones, W. A., and Friedlich, A. L.: External cardiac massage. N. Engl. J. Med. *265*:62, 1961.

Bellet, S., and Wasserman, F.: Indications and contraindications for the use of molar sodium lactate. Circulation *15*:591, 1957.

Birch, L.: The need for training, retraining, and testing trainees in cardiopulmonary resuscitation. *In* Gordon, A. S. (Ed.): Cardiopulmonary Resuscitation. Conference Proceedings. Washington, D.C., National Research Council, 1967.

Camarata, S., Weil, M. H., Shubin, H., and Hanashiro, P. K.: Hemodynamic documentation of cardiac arrest in 132 patients. (Abst.) Am. J. Cardiol. *26*:627, 1970.

Copley, D. P., Mantle, J. A., Rodgers, W. J., Russel, R. O., and Rackley, C. E.: Improved outcome for prehospital cardiopulmonary collapse with resuscitation by bystanders. Circulation *56*:901, 1977.

Druss, R. G., and Kornfeld, D. S.: Survivors of cardiac arrest. J.A.M.A. *201*:291, 1967.

Editorial: Complications of cardiac massage. Brit. Med. J. *1*:68, 1969.

Editorial: EEG signs of death. Brit. Med. J. *2*:318, 1968.

Elain, J. O.: Principles and practice of cardiopulmonary resuscitation. *In* Gordon, A. S. (Ed.): Cardiopulmonary Resuscitation. Conference Proceedings. Washington, D.C., National Research Council, 1967.

Flynn, R. L., and Fox, S. M.: Coronary care unit programs in the United States. Israel J. Sci. *3*:279, 1967.

Guzman, S. V., DeLeon, A. C., Jr., West, J. W., and Bellet, S.: Cardiac effects of isoproterenol, norepinephrine and epinephrine in complete A-V heart block during experimental acidosis and hyperkalemia. Circ. Res. *7*:666, 1959.

Hollingsworth, J. H.: The results of cardiopulmo-

nary resuscitation: A 3-year university hospital experience. Ann. Int. Med. *71*:459, 1969.

Johnson, A. L., Tanser, P. H., Ulan, R. A., and Wood, T. E.: Results of cardiac resuscitation in 552 patients. Am. J. Cardiol. *20*:831, 1967.

Jude, J. R.: Cardiopulmonary arrest and resuscitation. *In* Gibbon, J. H., Jr., Sabiston, D. C., Jr., and Spencer, F. C. (Eds.): Surgery of the Chest. Philadelphia, W. B. Saunders, 1969.

Killip, T., III, and Kimball, J. T.: Treatment of myocardial infarction in a coronary care unit. A two year experience with 250 patients. Am. J. Cardiol. *20*:457, 1967.

Lemire, J. G., and Johnson, A. L.: Is cardiac resuscitation worthwhile? N. Engl. J. Med. *286*:970, 1972.

Linko, E., Koskinen, P. J., Siitonen, L., and Ruosteenoja, R.: Resuscitation in cardiac arrest. An analysis of 100 successive medical cases. Acta Med. Scand. *182*·611, 1967.

Lund, I., and Skullberg, A.: Cardiopulmonary resuscitation by lay people. Lancet *2*:702, 1976.

Medical Tribune: Electrocerebral silence 24 hours is held proof. May 12, 1969.

Myerburg, R. J., Conde, C., Sheps, D. S., Appel, R. A., Kiem, I., Sung, R. J., and Castellanos, A.: Antiarrhythmic drug therapy in survivors of prehospital cardiac arrest. Circulation *59*:885, 1979.

Nelson, D. A., and Ashley, P. F.: Rupture of the aorta during closed-chest cardiac massage. J.A.M.A. *193*:681, 1965.

Paaske, F., Hanse, J. P. H., Koudahl, G., and Olsen, J.: Complications of closed-chest cardiac massage in a forensic autopsy material. Dan. Med. Bull. *15*:225, 1968.

Redding, J. S.: Cardiopulmonary resuscitation: An algorithm and some common pitfalls. Am. Heart J. *98*:788, 1979.

Ruth, H., Bukley, M. L., and Keown, K.: Cardiac asystole. J.A.M.A. *164*:831, 1957.

Semler, H. J., Lauer, K. E., Smith, L. D.: Stat-electrocardiography in cardiac arrest. Am. J. Cardiol. (Abst.) *26*:668, 1970.

Seppala, K., and Yli-Uotila, R.: Cardiac arrest. Resuscitation results. Acta Med. Scand. *181*:385, 1967.

Stephenson, H. E.: Cardiac Arrest and Resuscitation. 3rd ed., St. Louis, C. V. Mosby, 1969.

Thompson, R. G., Hallstrom, A. P., and Cobb, L. A.: Bystander initiated cardiopulmonary resuscitation in the management of ventricular fibrillation. Ann. Int. Med. *90*:737, 1979.

INDEX

Note: Page numbers in *italic* type refer to illustrations;
page numbers followed by (t) refer to tables.

Pericardial disease, arrhythmias associated
with, 233
Pericarditis, acute, 240
chronic constrictive, 240
Phenytoin. See *Diphenylhydantoin.*
Polyuria, in paroxysmal supraventricular
tachycardia, 76
Postural atrial tachycardia, *306*
Posture, changes of, effects of on heart rate,
A-V conduction, and ectopic rhythm, 305, *306*
Potassium, factors modifying tolerance to, 282
in treatment of digitalis toxicity, 270
in treatment of ventricular tachycardia, 154
serum, imbalance of, 276
Potassium equilibrium potential, 17
Potassium salts, and sinoatrial heart block, 61
Pre-excitation syndromes, in infants, children,
and fetuses, 244
indications for His bundle
electrocardiography in, 207
Premature atrial complexes, in mitral valve
prolapse, 234
Premature beats, and re-entry via bypass tract,
190
hypokalemia induced, 281
re-entry circuits generated by, 189, *189*
vs. aberrant complexes, in differential
diagnosis, 125
Premature complexes, quinidine administration
in, 313
Premature ventricular beats, effect on character
of systolic murmur, 139, *139*
Premature ventricular contractions, treatment of,
223
Procainamide, and A-V dissociation, 129
and widening of QRS complex, 118
dosage and administration of, 314
effects of, direct cardiac pharmacologic, 314
electrophysiologic, 313, 313(t)
on electrocardiograms, 314
on refractory period of bypass tracts, 189(t)
in antiarrhythmic therapy, 222
in post-countershock therapy, 358
in treatment of Lown-Ganong-Levine
syndrome, 193
in treatment of premature ventricular
contractions, 224
in treatment of ventricular premature beats,
143
in treatment of ventricular tachycardia, 154
indications for and contraindications to, 316
pharmacology of, 314, 315(t)
toxic manifestations of, 315, 315(t)
Programmed ventricular stimulation, 208
Propranolol, contraindications to use of, 324
doses and methods of administration of, 323
effects of, electrophysiologic, 322, 322(t)
on conduction, 322(t)
on electrocardiogram, 322(t)
on refractory periods of bypass tracts, 189(t)
in treatment of atrial fibrillation, 104
in treatment of atrial flutter, 92, 93
in treatment of digitalis induced arrhythmias,
271
in treatment of Lown-Ganong-Levine
syndrome, 193

Propranolol (*Continued*)
in treatment of ventricular tachycardia, 154
indications for use of, 322
pharmacology of, 322, 323(t)
side effects of, 323
Proximal conducting system, diagrammatic view
of, *10*
Pseudobigeminy, 89
Pulmonary heart disease, effect on cardiac
glycosides, 257
Pulmonary trunk, 3
Pulmonary valve, 2
Purkinje fibers, *2, 3*
changes of conductance of, for various ions
during action potential and during slow
diastolic depolarization, 19, *19*
effect of digitalis on, 262
in bundle branches, 11–12

Quinidine, and A-V dissociation, 129
and widening of QRS complex, 118
direct pharmacologic effects on heart, 310
dosage and administration of, 312
effects of, electrophysiologic, 309, 309(t)
on electrocardiogram, 310
on refractory periods of bypass tracts, 189(t)
in antiarrhythmic therapy, 222
in post-countershock therapy, 358
in treatment of atrial fibrillation, 105
in treatment of atrial flutter, 92, 93
in treatment of Lown-Ganong-Levine
syndrome, 193
in treatment of ventricular premature beats,
143
in treatment of ventricular tachycardia, 154
indications for and contraindications to, 313
pharmacology of, 310, 311(t)
toxic manifestations of, 311(t), 312
with propranolol, in treatment of arrhythmias
of sick sinus syndrome, 72
Quinidine sulfate, and sinoatrial heart block, 61
Quinidine toxicity, treatment of, 313
QRS complex, alterations in width of, 123, *123*
in A-V junctional rhythm, 112
paradoxical narrowing with short cycle, 123
widened, narrowing after long pause, *121*
widening of, aberration and, 120
at slow rates, 122
factors affecting, 118
mechanisms of, 121
rate independent, 122
QRS prolongation, classification of, 120
Q-T interval, shortened, in hypercalcemia,
282

Radioelectrocardiography, fetal, *250*
Reciprocal beats, *118*
atrial, *117*
definition of, 117
in patient with A-V junctional rhythm, *117*